# Oculoplastic Surgery

## Brian Leatherbarrow FRCS FRCOphth

*Consultant Ophthalmologist and Ophthalmic Plastic Surgeon*
*Manchester Royal Eye Hospital*
*Manchester*
*UK*

**MARTIN DUNITZ**

ISBN 1-85317-942-6

Distributed in the USA by
Fulfilment Centre
Taylor & Francis
7625 Empire Drive
Florence, KY 41042, USA
Toll Free Tel.:     +1 800 634 7064
E-mail:  cserve@routledge_ny.com

Distributed in Canada by
Taylor & Francis
74 Rolark Drive
Scarborough, Ontario M1R G2, Canada
Toll Free Tel.:     +1 877 226 2237
E-mail:  tal_fran@istar.ca

Distributed in the rest of the world by
ITPS Limited
Cheriton House
North Way
Andover, Hampshire SP10 5BE, UK
Tel.:     +44 (0)1264 332424
E-mail:  reception@itps.co.uk

Composition by Scribe Design, Gillingham, Kent, UK
Printed and bound in China by Imago

This book is due for return on or before the last date shown below.

# Oculoplastic Surgery

# Dedication

Affectionately dedicated to my wife Angela,
my son Michael and my daughter Erin

# Contents

# Preface

This book has been written with the intention of providing the reader with a pragmatic approach to the diagnosis and management of patients presenting with a broad range of oculoplastic, orbital and lacrimal problems. Although aimed primarily at the ophthalmologist, it should prove very useful to clinicians of all grades and experience in a number of other specialties that share an interest in the field of ophthalmic plastic and reconstructive surgery:

- plastic surgeons
- maxillofacial surgeons
- ENT surgeons
- dermatologists
- radiologists

The reader should already have acquired a basic knowledge of periocular anatomy and should seek to expand this knowledge as much as possible. As the eye, periocular area and orbit represent a major crossroads of surgical anatomical dissection, the surgeon who wishes to contribute to this field should acquire a detailed knowledge of the anatomy of adjacent structures. Applied anatomy relevant to each disorder is presented throughout the text and the operative procedures described are based on anatomical principles.

Important principles are highlighted in the text in boxes. Pertinent clinical signs, investigations, surgical indications, important technical considerations and complications receive appropriate emphasis in each chapter. The surgical techniques and procedures described are not exhaustive but represent those most commonly used in the author's own surgical practice. The text is accompanied by a considerable number of high-quality colour photographs and complementary original illustrations. References have not been cited throughout the text; instead, further reading lists have been provided at the end of each chapter to serve as a starting point for those who may wish to pursue additional information.

Brian Leatherbarrow

# Acknowledgements

I wish to convey my sincere gratitude to a number of people without whose assistance, time, influence, support and encouragement I would not have been able to complete this work:

My wife, Angela, has shown enormous patience and forbearance in allowing me to write this book in my 'spare' time and during our holidays over a period of 2 years.

My medical illustrator, Philip Jones, has devoted a great deal of time to this work. I am grateful not only for his skill and his patience but also for his desire to achieve accuracy and effect in the many detailed drawings.

My anaesthetist and close friend, Roger Slater, has taken many of the intraoperative photographs for me. I am grateful not only for the skill he has demonstrated in this task but for the dedication, patience and forbearance he has displayed to me and my team over the last 8 years during our very lengthy operating sessions together.

I am obliged to my colleagues in the Department of Medical Illustration at Manchester Royal Eye Hospital for their help with many of the photographs used in this book. I am particularly grateful to my friends and colleagues in the Department of Ocular Prosthetics at Manchester Royal Eye Hospital and to my dedicated nursing team who have lent me such support with my work over many years.

Saj Attaulah and Simon Taylor, both oculoplastic and orbital fellows at Manchester Royal Eye Hospital at the time of completion of this book, have given generously of their time in reviewing the manuscripts for this volume. I have appreciated their helpful suggestions, and criticisms.

I am hugely indebted to my preceptors Mr JRO Collin, Dr JA Nerad and Dr KD Carter from whose outstanding teaching and exemplary clinical and surgical skills I have benefited so much. They have greatly influenced the treatment philosophies and surgical approaches outlined in this text.

I wish to acknowledge the multitude of patients who have so kindly agreed to the use of their photographs for this book. I am also particularly grateful to so many colleagues throughout the UK and in many countries throughout the world who have referred so many challenging patients without whom this book would not have been possible.

I am particularly grateful to my parents, Jean and Stan, not only for their lifelong support in my endeavours but also for the many hours they devoted to helping me sort through thousands of my slides.

Brian Leatherbarrow

# 1

# Basic principles

## Introduction

The fundamental principles and techniques essential to success in ophthalmic plastic surgery are similar to those which underlie other branches of surgery. Careful attention to detail, meticulous surgical technique and an utmost respect for the functional requirement of the eye are of paramount importance. The surgeon who is well versed in fundamental surgical principles and techniques will avoid unnecessary complications and the requirement for secondary procedures. The following basic principles should be considered:

1. Preoperative patient evaluation
2. Documentation
3. Selection of the appropriate surgical procedure
4. Surgical planning
5. Selection of the most appropriate type of anaesthesia
6. Surgical instrumentation
7. Surgical incision and exposure
8. Haemostasis
9. Wound closure
10. Postoperative pain management
11. Postoperative care

## Preoperative patient evaluation

The surgeon should develop a routine for questioning and examining patients in order not to omit important questions or crucial aspects of the examination. Obtaining a careful detailed history about the presenting problem from the patient is essential. Details should also be obtained about the past ophthalmic history, past medical and surgical history, current medications, allergies, family and social history. Time spent taking the history has additional benefits:

- It provides the surgeon with information about the patient's potential expectations.
- It provides an opportunity for the surgeon to establish a rapport with the patient.
- It allows the surgeon to simply observe the patient and detect subtle physical signs which may otherwise be overlooked, e.g. signs of aberrant reinnervation of the facial nerve, blepharospasm, hemifacial spasm, an abnormal head posture, frontalis overaction and facial asymmetries.

The examination of the patient should be methodical. A record of the patient's corrected visual acuity and a basic ophthalmic examination should form part of the assessment of every patient presenting with an eyelid, orbital or lacrimal disorder. The detailed examination methods for various conditions are discussed in the ensuing chapters. Any ancillary laboratory or imaging investigations should be selected on the basis of the clinical evaluation of the patient and not simply performed as a blind 'work-up'.

It may be helpful to obtain copies of patient records from other institutions where the patient has previously been treated. The details of previous surgical procedures, the results of previous investigations and imaging, and original histology slides should be sought wherever this is relevant.

## Documentation

The surgeon must ensure careful and accurate documentation of the history and examination findings as well as the diagnosis, management plan and preoperative discussion with the patient.

Preoperative photographs are essential for the vast majority of patients who are to undergo ophthalmic plastic and reconstructive surgery. They serve a number of useful purposes:

- A learning and teaching aid for the surgeon
- A verification of the patient's disorder for health care insurance companies

- An aid to defence in a medicolegal claim
- An aid to the patient in legal proceedings following accidents and assaults
- To jolt the postoperative memory of the forgetful patient

> Written patient consent should be obtained before the photographs are taken. It should be made clear to the patient how the photographs may be used.

The treatment options should be discussed with the patient. The advantages, disadvantages, risks and potential complications should be discussed with the patient and relatives. The risks and the incidence of complications need to be outlined in an open and honest manner. The consequences of complications and their management should also be outlined. Any surgical procedure can have serious complications. The surgeon should therefore avoid describing any periocular procedure as 'basic', 'straightforward', 'simple', 'minor' or 'routine'. If the patient expresses the wish not to be given this information, this must be documented.

> For purely elective procedures the patient should be encouraged to consider the information carefully before making a decision to proceed. This may necessitate a further consultation or an attendance at a preadmission clinic to obtain fully informed consent and to answer any residual queries. The patient should not be asked to sign a consent form for an elective procedure on the day of surgery. The risks and potential complications that have been discussed should be documented in the patient's records.

## Selection of the appropriate surgical procedure

The surgical procedure that is best suited to the individual requirements of the patient should be selected, e.g. a patient whose other eye is not functional should not be subjected to a Hughes procedure for the reconstruction of a lower eyelid defect. An alternative surgical procedure should be selected.

An operation which is not indicated will not benefit a patient no matter how skilfully it is performed, e.g. a patient whose blepharoptosis is due to giant papillary conjunctivitis which has been overlooked by the failure to evert the upper eyelid will not benefit from any surgical procedure.

The patient's age and general health must be taken into consideration. It must also be borne in mind that under certain circumstances the patient's best interests may be served by advising against surgical intervention.

# Surgical planning

Each procedure should be planned carefully. Preoperative planning ensures that the surgical team is aware of the required instrumentation and materials. The scrub nurse needs to be aware of the required preparation and draping of the patient, e.g. the proposed site for the harvesting of a skin graft or dermis fat graft. This ensures that the procedure can be performed efficiently, minimizing tissue exposure, operating and anaesthetic time and thereby minimizing risks to the patient. Preoperative planning is essential when operating as a team with other surgical disciplines.

The details of the planned surgical approach should be communicated to the anaesthetist. The anaesthetist is an essential member of the team and should know details about the following:

- The anticipated duration of the operation
- Special positioning of the patient, e.g. to harvest a dermis fat graft from the buttock
- The potential sites for harvesting autologous tissue, e.g. upper inner arm which may affect the siting of intravenous lines and blood pressure cuffs
- The requirement for hypotensive anaesthesia
- The potential blood loss
- The potential risk of an oculocardiac reflex, e.g. during an enucleation or secondary orbital implant procedure
- Vasoactive agents to be used intraoperatively, including their concentration and volume, e.g. subcutaneous local anaesthetic agent injections with adrenaline, topical intranasal cocaine solution
- The potential for postoperative pain, e.g. severe pain may be experienced following an enucleation with placement of an orbital implant requiring opiate analgesia, whereas severe pain following a lateral orbitotomy may indicate a retrobulbar haemorrhage which should be investigated and not merely suppressed with opiates.
- The requirement for a throat pack
- The requirement to position the endotracheal tube in a specific location, e.g. to one side of the mouth or intranasally when harvesting a mucous membrane graft

The timing of surgical intervention may be crucial to the outcome, e.g. an orbital floor blowout fracture with signs of orbital tissue entrapment in a child should be managed without delay in contrast to the same clinical scenario in an adult where a delay of 10–14 days is usually advisable. Any significant delay in the management of the child could result in an ischaemic contracture of the inferior rectus muscle with a poor prognosis for the restoration of a satisfactory binocular field of vision.

## Selection of the most appropriate type of anaesthesia

The types of anaesthesia available are:

1. Topical anaesthesia
2. Local anaesthesia

3. Local anaesthesia with sedation
4. Regional anaesthesia
5. General anaesthesia

The selection of the type of anaesthesia for an individual patient depends on:

- The age of the patient
- The general health and emotional status of the patient
- The extent and anticipated duration of the surgery
- The requirement for intraoperative patient cooperation

The type of anaesthetic should allow the surgeon to complete the surgery in a safe and controlled manner while providing the best possible degree of comfort for the patient.

## Topical anaesthesia

Local anaesthesia may be applied topically, e.g. amethocaine by pledget in the inferior fornix in order to perform a forced duction test. It should be borne in mind that topical anaesthetic agents last for a short period of time and should be instilled at regular intervals during surgery on the conscious patient.

## Local anaesthesia

Local anaesthesia may be applied topically, e.g. amethocaine by pledget in the inferior fornix in order to perform a forced duction test. Local anaesthesia is most commonly achieved by local infiltration with bupivacaine (0.5% for adults and 0.25% for children) containing 1:200,000 units of adrenaline. A period of 5 min should be allowed for the bupivacaine to take effect. Its duration of action is approximately 2–3 hours. The amount of local anaesthetic agent used in relation to the age and body weight of the patient should be noted and care taken not to exceed safe levels.

Subcutaneous injections in the eyelid should be placed just beneath the skin, avoiding injections into the orbicularis muscle. This reduces the risk of causing a haematoma which can distort the tissue planes and cause a mechanical ptosis in the upper eyelid, making ptosis surgery more difficult to perform. A 25-gauge 24-mm needle is used to avoid the need for multiple injections, which further predispose to bleeding and haematoma. Injections into the eyelid should be performed from the temporal side of the patient, with the needle parallel to the eyelid. This reduces the risk of perforation of the globe in the event of sudden inadvertent movement of the patient. Immediate pressure and massage should be applied over the injection site for 5 min.

## Local anaesthesia with sedation

Many oculoplastic procedures can be safely and satisfactorily performed with the use of a combination of local anaesthesia, and neuroleptic sedation. An anaesthetist can provide monitored anaesthesia, care managing and monitoring a variety of medical conditions, e.g. hypertension, arryhthmias, while providing safe sedation which can be titrated and rapidly reversed. This is ideal for the anxious patient who requires a levator aponeurosis advancement procedure. The patient is sedated during the administration of the injections but is fully cooperative during the intraoperative assessment and adjustment of the eyelid height and contour.

## Regional anaesthesia

Regional nerve blocks are useful to supplement the effects of subcutaneous injections for a limited number of surgical procedures under local anaesthesia. An infratrochlear block can be combined with local infiltration and intranasal cocaine for an external dacryocystorhinostomy (DCR). A retrobulbar injection of bupivacaine with 1:200,000 units of adrenaline mixed with hyaluronidase is ideal for an enucleation or an evisceration procedure.

## General anaesthesia

General anaesthesia is required for children and uncooperative patients and is indicated for longer and more extensive surgical procedures, e.g. lateral orbitotomy. It is required for patients undergoing procedures that result in bleeding from the nose or mouth in order to protect the airway. The patient's general health will determine the suitability of the patient for general anaesthesia. The patient with a history of general medical disorders who is to undergo elective surgery should be identified to the anaesthetist at the preadmission clinic.

Local anaesthetic injections containing adrenaline (1:200,000 units) are used in combination with general anaesthesia to assist haemostasis and to provide immediate postoperative pain relief. The use of such injections prior to enucleation or evisceration surgery can be effective in blocking the effects of the oculocardiac reflex. The anaesthetist should be aware of the potential for such a reflex, which can cause severe bradycardia and, rarely, asystole.

## Surgical instrumentation

The variety of delicate surgical instruments used in ophthalmic plastic surgery attests to the special demands of surgery in this region.

A basic ophthalmic plastic surgery instrument set should be available for oculoplastic cases (Figure 1.1).

Separate instrument sets should be available for enucleation/evisceration (Figure 1.2), external DCR (Figure 1.3), endoscopic DCR and endoscopic brow lift surgery (Figure 1.4), and orbital surgery (Figure 1.5). A variety of accessory instruments should be readily available (Figure 1.6). These instruments must be kept in good repair and should be respected and used appropriately. Inappropriate use of instruments can result in damage to delicate instruments and damage to tissues. The nurse assistant should ensure that dried blood, tissue and char are removed from the instruments as these are handed back during surgery. The surgeon should ensure that the instruments are carefully handed to the nurse assistant, avoiding injury from sharp blades and needles. *The surgeon should ensure that instruments are never handed across the patient's face.*

A number of basic principles apply to the use of ophthalmic instruments. Toothed forceps or skin hooks should be used to avoid crushing and damaging tissue. A variety of forceps of varying size are available and should be selected according to the type of tissue to be handled. Skin hooks must be handled with great care to avoid inadvertent injury to the globe. The eyelid skin is very delicate and it is preferable to hold the underlying orbicularis muscle when lifting the skin to dissect underlying tissue planes.

A variety of scissors may be used during surgery. These are curved, straight, sharp or blunt-tipped. Curved blunt-tipped Westcott scissors are used for the dissection of tissue planes in eyelid surgery and conjunctival surgery. They should not be used to blunt dissect tissue, planes. They should not be used for the dissection of thicker tissue, e.g. a glabellar flap, and should not be used for cutting sutures. Sharp-tipped Westcott scissors are used

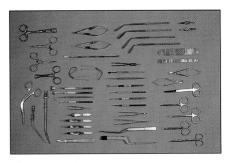

**Figure 1.1**
A basic oculoplastic instrument set (duplicate instruments, e.g. artery clips, have been omitted).

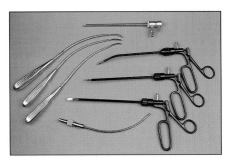

**Figure 1.4**
Endoscopic brow lift instruments.

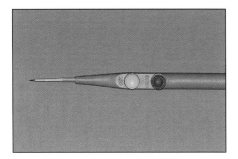

**Figure 1.7**
A Colorado needle.

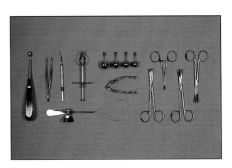

**Figure 1.2**
An enucleation/evisceration instrument set used in conjunction with a basic oculoplastic set.

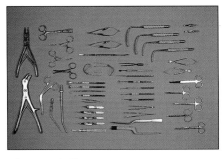

**Figure 1.5**
A basic orbitotomy instrument set.

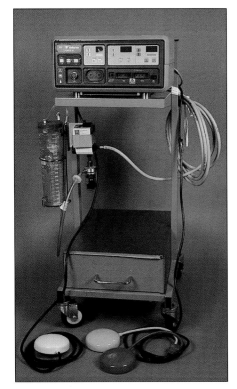

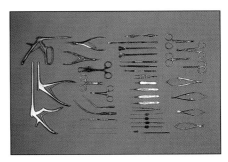

**Figure 1.3**
An external DCR instrument set.

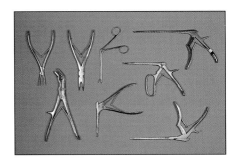

**Figure 1.6**
A variety of accessory bone rongeurs and forceps for orbital surgery.

**Figure 1.8**
A Valley Lab diathermy machine.

for punctal surgery, e.g. a three-snip procedure, and for the removal of the posterior eyelid margin in a lateral tarsorrhaphy.

The separation of tissue planes should be accomplished with blunt-tipped Stevens scissors which minimize the risk of bleeding or perforation, e.g. they are used to blunt dissect Tenon's fascia from the globe in an enucleation. Sharp-tipped iris scissors are used for performing eyelid wedge resections. Small suture scissors should be used for cutting sutures.

A Colorado needle is an efficient instrument for the precise delicate bloodless dissection of tissue planes in the eyelids in the hands of a skilled oculoplastic surgeon. An earthing plate must first be attached to the patient. The needle has both cutting and monopolar coagulation modes (Figure 1.7). It is used in conjunction with a Valley Lab diathermy machine (Figure 1.8). The author uses this instrument ubiquitously in his practice. Its use requires a dry surgical field. The tissues to be dissected should be held under some tension.

Artery clips are used routinely to fixate traction sutures and Jaffe retractor bands to the surgical drapes. It is preferable to use curved clips that lie flat against the surface of the drapes unlike straight clips. To fixate the suture or bands, one limb of the clips should lie beneath a fold of the drapes before the clips are closed.

Enucleation scissors in a variety of curvatures and sizes should be available and used whenever the use of a snare is inappropriate, e.g. where a long piece of optic nerve is required, a soft globe, previous corneal section or penetrating keratoplasty. A snare is otherwise very useful for enucleation surgery and its use is associated with minimal bleeding (Figure 1.9).

Needle holders are available in a variety of sizes and may be curved or straight. These are selected according to the size of needle. Needle holders designed to hold small needles, e.g. 7.0 Vicryl, will be damaged if used inappropriately to hold larger needles. The Castroviejo needle holders are preferred as these have a simple locking mechanism that permits the needle to be loaded securely and held between suture passes.

A variety of bone punches are available for bone removal, e.g. for an external DCR (see Figure 1.6). It is important that these are used appropriately. The delicate bone of the lacrimal fossa floor can be removed using a fine punch, e.g. a sella punch. This should then be replaced by progressively larger Kerrison rongeurs for the removal of the anterior lacrimal crest and nasal bone. The continued use of the delicate sella punch for the thicker bone will result in damage to this instrument.

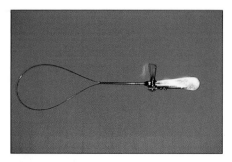

**Figure 1.9**
An enucleation snare.

# Surgical incision and exposure

Incisions should be planned preoperatively to provide adequate surgical access and yet result in a minimally conspicuous scar. Wherever possible, skin incisions should be planned to follow the relaxed skin tension lines (RSTL). These lines lie within normal skin creases or folds, enabling incisions to be hidden or disguised (Figure 1.10). The lines correspond to the directional pull existing in relaxed skin; this is determined by the underlying structures and the depth of subcutaneous tissue and fat. Incisions that run parallel to the RSTL tend to remain narrow after wound closure in contrast to those running perpendicular to them, which are more likely to gape.

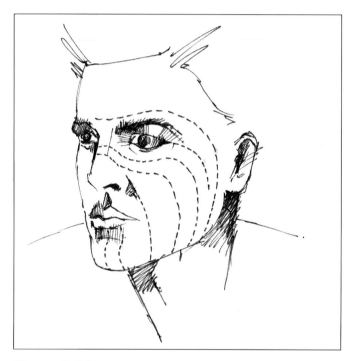

**Figure 1.10**
Relaxed skin tension lines.

Incisions which interrupt lymphatic drainage should be avoided, as these can lead to persistent postoperative lymphoedema, e.g. incisions directly over the infraorbital margin.

Skin incisions should be marked prior to the injection of the local anaesthetic agent as this may obscure anatomic landmarks, e.g. the upper eyelid skin crease. Marking is best achieved with the use of a cocktail stick inserted into a gentian violet marker block (Figure 1.11). This results in a fine line (Figure 1.12). Grease on the skin surface should first be removed with a small alcohol wipe.

In very young patients or in patients who are prone to hypertrophic or keloid scar formation (Figure 1.13) skin incisions may be avoided for certain procedures, e.g. a DCR may be performed endoscopically, an orbital floor blow-out fracture may be approached via a conjunctival incision.

Skin incisions which are commonly used in ophthalmic plastic surgery are shown in Figure 1.14.

Skin incisions should be made perpendicular to the skin surface, except in the eyebrow region where the incision should

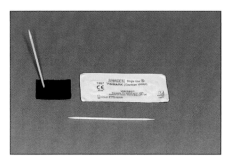

**Figure 1.11**
A gentian violet pad used with a cocktail stick.

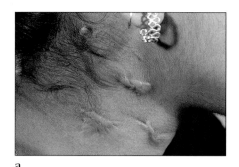

a b

**Figure 1.13**
(a) Keloid scarring in an Asian patient. (b) A lower eyelid hypertrophic scar.

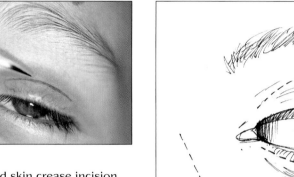

**Figure 1.12**
An upper eyelid skin crease incision being marked with a cocktail stick which has been inserted into a gentian violet marker pad.

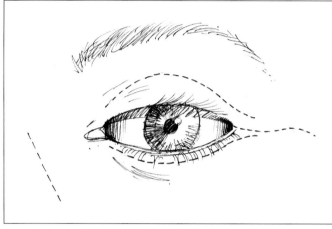

**Figure 1.14**
Periocular incisions commonly used in ophthalmic plastic surgery.

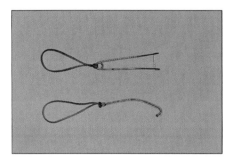

**Figure 1.15**
Jaffe retractors.

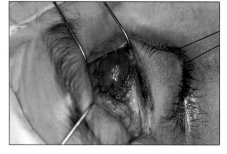

**Figure 1.16**
Jaffe retractors aiding exposure of a large conjunctival cyst.

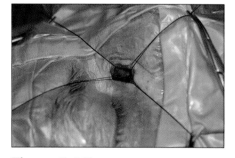

**Figure 1.17**
Traction sutures.

be bevelled. For eyelid skin incisions the Colorado needle is a very effective alternative to the use of a No. 15 Bard Parker blade. It results in less bleeding and permits a layer-by-layer-dissection of the tissues, allowing identification of blood vessels which can be cauterized before they are cut.

When making a skin incision with either a blade or the Colorado needle, the incision should be made with a continuous motion to avoid jagged wound edges. The skin should be held taut. Skin incisions in the eyelids are aided by the use of 4.0 silk traction sutures placed through the grey line. A 4.0 black silk suture on a reverse-cutting needle is passed into the grey line of the eyelid and the curvature of the needle followed until the needle emerges from the grey line again. The delicate eyelid skin should be held with fine-toothed forceps, e.g. Bishop Harmon

forceps. Skin hooks should be used with great care in the periocular region because of the risk of inadvertent injury to the globe.

Incisions along the grey line of the eyelids, e.g. a grey line split in the upper eyelid as part of an upper eyelid entropion procedure or in both eyelids as part of a tarsorrhaphy procedure, should be made with a Beaver micro-sharp blade (7530) on a Beaver blade handle.

Surgical exposure is aided by the use of retractors or traction sutures. In levator surgery or orbital floor fracture repair the use of self-retaining Jaffe retractors enables the surgeon to operate without the requirement for a surgical assistant in contrast to Desmarres retractors (Figures 1.15 and 1.16).

Traction sutures not only improve surgical exposure but also assist in haemostasis, e.g. in an external DCR (Figure 1.17).

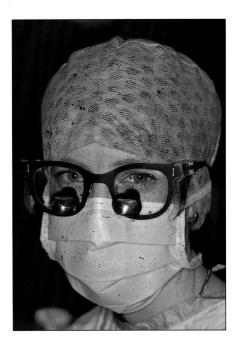

**Figure 1.18** Designs for Vision surgical loupes with side shields, offering ocular protection from sudden unexpected bleeding.

Safe surgical dissection is greatly facilitated by adequate magnification and illumination of the surgical field. The surgeon should wear surgical loupes, which do not unduly restrict the visual field. The loupes should be comfortable and should not require adjustment; typically, they provide 2.5 × magnification, and should be fitted with protective side shields (Figure 1.18).

The use of a headlight offers a number of advantages over an overhead operating lamp. The light is always focused on the surgical field, which is not placed in shadow by the surgeon's or assistant's hands. The use of a headlight is essential in surgery within cavities, e.g. external DCR.

# Haemostasis

Meticulous attention to haemostasis is essential in ophthalmic plastic surgery. The process of haemostasis begins preoperatively and continues postoperatively. Intraoperative bleeding can obscure and distort tissue planes, making surgical dissection difficult and prolonging the operative procedure. Eyelid haematoma formation can prevent accurate intraoperative assessment of eyelid height and contour in levator surgery. Haematomas retard healing, promote scarring and act as a nidus for the growth of microorganisms. Postoperative bleeding in the orbit can result in a compressive optic neuropathy and blindness.

## *Preoperative evaluation*

A careful medical history should be taken to identify medical conditions which predispose the patient to intraoperative and postoperative bleeding, e.g. systemic hypertension. Steps should be taken to ensure that this is adequately controlled before surgery is undertaken, particularly for elective procedures. The patient should be questioned about any history of a bleeding disorder, a tendency to bruise easily or a prior history of intraoperative bleeding.

It is important to identify patients who have a cardiac pacemaker, as the use of a radiofrequency device is contraindicated in such patients. The use of sympathomimetic agents, e.g. adrenaline and cocaine, may be contraindicated in patients with a history of cardiac arryhthmias, myocardial infarction, cerebrovascular accident (CVA) or hypertension.

A careful drug history should be taken. The use of aspirin, nonsteroidal anti-inflammatory agents and other antiplatelet agents should be discontinued at least 10 days prior to surgery unless this is contraindicated. Patients should be specifically asked about the use of aspirin, as this information is rarely volunteered. It is preferable to liaise with a haematologist for the management of patients who are taking anticoagulants. Patients taking warfarin who have undergone heart valve surgery should be admitted and converted to heparin preoperatively.

## *Preoperative injection*

The subcutaneous/submucosal injection of local anaesthetic agents containing adrenaline (1:200,000 units) is very helpful in minimizing intraoperative bleeding. Five minutes should be spent by the surgeon scrubbing, and a further 5 min should be spent prepping and draping the patient. This allows 10 min for the adrenaline to work. The anaesthetist must be informed prior to the use of any adrenaline.

## *Nasal packing*

For operations involving the nose, e.g. external or endoscopic DCR, the nose should be packed prior to surgery with small patties or a nasal epistaxis tampon, which are moistened with 5% cocaine solution. This is very effective in decongesting the nasal mucosa. Its use may be contraindicated, e.g. in children, patients with cardiovascular disease. For these patients, oxymetazoline should be substituted. Small patties moistened in 1:10,000 units of adrenaline may be placed directly over bleeding nasal mucosa in patients without a contraindication to the use of adrenaline.

## *Positioning of the patient*

Correct positioning of the patient can aid in achieving haemostasis. A gentle head-down position allows identification of the external angular vessels prior to marking the proposed skin incision in an external DCR procedure. The patient should then be placed into a reverse Trendelenburg position as soon as this is permitted by the anaesthetist. This reduces venous pressure within the head and face and can significantly reduce bleeding.

## Surgical technique

A meticulous gentle surgical technique is essential to avoid bleeding. The surgeon must be familiar with vascular anatomy of the periocular and orbital region (Figure 1.19). The vessels which are commonly encountered in ophthalmic plastic surgery are:

1.  The marginal and peripheral eyelid arcades in eyelid surgery
2.  The angular vessels in an external DCR
3.  Branches of the infraorbital vessels in orbital floor blowout surgery/orbital decompression surgery

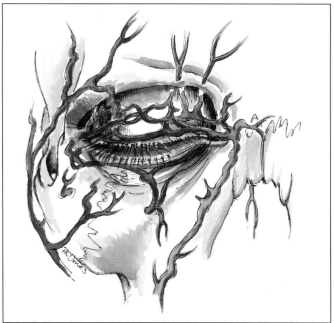

a

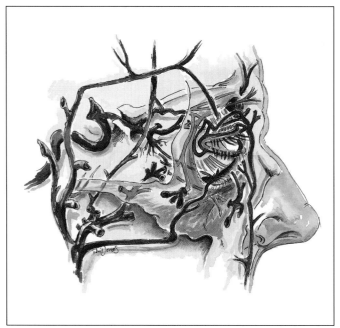

b

**Figure 1.19**
Vascular anatomy of the periocular and orbital region.

4.  The anterior and posterior ethmoidal vessels in an orbital exenteration, a medial orbital wall decompression/fracture repair
5.  The zygomaticofacial and zygomaticotemporal vessels in a lateral orbitotomy/lateral orbital wall decompression
6.  The supraorbital/supratrochlear vessels in endoscopic brow lift surgery

The use of the Colorado needle aids meticulous surgical dissection with ready identification of tissue planes. The tissue must be handled with great care to avoid tearing and maceration. It is essential to avoid traction on orbital fat, which can risk rupture of deeper orbital vessels. The surgical dissection should be restricted to that required to expose the area of interest.

Blunt dissection can avoid unnecessary intraoperative bleeding; e.g. in secondary orbital implant surgery, blunt dissection of deep orbital fibrous bands with blunt-tipped Stevens tenotomy scissors, also aided by digital dissection, is preferred.

## The application of external pressure

Intraoperative pressure tamponade is useful to assist haemostasis prior to the application of cautery. It is particularly useful following enucleation. Postoperatively capillary oozing may be limited by the application of a pressure dressing. This is particularly useful following anophthalmic socket surgery. It must be used with great caution, however, in situations where postoperative bleeding may lead to compressive optic neuropathy, e.g. following an upper eyelid retractor recession for thyroid eye disease.

## Suction

Suction is an important aid to haemostasis and must be used appropriately. There are a number of different suction tips available which should be selected according to the surgery to be undertaken, e.g. a small Baron sucker is appropriate to use in the non-dominant hand when performing dissection with a Freer periosteal elevator held in the dominant hand during an external DCR procedure. It is helpful to apply a moistened swab or neurosurgical cottonoid over orbital fat to prevent this from being drawn into the sucker. Suction can then be applied to the swab or cottonoid.

## Instrumentation

Haemostasis can be greatly influenced by the choice of instrumentation. For example, haemostasis is aided in enucleation surgery by the use of a snare. Contraindications to the use of a snare must, however, be observed, e.g. a soft globe, a previous corneal section or penetrating keratoplasty.

## *Cautery*

A Colorado needle has both a cutting mode and a monopolar cautery facility. This is very useful for cauterizing fine vessels in the eyelids. For larger vessels bipolar cautery is used. Fine-tipped jeweller's forceps limit tissue destruction to the zone between the tips of the instrument. A bayonet style of forceps is used for cautery of vessels at deeper levels within the orbit or socket. The forceps should be gently approximated until cauterization of tissue is seen to occur. A common error is to grasp tissue too firmly with the opposing tips of the forceps forced against each other. The surgeon should ensure that he/she is familiar with the required settings on the machine before using bipolar or monopolar cautery. Charred tissue should not be allowed to accumulate on the tips.

Cautery should be used with great care. Overuse of cautery may compromise the blood supply to periorbital flaps. The underuse of cautery may place a skin graft at jeopardy. If bleeding occurs beneath a skin graft, or mucosal graft the graft may fail.

A larger cutting diathermy blade (Figure 1.20) is used for fast bloodless incisions in the periorbital area, e.g. to aid in exenteration surgery. The blade can also be used in a fulgurate mode to prevent bleeding from bone.

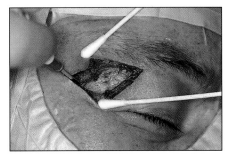

**Figure 1.20**
Cutting diathermy blade.

The use of disposable thermal hot-wire cautery should be avoided close to the eye or within the orbit. It is useful in the treatment of simple periocular skin lesions in a clinic setting.

Bleeding should first be stopped by the application of pressure. Small bleeding vessels are rolled with a cotton-tipped applicator until the vessel can be identified and cauterized. The applicators should not be wiped across the tissue, which removes clot and provokes more bleeding. For more profuse bleeding a gauze swab should be applied and gently removed until the vessels can be identified.

There is little justification for the use of a $CO_2$ laser to aid in haemostasis in ophthalmic plastic surgery. Most of the advantages of the $CO_2$ laser are also gained by the use of the Colorado needle without the numerous disadvantages of the $CO_2$ laser: significant expense, the requirement for nonflammable drapes, the risks of inadvertent injury to adjacent structures, the requirement for nonreflective instrumentation, the need to avoid supplemental oxygen, and the need for the operating room personnel to use protective eyewear.

## *Topical haemostatic agents*

The topical haemostatic agents commonly used during ophthalmic plastic surgery are:

- Adrenaline
- Thrombin
- Surgicel
- Bone wax

The application of 1:1000 units of adrenaline to the donor site of a mucous membrane or hard palate graft on a cottonoid is particularly useful prior to the use of cautery. This prevents mucosal capillary oozing and allows a more conservative use of bipolar cautery with less tissue destruction.

Thrombin is a protease that facilitates the clotting cascade by converting fibrinogen to fibrin. It is applied to tissue with gelfoam, an absorbable sponge, as a carrier. This is particularly useful to stop oozing from nasal mucosa or from a tumour bed in the orbit following an incisional biopsy.

Surgicel is oxidized cellulose that is applied dry to produce a local reaction with blood, promoting the formation of an artificial clot. It is nontoxic and creates very little local tissue reaction. Although it can be left *in situ* it is preferable to remove Surgicel at the completion of surgery as it can promote local swelling and a compartment syndrome in the orbit.

Bone wax is used to arrest bleeding from small perforating vessels in bone. The wax is applied on a cotton-tipped applicator or on the blunt end of a Freer periosteal elevator to plug the bleeding sites. It is important to dry the surrounding bone to enable the wax to adhere.

## *Postoperative haemostasis*

The maintenance of a head-up position overnight following surgery can help to prevent postoperative bleeding. Restriction on activity postoperatively can also be important. The patient should be instructed to avoid blowing the nose following a DCR procedure. The use of a surgical drain may be indicated following certain procedures, e.g. it can prevent the occurrence of a haematoma following a Mustardé cheek rotation procedure.

## Wound closure

Meticulous wound closure is essential to obtain good cosmetic and functional results. A number of factors are important in successful wound closure:

- The proper anatomical realignment of tissues
- The avoidance of undue wound tension
- Atraumatic tissue handling
- The elimination of 'dead space'
- Appropriate selection of needles
- Appropriate selection of suture materials

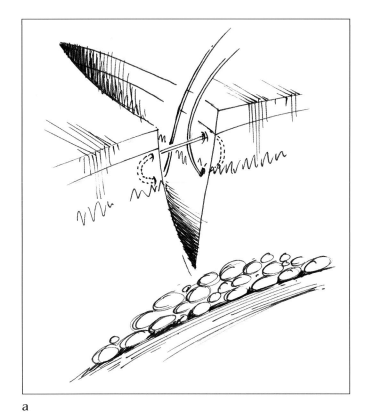
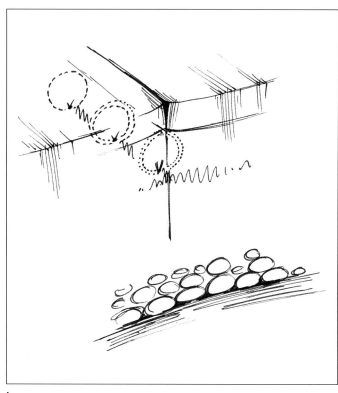

a                                                                                      b

**Figure 1.21**
(a) Buried subcutaneous suture. (b) Technique of suture placement ensures that the knots are buried deep in the wound.

'Dead space' within a wound must be eliminated as this may act as a reservoir for haematoma and microorganisms; it may prevent anatomical realignment of the tissues and may delay or impair wound healing. The appropriate deep closure of wounds reduces tension on the cutaneous wound, reducing the risk of wound breakdown or widening of the scar.

Deep wounds should be closed with 5.0 or 4.0 Vicryl (polyglactin 910) sutures, e.g. in the thigh following harvesting of autogenous fascia lata the subcutaneous tissues are realigned with interrupted 4.0 Vicryl sutures. The suture should be placed while everting the wound edge. The needle is inserted into the subcutaneous tissue so that the needle reaches 2–3 mm back from the wound edge. The sutures' knots are buried to prevent interference with skin closure or postoperative erosion of the sutures through the skin wound. To bury the knot, the needle is first passed from the deep to superficial in the wound and then from superficial to deep. Both ends of the suture should lie on the same side of the loop and the suture should be tied by pulling its ends along the line of the wound (Figure 1.21).

## *Selection of suture needles*

Suture needles are selected according to their size, curvature and cutting characteristics and the characteristics and location of the tissues to be sutured. The needles commonly used in ophthalmic plastic surgery are:

- Cutting (Figure 1.22)
- Reverse cutting (Figure 1.23)
- Spatula (or side-cutting) (Figure 1.24)
- Taper (Figure 1.25)

The needles are most commonly 1/4 or 1/2 circle: 1/4 circle needles are more commonly used, e.g. 5.0 Vicryl, for the reattachment of the levator aponeurosis to the tarsus; a 1/2 circle needle is used in a more confined space, e.g. 5.0 Vicryl, for the closure of mucosal flaps in external DCR surgery. Cutting and reverse cutting needles pass through tissue very easily and are particularly suited to skin closure and general purpose use.

Reverse cutting needles are the most frequently used needles in ophthalmic plastic surgery. The reverse cutting needle has a third cutting edge located on the outer convex curvature of the needle. This offers several advantages:

- Reverse cutting needles have more strength than similar-sized conventional cutting needles
- The danger of tissue cut out is greatly reduced
- The hole left by the needle leaves a wide wall of tissue against which the suture is to be tied

The side cutting edges of spatulated needles are designed for ophthalmic surgery. They permit the needle to separate or split through the thin layers of tissue, e.g. sclera. They are suited to partial-thickness passage through tarsus.

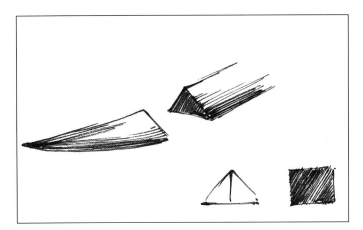

**Figure 1.22**
Conventional cutting needle.

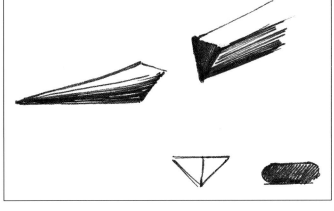

**Figure 1.23**
Reverse cutting needle.

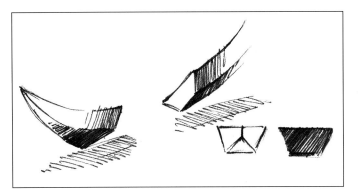

**Figure 1.24**
Spatulated needle.

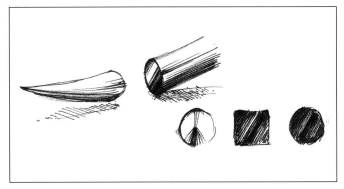

**Figure 1.25**
Taper needle.

Taper needles are designed to limit the cutting surface to the tip, making them more suitable for passage through more vascular tissues, e.g. extraocular muscles. They cause the smallest possible hole in the tissue and the minimum cutting of tissue. This needle is therefore most suited for use as a superior rectus bridle suture.

The actual placement of the needle in the patient's tissue can cause unnecessary trauma if performed incorrectly. The following principles should be borne in mind:

1. Force should be applied in the same direction as the curve of the needle.
2. Excessively large bites of tissue should not be taken with a small needle.
3. A blunted needle should not be forced through tissue. It should be replaced.
4. The needle should not be forced or twisted in an effort to bring the point through the tissue.
5. The needle should not be used to bridge or approximate tissues for suturing.
6. If the tissue is tougher than anticipated a heavier gauge needle should be used.
7. If a deep confined area prevents ideal placement of the needle, then it should be exchanged for a heavier gauge needle or a different curvature.

# Selection of suture materials

Suture materials are selected according to the type of tissue to be sutured, its physical location, the degree of wound tension and the suitability of the patient for suture removal. The size denotes the diameter of the suture material. In general the smallest diameter suture that will adequately support the wound is chosen to minimize trauma caused by passage of the suture through the tissue. Suture size is denoted numerically: as the number of 0's in the suture size increases, the diameter of the suture decreases, e.g. size 7/0 is smaller than size 6/0.

Sutures are classified according to the number of strands of which they are comprised. *Monofilament* sutures are made of a single strand of material. They encounter less resistance than *multifilament* sutures as they pass through tissue. They also resist harbouring microorganisms which may cause suture line infection. The sutures tie easily but crushing or crimping of this suture type can create a weak spot, predisposing to breakage. Multifilament sutures consist of several filaments braided together. This provides greater tensile strength, pliability and flexibility. They may be coated to assist in passage through tissues.

Sutures may be *absorbable* or *nonabsorbable*. Natural absorbable sutures are digested by body enzymes. Synthetic absorbable sutures are hydrolysed. Synthetic sutures result in a lesser degree of tissue reaction. Nonabsorbable sutures are not

**Table 1.1** Suture materials used in ophthalmic plastic surgery

| Suture material | Colour code of packet (Ethicon) |
| --- | --- |
| *Natural absorbable* | |
| Plain catgut | Yellow |
| Chromic catgut | Beige |
| *Synthetic absorbable* | |
| Coated Vicryl (polyglactin 910) | Violet |
| *Non-absorbable* | |
| Silk | Light blue |
| Ethibond (extra polyester fibre suture) | Orange |
| Ethilon (nylon) | Mint green |
| Prolene (polypropylene) | Deep blue |

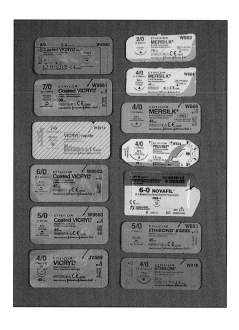

**Figure 1.26** Sutures most commonly used in oculoplastic surgery.

subject to enzymatic digestion or hydrolysis. The suture materials commonly used in ophthalmic plastic surgery are given in Table 1.1 and Figure 1.26.

Plain catgut is rapidly absorbed. Tensile strength is maintained for only 7–10 days postoperatively. Absorption is complete within 70 days; 4/0 plain catgut is used for lower eyelid transverse or everting sutures for involutional entropion.

Chromic catgut is treated with a chromium salt solution which resists body enzymes, prolonging absorption time to over 90 days. These sutures cause less tissue reaction than plain catgut. Tensile strength may be maintained for 10–14 days with some measurable strength for up to 21 days; 3/0 chromic catgut is used to reapproximate the bone fragment following a lateral orbitotomy.

Coated Vicryl sutures facilitate easy tissue passage, precise knot placement, a smooth tie down and a decreased tendency to incarcerate tissue; they are usually dyed violet. Approximately 65% of the tensile strength of coated Vicryl remains after 14 days and approximately 40% is retained at 21 days for suture sizes 6/0 and larger, whereas 30% is retained for suture sizes 7/0 and smaller. Absorption is minimal until 40 days postoperatively, and is essentially complete between 55 and 70 days.

4/0 Vicryl is used for subcutaneous wound closure in the thigh, e.g. following fascia lata removal, in the abdominal wall, e.g. following dermis fat graft removal, or in the brow, e.g. following a direct brow lift.

5/0 Vicryl is used for subcutaneous wound closure in the periocular region and for the attachment of the levator aponeurosis to the tarsus. It is used to reapproximate the mucosal flaps in external DCR surgery and for the attachment of the extraocular muscles to an orbital implant.

7/0 Vicryl is typically used for eyelid skin wound closure. It may be removed in adults but in uncooperative patients or children it can be left to disintegrate spontaneously aided by the application of warm saline compresses and the application of antibiotic ointment. They do not cause an inflammatory reaction or leave visible suture tracks. Although more expensive, Vicryl rapide is preferable for use in children.

8/0 Vicryl is typically used for conjunctival wound closure.

Silk sutures are usually dyed black for easy visibility in tissue. 6/0 silk is used to close an eyelid margin defect, whereas 2/0 or 4/0 silk sutures are used for eyelid traction sutures or to assist in wound exposure.

Ethibond extra sutures comprise untreated fibres of polyester closely braided into a multifilament strand. The suture does not weaken when wetted prior to use, causes minimal tissue reaction, retains its strength for extended periods and gradually becomes encapsulated in fibrous connective tissue. The coating of the suture allows easy passage through tissue and provides pliability, good handling qualities and a smooth tie down. The suture is available in white or dyed green: 5/0 Ethibond on a 1/2 circle needle is typically used to attach a lateral tarsal strip to the periosteum of the lateral orbital wall.

Ethilon sutures are particularly suited to skin closure because of their elasticity. Monofilament nylon sutures have a tendency to return to their original straight extruded state (a property referred to as 'memory'). More throws are therefore required to securely hold monofilament nylon sutures. 4/0 Ethilon is used as a Frost suture and for wound closure under tension, e.g. a thigh skin wound following the removal of a fascia lata graft, whereas 6/0 Ethilon is used for facial skin wound closure.

Polypropylene, unlike nylon, does not degrade over a number of years and can be considered permanent. 4/0 Prolene is the ideal material to be used in brow suspension surgery for patients at risk of exposure keratopathy as it can be cut easily and the eyelid position instantly reversed.

## Skin suturing techniques

Most skin wounds should be closed with a slight eversion of the skin edges to prevent an inverted wound. The exception to this is where skin wounds are to be hidden within a natural skin crease, in which case a slight inversion of the wound is desirable.

The skin wound edges should not be under undue tension. If this cannot be achieved, undermining of the tissues may be required. Overly tight sutures should be avoided, as these will cheese-wire through the tissues or impair the vascular supply of the tissues, resulting in wound breakdown.

The surgeon should use a needle holder that is appropriate to the size of the needle. The self-locking Castroviejo needle holders are the most appropriate for use. The needle holder should be armed properly. The needle should be grasped at the junction of the proximal 2/3 with the distal 1/3 with approximately 1 mm of the needle holders overlapping the needle (Figure 1.27).

The curvature of the needle should be followed as it is passed through the tissue. The tip of the needle should be avoided when grasping the needle to remove it from the tissues. For speed, the needle can be re-grasped with the needle holders so that the surgeon is ready for the next pass of the needle.

Interrupted percutaneous standard sutures are useful to approximate skin edges in small wounds that are not under tension. The needle should be inserted at a slight outward angle to achieve a slight eversion of the wound edges (Figure 1.28).

In the upper eyelid these sutures should incorporate a bite of the levator aponeurosis to recreate a skin crease.

A running percutaneous suture is useful to close a longer wound that is not under tension, e.g. a lower eyelid subciliary incision (Figure 1.29).

An interlocking running percutaneous suture is useful for efficient fast wound closure, e.g. for a postauricular wound under moderate tension following the removal of a skin graft (Figure 1.30).

A running intracuticular suture, e.g. 6.0 Ethilon, is useful for wounds under minimal tension where the dermis is relatively thick, e.g. the forehead, brow. Such a suture is used in conjunction with buried subcutaneous sutures for deep closure. The suture can be supplemented with the use of sterile adhesive tape.

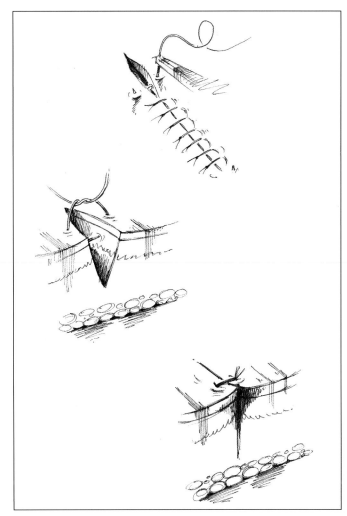

**Figure 1.28**
Technique of simple interrupted suture placement.

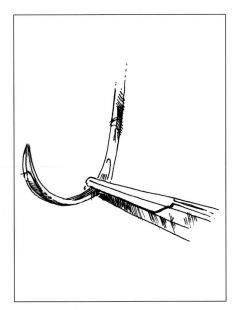

**Figure 1.27**
Correct arming of needle holder.

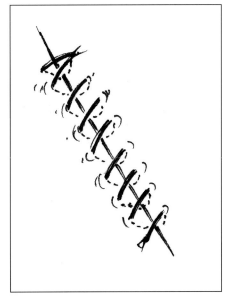

**Figure 1.29**
A continuous percutaneous suture.

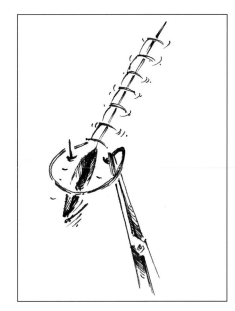

**Figure 1.30**
A continuous interlocking percutaneous suture.

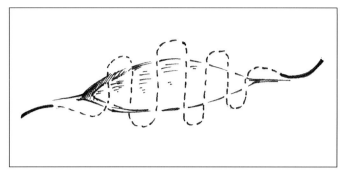

a

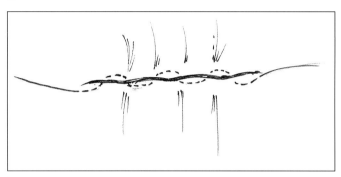

b

**Figure 1.31**
(a) Placement of a continuous intracuticular suture. (b) The wound edges are approximated by pulling on both ends of the suture.

The needle should be inserted through the skin approximately 1 cm beyond one end of the incision. It is brought into the wound and an artery clip attached to the free end of the suture to prevent the suture from being inadvertently pulled through the wound. The needle is then passed into the edge of the skin while everting the wound edges slightly with toothed forceps. The needle is curved through the skin for an arc of approximately 1 cm. The entire course of the suture is within the skin. The skin is then entered on the opposite side at the same point it exited the first side. The sides are alternated in this fashion until the end of the wound is reached. The wound is exited as it was entered. (Figure 1.31).

The suture ends are attached to the skin with sterile adhesive tape. For long wounds it is wise to bring the suture out to the skin every 8 cm in order to facilitate suture removal.

Vertical mattress sutures provide both superficial and deep support of the wound and assist in everting the skin edges. This technique is good for closing an external DCR wound with 7/0 Vicryl sutures but elsewhere on the face may leave unnecessary suture marks. Such a closure is very useful in the upper inner arm following the removal of a skin graft after undermining the skin edges (Figure 1.32).

The sutures should be tied correctly. The desired tension should be obtained with an initial double throw of the suture. It is important to avoid tying sutures for tissue approximation too tightly, as this may contribute to tissue strangulation: *'approximate – do not strangulate'*. Additional single throws are used to

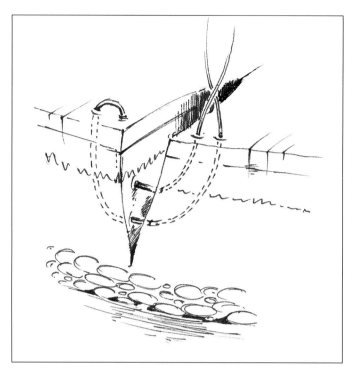

a

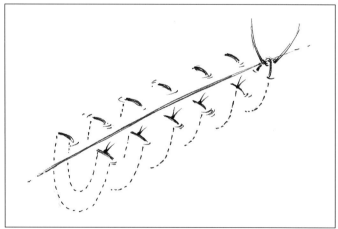

b

**Figure 1.32**
(a) Placement of a vertical mattress suture. (b) Wound closed with series of interrupted vertical mattress sutures.

maintain this tension. The tension should not be adjusted by the additional throws. The suture should be pulled through leaving a short end to grasp. This avoids unnecessary wastage of suture material and avoids an annoying loop of suture when attempting to tie the knots. Extra throws do not add to the strength of a properly tied knot, only to its bulk.

The timing of suture removal depends on the suturing technique which has been used, the type of sutures used, and the tension of the wound, e.g. eyelid margin sutures are removed after 14 days. An intracuticular suture can usually be removed after 5–7 days with the wound further supported by the use of sterile adhesive tape.

# Flap techniques

Flap techniques mobilize local tissue to close tissue defects and, where necessary, to add tissue bulk. Flap techniques can be faster than the use of a skin graft, require a shorter period of time for a compressive dressing postoperatively and are preferred in a situation where the recipient bed is unlikely to allow the survival of a graft.

Flaps used in ophthalmic plastic surgery are either 'random' or 'axial'. The random flap receives its blood supply from the underlying dermal plexus, whereas the axial flap is based upon a direct cutaneous artery. The midline forehead flap is an example of an axial flap, based upon the frontal branch of the ophthalmic artery.

Local flaps may also be classified as:

- Advancement flaps
- Rotation flaps
- Transpositional flaps

An advancement flap is usually rectangular in shape and is advanced directly into a defect. An example is the lower eyelid advancement flap which is used in conjunction with an upper eyelid tarsoconjunctival flap for the reconstruction of a lower eyelid defect. This is usually combined with the excision of Burow's triangles (Figure 1.33).

A rotation flap rotates about a pivot point and is rotated into an adjacent tissue defect. An example is the Mustardé cheek rotation flap (Figure 1.34)

A transposition flap is mobilized into a nonadjacent tissue defect. An example is the Limberg rhomboid flap. This is a very versatile flap which is particularly useful in the closure of defects lateral to the lateral canthus and of medial canthal defects (Figure 1.35).

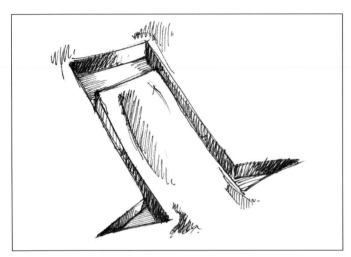

**Figure 1.33**
An advancement flap with the excision of Burow's triangles.

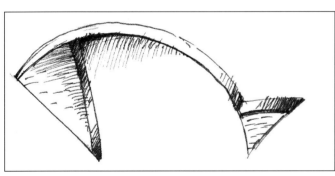

a

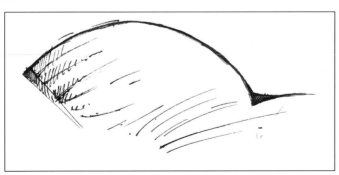

b

**Figure 1.34**
(a) A rotation flap being mobilized. (b) The rotation flap completed.

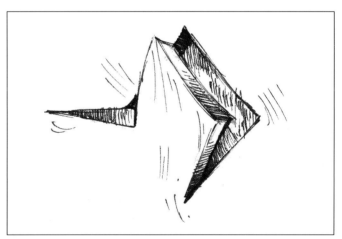

a

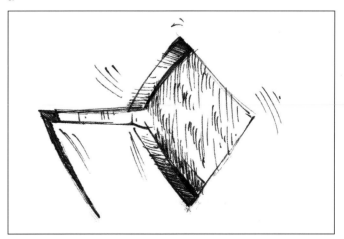

b

**Figure 1.35**
(a) A rhomboid flap dissected. (b) The flaps transposed.

The Z-plasty very rarely finds practical application in ophthalmic plastic surgery. This technique is based upon the transposition of two triangular flaps. Its aims are to lengthen skin in the direction of a linear scar, to achieve a cosmetic improvement in the scar by redirecting it within the relaxed skin tension lines and to reduce the effects of traction by the scar, e.g. a lower lid ectropion, lagophthalmos, limitation of ocular movement due to a linear conjunctival scar. The angles of each limb of the Z to the central scar are usually 60 degrees (Figures 1.36 and 1.37).

Free flaps, used for the reconstruction of large defects, e.g. the radically exenterated socket, are removed from one site and transplanted into the defect where the feeding artery and draining vein are attached to local blood vessels, e.g. the superficial temporal vessels. Examples are the rectus abdominis and radial forearm free flaps.

Flaps should be handled with great care as they have a delicate blood supply. Care should be taken in the use of cautery, in placing sutures without undue tension at appropriate intervals and in ensuring that there is no kinking of the pedicle of the flap. Excessive pressure from dressings should also be avoided.

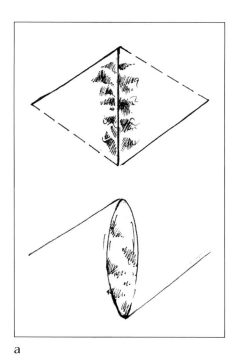

a

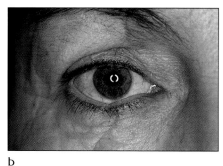

b

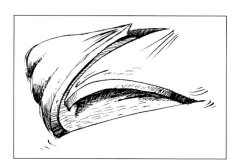

c

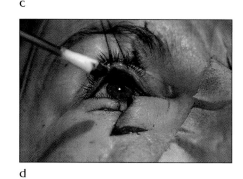

d

**Figure 1.36**
(a) The Z-plasty is marked out based on the vertical scar. (b) A patient with a vertical scar causing a lower eyelid malposition with epiphora. (c) The scar is excised and the flaps dissected. (d) The patient's vertical scar and eyelid notch have been excised and the flaps dissected.

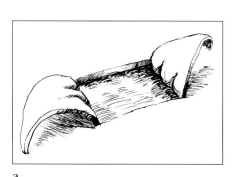

a

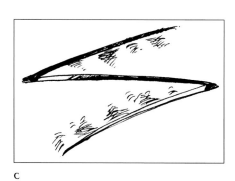

c

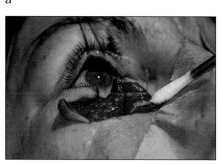

b

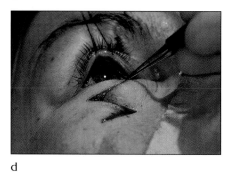

d

**Figure 1.37**
(a) The flaps are mobilized. (b) The Z-plasty skin–muscle flaps have been mobilized. (c) The flaps are transposed. (d) The Z-plasty flaps have been transposed and the eyelid raised.

# The dog-ear deformity

A dog-ear deformity typically occurs when a circular or elliptical defect is closed directly or when one side of an elliptical defect is longer than the other. The deformity is managed by elevating the dog ear, incising along one side of the dog ear following the line of the original incision, and elevating the resulting flat triangle of skin, which is then incised along its base (Figure 1.38).

Dog ears can be avoided in a number of situations by incorporating small triangular excisions into the wound closure, e.g. Burow's triangles (see Figure 1.33).

The principle of halving can be employed in closing an elliptical wound where one edge is longer than the other, e.g. an upper eyelid blepharoplasty wound. The wound is bisected with sutures until it is closed. Traction applied to both ends of the ellipse aids this closure.

An alternative method is to attempt to equalize the length of the wound edges by excising a triangle, e.g. the lower skin edge of a subciliary incision following a lower eyelid wedge resection procedure (Figure 1.39).

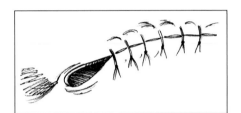

a

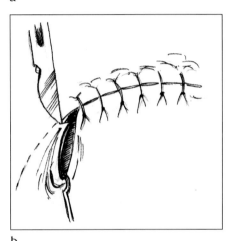

b

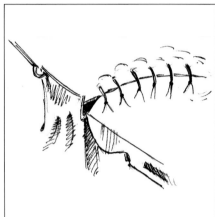

c

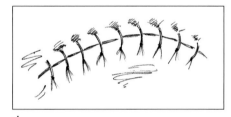

d

**Figure 1.38**
(a) A dog-ear deformity. (b) The apex of the dog ear is drawn away from the line of the wound with a skin hook and an incision is made along the line of the wound. (c) The triangle of skin and subcutaneous tissue is laid across the wound and the excess tissue is trimmed away. (d) The wound is closed.

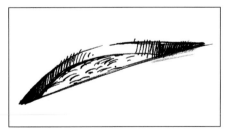

a

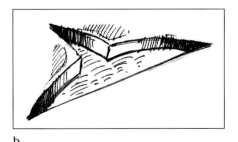

b

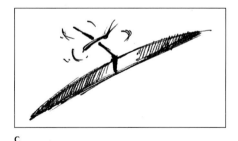

d

**Figure 1.39**
(a) Elliptical wound. (b) Removal of triangular piece of tissue from apex of ellipse. (c) Closure of triangular skin wound. (d) Closure of remaining wound.

# Postoperative pain management

The majority of the procedures undertaken by the ophthalmic plastic surgeon rank low on the pain scale. There are a few notable exceptions, e.g. enucleation with an orbital implant, secondary orbital implant surgery. Careful surgery with the minimal degree of iatrogenic tissue trauma reduces postoperative pain.

> Pain following eyelid and orbital surgery should be investigated immediately and not merely suppressed with analgesic agents as this may indicate a sight-threatening orbital haemorrhage. It is important to communicate the anticipated level of postoperative pain to the anaesthetist who is normally responsible for the prescription of postoperative analgesia regimens for the duration of the inpatient stay. It is also important to ensure that the nursing staff responsible for the administration of postoperative analgesia is aware of the potential significance of postoperative pain in an individual patient depending on the procedure which has been performed.

Postoperative analgesia should be prescribed to provide adequate relief of postoperative pain without the risk of significant side effects. It should be noted that older patients or those with systemic disorders may require lower doses of analgesia. In general, patients who are anxious require more postoperative analgesia.

The application of crushed ice packs in the first 24–48 hours following surgery helps to reduce swelling and bleeding. This is not practical, however, in the case of children or where compressive dressings have been applied. Great care should be taken to avoid excessive application of ice packs, however, as these can cause cryogenic burns, especially where the effects of local anaesthesia have not worn off.

For procedures undertaken under general anaesthesia, the use of a further injection of a longer-acting local anaesthetic agent, e.g. bupivacaine, as a local infiltration or a regional block is very helpful. Following an enucleation with an orbital implant or a secondary orbital implant procedure a retrobulbar injection of bupivacaine is recommended.

Moderate to severe pain is normally controlled postoperatively with narcotic agents, e.g. morphine, or nonsteroidal anti-inflammatory agents (NSAIAs) such as ketorolac. NSAIAs avoid the side effects of opiate agents but may cause gastrointestinal irritation and decreased renal function. Intramuscular ketorolac is very effective for immediate postoperative pain relief for day case procedures performed under general anaesthesia. This can be continued orally on discharge for 4–5 days. For mild postoperative pain codeine and paracetamol (Kapake) are usually adequate.

> Any drug allergies, interactions, contraindications and systemic disorders should always be considered before prescribing any analgesic agents.

# Postoperative care

The nursing staff should be carefully instructed about:

- Topical and systemic antibiotic treatment
- Dressings
- Drains
- Head positioning
- Visual monitoring
- Management of bleeding
- Activity restrictions
- Postoperative wound care
- Timing of suture removal
- Dietary restrictions
- Use of ice packs
- Postoperative analgesia

Clear effective communication is essential.

Patients should also be given clear written instructions about their aftercare on discharge from hospital. Postoperative instruction sheets for specific operations are particularly useful. A successful outcome without complications depends on good quality aftercare.

Topical antibiotic ointment should be applied to wounds at the end of surgery after rechecking the patient's allergy history with the nursing staff. This is also instilled into the conjunctival sac where ocular protection is required. The use of systemic antibiotics should be restricted to those cases for which there are specific indications, e.g. patients with diabetes undergoing lacrimal drainage surgery.

A Frost suture may be used in children following ptosis surgery: 4/0 nylon should be used, as this is more easily removed. If eyelid traction sutures are to be left in place for longer than 48 hours, they should be placed over small rubber bolsters. The suture is taped to the forehead with sterile adhesive tape.

Dressings may be left in place for a variable period of time depending on the operative procedure. Where firm compression is required, e.g. following an enucleation, it is preferable to apply tincture of benzoin to the forehead and cheek. Vaseline gauze should be placed over the wounds before eye pads are applied. Micropore tape is applied followed by a bandage.

Drains are rarely used in ophthalmic plastic surgery. They are mainly used following the drainage of subperiosteal abscesses or following a Mustardé cheek rotation flap. They are removed once the drainage from them has ceased.

It is preferable to advise patients to keep the head elevated following ophthalmic plastic surgery: this helps to reduce postoperative oedema.

It is important to perform regular postoperative visual checks following certain procedures where there is a risk of a postoperative orbital haemorrhage, e.g. a lateral orbitotomy and excision of an orbital tumour. It is important to ensure that the nursing staff is aware of the required frequency of these checks and the protocol to be followed. Dressings may have to be removed and reapplied frequently.

Postoperative bleeding may be anticipated following certain procedures, e.g. following an endoscopic DCR. Restricting activity for the first few hours following this operation reduces the risk

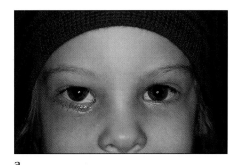
a

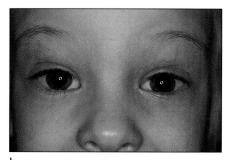
b

**Figure 1.40**
(a) Right lower eyelid retraction following wound repair in a child. (b) Satisfactory position of lower eyelid after 3 months of regular massage.

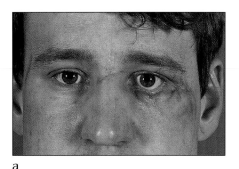
a

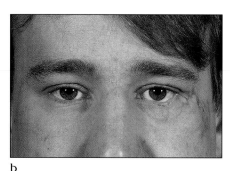
b

**Figure 1.41**
(a) Periocular scarring and a left lower eyelid retraction following a poor repair of irregular lacerations in a young adult. (b) Appearances after 3 months of regular wound massage.

of bleeding. Other restrictions should be made clear to the patient: e.g. patients should be instructed not to blow the nose following a DCR with placement of a stent or following an orbital decompression procedure.

Dietary restrictions are required following the removal of mucous membrane or hard palate grafts. The patient should be restricted to a bland soft diet for a few days and should be prescribed an antiseptic oral mouth wash such as Difflam.

Careful instructions on the use of ice packs postoperatively should be given to ensure that these are not overused with the risk of a cryogenic burn.

Postoperative wound care can greatly influence the outcome of surgery. Patients must be instructed on the necessity for thorough handwashing prior to touching any wounds. All debris should be gently soaked away with cotton wool moistened with boiled water or sterile saline. The patient should be instructed on the use of postoperative wound massage with ointment/ Vaseline. This reduces wound oedema, softens scars and prevents wound contracture (Figures 1.40 and 1.41). This can very successfully obviate the need for further surgery, e.g. postoperative massage commenced within 48 hours of a lower lid dissection for the management of a blowout fracture can prevent eyelid retraction.

# Conclusion

Although the fundamental principles and techniques essential to success in ophthalmic plastic surgery are similar to those which underlie other branches of surgery, the functional requirements of the globe and the ocular adnexal tissues and their delicate anatomical structure demand precise attention to detail, and a meticulous surgical technique. The surgeon who is well versed in fundamental surgical principles as well as specific surgical techniques will achieve successful results, avoiding unnecessary complications and the requirement for secondary procedures.

# Further reading

1.  Bartley GB. Oculoplastic surgery in patients receiving warfarin: suggestions for management. *Ophthal Plast Reconstr Surg* (1996) 12:229–30.

2.  Biswas S, Bhatnagar M, Rhatigan M, Kincey J, Slater R, Leatherbarrow B. Low-dose midazolam infusion for oculoplastic surgery under local anesthesia. *Eye* (1999) 13(Pt 4):537–40.

3.  Christle DB, Woog JJ. Basic surgical techniques, technology, and wound repair. In: Bosniak S, ed., *Principles and practice of ophthalmic plastic and reconstructive surgery.* Philadelphia: WB Saunders, 1996, pp. 281–93.

4.  Linberg JV, Mangano LM, Odoni JV. Comparison of nonabsorbable and absorbable sutures for use in oculoplastic surgery. *Ophthal Plast Reconstr Surg* (1991) 7:1–7.

5.  McCord C Jr, Codner MA. Basic principles of wound closure. In: McCord C, ed., *Eyelid surgery: principles and techniques,* 3rd edn. Philadelphia: Lippincott-Raven, 1995, pp. 23–8.

6.  Parkin B, Manners R. Aspirin and warfarin therapy in oculoplastic surgery. *Br J Ophthalmol* (2000) 84:1426–7.

7.  Sherman DD, Dortzbach RK. Monopolar electrocautery dissection in ophthalmic plastic surgery. *Ophthal Plast Reconstr Surg* (1993) 9:143–7.

8.  Tanenbaum M. Skin and tissue techniques. In: McCord CD, Tanenbaum M, Nunery WR, eds, *Oculoplastic surgery,* 3rd edn. New York: Raven Press, pp. 1–49.

# 2

# Blepharoptosis

## Introduction

Ptosis of the upper eyelid can affect all age groups and may be *congenital or acquired*. The causes of ptosis are numerous. It is important to appreciate that *ptosis itself is merely a physical sign, not a diagnosis*, and before therapeutic decisions are made it is essential to make every effort to determine the underlying cause. In considering the causes, it is useful to use a classification of ptosis which is based upon aetiological factors (Table 2.1).

## Classification

The classification of ptosis aims to provide some insight into the pathological processes involved.

## Pseudoptosis

Pseudoptosis (Table 2.2) refers to a condition that mimics a true ptosis. True ptosis may result from neurological disorders or from specific defects in the innervation of the levator palpebrae superioris muscle, from disorders affecting the levator muscle itself, from defects in the levator aponeurosis or in the attachment of the aponeurosis to the tarsal plate, or from mechanical factors which restrict normal movement of the eyelid. These aetiological mechanisms may be found in all age groups but with varying frequency. *Congenital 'dystrophic' ptosis and involutional aponeurotic ptosis are by far the commonest types of ptosis to be encountered.*

> It is particularly important that a pseudoptosis is clearly recognized and that a neurological cause of ptosis requiring further evaluation or an alternative therapeutic approach is excluded before ptosis surgery is embarked upon.

**Table 2.1**  Classification of ptosis

Pseudoptosis
True ptosis
    Neurogenic
    Myogenic
    Aponeurotic
    Mechanical

**Table 2.2**  Pseudoptosis

Contralateral eyelid retraction
Hemifacial spasm
Aberrant reinnervation of the facial nerve
Post enucleation socket syndrome
Double elevator palsy
Dermatochalasis/brow ptosis
Duane's retraction syndrome

## *Contralateral eyelid retraction*

Contralateral upper eyelid retraction may lead to diagnostic confusion, with the normal eyelid appearing to be ptotic (Figure 2.1).

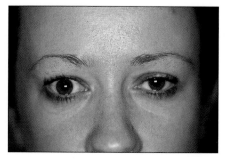

**Figure 2.1** Patient with right upper eyelid retraction who complained of a left ptosis. The patient had previously undiagnosed thyrotoxicosis.

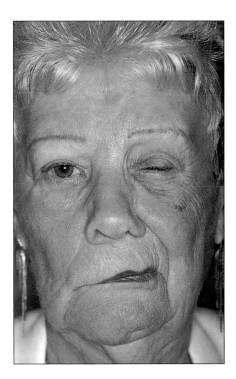

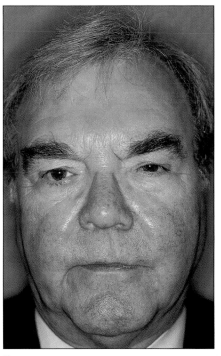

a

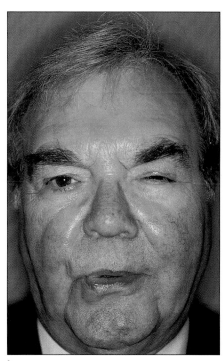

b

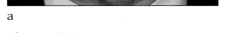

**Figure 2.2**
Patient with left hemifacial spasm.

**Figure 2.3**
(a) Patient following recovery from a Bell's palsy. There is an apparent left ptosis. The lower eyelid position is also high, further narrowing the palpebral aperture. (b) The patient demonstrating marked aberrant reinnervation of the facial nerve.

## Hemifacial spasm

This condition is characterized by unilateral involuntary intermittent irregular contractions of the muscles of facial expression (Figure 2.2). The orbicularis muscle is usually the first facial muscle to be involved. In some cases the cause is compression of the facial nerve in the posterior fossa by an aberrant artery. In these cases neurosurgical decompression of the nerve may be successful. Local injections of botulinum toxin can be very successful in controlling the associated blepharospasm.

## Aberrant reinnervation of the facial nerve

Aberrant reinnervation may occur following a peripheral lower motor neuron facial nerve palsy. This condition is characterized by involuntary eyelid closure stimulated by the use of other facial muscles, e.g. on smiling or whistling (Figure 2.3). The involuntary eyelid closure may be controlled by local injections of botulinum toxin. *It is important to exclude the possibility of aberrant regeneration in any patient referred with an acquired ptosis who gives a prior history of a facial palsy.* Ptosis surgery is contraindicated. Botulinum toxin treatment can be offered in severe cases, but the patient must then accept a secondary lagophthalmos and the frequent use of topical lubricants to avoid exposure keratopathy.

## Post enucleation socket syndrome

Ptosis (or indeed eyelid retraction) may be seen as one of the features which typify the post enucleation socket syndrome (Figure 2.4). It is thought to be due to the loss of the fulcrum for the action of the levator palpebrae superioris. This is corrected by replacement of a socket volume deficit by means of an orbital implant.

## Double elevator palsy

A ptosis which occurs in conjunction with a hypotropic eye may resolve completely once the eye has been elevated surgically. A cover test should be performed on all patients presenting with a history of a congenital ptosis to exclude this possibility (Figure 2.5).

## Dermatochalasis/brow ptosis

Excess upper eyelid skin and/or a brow ptosis may mimic an upper lid ptosis that resolves once a blepharoplasty and/or a brow lift have been performed (Figure 2.6).

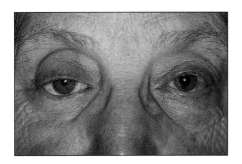

**Figure 2.4**
Patient demonstrating right post enucleation socket syndrome.

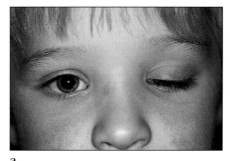

a

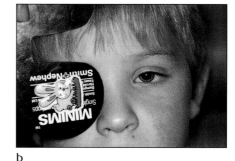

b

**Figure 2.5**
(a) Child with an apparent left ptosis. The underlying globe is hypotropic. (b) On cover testing, the left eye is forced to take up fixation. The apparent ptosis has resolved. The right eye under the occluder is now in a hypertropic position. The patient has a left double elevator palsy.

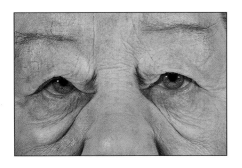

**Figure 2.6**
Patient demonstrating marked dermatochalasis.

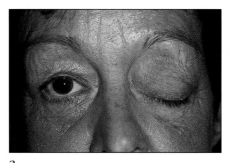

a

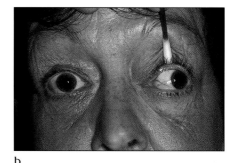

b

**Figure 2.7**
(a) Patient with left oculomotor nerve palsy. (b) Patient demonstrating failure of depression of left eye on attempted downgaze.

## Duane's retraction syndrome

Narrowing of the palpebral fissure may be associated with ocular movements. Patients may present with a complaint of ptosis, but a careful examination of the ocular motility reveals the true diagnosis.

## True ptosis
## Neurogenic ptosis

For classification of neurogenic ptosis see Table 2.3.

## Oculomotor nerve palsy

Oculomotor nerve palsy is characterized by a variable degree of ptosis associated with deficits of adduction, elevation, and depression of the eye due to weakness of the levator muscle, the superior, inferior and medial rectus muscles and the inferior oblique muscle (Figure 2.7). The pupillary fibres of the oculomotor nerve may be affected or spared depending on the underlying cause. Lesions confined to the superior division of the oculomotor nerve result in a ptosis and weakness of the superior rectus muscle only. Myasthenia may mimic an oculomotor nerve palsy when the pupil is spared. *The Bell's phenomenon is typically absent or poor.*

Cyclic oculomotor nerve palsy is a rare phenomenon characterized by alternating paresis and spasm of the extraocular and intraocular muscles. These cyclic phenomena are usually noted in early childhood and may be evident at birth.

An oculomotor nerve palsy may be caused by neoplastic, inflammatory, vascular or traumatic lesions, any of which may

---

**Table 2.3**  Neurogenic ptosis

Oculomotor nerve palsy
Horner's syndrome
Myasthenia gravis
Synkinetic ptosis
    Marcus Gunn jaw-winking phenomenon
    Aberrant reinnervation of the oculomotor nerve
Guillain–Barré syndrome
Cerebral ptosis
Botulism

affect the nerve in its course from the midbrain to the orbit. Associated symptoms and signs help to localize the underlying lesion.

*Treatment of the ptosis is problematic due to the impaired Bell's phenomenon with a risk of exposure keratopathy.* A frontalis suspension procedure may be undertaken after strabismus surgery has been performed to realign the globe in the primary position. A frontalis suspension procedure may be undertaken prior to strabismus surgery in infants to treat amblyopia. It is wise to use a polypropylene suture for the frontalis suspension as this can easily be removed and the procedure reversed if the patient develops exposure keratopathy.

# Horner's syndrome (oculosympathetic paresis)

Horner's syndrome is characterized by a ptosis of 1–2 mm with good levator function and a raised skin crease, miosis, an apparent enophthalmos, and is occasionally associated with facial anhidrosis (Figure 2.8). The features are due to interference with the sympathetic nerve supply to Müller's muscle in the upper eyelid and to its smooth muscle counterpart in the lower eyelid, and to the dilator pupillae muscle. The resultant anisocoria is accentuated in dim illumination. The apparent enophthalmos is due to the decrease in size of the palpebral aperture.

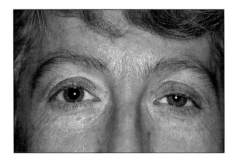

**Figure 2.8**
Patient demonstrating a left Horner's syndrome.

Horner's syndrome may be caused by a lesion which interrupts the course of the sympathetic neurons anywhere from the origin in the hypothalamus to the orbit. There are three orders of neuron carrying the sympathetic innervation to the orbit. The first neuron commences in the hypothalamus and synapses, with the second neuron in the intermediolateral cell column of the lower cervical and upper thoracic spinal cord. The second (preganglionic) neuron travels from the thorax across the neck of the first rib and ascends behind the carotid sheath, synapsing with the third neuron in the superior cervical ganglion, which lies in front of the lateral mass of the atlas and axis. The third (postganglionic) neuron travels along the internal carotid artery to innervate the smooth muscle of the upper and lower eyelids, the dilator pupillae muscle, and the sweat glands, hair follicles and blood vessels of the head and neck.

The diagnosis of Horner's syndrome is made clinically but may be confirmed by the instillation of *5% cocaine* solution into both

eyes. Cocaine blocks the reuptake of catecholamines by the nerve ending. The Horner's pupil, in contrast to the normal pupil, will fail to dilate as there is less free noradrenaline present at the synapse. The use of hydroxyamphetamine solution can assist in the differentiation of a preganglionic lesion from a postganglionic lesion. Hydroxyamphetamine displaces catecholamines from the nerve terminal. It will therefore dilate the pupil only if the third-order neuron is intact. In a postganglionic lesion, therefore, the pupil will fail to dilate. The differentiation between a first- and second-order neuron lesion is based upon the neurological signs associated with a first-order neuron lesion. The instillation of a weak solution of phenylephrine (1%) may demonstrate denervation hypersensitivity, resulting in a temporary resolution of the ptosis and restoration of a normal skin crease.

> It is important to differentiate a preganglionic from postganglionic Horner's syndrome because lesions which result in a postganglionic Horner's syndrome are usually benign in contrast to those resulting in a preganglionic Horner's syndrome.

The ptosis may be treated surgically either by means of a Fasanella–Servat procedure (see below), a Müller's muscle resection or by means of a levator aponeurosis advancement procedure.

## Myasthenia gravis

Myasthenia gravis is an autoimmune disorder caused by antibodies to the acetylcholine receptors of the motor endplate of voluntary muscle. The antibodies block access of the neurotransmitter acetylcholine to the receptors. The hallmarks of the disorder are variable muscular weakness and fatigue on exercise. Myasthenia may be generalized and may threaten the muscles of respiration, or it may be localized to the eyes (ocular myasthenia). Approximately 30% of patients present with ocular signs and symptoms (ptosis and diplopia), whereas 80–90% of patients have ocular signs at the time of diagnosis. If the symptoms and signs remain confined to the eyes for 3 years, progress to generalized myasthenia is unlikely. Ptosis is the most common clinical manifestation of myasthenia. It may be unilateral or bilateral. Exercise of the levator or sustained upgaze may provoke or worsen a ptosis. Attempted rapid saccades from downgaze to the primary position may provoke an overshoot of the upper eyelid above the superior limbus with a gradual fall of the lid to its original position (Cogan's twitch sign). There may be an associated weakness of the orbicularis oculi muscle and the Bell's phenomenon may be poor.

*The diagnosis of myasthenia should be contemplated in any patient with an acquired ptosis and normal pupils.* The diagnosis may be confirmed by means of a Tensilon test (edrophonium chloride) (Figure 2.9). Tensilon is a short-acting anticholinesterase agent that increases the amount of acetylcholine available at the motor endplate when given intravenously. In the majority of cases it will temporarily overcome the muscle weakness of

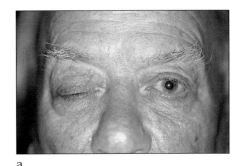
a

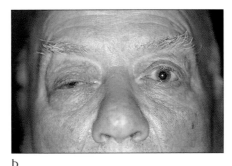
b

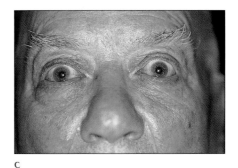
c

**Figure 2.9**
(a) Patient referred with history of acquired variable ptosis and diplopia. (b) Patient following test dose of Tensilon.
(c) Patient following injection of 10 mg of Tensilon.

myasthenia. Failure to do so, however, does not exclude the diagnosis. Other confirmatory tests can be performed, such as an acetylcholine receptor antibody assay and repetitive stimulation electromyography showing decremental responses.

Precautions should be taken prior to performing the Tensilon test. Resuscitation equipment should be available and an intravenous cannula placed for venous access. Monitoring of vital signs should be performed prior to and during the test. Atropine should be drawn up ready to counteract any adverse systemic cholinergic effects. A small intravenous test dose (2 mg) of Tensilon should be given and the response observed prior to injection of a further 8 mg to ensure there is no improvement in myasthenic signs nor any adverse side effects.

The treatment of the patient with myasthenia is best undertaken by a neurologist. The treatment may involve the use of anticholinesterase agents, systemic steroids, immunosuppressants or plasmapheresis. Thymectomy may be beneficial in some cases. The ophthalmologist plays a role in the management of ptosis and/or diplopia unresponsive to medical therapy. The ptosis may be treated by the use of ptosis crutches if the Bell's phenomenon is

absent and if the orbicularis function is poor. Patients with normal orbicularis function rarely tolerate ptosis crutches. The surgical management depends upon the levator function. If this is better than 4–5 mm, a levator aponeurosis advancement procedure may be used. If the levator function is less than 4 mm, a frontalis suspension procedure will be required. *The risk of exposure keratopathy must be considered carefully before embarking on such surgery.*

## Synkinetic ptosis

A synkinesis is simultaneous movement of muscles supplied by different nerves or by separate branches of the same nerve. It can be congenital or acquired.

**Marcus Gunn Jaw Wink Phenomenon (congenital trigemino-oculomotor synkinesis).** In this disorder there is a central anomalous innervational pattern between the oculomotor and trigeminal nerves. The phenomenon is characterized by eyelid synkinesis with jaw movement (Figure 2.10) Character-

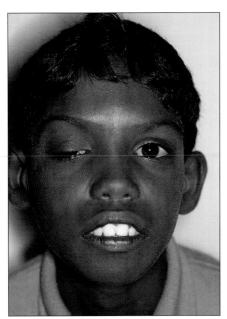
a

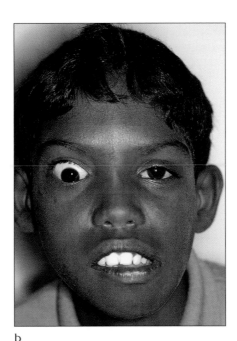
b

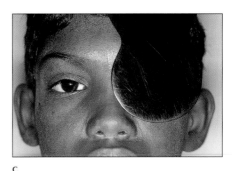
c

**Figure 2.10**
(a) Patient with a right ptosis and hypotropia. (b) Patient demonstrating external pterygoid–levator synkinesis on moving the mandible to his left. (c) The ptosis in the resting position resolves on occluding the fellow eye.

istically, a unilateral ptosis of variable degree is noted shortly after birth. The ptotic eyelid is noted to open and close as the infant feeds. The phenomenon accounts for approximately 5% of congenital ptosis cases, and may be associated with amblyopia, anisometropia and strabismus. *It may also be associated with a superior rectus palsy or a double elevator palsy.*

There are two major groups of trigemino-oculomotor synkinesis:

1. External pterygoid-levator synkinesis in which the lid elevates when the jaw is thrust to the opposite side, when the jaw is projected forward, or when the mouth is widely opened
2. Internal pterygoid-levator synkinesis in which the lid elevates on teeth clenching

In some patients the abnormal movements are only provoked by sucking.

A rare condition in which the lid falls as the mouth opens has been referred to as the inverse Marcus Gunn phenomenon.

The treatment of this phenomenon is difficult. It is important to ascertain whether the wink, the ptosis or both is of concern to the patient. If the wink is mild and not of major concern, the ptosis can be treated according to the usual criteria applied to the management of ptosis, i.e. determined by the degree of levator function. If the wink is of concern this can be treated either by an extirpation of the levator and a frontalis suspension procedure, performed unilaterally or, more controversially, bilaterally, or by means of a Lemagne procedure.

**Aberrant reinnervation of the oculomotor nerve.** In this disorder there is an innervational anomaly within the neural sheath between the eyelid and other targets of the oculomotor nerve. It is characterized by inappropriate eyelid and extraocular muscle synkinesis. The disorder typically follows trauma or compression of the oculomotor nerve. The management of this disorder is particularly difficult.

## Guillain–Barré syndrome

This rare disorder, which may be generalized or may present as a bulbar variant, usually follows a febrile illness. Ptosis, which is usually of mild degree, is symmetrical and occurs in the context of a rapidly progressive bilateral ophthalmoplegia and facial diplegia. Classically, the cerebrospinal fluid (CSF) shows a raised protein level in the absence of a cellular response. A more limited form of Guillain–Barré syndrome, the Fisher variant, consists of bilateral ptosis and ophthalmoplegia associated with ataxia and areflexia but with no systemic weakness.

## Cerebral ptosis

A moderate to severe bilateral ptosis may be seen following acute damage to the right cerebral hemisphere. The ptosis may be asymmetric. A conjugate ocular deviation is also seen in this condition (Figure 2.11).

## Botulism

Botulinum toxin blocks neuromuscular transmission and is commonly used therapeutically in the treatment of essential blepharospasm. Botulism, acquired through food poisoning, is a very rare neurological disorder characterized by ptosis and ophthalmoplegia, followed by dysarthria and dysphagia and then by weakness of the extremities.

# *Myogenic ptosis*

For classification of myogenic ptosis see Table 2.4.

| **Table 2.4**  Myogenic ptosis |
| --- |
| Congenital 'dystrophy' of the levator muscle<br>Myotonic dystrophy<br>Chronic progressive external ophthalmoplegia<br>Traumatic |

## Congenital 'dystrophy' of the levator muscle

In this condition the levator muscle is replaced to a variable extent by fibrous tissue. The levator function varies from good to fair to poor. The degree of ptosis can vary from minimal to

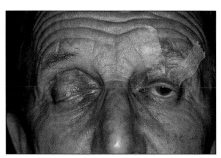
a

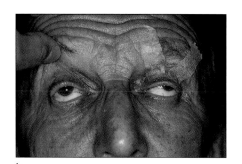
b

**Figure 2.11**
Patient with cerebral ptosis.

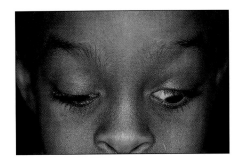

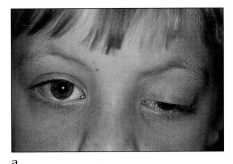

a                    b

**Figure 2.12**
Patient with congenital 'dystrophic' ptosis, demonstrating left lid lag on downgaze.

**Figure 2.13**
(a) Patient with a left congenital 'dystrophic' ptosis. (b) Patient demonstrating associated left superior rectus weakness.

severe and may interfere with visual development. The eyelid typically shows lag on downgaze (Figure 2.12).

A congenital 'dystrophic' ptosis may occur in isolation (simple congenital dystrophic ptosis) or it may be associated with a weakness of the superior rectus muscle (Figure 2.13). It may also be seen in the blepharophimosis syndrome or in the congenital ocular fibrosis syndrome. The blepharophimosis syndrome comprises bilateral ptosis, usually with poor levator function, blepharophimosis, telecanthus, epicanthus inversus and high arched eyebrows (Figure 2.14). Patients may also have a lower lid ectropion. Such patients require a bilateral frontalis suspension procedure usually following surgery to address the telecanthus.

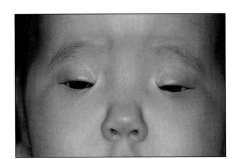

**Figure 2.14**
Patient with blepharophimosis syndrome.

## Myotonic dystrophy

Myotonic dystrophy is a rare myopathic process that may be associated with a mild degree of symmetrical ptosis with a fair to poor degree of levator function. It is characterized by progressive symmetrical external ophthalmoplegia, myopathy with atrophy affecting the musculature of the face, neck and limbs, and classical cataracts (Figure 2.15). These consist of small, coloured crystalline opacities, or posterior, subcortical and spoke-like opacities. Classically, these patients demonstrate myotonia, a delayed relaxation after contraction, which is most noticeable on hand shaking. Males may show frontal balding and testicular atrophy. *Affected patients typically have a poor Bell's phenomenon and orbicularis weakness. These patients are at particular risk of exposure keratopathy following surgery.* They are more likely than other patients to tolerate ptosis props as their orbicularis muscle is weakened. Other ocular signs of myotonic dystrophy include pupillary light-near dissociation, ocular hypotonia, dry eyes and a retinal pigmentary degeneration.

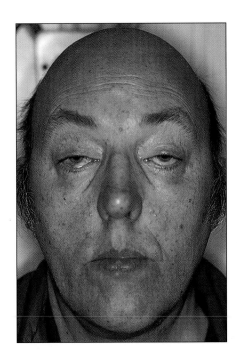

**Figure 2.15**
Patient with myotonic dystrophy.

## Chronic progressive external ophthalmoplegia (CPEO)

This condition, which is now regarded as a neurogenic disorder, is characterized by a progressive, symmetric paralysis of the extraocular muscles which do not respond to oculocephalic movements or to caloric stimulation. The levator muscle is also affected, resulting in a degree of ptosis related to the degree of severity of the disorder (Figure 2.16). *The levator function is usually poor, as is the Bell's phenomenon. The orbicularis function, however, is usually good but may be compromised.*

Muscle biopsy material may reveal characteristic 'ragged-red' muscle fibres on light microscopy, and electron microscopy typically demonstrates strikingly abnormal mitochondria.

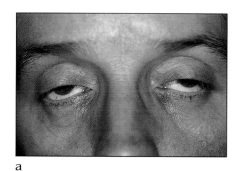 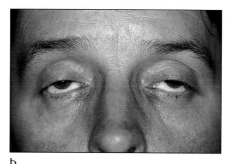 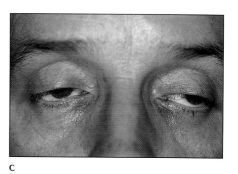

a                    b                    c

**Figure 2.16**
(a) Patient with chronic progressive external ophthalmoplegia (CPEO). (b) Patient attempting upgaze. (c) Patient attempting to left gaze.

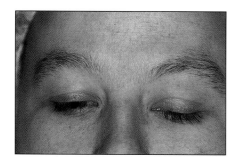 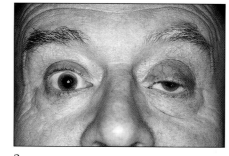 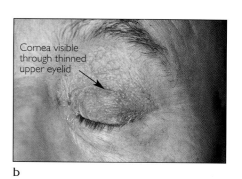

a                    b

**Figure 2.17**
Patient with a left levator aponeurosis dehiscence following contact lens wear demonstrating a raised skin crease and typical lid drop in downgaze.

**Figure 2.18**
(a) Patient with a left levator aponeurosis disinsertion demonstrating a raised skin crease. (b) The eyelid in this patient is so thin that the cornea is clearly visible through it.

The term *ophthalmoplegia plus* has been used to refer to a range of abnormalities which may be found with chronic progressive ophthalmoplegia. These abnormalities may be manifestations of associated neurodegenerative disorders. The Kearns–Sayre syndrome refers to a condition characterized by chronic progressive ophthalmoplegia, a retinal pigmentary degeneration, cardiac conduction defects often leading to complete heart block, and elevated CSF protein. It is important to identify the cardiac conduction defect by means of an electrocardiogram (ECG), as a cardiac pacemaker may be life-saving. Oculopharyngeal muscular dystrophy is an hereditary condition, with affected individuals typically demonstrating ptosis, difficulty in swallowing and a progressive external ophthalmoplegia. A large number of such patients are of French-Canadian descent.

The management of the ptosis is similar to that of ptosis-complicating myasthenia (see above).

A levator aponeurosis advancement procedure for CPEO is best performed via a posterior eyelid approach. This affords a greater control of the final eyelid position and offers greater protection of the cornea in the early postoperative period as the eyelid is initially low and the degree of postoperative lagophthalmos less than with an anterior approach.

## Traumatic

A myogenic ptosis can occur following eyelid or orbital trauma e.g. a 'blow-in' fracture of the orbital roof. Where the levator muscle has previously been transected following penetrating trauma resulting in complete ptosis with no levator function, it can be very difficult to differentiate a neurogenic ptosis from a myogenic ptosis.

## *Aponeurotic ptosis*

For classification of aponeurotic ptosis see Table 2.5.

**Table 2.5** Aponeurotic ptosis

Involutional
Post surgical, e.g. cataract surgery
Post eyelid trauma
Post eyelid oedema
Post contact lens wear

Aponeurotic ptosis is the result of a defect in the aponeurotic linkage between the levator muscle and the tarsal plate. It may be the result of a frank disinsertion of the aponeurosis from the tarsal plate, or a dehiscence in the aponeurosis, or involutional stretching and redundancy of the aponeurosis. The typical features of an aponeurotic ptosis are a ptosis that is constant in all positions of gaze, a lid drop as opposed to a lid lag on downgaze (Figure 2.17), good levator function, a high skin crease, an upper lid sulcus and thinning of the eyelid (Figure 2.18). Patients typically notice worsening of the ptosis towards the end of the day and this history of variability may lead to the suspicion of myasthenia.

## *Mechanical ptosis*

For classification of mechanical ptosis see Table 2.6.

A variety of eyelid lesions can result in a secondary mechanical ptosis (Figure 2.19), the management of which depends on the nature of the lesion, e.g. an upper lid capillary haemangioma. Orbital lesions may present with a secondary mechanical ptosis. Adhesions between the eyelid and the globe, e.g. in mucous membrane pemphigoid, may also result in a mechanical ptosis (Figure 2.20). *It is essential to palpate around the eyelids, to evert the lids and to examine the superior fornices to exclude such possibilities.*

# Patient assessment

The purpose of a careful assessment of the patient by means of a good history and physical examination, in some cases followed by specific investigations/diagnostic tests, is to determine the diagnosis and classification of the ptosis and thereby decide on the most appropriate therapeutic intervention.

## *History*

One should establish the age of onset of the ptosis, the presence of any known predisposing factors, e.g. trauma, previous ocular or eyelid surgery, any variability, associated symptoms, e.g. jaw-winking, diplopia, muscle weakness, dysphagia, and any family history (Table 2.7). A past ophthalmic history, including contact lens wear, and a past medical and surgical history are not to be overlooked.

## *Examination*

A complete ophthalmic examination should be undertaken. Where appropriate, a general physical and neurological examination should also be performed. In all cases the following specific features should be noted:

| **Table 2.6** Mechanical ptosis |
| --- |
| Eyelid tumours<br>Orbital lesions<br>Cicatrizing conjunctival disorders |

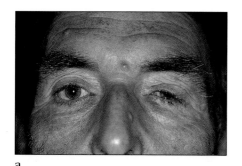
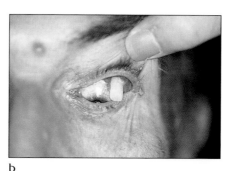

a    b

**Figure 2.19**
(a) Patient referred with a left ptosis.
(b) Raising of the left upper lid revealed an extruding retinal explant to be the cause of the ptosis.

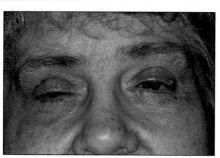
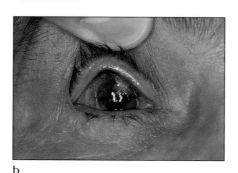

a    b

**Figure 2.20**
(a) Patient referred with a right ptosis.
(b) Raising of the right upper lid revealed symblepharon.

| **Table 2.7** History | |
|---|---|
| *Parameter* | *Ptosis category* |
| Age of onset | Congenital vs acquired |
| Any known abnormal lid movements | Jaw wink |
| Previous ocular surgery | Aponeurotic ptosis |
| Variability | Myasthenia |
| Diplopia, muscle weaknesses | Myasthenia |
| Previous contact lens wear | Aponeurotic ptosis or mechanical ptosis from giant papillary conjunctivitis (GPC) |
| Previous trauma | Aponeurotic ptosis |
| Atopy | Mechanical ptosis from GPC |
| Previous facial palsy | Aberrant reinnervation/brow ptosis |

I. The *palpebral apertures* should be measured in the primary position to determine the degree of ptosis (Figure 2.21). If the lower lid is abnormally positioned, however, the degree of ptosis can instead be measured using the difference between the corneal light reflex and upper lid margin (the upper eyelid margin reflex distance – MRD). *Beware contralateral lid retraction.* Prevent frontalis overaction by the patient by applying direct pressure over the brows. Frontalis action can be marked in some patients, particularly those with bilateral ptosis.

In unilateral cases, the ptotic lid should be manually elevated and the contralateral eyelid observed. The contralateral eyelid may be seen to drop spontaneously following Hering's law (Figure 2.22). This procedure may unmask a bilateral asymmetric ptosis. It is particularly seen in aponeurotic ptoses and it is important that the patient's attention is drawn to this preoperatively. Failure to observe this phenomenon can lead to unexpected postoperative disappointment and a 'see-saw' effect.

2. Perform a *cover test* to exclude a hypotropia and pseudo-ptosis and observe *any abnormal head posture.* It is important to ensure an infant with a congenital ptosis undergoes a complete orthoptic evaluation and a refraction. Most infants with a ptosis develop amblyopia from undetected strabismus and untreated refractive errors (Figure 2.23): 20% of infants with a congenital ptosis will have concurrent strabismus, of which 50% have a concurrent vertical deviation.

3. The *levator function* should be very carefully assessed. This will not usually be possible to do in infants below the age of 4 years. The maximum excursion of the lid margin from downgaze to upgaze is measured, ensuring that the frontalis muscle is prevented from assisting the lid movement by pressing on the brow with a thumb (Figure 2.24). Normal levator function is approximately 15–18 mm. *Levator function is graded as good (8–18 mm), fair (5–8 mm), poor (1–4 mm) and absent (0 mm).*

4. The *lid position on downgaze* is noted. This will demonstrate *lid lag* in congenital dystrophic ptosis in which the 'dystrophic' muscle will neither contract nor relax normally (Figure 2.25). Lid lag may also be seen where previous surgery has been performed or where there has been previous trauma with adhesions.

5. The *skin crease height* above the lid margin should be measured. The presence of a good skin crease in an infant with ptosis is a guide to the presence of at least fair levator function; conversely, the absence of a skin crease suggests poor levator function (Figure 2.26). A high skin crease suggests an aponeurotic defect. In adults, any excess upper lid skin and any degree of eyebrow ptosis should be noted.

6. The *Bell's phenomenon* should be assessed. Its absence should be taken into consideration in recommending ptosis surgery, as the risk of postoperative corneal exposure is increased. At the same time the orbicularis function should be

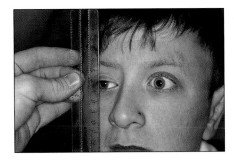

**Figure 2.21**
Patient undergoing measurement of palpebral aperture.

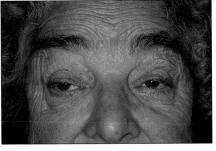
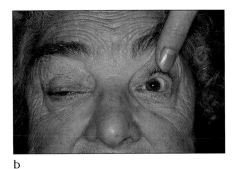

a                                                    b

**Figure 2.22**
Patient demonstrating phenomenon of contralateral lid drop.

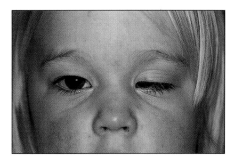

**Figure 2.23**
Patient with congenital ptosis and a left esotropia.

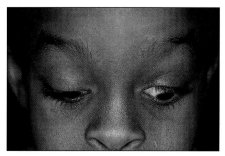

**Figure 2.25**
Patient with congenital 'dystrophic' ptosis, demonstrating left lid lag on downgaze.

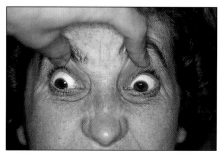

**Figure 2.27**
Patient with myotonic dystrophy demonstrating poor orbicularis function on attempted forced closure of the eyelids and an absent Bell's phenomenon.

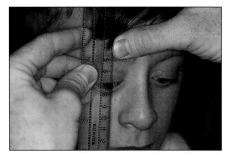

a

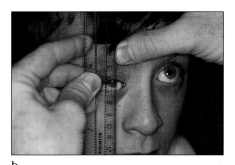

b

**Figure 2.24**
Patient undergoing measurement of levator function.

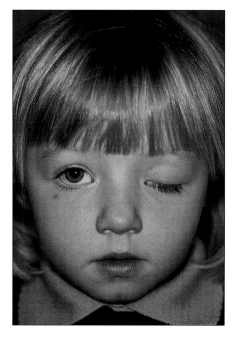

**Figure 2.26**
Patient with left congenital 'dystrophic' ptosis with very poor levator function. Note the absence of any skin crease.

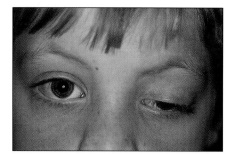

a

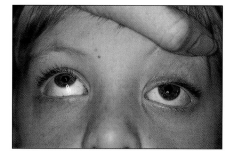

b

**Figure 2.28**
Patient with left superior rectus underaction.

determined and the extent of any lagophthalmos recorded (Figure 2.27).

7. The *ocular movements* should be assessed, looking specifically for a superior rectus weakness or aberrant eyelid movements (Figure 2.28).

8. *Jaw winking* should be looked for by asking the patient to open and close the mouth, and to thrust the jaw from side to side. An infant can be observed feeding and a child can be observed sucking a sweet. In some patients the phenomenon is only manifest when sucking (Figure 2.29).

9. The *pupils* should be examined to exclude the possibility of a Horner's syndrome.

10. *Myasthenia* should always be considered in acquired ptosis. Examine for fatigability, and a Cogan's twitch. Consider a Tensilon test where appropriate (after informed consent has been obtained and all necessary safety precautions taken).

11. *Evert the upper eyelid* and examine the tarsus. Document the height of the tarsal plate and exclude any giant papillary conjunctivitis, amyloid lesions, etc. (Figures 2.30–2.34). Undue laxity of the upper eyelid with a papillary conjunctivitis should raise the suspicion of a 'floppy eyelid syndrome'.

> In a patient with a prior history of facial palsy, ask the patient to purse the lips and blow as if to whistle and to smile to detect signs of aberrant reinnervation.

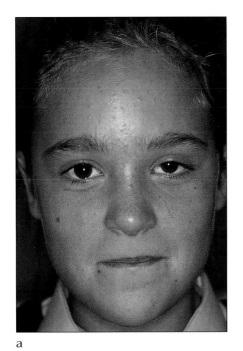
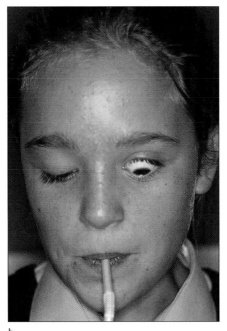

a                                            b

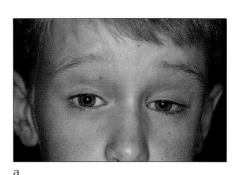

a

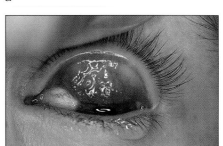

b

**Figure 2.29**
(a) Patient referred with mild ptosis. (b) Synkinetic movements provoked by sucking.

**Figure 2.30**
(a) Patient referred with a bilateral ptosis. (b) Eyelid eversion revealed vernal catarrh.

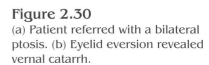

**Figure 2.31**
(a) Patient referred with a left acquired ptosis with a palpable upper lid mass. (b) A 'salmon patch' lesion was visible in the superior fornix. Biopsy of the lesion confirmed the diagnosis of lymphoma.

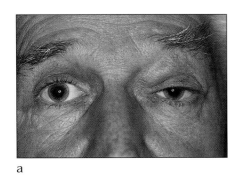
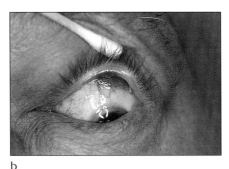

a                                            b

**Figure 2.32**
A patient with a left ptosis and a complaint of an irritable eye with a mucoid discharge.

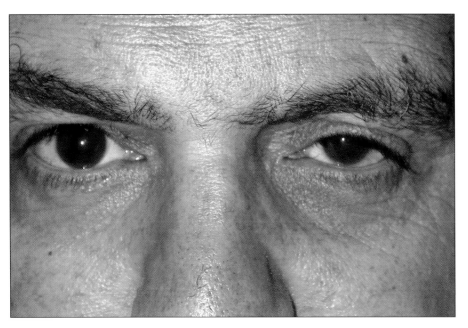

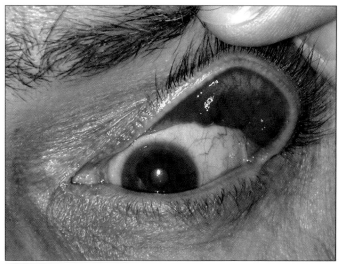

a

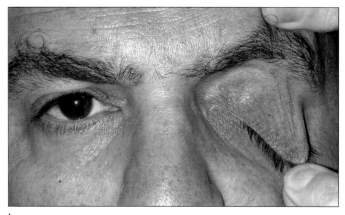

b

**Figure 2.33**
(a) The left upper eyelid everts very easily and demonstrates subtarsal papillary conjunctivitis. (b) The eyelid has extreme laxity. The patient has a 'floppy eyelid syndrome'. This should be managed by means of an upper eyelid wedge resection.

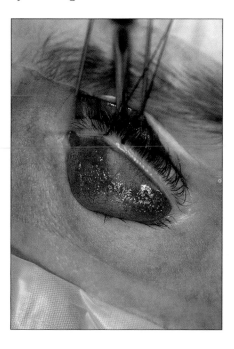

**Figure 2.34**
Multiple 'pseudo-papillae' in a patient referred with a unilateral acquired ptosis: this is localized conjunctival amyloidosis and was a cause of spontaneous bleeding from the eyelid.

12. *Examine the superior fornix* and exclude any symblephara, salmon patch lesions, etc.

13. *Palpate the upper lid* and lacrimal gland to exclude any masses (Figure 2.31).

14. Examine the *fundi* for pigmentary retinopathy seen in some of the ophthalmoplegias.

15. Determine the presence of normal *corneal sensation* (prior to any instillation of topical anaesthetic agent for tonometry) and *exclude a dry eye*, which will be aggravated by ptosis surgery.

16. Consider a *phenylephrine test:* 2.5% phenylephrine is instilled into the affected eye. A good response to this will help determine whether or not the patient will respond to Müller's muscle surgery.

# Management

*The major determining factor in deciding the most appropriate surgical procedure for the correction of ptosis is the degree of levator function* (Table 2.8). Most cases of ptosis can be adequately managed by means of a levator aponeurosis advancement procedure. This should be performed under local anaesthesia in adults, as this permits the most accurate results. In children, the extent of advancement of the aponeurosis, or of resection of the levator muscle, is determined by various formulae advocated by different surgeons over the years. Where the levator function is good and the extent of the ptosis is 2 mm or less, a Fasanella–Servat procedure or a Müller's muscle resection may be performed. For children with borderline levator function (3–4 mm) a Whitnall's sling procedure can be considered. For patients with poor levator function, a frontalis suspension procedure is required using either autogenous (usually fascia lata) or nonautogenous materials (e.g. polypropylene, supramid, Gore-Tex, mersilene mesh).

**Table 2.8** Surgical procedures for ptosis

Fasanella–Servat procedure
Müller's muscle resection
Levator aponeurosis advancement procedure
Levator muscle resection
Whitnall's sling procedure
Frontalis suspension procedure
Lemagne procedure

For patients in whom ptosis surgery would be dangerous, e.g. myotonic dystrophy with an absent Bell's phenomenon, poor orbicularis function and a dry eye, ptosis props should be considered.

It is important to document the ptosis with photographs in the primary position and in up and downgaze prior to surgery.

## Applied anatomy

See Chapter 21: blepharoplasty.

## Fasanella–Servat procedure

This procedure has been advocated for minimal degrees of ptosis in patients with good levator function, e.g. Horner's syndrome. *The Fasanella–Servat procedure is a simple but crude*

*procedure that is best avoided as it sacrifices both a portion of the tarsal plate, which is important for the structural integrity of the upper eyelid, and conjunctival tear secretor glands.* It has the disadvantage that it does not allow for graded adjustment. It does not take into account the variable height of the tarsal plate and is often used in inappropriate cases by general ophthalmic surgeons because of its simplicity. The recurrence rate is high. It may cause corneal problems from exposed posterior sutures. It can be difficult to correct postoperative contour defects and aponeurotic surgery is more difficult to perform later because of the loss of a portion of the tarsal plate.

Two curved artery clips are placed at least 4 mm from the eyelid margin to include equal amounts of tarsus and palpebral conjunctiva (Figure 2.35). These are angulated slightly away from the eyelid margin. A 6/0 nylon suture is passed through the eyelid medially and run above the artery clips taking 5–6 bites (Figure 2.36). It is brought out of the eyelid laterally after cutting along the crush marks with Westcott scissors. The ends of the suture are taped to the skin and removed after 7 days.

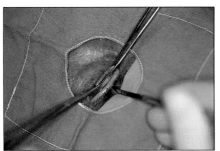

a

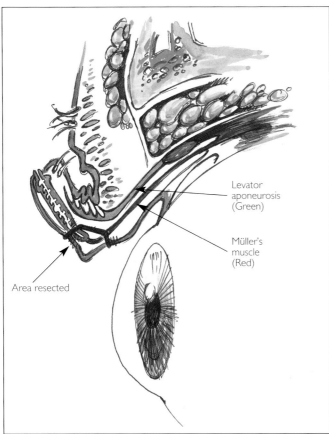

b

**Figure 2.35**
(a) Fasanella–Servat procedure demonstrating placement of curved artery clips. (b) Diagram demonstrating the tissue resected in a Fasanella–Servat procedure. This does not include the levator aponeurosis.

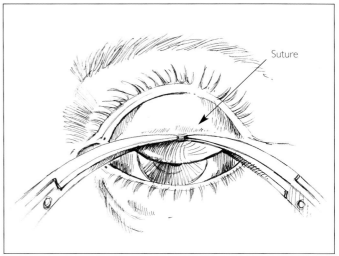

a

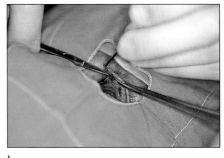

b

**Figure 2.36**
(a) Diagram demonstrating suture placement above the artery clips. (b) Each artery clip is removed and Westcott scissors used to cut along the crush marks.

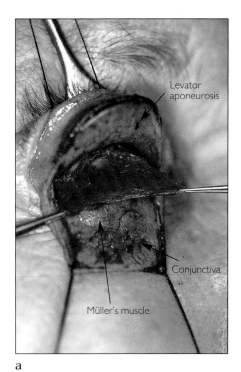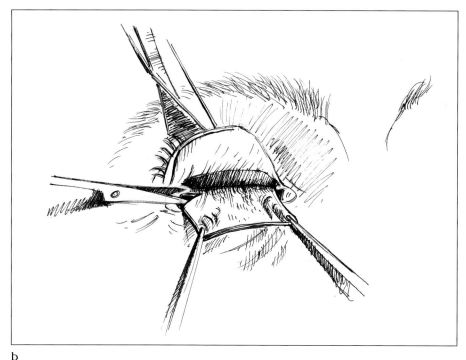

a                          b

**Figure 2.37**
(a) Müller's muscle dissected from the overlying levator aponeurosis. (b) Diagram demonstrating resection of a portion of Müller's muscle.

# Müller's muscle resection

This posterior lamella procedure is particularly useful for minimal ptosis surgery. It is preferable to the Fasanella–Servat procedure as only a portion of Müller's muscle is excised, leaving the rest of the upper eyelid anatomy intact. It is useful to apply the 2.5% phenylephrine eyedrop test preoperatively to determine patient suitability for this procedure.

The procedure (modified) is performed as follows:

1. 1–1.5 ml of 0.5% Marcain (bupivacaine) with 1:200,000 units of adrenaline are injected subcutaneously into the upper eyelid.
2. A 4/0 silk suture is placed through the grey line of the upper eyelid and the eyelid is everted over a large Desmarres retractor.
3. A further 1 ml of 0.5% Marcain with 1:200,000 units of adrenaline are injected subconjunctivally.
4. A conjunctival incision is made with a No. 15 Bard Parker blade just below the superior aspect of the tarsus.
5. An incision is made with Westcott scissors through Müller's muscle, exposing the avascular space between Müller's muscle and the levator aponeurosis. This plane is dissected with Westcott scissors.
6. Müller's muscle is then separated from the underlying conjunctiva (Figure 2.37).
7. The desired amount of Müller's muscle is resected (usually 5–6 mm).
8. A 4–5 mm strip of conjunctiva is then resected.
9. The wound is left unsutured.

A postoperative overcorrection or contour defect can be managed by eyelid massage.

# Levator aponeurosis advancement procedure

> It is important to have a very good understanding of eyelid and orbital anatomy before embarking upon surgery on the levator muscle or its aponeurosis.

## Anterior approach

This is the most common type of ptosis surgery performed. It involves either a repair of a levator aponeurosis dehiscence or a small resection of the levator aponeurosis. It can be combined with an upper lid blepharoplasty if necessary. *In adults, wherever possible, the procedure should be performed under local anaesthesia, with or without sedation, in order to achieve a greater degree of accuracy in adjusting the height and contour of the upper eyelid.* Short-acting intravenous sedation is particularly useful to avoid problems when patient cooperation is required during the adjustment of the eyelid. The patient should be advised that an intraoperative overcorrection of the lid height will be the goal, as the lid position will drop postoperatively, and that postoperative topical lubricants will be necessary to avoid exposure keratopathy until the denervated orbicularis regains normal function.

The procedure is performed as follows:

1. A skin crease incision is marked at the desired level in the upper eyelid using gentian violet and a cocktail stick after cleansing the skin with an alcohol wipe.
2. 1–1.5 ml of 0.5% Marcain with 1:200,000 units of adrenaline are injected subcutaneously into the upper eyelid. It is important to avoid a deeper injection in order to prevent a haematoma and to minimize the effect on the levator function.
3. A 4/0 silk traction suture is placed through the grey line of the upper lid at the desired location of the peak of the eyelid and fixated to the face drapes using a small haemostat (Figure 2.38).
4. An upper eyelid skin crease incision is made using a Colorado needle (Figure 2.39).
5. The Colorado needle is used to dissect down through the orbicularis oculi muscle to the orbital septum. The orbicularis is dissected from the orbital septum superiorly to avoid inadvertent injury to the levator aponeurosis.

6. The orbital septum is then opened with the Colorado needle throughout the entire length of the incision and the preaponeurotic fat exposed (Figure 2.40).
7. The preaponeurotic fat is dissected from the underlying levator aponeurosis.
8. A Jaffe lid speculum is then placed in the incision site to provide complete exposure of the levator aponeurosis (Figure 2.41).
9. Two skin hooks are then placed under the orbicularis muscle inferiorly and the upper 1/3 of the tarsus is bared using the Colorado needle.
10. If a dehiscence in the aponeurosis is identified, this is repaired with a 5/0 Vicryl suture; otherwise, the edge of the levator aponeurosis is identified and dissected off the tarsus throughout the entire length of the incision, avoiding the superior tarsal vascular arcade.
11. The levator aponeurosis is dissected from the underlying Müller's muscle, taking care not to damage the levator horns or Whitnall's ligament (Figure 2.42). The dissection is kept to a minimum, with the aim of disrupting normal structures as little as possible.

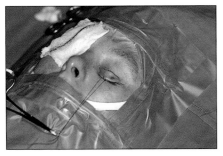

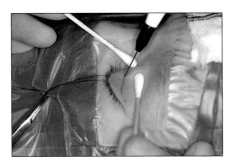

**Figure 2.39**
A Colorado needle being used to make a skin crease incision. Placing the eyelid on traction straightens the incision, making this procedure easier.

**Figure 2.38**
The basic set up for a levator aponeurosis advancement procedure.

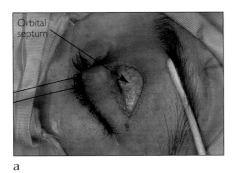

a

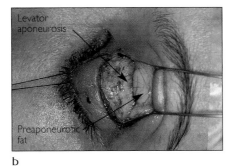

b

**Figure 2.40**
(a) Orbital septum exposed. (b) Preaponeurotic fat exposed.

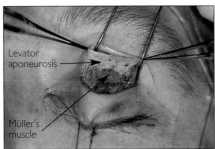

**Figure 2.41**
Placement of Jaffe lid retractor.

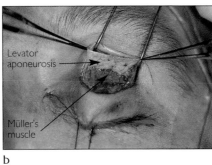

a                b

**Figure 2.42**
(a) The levator aponeurosis dissected free. (b) The levator aponeurosis elevated to demonstrate the avascular plane between the levator aponeurosis and the underlying Müller's muscle.

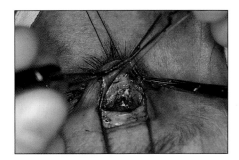

**Figure 2.43**
Suture being passed in lamellar
fashion through the tarsus.

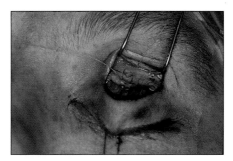

**Figure 2.44**
Suture being passed through the
levator aponeurosis.

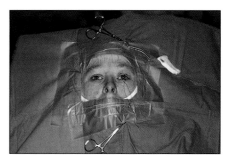

**Figure 2.45**
Eyelid height and contour being
checked with patient in sitting position.

12. A double-armed 5/0 Vicryl suture is passed in a lamellar fashion through the tarsus at the junction of the upper 1/3 with the lower 2/3 of the tarsus in a transverse orientation taking care to protect the underlying globe (Figure 2.43). This initial suture is placed just above the silk traction suture to ensure the maximum peak is at this position.

13. Both arms of the 5/0 Vicryl suture are passed through the levator aponeurosis at a variable distance from the tarsus and tied in a loop fashion (Figure 2.44). The height and contour of the lid is checked with the patient placed into a sitting position. The eyelid should be overcorrected by 1–1.5 mm.

14. Excess levator aponeurosis is excised and two additional 5/0 Vicryl sutures are passed through the tarsus and through the aponeurosis in a vertical fashion, and the lid position is checked again (Figure 2.45).

15. Once the height and contour are found to be acceptable, the skin edges are reapproximated using interrupted 7/0 Vicryl sutures, incorporating the levator aponeurosis to reform the skin crease.

It is preferable to place a lower lid Frost suture and apply a compressive dressing for 48 hours but, if this is not tolerated, ice packs should be applied intermittently for 24 hours. An alternative to the use of a Frost suture is the injection of air into the lower eyelid, which raises the lower eyelid temporarily and affords protection of the cornea until the effects of the local anaesthetic on the orbicularis muscle have worn off.

Postoperative adjustments for unsatisfactory height and contour can be made within the first few days after surgery but are rarely necessary with attention to detail at the primary procedure. Postoperative eyelid massage can be commenced 2 weeks after surgery for any residual minor overcorrection. There is no requirement to remove any sutures. The skin crease is cleaned with sterile saline solution twice a day and antibiotic ointment applied. The sutures drop out in 2–3 weeks.

## Posterior approach

This alternative approach requires far greater assistance in its execution and is associated with a great deal more aftercare on the part of the patient. *It should be avoided in patients with dry eyes, contact lens wearers and patients with a tarsus with a small vertical dimension*. For these reasons the anterior approach is preferable in the author's opinion.

# *Levator muscle resection*
## Anterior approach

The anterior approach is performed for congenital 'dystrophic' ptosis where the levator function is between 5 and 8 mm. This procedure differs from a levator aponeurosis advancement in that the levator aponeurosis is dissected along with Müller's muscle from the conjunctiva and the levator muscle is exposed above Whitnall's ligament. The horns of the levator are cut and the levator muscle is advanced beneath Whitnall's ligament if possible and a variable amount of levator muscle resected. This procedure is rarely necessary if the eyelid dissection is kept to a minimum and Whitnall's ligament is preserved. A maximal levator aponeurosis advancement is then usually sufficient, which avoids potential complications associated with more extensive eyelid dissection, e.g. conjunctival prolapse.

## Posterior approach

*The posterior approach is technically demanding but offers particular advantages to patients at risk of exposure keratopathy, e.g. patients with chronic progressive external ophthalmoplegia*. Such patients are also exquisitely sensitive to the effects of local anaesthetic agents, which cause a marked decline in levator function intra-operatively, making eyelid height adjustments via the anterior approach under local anaesthesia particularly difficult. This approach does not involve an incision that transects the orbicularis muscle and its motor innervation and does not therefore cause the same degree of postoperative lagophthalmos associated with the anterior approach. In addition, the eyelid height is lower in the immediate postoperative period, with a gradual rise in the eyelid height occurring over the first few days, which also affords greater corneal protection. The wound can be manipulated by the patient very early in the postoperative period to adjust the height and contour of the eyelid. It does not, however, permit any adjustment of the skin crease position.

The procedure is performed as follows:

1. A skin crease incision is marked at the desired level in the upper eyelid using gentian violet and a cocktail stick after cleansing the skin with an alcohol wipe.
2. 1–1.5 ml of 0.5% Marcaine with 1:200,000 units of adrenaline is injected subcutaneously into the upper eyelid.
3. A 4/0 silk traction suture is placed through the grey line of the upper lid at the desired location of the peak of the eyelid and the lid everted over a Desmarres retractor. The anaesthetic solution is injected subconjunctivally above the tarsal plate.
4. The conjunctiva is incised along the upper margin of the tarsus with a No. 15 blade.
5. The conjunctiva and Müller's muscle are dissected from the levator aponeurosis until a white line is located (Figure 2.46). This is opened with Westcott scissors, exposing the levator aponeurosis and the preaponeurotic fat pad (Figure 2.47).
6. Müller's muscle is dissected from the conjunctiva and both the levator aponeurosis and Müller's muscle are advanced from beneath Whitnall's ligament after releasing the horns of the levator.
7. Three double-armed 6/0 silk sutures are placed through the edge of the conjunctiva, the levator and Muller's muscle and attached to the upper end of the tarsus and brought through into the skin crease. These are tied over cotton wool bolsters.
8. The height and contour of the lid are inspected. If these are unsatisfactory, the sutures are replaced in a different location through the eyelid retractors. Once the result is satisfactory, the redundant Müller's muscle and levator muscle are resected.
9. A lower lid Frost suture is placed and a compressive dressing applied for 48 hours.

The eyelid sutures are removed after 6–7 days and eyelid traction/massage commenced if the eyelid rises above its desired level (Figure 2.48).

# Whitnall's sling procedure

The Whitnall's sling procedure is a potential advantage for the child with a 'borderline' levator function (3–5 mm) where a frontalis suspension is not desired. In this procedure the eyelid is very carefully dissected to ensure that Whitnall's ligament attachments, particularly medially, are maintained intact (Figure 2.49). The tarsus is sutured directly to Whitnall's ligament after resecting redundant levator aponeurosis and Müller's muscle (Figure 2.49). This is associated with a rather static eyelid with marked lag on downgaze (Figure 2.50).

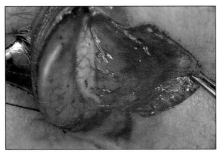

**Figure 2.46**
Anatomy seen during a posterior eyelid dissection (in this example a tarso-conjunctival flap is being dissected to be used for a lower eyelid reconstruction).

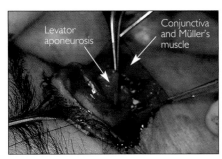

**Figure 2.47**
The levator aponeurosis is drawn forward after opening along the 'white line'.

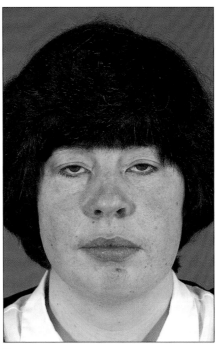
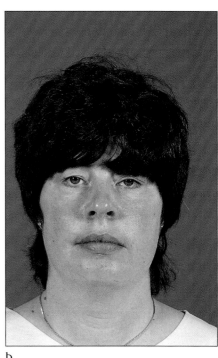
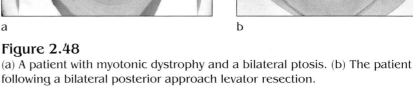

a                                    b

**Figure 2.48**
(a) A patient with myotonic dystrophy and a bilateral ptosis. (b) The patient following a bilateral posterior approach levator resection.

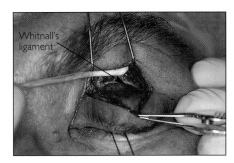

**Figure 2.49**
Whitnall's ligament exposed.

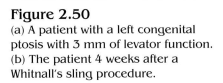

**Figure 2.50**
(a) A patient with a left congenital ptosis with 3 mm of levator function. (b) The patient 4 weeks after a Whitnall's sling procedure.

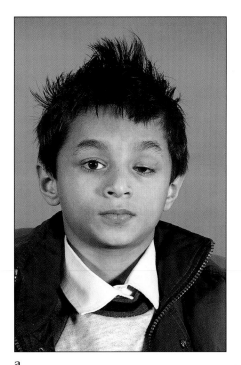

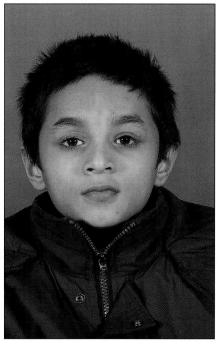

a                                                   b

# *Frontalis suspension procedure*

The purpose of a frontalis sling procedure is to harness the action of the frontalis muscle to elevate the eyelid(s). The normal frontalis muscle has 10–15 mm of action, which can be transferred directly to the eyelid if it is connected to the eyelid with either autogenous or nonautogenous tissue. It can yield very good functional and cosmetic results when performed bilaterally but is less successful if the procedure is performed unilaterally for a unilateral ptosis.

Autogenous materials such as fascia lata are preferable for this procedure but nonautogenous materials can be used: e.g. in infants, if the ptosis is so marked as to cause amblyopia; in older patients in whom it is less desirable to harvest fascia lata; and in patients with myopathies in whom it is desirable to avoid a general anaesthetic. There is a variety of nonautogenous suspensory material (Table 2.9) which can be used, but all materials have the disadvantages of potential infection, extrusion, breakage and foreign body granuloma formation. Silicone with the use of an adjustable Watzke sleeve is an advantage in patients with muscular dystrophies, as the degree of lagophthalmos is not as great. Polypropylene has the advantage of being very quick and easy to insert and to remove if necessary in contrast to Mersilene mesh. It does not biodegrade. Other autogenous materials have been used, e.g. temporalis fascia, palmaris longus tendon, but fascia lata remains the most popular choice.

## Surgical techniques

- The Fox pentagon is one of the simplest techniques which requires the least material and is preferred for nonautogenous material.
- The Crawford technique gives the best control of the eyelid contour and height and is usually used with autogenous fascia lata. It gives the best long-term results.

### Trapezoid-pentagon (Fox) technique
The procedure is performed as follows:

1. Two small incisions are marked 1–2 mm above the lash line 1 mm medial to the medial and 1 mm lateral to the lateral limbus.
2. Three small brow incisions are marked in the forehead, as shown in Figure 2.51. 0.2 ml of 0.5% Marcain with 1:200,000 units of adrenaline is injected subcutaneously at each mark.

**Table 2.9** Examples of nonautogenous materials used for frontalis suspension

| Material | Description |
| --- | --- |
| 1. Stored fascia lata | Irradiated or lyophilized |
| 2. Prolene | Monofilament polypropylene |
| 3. Supramid | 4/0 nylon polyfilament cable-type suture |
| 4. Mersilene mesh | Flexible interwoven polyester fibre mesh |
| 5. Silicone | Silicone cord or 240 retinal band |
| 6. Gore-Tex | Polytetrafluoroethylene (PTFE) |

3. The brow incisions are made as stab incisions using a No. 15 blade.
4. The eyelid incisions are made as careful nicks with the blade down to the tarsus.
5. When using a polyproylene suture, the needle is passed through the lid incisions, engaging partial thickness of the tarsal plate, and *taking care to protect the globe*. The needle is removed and the suture is passed from the lid to the brow incisions behind the orbital septum in a pentagonal fashion using a Wright needle (Figure 2.51). When using a Supramid suture the ski needles are used to engage the tarsus and to pass the suture from the lid to the brow. When using Mersilene mesh or stored fascia lata, the material is threaded subcutaneously in the eyelid using a Wright needle and then behind the orbital septum.
6. The lid is brought to a height corresponding to the superior limbus and the contour adjusted. The suture is tied using a surgeon's knot. The knot is carefully buried subcutaneously.
7. The forehead wounds are closed using interrupted 7/0 Vicryl sutures.
8. A lower eyelid Frost suture is placed and a compressive dressing applied.

**The double triangle (Crawford) technique.** The Crawford technique is a very popular procedure that uses autogenous fascia lata. The technique can be performed in children or adults but a child has to be sufficiently developed to harvest the fascia (usually over 4 years of age).

The procedure is performed as follows:

1. Three small incisions are marked 1–2 mm above the lash line 1 mm medial to the medial and 1 mm lateral to the lateral limbus and one centred over the pupil.
2. Three small brow incisions are marked in the forehead (Figure 2.52).
3. 0.2 ml of 0.5% Marcain with 1:200,000 units of adrenaline is injected subcutaneously at each mark.
4. The brow incisions are made as stab incisions using a No. 15 blade.
5. A 4/0 silk traction suture is placed through the grey line of the upper lid and fixated to the face drape.
6. The eyelid incisions are made as careful nicks with the blade down to the tarsus.
7. The fascia lata material is threaded subcutaneously in the eyelid using a Wright's ptosis needle and then behind the orbital septum to the medial and lateral brow incisions, *taking care to protect the globe*.
8. The lid is brought to a height corresponding to the superior limbus or until the eyelid comes away from the globe and the contour adjusted. The fascia is tied using a surgeon's knot and the knot reinforced with a 5/0 Vicryl suture (Figure 2.52). The longest remaining strips of fascia are brought through the central brow incision and again tied and reinforced.
9. The knots are carefully buried subcutaneously.
10. The forehead wounds are closed using interrupted 7/0 Vicryl sutures.
11. A lower eyelid Frost suture is placed and a compressive dressing applied.

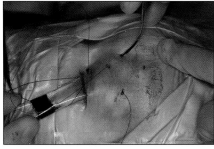

a

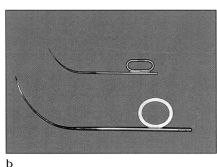

b

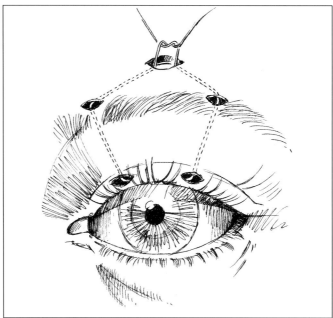

c

**Figure 2.51**
(a) A polypropylene frontalis suspension using a Fox pentagon technique. The globe is protected with an eyelid guard lubricated with ointment. A Wright's ptosis needle is used to withdraw the suture from the eyelid to the brow incisions.
(b) Wright's ptosis needles – adult and paediatric sizes. (c) The suture is tied and adjusted to ensure an adequate eyelid height and satisfactory contour.

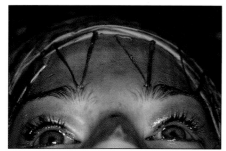

a

**Figure 2.52**
(a) An autogenous fascia lata brow suspension using the Crawford technique. (b) Diagram demonstrating reinforcement of the knots in the fascia.

b

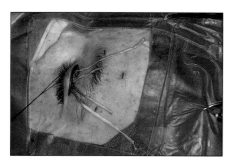

**Figure 2.53**
Fascia lata strips sutured directly to the tarsus.

**Figure 2.54**
(a) Patient with a bilateral congenital ptosis with poor levator function and frontalis overaction. (b) Patient following a bilateral autogenous fascia lata brow suspension using the alternative skin crease approach.

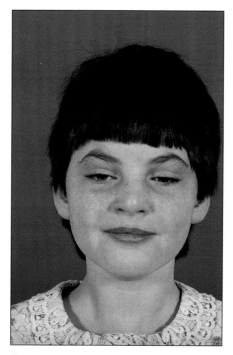

a

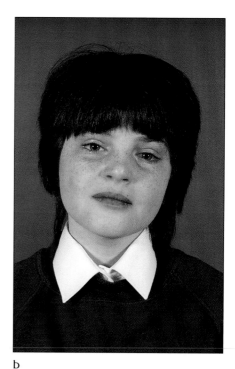

b

An alternative technique involves making a skin crease incision and exposing the tarsus to which the fascia is directly sewn. Although more time consuming, this technique permits the creation of a more natural skin crease that can be adjusted with a small additional blepharoplasty if necessary (Figures 2.53 and 2.54). The original technique creates a very low skin crease that cannot be easily adjusted.

# Harvesting autogenous fascia lata

The procedure is performed as follows:

1. A 3 cm incision is marked over the lateral aspect of the left thigh just above the lateral condyle of the knee along an imaginary line connecting the head of the fibula and the anterior superior iliac spine (Figure 2.55).

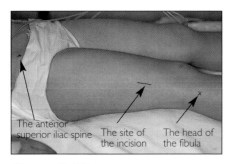

**Figure 2.55**
The incision for the removal of fascia lata lies on a line running between the anterior superior iliac spine and the head of the fibula.

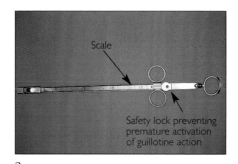

a

**Figure 2.56**
A Crawford fascia lata stripper.

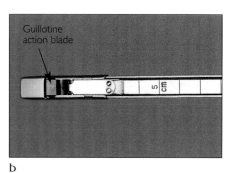

b

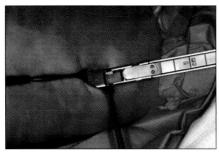

a

**Figure 2.57**
(a) The cut inferior end of the fascia is inserted into the fascia lata stripper.
(b) The 1 cm × 15 cm strip of fascia is removed

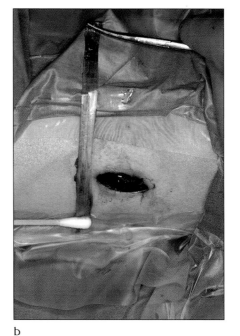

b

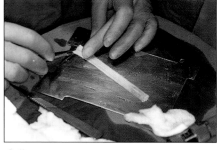

**Figure 2.58**
The fascia being cleaned on a graft board before being divided into 2 mm strips.

2. A 5 ml subcutaneous injection of 0.5% Marcain with 1:200,000 units of adrenaline is given.
3. A skin incision is made using a No. 15 blade.
4. Blunt dissection is used to expose the fascia lata.
5. Horizontal fascia overlying the fascia lata is bluntly dissected away with toothed forceps.
6. Two vertical incisions are made in the fascia lata 10 mm apart with long straight blunt-tipped scissors (Nelson scissors) if a Moseley fasciotome is being used to remove the fascia. This step is unnecessary if a Crawford stripper is used. The Crawford stripper has a side cutting mechanism and also has the advantage of offering a scale to measure the length of fascia to be removed (Figure 2.56).
7. The fascia is then cut across at the inferior aspect of the wound and inserted into the fascia lata stripper which is passed up the thigh 15 cm towards the anterior superior iliac crest (Figure 2.57).

8. The stripper guillotine mechanism is activated and the fascia removed.
9. The leg wound is then closed with subcutaneous 4/0 Vicryl sutures and the skin closed using interrupted 4/0 nylon vertical mattress sutures.
10. The fascia is cleaned of any fat and carefully divided into four symmetric lengths and kept moistened with saline (Figure 2.58).

## *Lemagne procedure*

This is a two-stage unilateral procedure for the treatment of patients with a significant ptosis and aberrant movements of the eyelid. Muscular neurotization occurs in the transposed levator muscle from the underlying frontalis muscle, permitting some

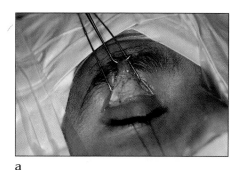

a

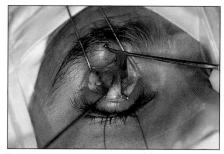

b

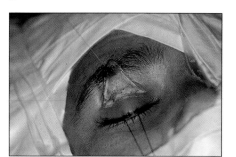

c

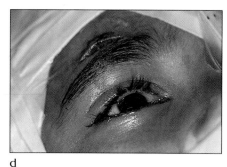

d

**Figure 2.59**
A Lemagne procedure. (a) The levator muscle is isolated and hooked with a strabismus hook. (b) The full length of the levator muscle is exposed. (c) The muscle is transected at the orbital apex and a double-armed 5/0 Vicryl suture placed. (d) A brow incision is made and the muscle transposed to the forehead.

levator function to be restored. The maximal degree of levator function may not be achieved for a period of 12 months following the first stage of surgery. The procedure is successful in abolishing aberrant eyelid movements. It requires a second-stage levator advancement procedure after 12 months to achieve a satisfactory improvement in the ptosis.

The levator muscle is isolated via an upper eyelid skin crease incision and a strabismus hook placed beneath it, ensuring that the superior rectus muscle is not inadvertently included (Figure 2.59a). The muscle is dissected to the orbital apex and transected (Figure 2.59b). A double-armed 5/0 Vicryl suture is placed through the cut end of the muscle (Figure 2.59c). The levator aponeurosis and Whitnall's ligament are left undisturbed. A 2 cm incision is made just above the central aspect of the eyebrow. This incision and the eyelid crease incision are joined by blunt dissection with Stevens tenotomy scissors. The levator muscle is transposed to lie above the frontalis muscle to which it is sutured (Figure 2.59d). A levator advancement is performed 12 months later.

# Complications of ptosis surgery

The majority of complications (Table 2.10) of ptosis surgery can be avoided by:

1. A thorough knowledge of eyelid anatomy
2. A careful preoperative evaluation of the patient
3. Selection of the most appropriate surgical technique
4. Preoperative counselling to avoid unrealistic patient expectations
5. Meticulous surgical technique
6. Good postoperative care

**Table 2.10** Complications of ptosis surgery

Undercorrection
Overcorrection
Lagophthalmos/exposure keratopathy
Eyelid contour defects
Skin crease defects
Conjunctival prolapse
Upper lid entropion/ectropion
Eyelash ptosis
Loss of eyelashes
Posterior lamellar granuloma/suture exposure
Extrusion/infection of frontalis suspension material
Diplopia
Haemorrhage

# *Undercorrection*

## Levator aponeurosis advancement/levator resection

An undercorrection may be the desired result in patients who are at high risk of exposure keratopathy. An unplanned undercorrection can have a variety of causes:

- An inadequate levator aponeurosis advancement
- Cheese-wiring of sutures placed too superficially in the tarsus
- Loosening of incorrectly tied sutures
- Placement of sutures through a very thinned levator aponeurosis
- Cheese-wiring of sutures following excessive eyelid oedema or haematoma

When this procedure has been performed in adults it is preferable to explore the levator aponeurosis within a week of surgery and readvance the aponeurosis under local anaesthesia. In children this will require another general anaesthetic. If there is excessive postoperative oedema or haematoma, however, it is preferable to await resolution and perform a formal reoperation at a later date.

## Whitnall's sling

An undercorrection may be cosmetically and functionally acceptable and preferable to a unilateral frontalis suspension. An unsatisfactory result will usually require a frontalis suspension.

## Frontalis suspension

An undercorrection following a frontalis suspension procedure will usually require early reintervention as the slings are likely to have loosened or the knots undone. These can be explored and tightened only with prompt intervention; otherwise, a reoperation at a later date will be required.

## *Overcorrection*

Overcorrection is rarely encountered following surgery for congenital 'dystrophic' ptosis. In such cases it is likely that the lid position will improve spontaneously and lubrication of the cornea is all that is required. Overcorrection is more commonly encountered following surgery for aponeurotic ptosis, especially if this has been performed under general anaesthesia (Figure 2.60). Postoperative massage may be performed as soon as the sutures have been removed when the levator surgery has been performed via a posterior approach. Massage cannot be performed so soon following anterior approach surgery without risking a skin wound dehiscence. A period of weeks is usually required.

Overcorrections which do not respond to more conservative measures will require a levator tenotomy. The eyelid is everted over a Desmarres retractor and a transconjunctival incision made. The levator aponeurosis is dissected with Westcott scissors and the lid position inspected at intervals. The lid position should be slightly overcorrected to allow for postoperative wound contracture. No sutures are required. Massage is commenced as soon as the lid height is satisfactory to prevent a recurrence.

Overcorrection following a frontalis suspension is rarely encountered. If synthetic material has been used, this will have to be explored and adjusted. If silicone has been used with a sleeve, the sleeve can be adjusted. Such intervention, however, increases the risks of infection and extrusion. If autogenous material has been used, the bands can be divided above the skin crease once they have scarred into position after a few days. A grey line traction suture is placed and the lid stretched inferiorly. The bands are then easily palpated and divided with scissors.

## *Lagophthalmos/exposure keratopathy*

Patients should be warned preoperatively that their reflex blink will be incomplete following ptosis surgery and even voluntary eyelid closure may be compromised, albeit temporarily. Frequent lubrication should be used to prevent exposure keratopathy. In cases where conservative treatment fails to control the symptoms and signs of exposure, the eyelid(s) will have to be lowered as in the case of overcorrections. Patients who are at increased risk of exposure keratopathy, e.g. patients with CPEO with an absent Bell's phenomenon, should be monitored very closely following ptosis surgery (Figure 2.61). Overcorrections should be avoided.

## *Eyelid contour defects*

Eyelid contour defects usually occur from improper placement of tarsal sutures during levator surgery or from improper tightening of suspension material during a frontalis suspension procedure (Figure 2.62). Minor defects can respond to massage applied selectively to areas of overcorrection. More severe defects usually require surgical correction with proper placement of sutures to adjust the contour.

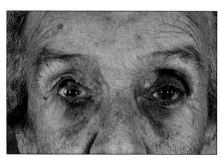

a

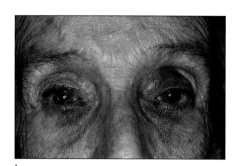

b

**Figure 2.60**
(a) Elderly patient with overcorrected levator advancement performed under general anaesthesia. (b) The patient following a levator recession performed under local anaesthesia.

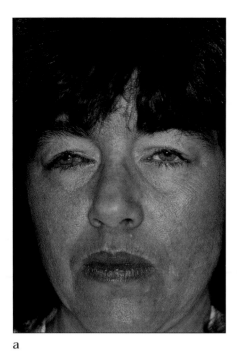

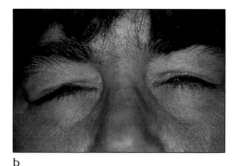

b

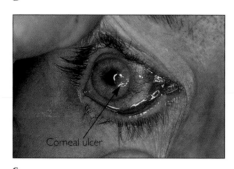

Corneal ulcer

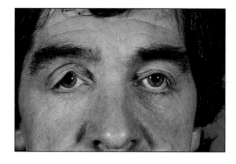

a                                         c

## Figure 2.61
(a) Patient with CPEO following bilateral autogenous fascia lata frontalis suspension with red right eye. (b) Same patient demonstrating lagophthalmos and an absent Bell's phenomenon. (c) Same patient demonstrating medial corneal ulcer of right eye. The ulcer perforated a few days later.

## Figure 2.62
Patient with a marked right upper eyelid contour defect following a levator advancement.

## Skin crease defects

Skin crease defects can mar an otherwise satisfactory result (Figure 2.63). They can occur for a variety of reasons:

- Failure to measure out and mark the new proposed skin crease prior to surgery (Figure 2.63)
- Failure to reform the skin crease by passing the interrupted skin sutures through the levator following levator surgery
- Failure to perform an upper lid blepharoplasty when there is excess upper lid skin
- A low skin crease is an inherent disadvantage of a frontalis suspension procedure performed via eyelid stab incisions (Figure 2.64)
- A lowering of the skin crease is an inherent disadvantage of the Fasanella–Servat procedure

An unsatisfactory skin crease can usually be addressed by a formal blepharoplasty. In some cases passing dissolvable sutures through the eyelid from the conjunctival surface at the upper border of the tarsus and tying them in the skin will create scarring and a skin crease (Pang sutures).

## Conjunctival prolapse

A conjunctival prolapse usually occurs in severe cases of congenital 'dystrophic' ptosis where the dissection has been taken above the superior fornix, causing the suspensory ligaments of the conjunctival fornix to be separated (Figure 2.65). It may also occur as a result of excessive postoperative oedema. Conservative treatment with simple topical lubrication may suffice. An

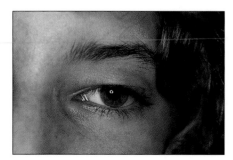

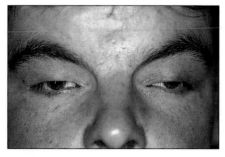

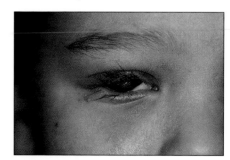

## Figure 2.63
Patient with a left skin crease defect following a levator advancement.

## Figure 2.64
Patient with a bilateral skin crease defect following a bilateral autogenous fascia lata frontalis suspension.

## Figure 2.65
A child with a postoperative conjunctival prolapse.

attempt to reposition the prolapsed conjunctiva can be made with the use of a muscle hook but if this fails Pang sutures can be passed through the prolapsed conjunctiva and tied in the skin crease. Rarely, if the prolapse is chronic, the prolapsed conjunctiva requires a formal excision.

## Upper lid entropion/ectropion

Entropion of the upper eyelid following ptosis surgery can occur in the following circumstances:

- Following excessive tarsal resection during a Fasanella–Servat procedure (Figure 2.66)
- Following excessive levator resections
- Following an autogenous fascia lata frontalis suspension procedure if the anterior lamellar dissection has been overly aggressive and the fascia has been sutured too low on the tarsus

Where an excessive tarsal resection has been performed a posterior lamellar graft may have to be undertaken. Following an excessive levator resection procedure, the eyelid position may improve with a release of the tarsal sutures. Otherwise, as in the case following frontalis suspension, a more formal upper eyelid entropion procedure may be required.

Ectropion of the upper eyelid following ptosis surgery is very rare. It can occur if the levator is advanced too far on the tarsus or if fascia is sutured too low on the tarsus following a frontalis suspension procedure. This malposition should normally improve with massage or suture release.

## Eyelash ptosis

An eyelash ptosis occurs following overly aggressive dissection of the tarsus with placement of the eyelid retractor too high on the tarsus (Figure 2.67). If the lash ptosis persists following resolution of pretarsal oedema, the retractor may need to be advanced on the tarsus. This may have to be combined with a grey line split.

## Loss of eyelashes

Loss of eyelashes is caused by an overly aggressive dissection of the tarsus (Figure 2.68). It is necessary only to bare the superior 1/3 of the tarsus during ptosis surgery.

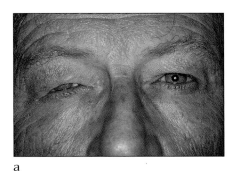
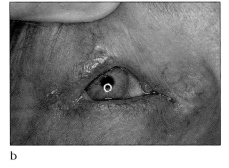
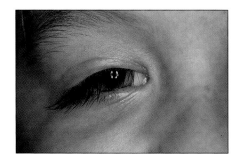

a      b

**Figure 2.66**
(a) Patient with a severe right upper eyelid entropion following a Fasanella–Servat procedure. (b) Close-up of the right upper eyelid with the brow elevated manually.

**Figure 2.67**
Patient with a severe right upper eyelid lash ptosis following a levator resection.

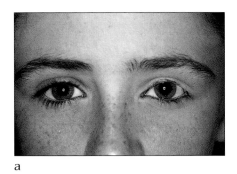
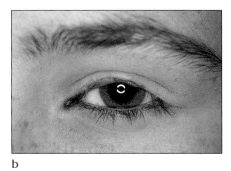
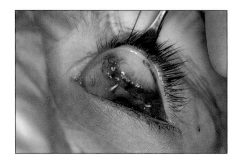

a      b

**Figure 2.68**
(a) Patient with an extensive area of loss of upper lid lashes following a levator resection. (b) Close-up of the patient's left upper eyelid.

**Figure 2.69**
Patient with an exposed Ethibond suture following a levator resection.

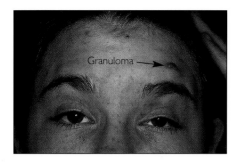

**Figure 2.70**
Patient with a foreign body granuloma following a Mersilene mesh frontalis suspension.

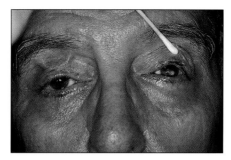

**Figure 2.71**
Patient with a visible silicone band in the right upper eyelid following a frontalis suspension. The left eye has had the band removed following severe exposure keratopathy

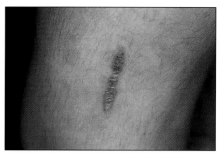

**Figure 2.72**
Patient with an unsightly leg scar following harvesting of fascia lata.

## *Posterior lamellar granuloma/suture exposure*

A foreign body granuloma is a common complication following posterior approach levator surgery. The granuloma can be removed and the base cauterized. Occasionally sutures erode through the conjunctiva if nondissolvable sutures have been used (Figure 2.69). The occurrence of a granuloma should provoke a search for such suture material.

## *Extrusion/infection of frontalis suspension material*

Infection, foreign body reaction, and extrusion are a risk whenever nonautogenous material is used for frontalis suspension (Figure 2.70). Once this has occurred, the material will usually have to be removed. Occasionally the postoperative scarring can itself assist in frontalis suspension, obviating the need for further surgery.

It is important to ensure that frontalis suspension material is buried and that the wounds are closed meticulously. A strictly aseptic surgical technique should be employed with the area prepped as for an intraocular procedure. It is also important to ensure that the material is passed posterior to the orbital septum or the material will be visible through the skin (Figure 2.71).

Although the results of autogenous fascia lata brow suspension are usually very good the patient should be also be warned that the scar on the leg may be unsightly as the wound tends to spread postoperatively (Figure 2.72).

## *Diplopia*

Diplopia should be an extremely rare complication following ptosis surgery. It is usually due to inadvertent injury to the superior rectus muscle or to the superior oblique tendon. Such a complication should not occur if the surgeon has an adequate knowledge of upper eyelid anatomy.

## *Haemorrhage*

Haemorrhage can seriously affect the outcome of ptosis surgery. Precautions should be taken to prevent intraoperative and postoperative haemorrhage:

- The patient should discontinue aspirin and any other antiplatelet drug at least 3 weeks prior to surgery
- Any patient on anticoagulants should undergo surgery in consultation with a haematologist
- Any patient with hypertension should take their usual antihypertensive agents on the day of surgery
- Local anaesthetic injections should be given subcutaneously and not into the orbicularis muscle or deeper
- Meticulous haemostasis should be performed at all stages of surgery
- A compressive dressing should be applied postoperatively wherever possible

## Further reading

1.  Anderson RL, Beard C. The levator aponeurosis. *Arch Ophthalmol* (1977) **95**:1437–41.
2.  Anderson RL, Dixon RS. Aponeurotic ptosis surgery. *Arch Ophthalmol* (1979) **97**:1123–8.
3.  Anderson RL. Age of aponeurotic awareness. *Ophthal Plast Reconstr Surg* (1985) **1**:77–9.
4.  Anderson RL, Jordan DR, Dutton JJ. Whitnall's sling for poor function ptosis. *Arch Ophthalmol* (1990) **108**:1628–32.
5.  Beard C. *Ptosis*, St. Louis: CV Mosby, 1981.
6.  Beard C. A new classification of blepharoptosis. *Int Ophthal Clin* (1989) **29**:214–16.
7.  Buckman G, Levine MR. Treatment of prolapsed conjunctiva. *Ophthal Plast Reconstr Surg* (1986) **2**:33–9.

8. Carroll RP. Preventable problems following the Fasanella–Servat procedure. *Ophthal Surgery* (1986) **11**:44–51.

9. Codere F, Tucker NA, Renaldi B. The anatomy of Whitnall ligament. *Ophthalmology* (1995) **102**:2016–19.

10. Collin JR. Complications of ptosis surgery and their management: a review. *J R Soc Med* (1979) **72**:25–6.

11. Dresner SC. Further modification of the Müller's muscle: conjunctival resection procedure for blepharoptosis. *Ophthal Plast Reconstr Surg* (1991) **7**:114–22.

12. Dutton JJ. *Atlas of clinical and surgical orbital anatomy*, Philadelphia: WB Saunders, 1994.

13. Edmunds B, Manners RM, Weller RO, Steart P, Collin JR. Levator palpebrae superioris fibre size in normals and patients with congenital ptosis. *Eye* (1998) **12**:47–50.

14. Fasanella RM, Servat J. Levator resection for minimal ptosis, with indications and reappraisal. *Int Ophthal Clin* (1970) **10**:117–30.

15. Ficker LA, Collin JR, Lee JP. Management of ipsilateral ptosis with hypotropia. *Br J Ophthalmol* (1986) **70**:732–6.

16. Frueh BR. The mechanistic classification of ptosis. *Ophthalmology* (1980) 87:1019–21.

17. Jordan DR, Anderson RL. The aponeurotic approach to congenital ptosis. *Ophthal Surg* (1990) 21:237–44.

18. Lane CM, Collin JR. Treatment of ptosis in chronic progressive external ophthalmoplegia. *Br J Ophthalmol* (1987) 71:290–4.

19. Leone CR Jr., Shore JW. The management of the ptosis patient: Part I. *Ophthal Surg* (1985) 16:666–70.

20. Manners RM, Tyers AG, Morris RJ. The use of Prolene as a temporary suspensory material for brow suspension in young children. *Eye* (1994) 8:346–8.

21. Manners RM, Rosser P, Collin JR. Moorfields Eye Hospital, London, UK. Levator transposition procedure: a review of 35 cases. *Eye* (1994) 10:539–44.

22. Martin JJ Jr., Tenzel RR. Acquired ptosis: dehiscences and disinsertions. Are they real or iatrogenic? *Ophthal Plast Reconstr Surg* (1992) 8:130–2; discussion 133.

23. McCord C, ed. Decision making in ptosis surgery. In: *Eyelid surgery principles and techniques*. Philadelphia: Lippincott-Raven, 1995, pp. 139–43.

24. McCord C, ed. Complications of ptosis surgery and their management. In: *Eyelid surgery principles and techniques*. Philadelphia: Lippincott-Raven, 1995, pp. 144–55.

25. Meyer DR, Linberg JV, Wobig JL, McCormick SA. Anatomy of the orbital septum and associated eyelid connective tissues. Implications for ptosis surgery. *Ophthal Plast Reconstr Surg* (1991) 7:104–13.

26. Putterman AM. Müllers muscle-conjunctival resection ptosis procedure. *Austral & NZ J Ophthalmol* (1985) 13:179–83.

27. Shore JW, Bergin DJ, Garrett SN. Results of blepharoptosis surgery with early postoperative adjustment. *Ophthalmology* (1990) 97:1502–11.

28. Striph GG, Miller NR. Disorders of eyelid function caused by systemic disease. In: Bosniak S, ed., *Principles and practice of ophthalmic plastic and reconstructive surgery*. Philadelphia: WB Saunders, pp. 72–93.

29. Woog JJ. Obstructive sleep apnea and the floppy eyelid syndrome, *Am J Ophthalmol* (1990) 110:314–16.

# 3

# Lower eyelid entropion

## Introduction

Lower eyelid entropion is an eyelid malposition in which the lower eyelid margin is turned inwards against the globe.

## Classification

1. Congenital entropion
2. Involutional entropion
3. Cicatricial entropion
4. Acute spastic entropion

## *Congenital entropion*

Congenital lower eyelid entropion is a rare condition. It differs from congenital epiblepharon, a much more common condition, by the fact that the tarsus is inverted (Figure 3.1). This eyelid malposition does not resolve spontaneously and requires surgical intervention to prevent corneal morbidity. It has been postulated that an abnormal insertion of the lower lid retractors is the underlying cause.

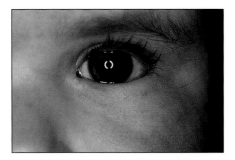

**Figure 3.1**
Congenital lower eyelid entropion.

## *Involutional entropion*

The majority of entropia are involutional and therefore seen in older patients. In the lower eyelid, involutional changes typically result in either a lower lid entropion or ectropion, whereas in the upper eyelid the same changes result in ptosis. A combination of factors has been proposed to account for the eyelid malposition. These are:

1. Laxity, dehiscence or disinsertion of the lower eyelid retractors (Figure 3.2a)
2. Over-riding of the preseptal orbicularis muscle over the pretarsal orbicularis (Figure 3.2b)
3. Horizontal eyelid laxity
4. Enophthalmos

Any surgical treatment should aim to address these factors with the exception of enophthalmos. Enophthalmos is no longer considered a significant factor in the aetiology of involutional lower eyelid entropion.

## *Cicatricial entropion*

Any condition that causes contracture of the conjunctiva can result in a cicatricial entropion (Figure 3.3). Such conditions include chemical burns, topical glaucoma medications, ocular cicatricial pemphigoid and Stevens–Johnson syndrome.

## *Acute spastic entropion*

This form of entropion is seen in susceptible individuals with blepharospasm that has been induced by ocular irritation. Although treatment of the underlying cause of ocular irritation may reverse the eyelid malposition, a permanent entropion may ensue which will require surgical intervention.

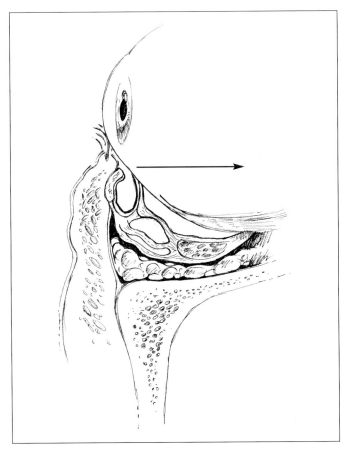

a

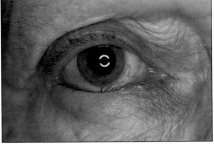

b

**Figure 3.2**
(a) Laxity of the lower eyelid retractors and over-riding of the preseptal orbicularis muscle over the pretarsal orbicularis, causing lower eyelid entropion. (b) A typical lower eyelid involutional entropion.

# Applied surgical anatomy

A thorough understanding of lower eyelid anatomy is essential to the surgical management of lower eyelid entropion (Figure 3.4). The lower eyelid can be considered to consist of three lamellae:

- Anterior – skin and orbicularis oculi muscle
- Middle – orbital septum and inferior eyelid retractors
- Posterior – tarsus and conjunctiva

The lower eyelid tarsus is approximately 3–4 mm in height and 1 mm in thickness. The tarsal conjunctiva is firmly adherent to the tarsus and cannot be dissected freely. The forniceal conjunctiva, in contrast, is very loosely attached to the underlying retractors. The lower eyelid skin crease is variable but usually situated approximately 4–5 mm below the eyelid margin. The lateral canthal angle normally sits approximately 2 mm higher than the medial canthal angle.

The lower eyelid retractor complex consists of an aponeurotic expansion from the inferior rectus muscle. This aponeurotic expansion, known as the capulopalpebral fascia, extends anteriorly to envelop the inferior oblique muscle, where it fuses with the inferior suspensory ligament (Lockwood's ligament). The fascia also contains fibres which insert into the inferior margin of the tarsus, the preseptal orbicularis muscle at the level of the lower lid skin crease and the inferior fornix. The fascia is also accompanied by some smooth muscle fibres. The orbital septum fuses with the fascia approximately 5 mm below the tarsus. The orbital septum extends from the arcus marginalis of the inferior orbital margin to the inferior border of the tarsus. Posterior to this lies the three lower lid fat pockets.

The anatomy of the lower eyelid resembles that of the upper eyelid. Although the tarsus is much smaller, the capsulopalpebral fascia is analogous to the levator aponeurosis. The smooth muscle fibres accompanying this fascia are analogous to Müller's muscle. Lockwood's ligament is analogous to Whitnall's ligament. The fat in the lower eyelid lies posterior to the septum but anterior to the capsulopalpebral fascia and is analogous to the upper lid preaponeurotic fat. There are three fat pads in the lower eyelid: medial, central and lateral. These lie between the capsulopalpebral fascia and the orbital septum. The inferior oblique muscle lies between the medial and central fat pads.

In the lower eyelid an anastomotic arterial arcade runs in the orbicularis oculi muscle plane approximately 4–5 mm below the eyelid margin.

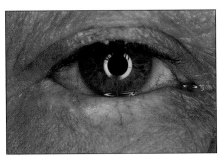

a

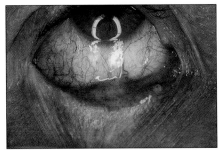

b

**Figure 3.3**
(a) A lower eyelid cicatricial entropion. The lower eyelid lashes have been removed by previous cryotherapy. (b) Eversion of the lower eyelid reveals conjunctival scarring.

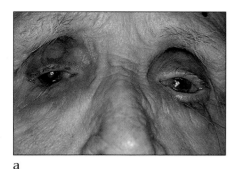
a

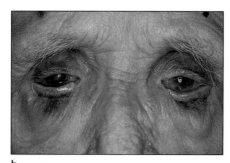
b

**Figure 3.7**
(a) An elderly patient with a right lower eyelid involutional entropion. Everting sutures have been placed in the left lower eyelid. (b) The sutures have been placed in both lower eyelids and tied tightly enough to produce a minimal degree of ectropion.

these sutures are passed through the eyelid from the conjunctival surface just below the tarsus and tied in the same manner.

**Lower lid retractor advancement with lateral tarsal strip.** A volume of 5 ml of 0.5% bupivacaine with 1:200,000 units of adrenaline are injected subcutaneously into the lower eyelid and into the lateral canthus. A 4/0 silk traction suture is placed through the grey line of the lower eyelid and fixated to the head drapes using a small haemostat. A skin incision is then made 3 mm below the eyelid margin using a Colorado needle. Haemostasis is obtained using bipolar cautery. The Colorado needle is then used to dissect through the orbicularis oculi muscle and to expose the orbital septum. The septum is opened with the Colorado needle or Westcott scissors 6–8 mm below the eyelid margin, exposing the preaponeurotic fat (Figure 3.8a). The inferior eyelid retractors are identified beneath the fat. The tarsus is not specifically identified. The retractors are then carefully dissected from the underlying conjunctiva with Westcott scissors avoiding the inferior tarsal vascular arcade (Figure 3.8b).

The retractors are then held and the patient instructed to look down (Figure 3.9). An inferior pull on the fascia should be felt. A 1 mm strip of fascia is removed, shortening the retractors vertically. Next, 2–3 interrupted 5/0 Vicryl sutures are used to reattach the lower lid retractors to the inferior border of the tarsus, avoiding the medial aspect of the eyelid to avoid creating a medial punctal ectropion (Figure 3.10). When these are tied, the lower eyelid should now have a minimal degree of central and lateral ectropion.

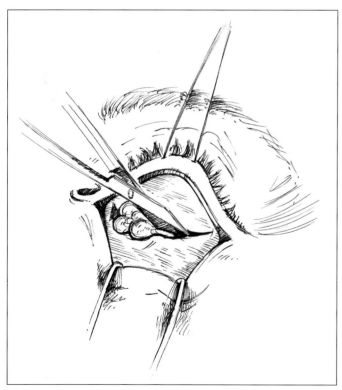
a

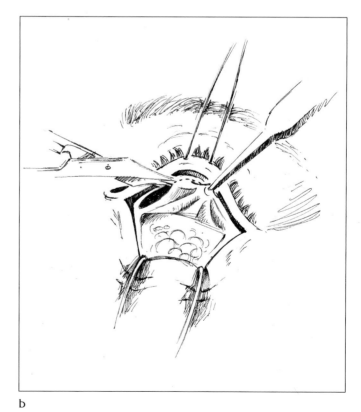
b

**Figure 3.8**
(a) The orbital septum is opened, exposing the preaponeurotic fat. (b) The lower eyelid retractors are dissected from the underlying conjunctiva.

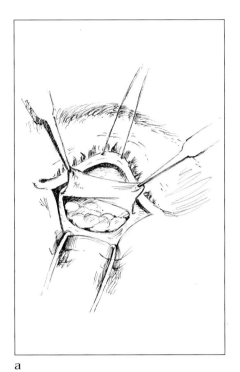

a

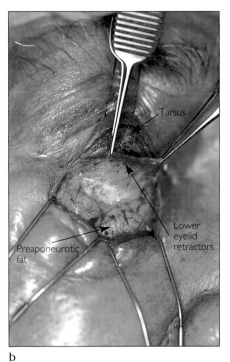

b

**Figure 3.9**
(a) The lower eyelid retractors are held and the patient is asked to look down. (b) The appearance of the lower eyelid retractors dissected from the underlying conjunctiva.

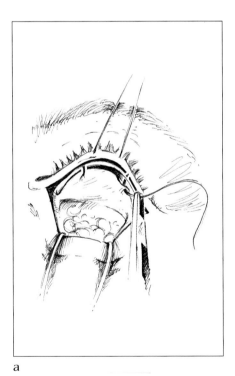

a

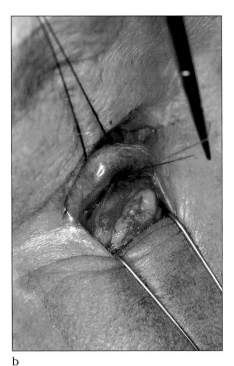

b

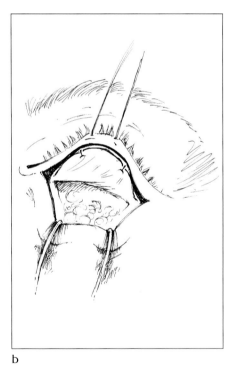

b

**Figure 3.10**
(a) The lower eyelid retractors are sutured to the inferior border of the tarsus. (b) The lower eyelid retractors have been sutured to the central area of the tarsus. (c) The retractor advancement has been completed.

Next a lateral tarsal strip procedure is performed, as described in Chapter 5 (Lower Eyelid Ectropion). This should be tightened sufficiently to bring the eyelid in apposition with the globe. The subciliary skin wound is then closed using a continuous 7/0 Vicryl suture.

A compressive dressing is applied for 3 days.

**Lower lid retractor advancement with lower lid wedge resection.** A volume of 3 ml of 0.5% bupivacaine and 1:200,000 units of adrenaline are injected subcutaneously in the lower eyelid. The retractor dissection proceeds in the same manner as described above to the point at which the lower lid retractors have been freed. Next a lower lid wedge resection is performed

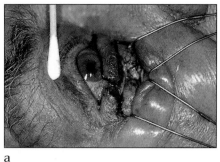
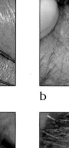
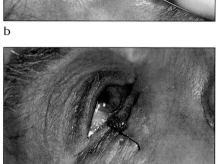

a

b

c

d

**Figure 3.11**
(a) The lower eyelid has been incised at the junction of the medial two-thirds with the lateral third. (b) The eyelid is overlapped to determine the amount of eyelid which can be safely removed without leaving the wound under undue tension and without causing lower eyelid retraction. (c) The uppermost Vicryl suture is used for traction, while the remaining Vicryl sutures are placed in the tarsus. (d) The appearance of the eyelid at the completion of surgery.

at the junction of the lateral third with the medial two-thirds of the eyelid (Figure 3.11a,b). The tarsus is repaired using interrupted 5/0 Vicryl sutures and the eyelid margin is repaired with 6/0 silk sutures passed along the lash line and along the line of the meibomian gland orifices (see also Figure 10.10c,d).

A 1 mm strip of fascia is removed, shortening the retractors vertically. Next 2–3 interrupted 5/0 Vicryl sutures are used to reattach the lower lid retractors to the inferior border of the tarsus, avoiding the medial aspect of the eyelid to avoid creating a medial punctal ectropion. When these sutures are tied, the lower eyelid should be in apposition to the globe without any ectropion.

The subciliary skin wound is then closed using a continuous 7/0 Vicryl suture. The eyelid margin sutures are removed in 14 days.

These procedures have an extremely low recurrence rate and minimal morbidity in the hands of an experienced oculoplastic surgeon. The many potential complications of these procedures can be avoided by careful patient selection, by a good knowledge of surgical anatomy, and by attention to appropriate haemostasis and meticulous surgical technique.

## Complications

1. Wound dehiscence
2. Haematoma
3. Infection
4. Granuloma
5. Ectropion
6. Lateral canthal discomfort
7. Overlapping of the upper eyelid
8. Eyelid notch
9. Trichiasis
10. Corneal ulcer

11. Recurrence of entropion
12. Lateral canthal angle deformity

A lateral canthal granuloma following a lateral tarsal strip procedure is avoided by ensuring that the Ethibond suture is completely buried. Before performing a wedge resection the surgeon should determine the precise amount of eyelid which can be safely sacrificed without leaving the wound under tension. If the eyelid wound is under too much tension or if the sutures are tied too tightly causing strangulation of the wound edges, the wound is more likely to break down. A notch and trichiasis are avoided by meticulous attention to the apposition of the wound edges and the use of vertical mattress sutures through the eyelid margin.

A haematoma or excessive postoperative oedema place the wound at risk of breakdown. These are avoided by the preoperative management of hypertension, the avoidance of antiplatelet agents, meticulous dissection and careful use of bipolar cautery, and by the postoperative use of a compressive dressing.

Great care needs to be taken over the placement of the Ethibond suture in the lateral tarsal strip procedure. This should engage periorbita just inside the lateral orbital wall at the junction with the upper eyelid to avoid anterior displacement of the eyelid from the globe and lateral canthal dystopia. If the upper eyelid is very lax, there may be an unsightly overlap of the upper eyelid over the lower eyelid if the lateral tarsal strip is overtightened.

## Congenital entropion

Congenital entropion (Figure 3.12) is managed under general anaesthesia. A subciliary incision is made with a Colorado needle 2 mm below the eyelid margin. A retractor advancement is combined with a conservative resection of skin and orbicularis.

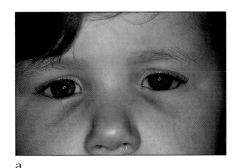
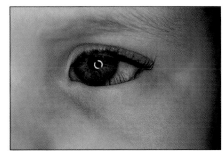

a

b

**Figure 3.12**
(a) A left lower eyelid congenital entropion. (b) A close-up photograph of the lower eyelid entropion. This should be differentiated from a lower eyelid congenital epiblepharon

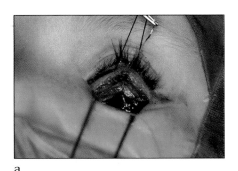
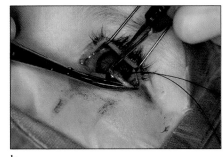

a

b

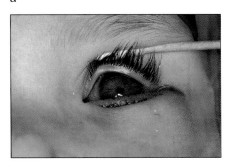
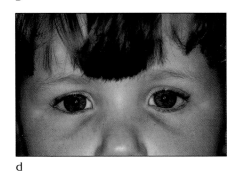

c

d

**Figure 3.13**
(a) The lower eyelid retractors are advanced and attached to the lower border of the tarsus. (b) A conservative skin–muscle blepharoplasty is performed. (c) The appearance of the eyelid at the completion of surgery. (d) The postoperative appearance of the eyelid 2 weeks after surgery

The lower eyelid retractors may be found to be disinserted. A simple advancement of the retractor will usually suffice without the need for any resection of the retractor. A very conservative resection of a strip of skin and orbicularis muscle may be required (Figure 3.13). No eyelid shortening is normally required.

## Cicatricial entropion

The choice of surgical procedure for the management of a lower lid cicatricial ectropion is dictated by the severity of the entropion and eyelid retraction and by the underlying cause. In the case of a cicatricial entropion caused by ocular cicatricial pemphigoid, surgery should be confined to the anterior lamella wherever possible to avoid exacerbating the conjunctival disease.

The surgical procedures that may be used are:

1. Retractor advancement
2. Tarsal fracture
3. Posterior lamellar graft

**Retractor advancement.** This procedure is particularly useful for patients with active conjunctival disease or ocular cicatricial pemphigoid. A retractor advancement is used alone without any horizontal eyelid shortening. The retractor advancement can be repeated if the entropion recurs.

**Tarsal fracture.** This procedure is indicated for patients with a mild cicatricial entropion with a minor degree of lower lid retraction.

A volume of 3–5 ml of 0.5% bupivacaine and 1:200,000 units of adrenaline are injected subcutaneously and subconjunctivally in the lower eyelid. A horizontal incision is made through the whole length of the tarsus just below its centre down to the deep surface of the orbicularis muscle. Three or four double-armed 5/0 Vicryl sutures are passed just below the incision from the conjunctival surface to the skin just below the lash line. These sutures are tied to produce a moderate ectropion; they are removed after 14 days.

**Posterior lamellar graft.** A posterior lamellar graft is indicated for the patient with a more severe degree of cicatricial entropion with more marked eyelid retraction.

The procedure is usually performed under general anaesthesia: 3–5 ml of 0.5% bupivacaine and 1:200,000 units of adrenaline are injected subcutaneously and subconjunctivally in the lower eyelid.

A 4/0 silk traction suture is inserted through the grey line and the eyelid everted over a Desmarres retractor. A horizontal incision is made through the whole length of the tarsus just below its centre down to the deep surface of the orbicularis with a No. 15 blade. The inferior margin of the tarsus is freed from the lid retractors and the orbital septum. The ensuing defect is measured and a slightly oversized hard palate graft is harvested and sutured between the cut edges of the tarsus with interrupted 7/0 Vicryl sutures. (See Chapter 26, The Use of Autogenous Grafts in Ophthalmic Plastic Surgery.) Three or four double-armed 5/0 Vicryl sutures are passed through the hard palate graft and tied just below the lash line to evert the eyelid margin and to maintain the graft in apposition to its bed. These sutures are removed after 14 days.

A number of alternative autogenous or nonautogenous materials exist for use as a posterior lamellar graft but none are as satisfactory as hard palate mucosa in this situation.

### Complications

1. Corneal abrasion
2. Corneal ulcer
3. Haematoma
4. Necrosis of the hard palate graft
5. Infection
6. Recurrence of the entropion

These complications can be largely avoided. The cornea should be protected intraoperatively. If suture abrasion is a concern, a bandage contact lens can be used. The graft should be firmly attached to its bed to prevent a haematoma from collecting beneath it. A haemotoma or movement of the graft can lead to graft failure.

# Epiblepharon

An epiblepharon is an excess fold of skin and orbicularis muscle in the medial aspect of the lower eyelid (Figure 3.14). Epiblepharon can cause the eyelashes to invert against the globe, and can be unilateral or bilateral. The management of this condition should be conservative, as spontaneous improvement typically occurs with age, and eyelashes in an infant tend to be very soft. If, however, the child suffers from tearing, photophobia and discomfort with corneal abrasion by the lashes, surgical intervention is warranted.

The procedure is performed under general anaesthesia: 3 ml of 0.25% bupivacaine and 1:200,000 units of adrenaline are injected subcutaneously in the lower eyelid. A 4/0 silk traction suture is inserted through the grey line and fixated to the head drapes with an artery clip. A subciliary incision is made along the medial two-thirds of the eyelid with a Colorado needle commencing below the inferior punctum. A skin–muscle flap is dissected from the orbital septum and extended some 4–5 mm inferiorly. The traction suture is released and the skin–muscle flap is draped over the eyelid margin and the excess skin and muscle is very carefully excised, taking great care not to excise too much tissue.

If the eyelid margin is still inverted the eyelid retractors can be dissected free, advanced and sutured to the lower border of the tarsal plate with a single 6/0 Vicryl suture until the eyelid margin is normally positioned. The skin edges are then reapproximated with interrupted 7/0 fast-absorbing Vicryl.

It may be necessary to perform the procedure bilaterally to achieve symmetry if only one eyelid is affected.

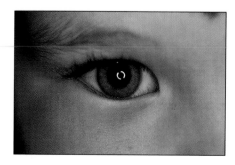

**Figure 3.14**
A congenital epiblepharon.

# Further reading

1. American Academy of Ophthalmology. *Basic and clinical science course: orbit, eyelids, and lacrimal system*, section 7. San Francisco: American Academy of Ophthalmology, 1998–99, pp. 148–56.
2. Anderson RL, Gordy DD. The tarsal strip procedure. *Arch Ophthalmol* (1979) **97**:2192–6.
3. Dutton JJ. *Atlas of clinical and surgical orbital anatomy*. Philadelphia: WB Saunders, 1994.
4. Hawes MJ, Dortzbach RK. The microscopic anatomy of the lower eyelid retractors. *Arch Ophthalmol* (1982) **100**:1313–18.
5. Jones LT, Rech MJ, Wobig JL. Senile entropion: a new concept for correction. *Am J Ophthalmol* (1972) **74**:327–9.
6. Kersten RC, Kleiner FP, Kulwin DR. Tarsotomy for the treatment of cicatricial entropion with trichiasis. *Arch Ophthalmol* (1992) **110**:714.
7. Martin RT, Nunery WR, Tanenbaum M. Entropion, trichiasis, and distichiasis. In: McCord CD, Tanenbaum M, Nunery WR, eds, *Oculoplastic surgery*, 3rd edn. New York: Raven Press, 1995, pp. 221–48.
8. Nerad JA. Eyelid malpositions. In: Linberg JV, ed., *Contemporary issues in ophthalmology, lacrimal surgery*. New York: Churchill Livingstone, 1988, pp. 62–89.
9. Wesley RE. Cicatricial entropion. In: Levine MR, ed., *Manual of oculoplastic surgery*, 2nd edn. Boston: Butterworth-Heinemann, 1996, pp. 129–34.
10. Wright M, Bell D, Scott C, Leatherbarrow B. Everting suture correction of lower lid involutional entropion. *Br J Ophthalmol* (1999) **83**:1060–3.

# 4

# Upper eyelid entropion

## Introduction

Upper lid entropion is an eyelid malposition in which the upper eyelid margin is turned inwards against the globe. It can be responsible for severe ocular morbidity. It is an uncommon condition in the Western World in contrast to a number of countries in the Third World, where trachoma is endemic. It has tended to receive very little attention in standard oculoplastic texts although its management can be difficult and challenging.

## Classification

Upper lid entropion may be classified as congenital or acquired. Acquired upper lid entropion can be further classified according to the underlying aetiology (Table 4.1). Any cause of conjunctival scarring can lead to an acquired upper lid entropion. The entropion may be further subclassified according to its severity as mild, moderate or severe.

A true congenital upper lid entropion is very rare. A horizontal tarsal kink is a similar but separate entity. The upper lid tarsus is frequently found to be abnormal and foreshortened (Figure 4.8).

**Table 4.1** Classification of upper eyelid entropion

**Congenital**

**Acquired**
- Trachoma (Figure 4.1)
- Chronic blepharoconjunctivitis
- Chemical burns
- Cicatrizing conjunctivitis
    topical glaucoma medications
    Stevens–Johnson syndrome (Figure 4.2)
    herpes zoster ophthalmicus (Figure 4.3)
    ocular cicatricial pemphigoid (Figure 4.4)
- Iatrogenic – e.g. a complication of the Fasanella–Servat procedure (Figure 4.5a)
- Chronic anophthalmic socket inflammation (Figure 4.5b)
- Eyebrow ptosis (Figure 4.6)
- Thyroid eye disease (Figure 4.7)

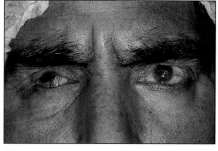

a

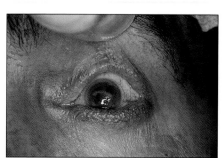

b

## Figure 4.1
(a) A left upper eyelid entropion as a consequence of trachoma in an Asian patient. The cornea is scarred. The extent of the entropion is masked by a brow ptosis. (b) Close-up of left side with brow elevated demonstrating the extent of the entropion.

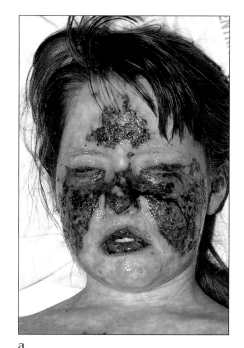

a

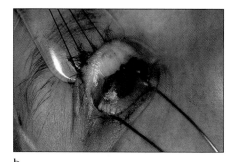

b

## Figure 4.2

(a) A patient with acute Stevens–Johnson syndrome. (b) A severe upper eyelid entropion developed with extensive keratinization of the posterior lamella.

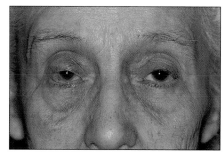

a

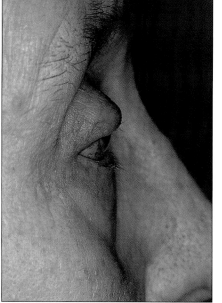

b

## Figure 4.3

(a) A right upper eyelid entropion as a consequence of herpes zoster ophthalmicus. (b) A side view of the right upper eyelid entropion.

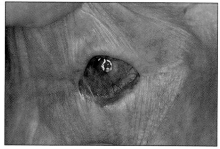

a

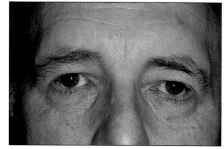

b

## Figure 4.4

(a) A right upper and lower eyelid entropion following ocular cicatricial pemphigoid. Extensive cryotherapy has removed all eyelashes.
(b) Extensive symblephara with obliteration of the fornices.

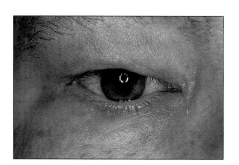

a

## Figure 4.5

(a) A right upper eyelid entropion occurring as a complication of a Fasanella–Servat procedure. (b) A right upper eyelid entropion in a child with a contracted anophthalmic socket.

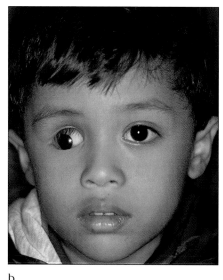

b

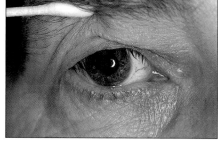

a

b

## Figure 4.6

(a) A bilateral upper eyelid entropion as a consequence of a marked bilateral ptosis. (b) A close-up of the right side demonstrating the proximity of the brow to the eyelid margin.

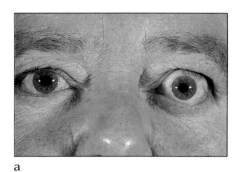 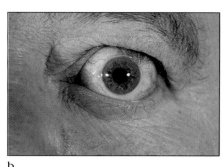

a                              b

**Figure 4.7**
(a) A left upper eyelid entropion as a consequence of thyroid eye disease. (b) A close-up of the left side demonstrating the upper eyelid entropion with marked upper eyelid retraction, proptosis and thickening of the sub-brow tissue

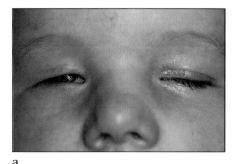 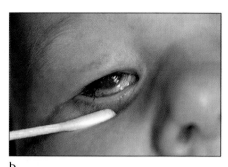

a                              b

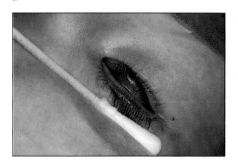 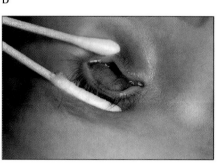

c                              d

**Figure 4.8**
(a) A congenital right upper eyelid entropion. (b) A close-up of the right upper eyelid entropion. (c) The right upper eyelid everted demonstrating a small tarsus. (d) The left upper eyelid everted demonstrating a normal tarsus.

# Patient assessment

A careful history and meticulous clinical examination are essential to determine the aetiology of the entropion. In addition to a complete ocular examination, the eyelid should be everted and the posterior lamella and the superior fornix examined. It is important to establish the presence of upper eyelid entropion and differentiate this from simple trichiasis. The presence of an early entropion is indicated by an apparent posterior migration of the meibomian gland orifices. It is important to determine whether or not there is any keratin present on the posterior lamella. The presence and degree of eyelid retraction and lagophthalmos should be determined. If an artificial eye is present, this should be removed and the superior fornix examined.

**Table 4.2** Factors influencing the surgical management of upper eyelid entropion

- The severity of the entropion
- The thickness of the tarsal plate
- The presence or absence of keratin on the posterior lamella
- The degree of eyelid retraction
- The degree of any lagophthalmos
- The underlying aetiology
- The presence of a corneal graft
- The planning of a future corneal graft
- The presence of an artificial eye

# Surgical management

A number of factors influence the operative management of this eyelid malposition (Table 4.2).

## Congenital upper lid entropion

In some cases the upper lid entropion resolves spontaneously but where this is causing distress or ocular complications the eyelid malposition should be corrected surgically.

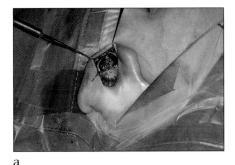
a

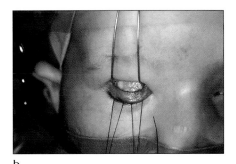
b

**Figure 4.9**
(a) An auricular cartilage graft has been harvested from the right ear.
(b) The graft has been placed over the infant's tarsus, extending superiorly onto the conjunctiva.

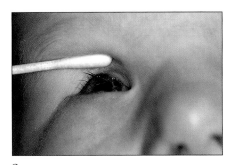
a

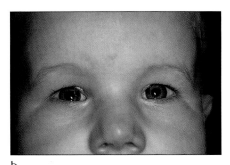
b

**Figure 4.10**
(a) The preoperative appearance of the right upper eyelid entropion.
(b) The appearance of the right upper eyelid 6 weeks after an auricular cartilage graft.

A skin crease incision is made and the patient's tarsus exposed down to the eyelash follicles, taking care not to damage these. The eyelid retractors are freed from the surface of the tarsus. An auricular cartilage graft, shaped to mimic a normal tarsus, is placed over the patient's tarsus, extending above its superior border onto the conjunctiva (Figure 4.9). The retractors are attached to the superior third of the cartilage graft with 5/0 Vicryl sutures. The skin crease is reformed as in a levator advancement procedure. The patient shown in Figures 4.8 and 4.9 is shown before and after this surgical procedure (Figures 10a and 10b).

## Acquired upper eyelid entropion

In contrast to the management of lower eyelid entropion, one of a number of different surgical procedures are selected for the individual patient based on the factors listed in Table 4.2 (see Table 4.3).

---

**Table 4.3**  The choice of operative procedures in the management of acquired upper eyelid entropion

- Anterior lamellar reposition with grey line split
- Tarsal wedge excision
- Lamellar split and posterior lamellar advancement
- Terminal tarsal rotation
- Posterior lamellar graft
- Auricular cartilage graft

---

## Anterior lamellar reposition with grey line split

This procedure is relatively simple to perform under local anaesthesia. It is used for patients with a mild upper lid entropion that is typically the result of chronic blepharoconjunctivitis (Figure 4.11).

An upper lid skin crease incision is marked with a cocktail stick dipped in gentian violet. The eyelid is injected subcutaneously with 0.5% bupivacaine and 1:200,000 units of adrenaline. A Beaver micro-sharp blade (7530) on a Beaver blade handle is used to create a grey line split to a depth of 1–2 mm (Figure 4.12). The incision should be made in a single sweep to avoid an irregular wound. Next, an upper lid skin crease incision is made with a Colorado needle and the superior half of the tarsus is exposed (Figure 4.13). The upper lid retractors are dissected from the superior border of the anterior surface of the tarsus and recessed approximately 5 mm.

A 5/0 Vicryl suture on a 1/4 circle needle is passed through the skin and orbicularis muscle just anterior to the grey line split and then passed horizontally in a lamellar fashion through the tarsus (Figure 4.14). The height of this suture placement determines the degree of eyelash eversion.

The suture is then passed anteriorly through the orbicularis muscle and skin 2–3 mm away from the initial suture pass and held with a bulldog clip (Figure 4.15). A series of additional sutures are placed along the length of the tarsus and then tied.

The skin crease is reformed, after removing a small strip of skin and orbicularis muscle from above the incision, by picking up the underlying levator aponeurosis (Figure 4.16). A lower lid Frost suture is inserted and a compressive dressing is applied for 2–3 days. The sutures should be removed after 4 weeks if still present.

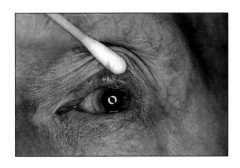

**Figure 4.11**
A mild left upper eyelid entropion resulting from chronic staphylococcal blepharitis.

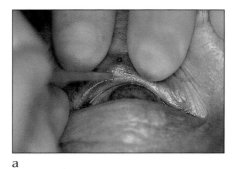

a                                    b

**Figure 4.12**
(a) A grey line split being performed with a micro-sharp blade. (b) The appearance of a grey line split.

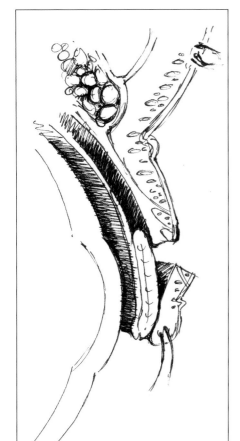

**Figure 4.13**
The anterior surface of the tarsus is exposed via a skin crease incision.

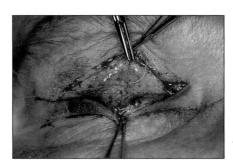

**Figure 4.14**
The upper lid retractors have been recessed. A 5/0 Vicryl suture is placed horizontally through the tarsus close to its upper border.

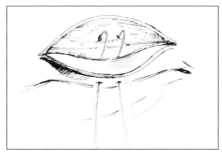

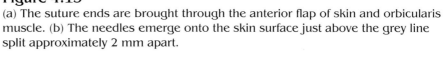

a                                    b

**Figure 4.15**
(a) The suture ends are brought through the anterior flap of skin and orbicularis muscle. (b) The needles emerge onto the skin surface just above the grey line split approximately 2 mm apart.

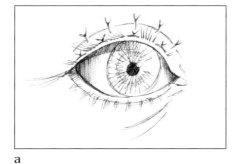

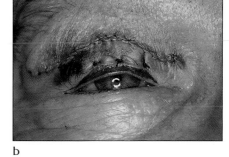

a                                    b

**Figure 4.16**
(a) A diagram demonstrating the position of the sutures. (b) In this patient the grey line split has been opened more than is usually required. A continuous suture was used to avoid a well-defined skin crease for better symmetry.

## Tarsal wedge excision

Tarsal wedge excision is typically used for patients with a greater degree of entropion with a thickened tarsus, an absence of posterior lamellar keratin and no lagophthalmos on voluntary eyelid closure. This condition is typically seen in the patient who has an upper lid entropion from trachoma.

The operation differs from the anterior lamellar reposition with grey line split only in that a horizontal wedge is removed with a blade from the anterior tarsal surface along the line of maximal thickening. The eyelid retractors are recessed to a greater degree to allow a posterior lamellar advancement to compensate for any eyelid retraction. Failure to recess the retractors will result in worsening of eyelid retraction postoperatively. The wedge resection is closed with interrupted sutures before the everting sutures are placed as in the anterior lamellar reposition with grey line split (Figure 4.17).

A lower lid Frost suture is inserted and a compressive dressing is applied for 2–3 days. The sutures should be removed after 4 weeks if still present.

## Lamellar split and posterior lamellar advancement

This procedure is typically used for patients with a greater degree of entropion with a thin tarsus, an absence of posterior lamellar keratin and no lagophthalmos on voluntary eyelid closure. This is typically seen in the anophthalmic patient who has an upper lid entropion.

In this procedure the upper eyelid is completely split into an anterior lamella of skin and orbicularis oculi muscle and a posterior lamella of tarsus and conjunctiva. The eyelid is injected subcutaneously with 0.5% bupivacaine and 1:200,000 units of adrenaline. A supersharp blade on a Beaver blade handle is used

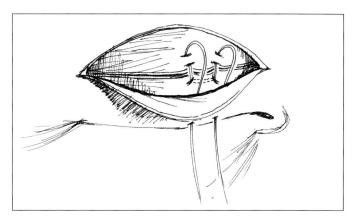

**Figure 4.17**
A small linear wedge has been removed from a thickened tarsus and the wedge closed with the Vicryl suture also used to open the grey line split.

to create a grey line split to a depth of 1–2 mm. The incision should be made in a single sweep to avoid an irregular wound. The incision is then deepened with Westcott scissors and the eyelid divided into an anterior and a posterior lamella as far as the superior fornix. The eyelid retractors are recessed and any subconjunctival scar tissue dissected from the conjunctiva to allow the posterior lamella to advance.

Next, four double-armed 4/0 Vicryl sutures are passed through the full thickness of the eyelid from the superior fornix to the desired position of the skin crease where they are tied. The posterior lamellar advancement should extend below the inferior margin of the anterior lamella by approximately 4 mm. The recessed edge of the anterior lamellar is sutured to the advanced tarsus with interrupted 7/0 Vicryl sutures. The raw surface of the tarsus is left to granulate (Figure 4.18).

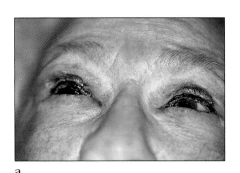
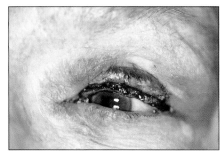

a

b

**Figure 4.18**
(a) A completed bilateral lamellar split and posterior lamellar advancement. (b) A close-up of the left eye.

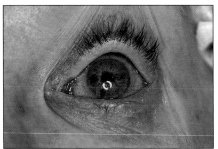
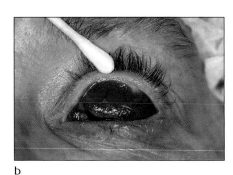

a

b

**Figure 4.19**
(a) The appearance of a keratinized right upper eyelid margin in a patient following a Stevens–Johnson syndrome episode. (b) Keratin is seen extending onto the inferior aspect of the tarsus.

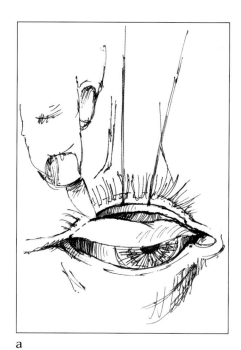

a

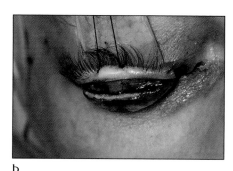

b

**Figure 4.20**
(a) An incision is made through the full thickness of the tarsus with a No. 15 Bard Parker blade. (b) The appearance of the incised tarsus.

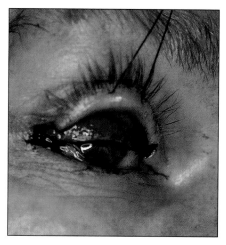

**Figure 4.21**
Relieving incisions are made through the eyelid margin medially and laterally.

A lower lid Frost suture is inserted and a compressive dressing is applied for 2–3 days. The sutures should be removed after 4 weeks.

## Terminal tarsal rotation

This procedure is used for patients with an upper lid entropion with keratin on the inferior aspect of the tarsus which typically occurs as a complication of Stevens–Johnson syndrome (Figure 4.19).

The eyelid is injected subcutaneously with 0.5% Marcain and 1:200,000 units of adrenaline. A 4/0 silk suture is placed through the grey line and the eyelid is everted over a Desmarres retractor. An incision is made with a No. 15 blade through the tarsus above the keratin (Figure 4.20).

The anterior surface of the tarsus and the conjunctiva up to the superior fornix are dissected using Westcott scissors until the posterior lamella will advance freely. A vertical relieving incision is made through the eyelid margin just lateral to the punctum and at the lateral aspect of the eyelid (Figure 4.21).

The anterior surface of the inferior tarsus is undermined until this fragment will rotate through 180 degrees (Figure 4.22a). Next, three double-armed 4/0 Vicryl sutures are passed through

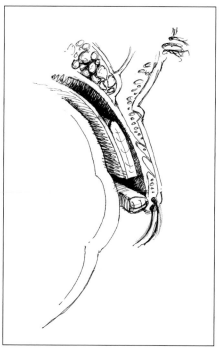

a

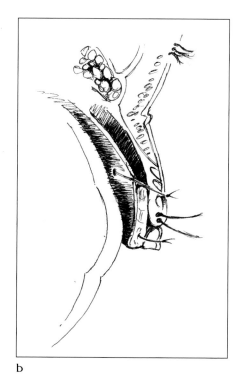

b

**Figure 4.22**
(a) The lower tarsal fragment is undermined anteriorly until it will rotate 180 degrees. (b) The terminal tarsal fragment has been rotated and sutured to the anterior tarsal surface.

the full thickness of the eyelid from the superior fornix to the desired position of the skin crease, where they are tied (Figures 4.22b, 4.23). The posterior lamellar advancement should extend below the inferior margin of the anterior lamella with its attached distal tarsal fragment by approximately 4 mm. The everted fragment of tarsus is sutured to the advanced anterior tarsal surface with interrupted 6/0 Vicryl sutures. The raw surface of the tarsus is left to granulate (Figure 4.23).

A lower lid Frost suture is inserted and a compressive dressing is applied for 2–3 days. The sutures should be removed after 4 weeks. Although the eyelashes are initially in an overcorrected position, these gradually return to a satisfactory position as the wound granulates (Figure 4.24).

## Posterior lamellar mucous membrane graft

A posterior lamellar mucous membrane graft is typically used for patients with a severe entropion with marked symblephara, severe lagophthalmos and eyelid retraction. A graft is indicated if the patient requires a subsequent penetrating keratoplasty. Amniotic membrane may be used as an alternative graft if the patient agrees to the use of donor material. It is preferable to avoid the use of a hard palate graft for use in the upper eyelid as the corneal surface, which is often already compromised, can be damaged by its rough surface.

The procedure is performed under general anaesthesia. A throat pack is placed and the anaesthetist is asked to position the endotracheal tube to one corner of the mouth. The eyelid is injected subcutaneously and subconjunctivally with 0.5% Marcain and 1:200,000 units of adrenaline. A 4/0 silk suture is placed through the grey line and the eyelid is everted over a Desmarres retractor. All symblephara are divided. The conjunctiva at the upper border of the tarsus is incised and dissected free of all subconjunctival scar tissue into the superior fornix and onto the bulbar surface of the globe. At the same time, the retractors are freed from the tarsus to correct eyelid retraction. Next, a template is taken of the conjunctival defect.

Next, the lower lip mucosa is injected with 0.5% Marcain and 1:200,000 units of adrenaline. Atraumatic Babcock's bowel clamps are used to evert the lower lip. The template is trans-

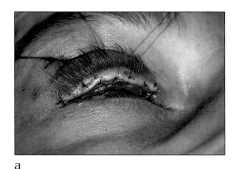
a

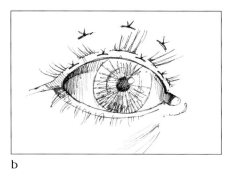
b

**Figure 4.23**
(a) The terminal tarsal fragment has been rotated 180 degrees and sutured to the anterior surface of the tarsus. (b) Three 4/0 Vicryl sutures are tied in the skin crease to hold the posterior lamella in an advanced position.

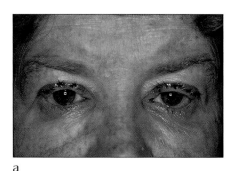
a

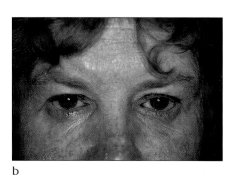
b

**Figure 4.24**
(a) The appearance of the eyelids 2 weeks postoperatively. (b) The appearance of the eyelids 6 months postoperatively.

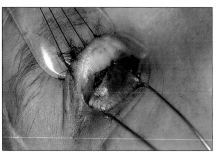
a

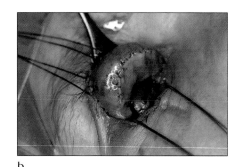
b

**Figure 4.25**
(a) Extensive keratinization of the posterior lamella of the upper eyelid with obliteration of the superior fornix following severe Stevens–Johnson syndrome. (b) The symblephara have been dissected, the keratinized area excised and a large mucous membrane graft sutured into place.

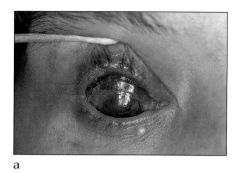
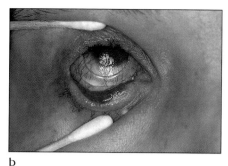
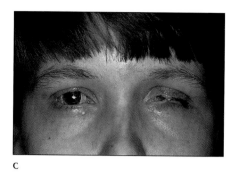

a      b      c

**Figure 4.26**
(a) The patient seen 6 weeks postoperatively with a symblepharon ring in place. (b) The symblepharon ring is seen on upgaze. (c) The right cornea has re-epithelialized. A left central tarsorrhaphy was required.

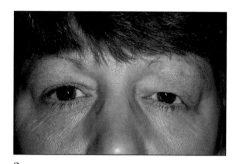
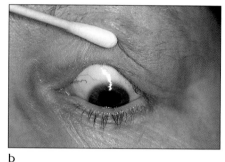

a      b

**Figure 4.27**
(a) A patient referred with a severe left upper eyelid entropion following an excessive resection of tarsus in a Fasanella–Servat procedure. (b) A close-up of the left upper eyelid entropion. Previous inappropriate cryotherapy has been performed for 'trichiasis'.

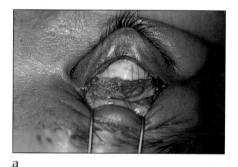
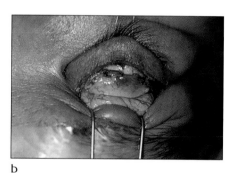

a      b

**Figure 4.28**
(a) An auricular cartilage graft has been scored vertically with a No. 15 Bard Parker blade to allow the graft to bend to a slightly convex configuration. It has been inserted to lie over the residual tarsal plate, extending inferiorly to a position just above the lash roots. (b) The levator aponeurosis has been attached to the auricular cartilage graft.

ferred to the lower lip mucosa, avoiding the vermillion border. This is outlined with gentian violet. The graft is harvested with a No. 15 Bard Parker blade and blunt-tipped Westcott scissors or with a mucotome. The bowel clamps are removed and the graft donor site is treated with topical 1:10,000 adrenaline on a swab.

The graft is shaped with Westcott scissors and sutured into place with interrupted 8.0 Vicryl sutures (Figure 4.25).

A symblepharon ring of suitable size and shape is inserted (Figure 4.26). A compressive dressing is applied for 7 days.

If the tarsal plate has atrophied this can be reconstructed in the same manner described above for the management of a congenital upper eyelid entropion using an auricular cartilage graft.

## Auricular cartilage graft

This procedure is typically required for patients with a moderate degree of entropion who have undergone an excessive excision of tarsal plate during eyelid reconstructive surgery or ptosis surgery (Figure 4.27). The procedure is performed in the same manner as that described above for the management of a congenital upper eyelid entropion (Figure 4.28).

## Further reading

1. Collin JRO. *A manual of systematic eyelid surgery.* New York: Churchill Livingstone, 1989.

2. Rhatigan MC, Ashworth JL, Goodall K, Leatherbarrow B. Correction of blepharoconjunctivitis-related upper eyelid entropion using the anterior lamellar reposition technique. *Eye* (1997) **11**(Part 1):118–20.

3. Yaqub A, Leatherbarrow B. The use of autogenous auricular cartilage in the management of upper eyelid entropion. *Eye* (1997) **11**(Part 6):801–5.

# 5

# Lower eyelid ectropion

## Introduction

Lower eyelid ectropion is an eyelid malposition in which the lower eyelid margin is turned away from its normal apposition to the globe. The condition may be classified into four categories according to the underlying aetiology.

## Classification

1. Involutional ectropion (Figure 5.1a)
2. Cicatricial ectropion (Figure 5.1b)
3. Paralytic ectropion (Figure 5.2a)
4. Mechanical ectropion (Figure 5.2b)

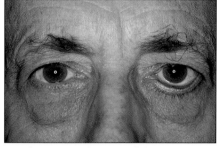

a

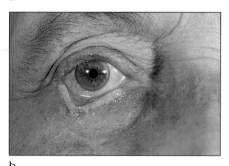

b

## Figure 5.1
(a) A left lower eyelid involutional ectropion. (b) A right lower eyelid cicatricial ectropion.

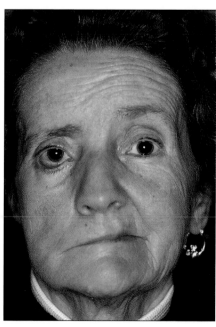

a

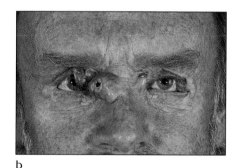

b

## Figure 5.2
(a) A right lower eyelid paralytic ectropion. (b) A left lower eyelid mechanical ectropion.

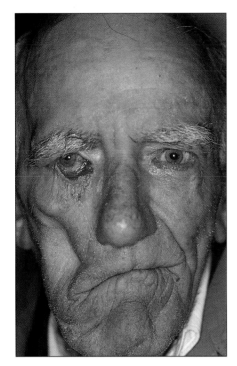

**Figure 5.3**
A right lower eyelid ectropion in a patient with a chronic lower motor neuron facial palsy. In this patient all the aetiological factors coexist and should be addressed in his management.

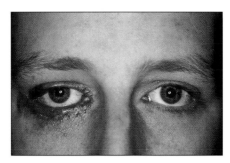

**Figure 5.4**
A disastrous result in from a K–Z procedure inappropriately performed on a patient who presented with epiphora and a medial ectropion. His mild cicatricial ectropion was due to eczema.

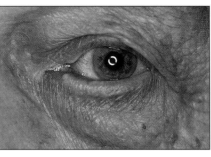

**Figure 5.5**
Punctal eversion of the left lower eyelid.

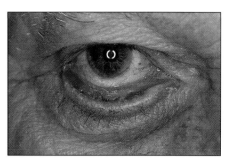

**Figure 5.6**
A chronic lower eyelid ectropion with keratinization of the exposed conjunctiva.

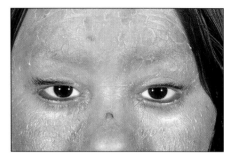

**Figure 5.7**
A bilateral lower eyelid cicatricial ectropion in a patient with lamellar ichthyosis.

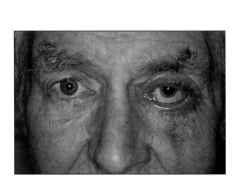

**Figure 5.8**
A patient with a left lower eyelid cicatricial ectropion. The patient was allergic to the topical glaucoma medication prescribed for the left eye only. The ectropion (and ptosis) resolved completely after a short course of topical steroid applied to the periocular skin.

It should be recognized, however, that more than one aetiological factor may be present in an individual patient: e.g. in a patient with a chronic facial palsy and a lower lid ectropion, all four aetiological factors may coexist (Figure 5.3).

It is important to be able to classify the type of ectropion that is seen so that the correct treatment is directed at the underlying cause. Involutional ectropion is by far the most common type of ectropion but a cicatricial cause of lower lid ectropion is often overlooked. Failure to recognize this leads to poor results from inappropriately selected surgical procedures (Figure 5.4).

The initial sign of a lower lid ectropion is inferior punctal eversion (Figure 5.5). This can lead to a vicious cycle of secondary events and needs to be addressed early. Eversion of the inferior punctum leads to exposure and drying of the punctum, which becomes stenosed. Epiphora ensues, which may lead to excoriation and contracture of the skin of the lower eyelid that further exacerbates the ectropion. In addition, the patient tends to continually wipe the lower eyelid, which in turn results in eyelid and medial canthal tendon laxity that further exacerbates the lower eyelid ectropion. If the condition is neglected, the tarsal conjunctiva becomes exposed and eventually thickened and keratinized (Figure 5.6). The patient's cornea may show exposure keratopathy.

## Patient evaluation

The patient's history may point to a number of dermatological disorders which may be responsible for a cicatricial ectropion, e.g. eczema, lamellar ichthyosis (Figure 5.7).

A drug history may reveal topical medications the patient may be taking to which there may be an allergy with a secondary chronic dermatitis, e.g. topical glaucoma medications (Figure 5.8).

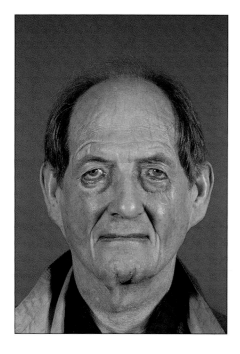

**Figure 5.9**
A patient with a bilateral lower eyelid ectropion. The patient has Ehlers–Danlos syndrome.

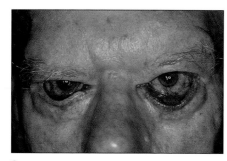

a                                    b

**Figure 5.10**
(a) A patient with a severe bilateral lower eyelid ectropion. He also has a bilateral brow ptosis. (b) An examination of his whole face reveals a severe bilateral lower facial weakness. He also had a bilateral abduction weakness of both eyes. The patient has Möbius syndrome.

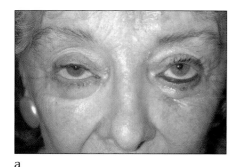

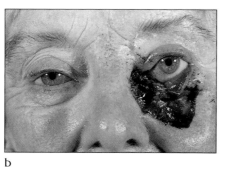

a                                    b

**Figure 5.11**
(a) This patient's left lower eyelid ectropion was due to a lower eyelid morphoeic basal cell carcinoma. (b) The patient's appearance following a Mohs' micrographic surgical excision of the tumour.

The inferior punctum

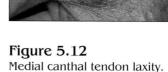

**Figure 5.12**
Medial canthal tendon laxity.

Patients who have previously undergone a lower eyelid blepharoplasty or laser skin resurfacing may be reluctant to divulge such information. When examining the patient the whole of the patient's face should be scrutinized for evidence of a dermatological disorder, connective tissue disorder, facial weakness, scars from previous surgery or trauma, or evidence of malignant cutaneous lesions (Figures 5.9–5.11).

The degree of eyelid laxity is assessed by drawing the eyelid away from the globe and releasing it (the 'snap back' test). The eyelid is drawn laterally and the position of the punctum is observed. If the punctum can be drawn lateral to the medial limbus with the globe in the primary position, the medial canthal tendon will probably require attention during the surgical repair of the ectropion (Figure 5.12). Rounding of the lateral canthus indicates lateral canthal tendon laxity or dehiscence.

If a cicatricial component of the ectropion is not obvious, the lower eyelid skin should be observed for tension lines seen when the patient blinks. The patient is asked to look up and to open the mouth to see whether or not these manoeuvres exacerbate the ectropion (Figure 5.13). *Failure to recognize a cicatricial component is a common cause of surgical failure in the management of lower lid ectropion.*

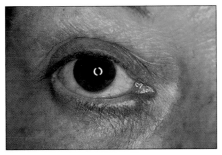

a

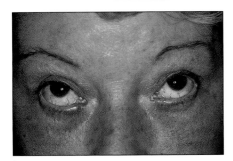

b

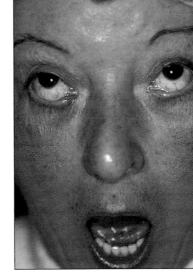

c

**Figure 5.13**
(a) A lower eyelid punctal ectropion in a patient referred with epiphora. (b) The punctal ectropion is exaggerated by asking the patient to look up. (c) The punctal ectropion is further exaggerated by asking the patient to open her mouth.

# Management

It is important to recognize dermatological causes of cicatricial ectropion that may be amenable to medical management alone, e.g. chronic contact or allergic dermatitis. Removal of the offending substance, e.g. replacement of a topical glaucoma medication with a preservative-free preparation along with a short course of a weak topical steroid, may be all that is required.

The choice of surgical procedure depends on a number of factors:

1. The degree of ectropion
2. The degree of laxity of the medial and lateral canthal tendons
3. The tone of the orbicularis muscle
4. The nature of any cicatricial forces
5. The presence of any mechanical force
6. The age and general health of the patient

The surgical procedure should be selected to address these factors in each individual patient. Although an abundance of surgical procedures has been described for the management of lower eyelid ectropion, the choice of procedure can in practice be made from a relatively small number:

1. Retropunctal cautery
2. Medial spindle
3. Medial spindle + medial wedge resection
4. Medial canthal tendon plication
5. Medial canthal resection
6. Lateral wedge resection
7. Lateral wedge resection with skin–muscle blepharoplasty
8. Lateral tarsal strip procedure
9. Z-plasty
10. Lateral wedge resection or lateral tarsal strip + skin graft
11. Posterior approach retractor reinsertion + medial spindle + lateral tarsal strip
12. Fascia lata sling

# Involutional ectropion

Involutional ectropion can be further classified into the following subtypes:

1. Punctal ectropion
2. Medial ectropion without horizontal eyelid laxity
3. Medial ectropion with horizontal eyelid laxity
4. Medial ectropion with medial canthal tendon laxity
5. Ectropion of the whole length of the lower eyelid
6. Complete tarsal ectropion

## Punctal ectropion

**Retropunctal cautery.** Where this is very early, it is simple to apply retropunctal cautery. Using a disposable cautery device, deep burns are applied to the conjunctiva 3–4 mm below the punctum. The effect on the punctal position is observed and titrated by the number of burns applied and the depth of the burn.

## Medial ectropion without horizontal eyelid laxity

**Medial spindle procedure.** Where the punctal ectropion is more pronounced, a medial spindle procedure is performed. It is

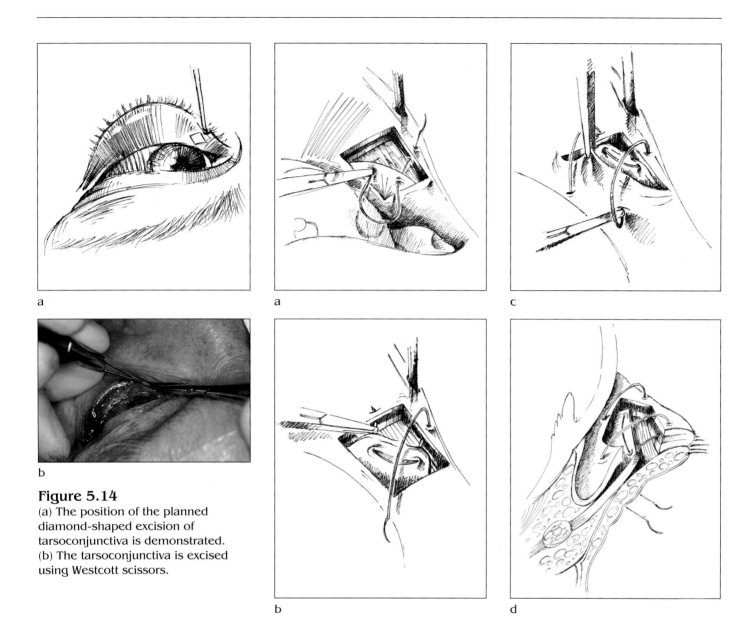

**Figure 5.14**
(a) The position of the planned diamond-shaped excision of tarsoconjunctiva is demonstrated. (b) The tarsoconjunctiva is excised using Westcott scissors.

**Figure 5.15**
(a) A double-armed 5/0 Vicryl suture on a 1/4-circle needle is passed from the lower eyelid retractors at the base of the wound to the superior apices of the diamond. (b) This suture advances the lower eyelid retractors towards the inferior punctum. (c) The suture is then passed back through the inferior apex of the diamond and out through the skin of the lower lid at the junction of eyelid and cheek skin. (d) The arrangement of the sutures is demonstrated in a lateral view of the eyelid.

usually necessary to dilate the punctum at the same time, as this is usually stenosed. It is not appropriate to perform any more invasive procedures on the punctum as this may resume its normal appearance once it has been repositioned against the globe.

A volume of 3 ml of 0.5% bupivacaine with 1:200,000 units of adrenaline is injected subcutaneously and subconjunctivally into the lower eyelid medially. A diamond-shaped excision of tarsoconjunctiva is performed in the posterior lamella of the lower eyelid just beneath the inferior punctum using Westcott scissors and a 0.3 toothed forceps (Figure 5.14).

A double-armed 5/0 Vicryl suture on a 1/4-circle needle is passed from the lower eyelid retractors at the base of the wound to the superior apices of the diamond. It is then passed back through the inferior apex of the diamond and out through the skin of the lower lid at the junction of eyelid and cheek skin (Figure 5.15). The effect of the suture is to attach the inferior retractors to the superior aspect of the wound to pull the punctum posteriorly against the globe and to close the wound. The tension on the suture is titrated against the effect on the position of the punctum that should be slightly overcorrected. The suture is removed after 2 weeks.

## Medial ectropion with horizontal eyelid laxity

**Medial spindle procedure with a medial wedge resection.** In this situation a medial spindle procedure is combined with a medial wedge resection of the lower eyelid (Figure 5.16). The wedge resection is positioned to remove thickened keratinized conjunctiva. It is important that sufficient eyelid is left medial to the resection to enable vertical mattress sutures to be placed across the eyelid margin without risking damage to the punctum or to the inferior canaliculus.

## Medial ectropion with medial canthal tendon laxity

In the majority of elderly patients with medial canthal tendon laxity, no specific measures are necessary. A moderate degree of lateral punctal displacement is well tolerated and it may be inappropriate to subject the patient to a longer operative procedure. Where the degree of medial canthal tendon laxity is very pronounced, however, this can be addressed with a medial canthal resection procedure. In general, medial canthal tendon plication procedures do not tend to achieve adequate long-lasting results.

**Medial canthal tendon plication.** A volume of 2 ml of 0.5% bupivacaine with 1:200,000 units of adrenaline is injected subconjunctivally into the lower eyelid medially. A conjunctival incision is made with Westcott scissors between the caruncle and the plica semilunaris and extended to the medial end of the inferior tarsal plate (Figure 5.17).

The scissors are used to dissect down to the posterior lacrimal crest that can be palpated with a Freer periosteal elevator. Small malleable retractors are used to aid visualization of the periosteum of the crest. A double-armed 5/0 Ethibond suture on a 1/2–circle needle is passed through the posterior lacrimal crest (Figure 5.18).

Next, each needle of the Ethibond suture is passed through the exposed medial aspect of the tarsal plate (Figure 5.19).

A 7/0 Vicryl suture is positioned across the conjunctival wound. The Ethibond suture is tied, bringing the eyelid into contact with the globe. The Vicryl suture is then tied to ensure that the Ethibond suture is not left exposed.

Tincture of benzoin is applied to the cheek skin and a firm compressive dressing is applied. Tape is applied to the cheek and

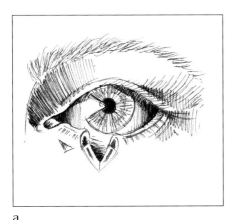
a

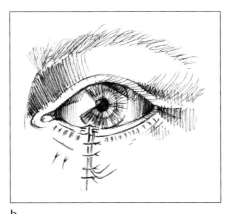
b

**Figure 5.16**
(a) A wedge resection is performed just lateral to the position of the medial spindle. (b) The wedge resection closure is performed after the closure of the medial spindle.

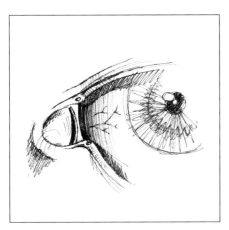

**Figure 5.17**
A conjunctival incision is made between the caruncle and the plica semilunaris.

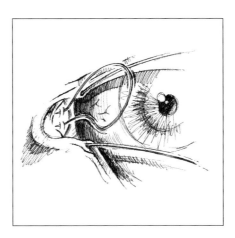

**Figure 5.18**
A double-armed 5/0 Ethibond suture on a 1/2-circle needle is passed through the posterior lacrimal crest.

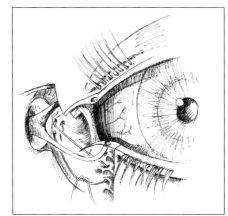

**Figure 5.19**
The Ethibond suture is passed through the medial aspect of the tarsal plate.

drawn superomedially to ensure that tension is reduced on the wound. The compressive dressing is maintained in place for a minimum of 5 days.

**Medial canthal resection.** A volume of 3 ml of 0.5% bupivacaine with 1:200,000 units of adrenaline is injected subcutaneously and subconjunctivally into the lower eyelid medially. A full-thickness vertical incision is made through the eyelid adjacent to the caruncle (Figure 5.20).

A conjunctival incision is made with Westcott scissors between the caruncle and the plica semilunaris. The scissors are used to dissect down to the posterior lacrimal crest, which can be palpated with a Freer periosteal elevator. Small malleable retractors are used to aid visualization of the periosteum of the crest. A double-armed 5/0 Ethibond suture on a 1/2-circle needle is passed through the posterior lacrimal crest. Next, a triangular section of medial eyelid is removed, sufficient to allow the wound to be closed without undue tension (Figure 5.21).

The canaliculus is opened and marsupialized into the conjunctiva sac using interrupted 8/0 Vicryl sutures. A monocanalicular silicone stent can be passed into the canaliculus. Next, each needle of the Ethibond suture is passed through the cut end of the tarsus and tied, bringing the eyelid into contact with the globe. The skin is then closed with interrupted 6/0 silk sutures to aid in support of the wound.

Tincture of benzoin is applied to the cheek skin and a firm compressive dressing is applied. Tape is applied to the cheek and drawn superomedially to ensure that tension is reduced on the wound. The compressive dressing is maintained in place for a minimum of 5 days.

# Ectropion of the whole length of the lower eyelid with lateral canthal tendon laxity

The choice of procedure for a more extensive lower eyelid ectropion depends on a consideration of the following factors:

1.   The degree of rounding of the lateral canthus
2.   The presence of excess lower eyelid skin
3.   The degree of upper eyelid laxity
4.   The general health of the patient

If there is significant lateral canthal tendon laxity with rounding of the lateral canthus and a narrowing of the horizontal palpebral aperture, a wedge resection of the lateral aspect of the eyelid will further exaggerate the problem and will not address the underlying anatomical abnormality. A lateral tarsal strip procedure is preferable for such a patient. A lateral strip procedure is also more convenient as this avoids the need for suture removal but may leave an unsatisfactory overlap of the upper lid at the lateral canthus if the upper eyelid is very lax. The lateral tarsal strip procedure is also more problematic to perform in the obese, hypertensive patient, or in the patient who is unable to discontinue the use of aspirin preoperatively. If the patient has excess lower eyelid skin, a lateral wedge resection can be combined with a lower lid skin–muscle blepharoplasty.

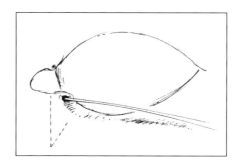

**Figure 5.20**
The extent of the excision in a medial canthal resection is demonstrated.

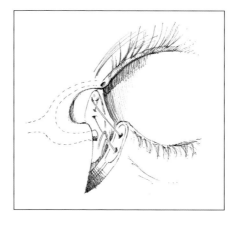

**Figure 5.21**
The suture placement in medial canthal resection procedure is demonstrated.

These procedures can also be combined with a medial spindle procedure for a punctal ectropion that is not corrected by a lateral eyelid-tightening procedure. The medial spindle procedure should be performed prior to completing the repair of any lateral eyelid-tightening procedure.

**Lateral wedge resection.** The wedge resection is performed at the junction of the lateral third with the medial two-thirds of the eyelid. It is important to ensure that a retraction of the lower eyelid is not caused by too aggressive a resection of eyelid tissue.

A volume of 3 ml of 0.5% bupivacaine and 1:200,000 units of adrenaline is injected into the eyelid subcutaneously. The eyelid margin is incised using a No. 15 Bard Parker blade at the junction of the lateral third with the medial two-thirds of the eyelid. A vertical incision is made with straight sharp-tipped scissors to the base of the tarsal plate. The amount of eyelid to be resected is carefully estimated by overlapping the edges of the eyelid with toothed forceps. The eyelid margin is again incised using a No. 15 Bard Parker blade and a second vertical incision is made with straight sharp-tipped scissors to the base of the tarsal plate. The wedge excision is then completed. Haemostasis is achieved using bipolar cautery.

The eyelid is then repaired in layers. The upper borders of the tarsal plate are reapproximated using an interrupted 5/0 Vicryl suture on a 1/2-circle needle. Care is taken to ensure that the suture lies beneath the surface of the conjunctiva posteriorly and just beneath the skin anteriorly. The suture is tied with a single throw and the alignment of the eyelid checked. If it is not satisfactory the suture is replaced. Once the alignment is satisfactory, the suture is loosened and used for traction by fixating it to the head drape using an artery clip.

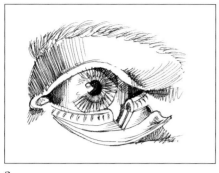
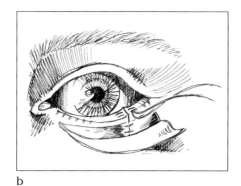

a

b

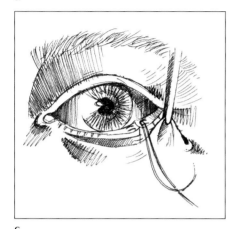
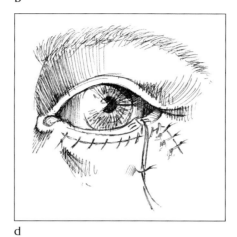

c

d

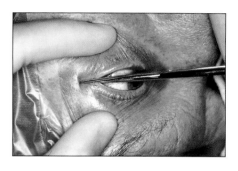

**Figure 5.22**
(a) A skin–muscle flap is raised and a lateral wedge resection performed. (b) The wedge resection is repaired. (c) The skin–muscle flap is drawn laterally and the excess skin and muscle are resected as a base-up triangle. (d) The lateral skin wound and the subciliary incision wound are closed with 7/0 Vicryl sutures.

**Figure 5.23**
A lateral canthotomy is performed using straight blunt-tipped scissors.

The rest of the tarsal plate edges and orbicularis edges are reapproximated using interrupted 5/0 Vicryl. Next, the initial 5/0 Vicryl suture is tied and cut. Then two interrupted 6/0 silk sutures are passed, one through the meibomian glands and the other through the lash line, in a vertical mattress fashion. The sutures are then tied to produce a slight eversion of the wound edges and cut long. The skin edges are then reapproximated using interrupted 7/0 Vicryl sutures passed in a vertical mattress fashion. The uppermost sutures incorporate the long ends of the silk sutures in order to keep the ends away from the cornea. The silk sutures are not removed for 2 weeks.

**Lateral wedge resection with skin–muscle blepharoplasty.** The vertical cutaneous scar created by a simple wedge resection can be avoided by creating a skin–muscle blepharoplasty flap and performing the wedge resection beneath this.

A volume of 3–4 ml of 0.5% bupivacaine and 1:200,000 units of adrenaline is injected into the eyelid subcutaneously along its entire length. A 4/0 silk traction suture is placed through the grey line and fixated to the head drapes using an artery clip. A subciliary skin incision is made with a Colorado needle extending inferolaterally at the lateral canthus in a skin crease. A skin–muscle flap is dissected inferiorly from the orbital septum approximately 8–9 mm and extended laterally. Next, a wedge resection of the underlying posterior lamella is performed. The

skin–muscle flap is drawn laterally and the excess skin and muscle are resected as a base-up triangle. The skin incision is closed with a continuous 7/0 Vicryl suture (Figure 5.22).

**Lateral tarsal strip procedure.** A volume of 3 ml of 0.5% bupivacaine with 1:200,000 units of adrenaline is injected into the lower eyelid and into the lateral canthus. A lateral canthotomy is performed using straight blunt-tipped scissors (Figure 5.23). The canthotomy is extended to the lateral orbital rim.

The lower eyelid is then lifted in a superotemporal direction and the inferior crus of the lateral canthal tendon is cut using blunt-tipped Westcott scissors (Figure 5.24). The septum is also freed until the eyelid becomes loose. Care is taken to avoid bleeding. It is easier to perform the initial steps of this procedure sitting at the head of the patient. It is then preferable to move to the side of the patient to complete the remainder of the procedure.

Once the lower eyelid is free of its canthal attachments, the anterior and posterior lamellae are split along the grey line using sharp-tipped scissors (Figure 5.25).

The lateral tarsal strip is then formed by cutting along the inferior border of the tarsus (Figure 5.26). Next, the superior border of the tarsus is excised (Figure 5.27).

The tarsal strip is then drawn to the lateral orbital margin to determine the extent of any redundant tarsal strip. This is then excised (Figure 5.28).

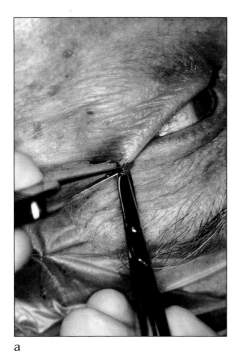
a

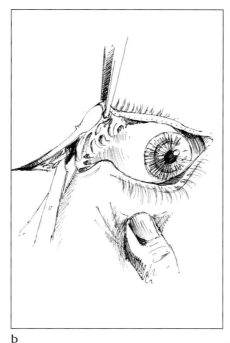
b

**Figure 5.24**

(a) The lower eyelid is then lifted in a superotemporal direction and the inferior crus of the lateral canthal tendon is cut using blunt-tipped Westcott scissors. (b) All residual attachments of the eyelid to the lateral orbital margin are released by cutting all tissues between the skin and the conjunctiva laterally.

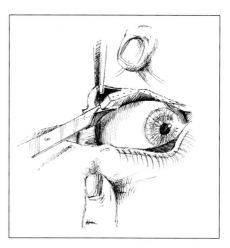

**Figure 5.26**

The lateral tarsal strip is formed by cutting along the inferior border of the tarsus.

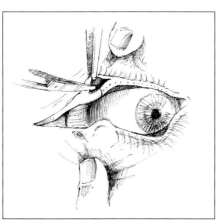
a

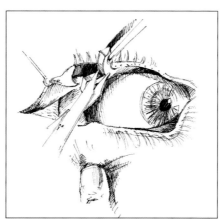
a

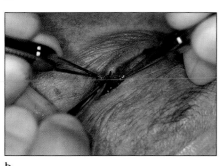
b

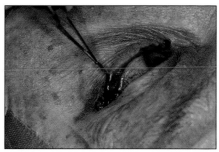
b

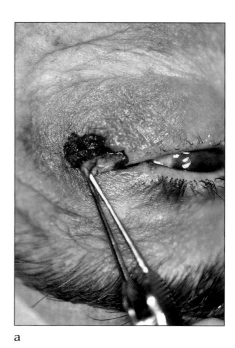
a

b

**Figure 5.25**

The anterior and posterior lamellae are split along the grey line using sharp-tipped scissors.

**Figure 5.27**

(a) The superior border of the tarsus is excised. (b) The appearance of the strip of superior tarsus being excised.

**Figure 5.28**

(a) The tarsal strip is drawn laterally to determine if some redundant tarsus needs to be excised. (b) The tarsal strip is shortened as required.

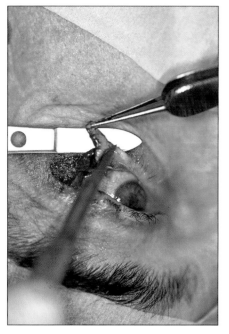

**Figure 5.29**
The tarsal strip is placed over the handle of a Paufique forceps and the conjunctiva scraped away.

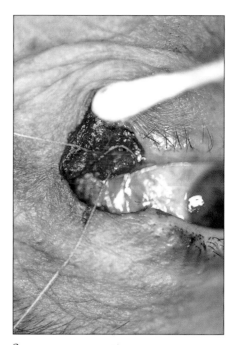

a

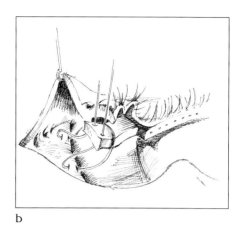

b

**Figure 5.30**
(a) A 5/0 double-armed Ethibond suture is used to anchor the tarsal strip to the lateral orbital margin. (b) The arrangement of the suture is demonstrated.

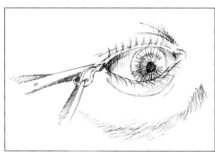
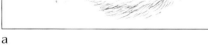

a

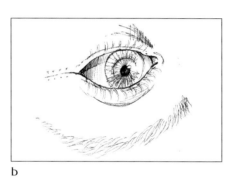

b

**Figure 5.31**
(a) The redundant anterior lamella is excised. (b) The lateral canthal wound is carefully closed to reform the lateral canthal angle.

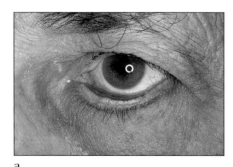
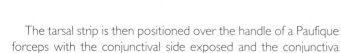

a

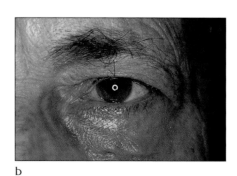

b

**Figure 5.32**
(a) A lower eyelid involutional ectropion. (b) The appearance 2 weeks following a lateral tarsal strip procedure.

The tarsal strip is then positioned over the handle of a Paufique forceps with the conjunctival side exposed and the conjunctiva scraped from the tarsal strip using a No. 15 blade (Figure 5.29).

Next, a double-armed 5/0 Ethibond suture on a 1/2-circle needle is passed through the periosteum of the lateral orbital wall, leaving a loop. The end of the tarsal strip is passed through the loop and the loop tightened, drawing the tarsal strip in a posterior direction (Figure 5.30).

The suture is tied and the redundant anterior lamella is excised. The lateral canthotomy wound is closed using interrupted 7/0 Vicryl sutures subcutaneously to ensure that the Ethibond suture is buried followed by interrupted 7/0 Vicryl sutures to the skin wound (Figures 5.31 and 5.32).

The lateral tarsal strip procedure can also be combined with a skin–muscle blepharoplasty procedure where necessary.

## Complete tarsal ectropion

This form of lower eyelid ectropion, in which the tarsal plate is completely everted, is rare. The diagnosis is reserved for those patients who have no cicatricial element and little horizontal eyelid laxity. The condition is thought to be due to disinsertion of the lower eyelid retractors from the lower border of the tarsal plate. The malposition is managed by a combination of a posterior approach retractor reinsertion, a medial spindle procedure and a lateral tarsal strip procedure.

**Posterior approach retractor reinsertion + medial spindle + lateral tarsal strip.** A volume of 5 ml of 0.5% bupivacaine with 1:200,000 units of adrenaline is injected subcutaneously and subconjunctivally into the lower eyelid. A 4/0 silk traction suture is placed through the grey line and the eyelid is everted over a Desmarres retractor. A conjunctival incision is made with a No. 15 Bard Parker blade extending from a point 2–3 mm lateral to the punctum to the lateral canthus. The conjunctiva is undermined inferiorly for 6–7 mm. The lower eyelid retractors are now visible and may be detached from the lower border of the tarsus. The retractors are dissected from the orbital septum and orbicularis muscle with Westcott scissors. Next, the retractors are reattached to the inferior border of the tarsal plate with interrupted 5/0 Vicryl sutures (Figure 5.33).

The conjunctival flap is repositioned and closed with inter-

rupted 7/0 Vicryl sutures, taking care to bury the sutures beneath the conjunctival wound (Figure 5.34).

Next, a medial spindle procedure is performed followed by a lateral tarsal strip procedure (Figure 5.35). A compressive dressing is applied for 3 days.

# Cicatricial ectropion

Cicatricial lower eyelid ectropion is caused by scarring or contracture of the skin and/or orbicularis muscle, causing a vertical shortening of the eyelid. The causes, are numerous:

1. Actinic damage from chronic sun exposure
2. Acute/chronic dermatitis, e.g. allergy to topical glaucoma medications, eczema
3. Morphoeic basal cell carcinoma of the lower eyelid/medial canthus
4. Tumour irradiation therapy
5. Thermal/chemical burns
6. Specific dermatological disorders, e.g. lamellar ichthyosis
7. Trauma
8. Iatrogenic, e.g. following lower lid blepharoplasty or laser skin resurfacing, blowout fracture repair with scarring of the orbicularis muscle/orbital septum to the orbital margin, over-correction of lower eyelid entropion (Figure 5.36)

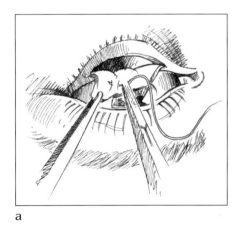
a

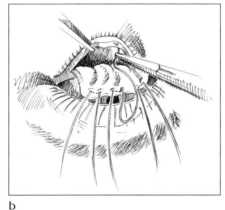
b

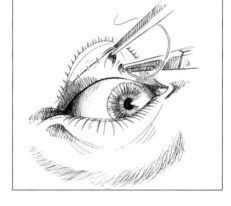

### Figure 5.33
(a) The lower eyelid retractors have been dissected free and sutures are placed through the edge of the retractors. (b) The sutures are then passed through the inferior border of the tarsus.

### Figure 5.34
The conjunctiva is reapproximated with interrupted 7/0 Vicryl sutures.

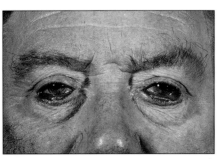
a

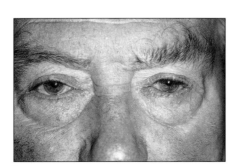
b

### Figure 5.35
(a) A bilateral tarsal ectropion. (b) The postoperative appearance following a posterior approach retractor advancement, a medial spindle procedure and a lateral tarsal strip procedure.

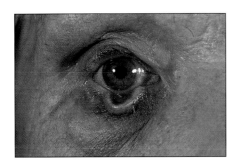

**Figure 5.36**
A marked cicatricial ectropion following the use of a Wies procedure for a lower eyelid involutional entropion.

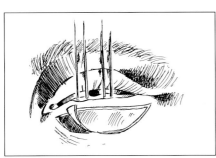

**Figure 5.37**
A template is taken of the lower eyelid skin defect using a piece of Steridrape.

Medical treatment alone may suffice for some of the many causes of cicatricial ectropion. Although some patients will benefit from soft tissue rearrangement techniques for a very specific localized scar, e.g. a Z-plasty, such situations are not encountered very frequently. A full-thickness skin graft is more often required. A small medial ectropion will usually require a small skin graft alone, although this can be combined with a medial spindle procedure. Where the ectropion is more extensive a horizontal eyelid-shortening procedure, either a wedge resection or a lateral tarsal strip, should be combined with the skin graft, to prevent a recurrence of the ectropion. A cicatricial ectropion affecting children is an exception to this rule.

A skin graft may be taken from a variety of sites:

1.  The upper eyelid
2.  The preauricular region
3.  The postauricular region
4.  The supraclavicular fossa
5.  The upper inner arm

Each site has its advantages and disadvantages. The upper eyelid skin provides the best quality skin. It provides a good colour match. It is easy to remove and has no subcutaneous fat. It is therefore very quick to prepare. The wound is simple to close. The upper lid, however, may not be a suitable site in some patients. It may show extensive actinic damage. There may be insufficient skin available to remove without risking a secondary lagophthalmos. It may leave an obvious asymmetry. It may exaggerate an associated brow ptosis.

The preauricular skin also provides a good colour match and is an easy site to access. The site may not, however, yield sufficient skin. It may also be affected by actinic damage. The postauricular site provides good skin but is unsuitable for patients who wear a hearing aid. The wound is difficult to close and may alter the position of the ear.

The supraclavicular fossa skin tends to be rather pale. It can leave an unsightly scar and is best avoided in female patients who wear open-necked clothing.

The upper inner arm skin is pale but can yield a good result if the grafts are placed bilaterally. The skin is protected from solar damage. It is easy to access and large grafts can be harvested. The wound edges can be undermined to effect easy closure. If the wound breaks down it can be left to heal by secondary intention. The scar is then unobtrusive. The additional advantage is that the skin graft harvest and the wound closure can be performed by a surgical assistant while the surgeon is working on the eyelid. This can save a great deal of valuable surgical time.

**Lateral wedge resection or lateral tarsal strip + skin graft.** A volume of 3–4 ml of 0.5% bupivacaine and 1:200,000 units of adrenaline is injected into the eyelid subcutaneously along its entire length; 7–10 ml of the same solution is injected subcutaneously at the skin graft donor site. Two 4/0 silk traction sutures are placed through the grey line and fixated to the head drapes using artery clips. A subciliary skin incision is made with a No. 15 Bard Parker blade from a point 2–3 mm medial to the punctum to a point 3–4 mm lateral to the lateral commissure. A skin flap is dissected inferiorly from the orbicularis muscle approximately 7–8 mm. The eyelid should now rise with the pull from the traction sutures. If there is scarring at a deeper level, however, the eyelid will remain in the same position. Westcott scissors are now used to dissect the scar tissue away from the eyelid retractors or from the conjunctiva if the retractors are scarred. Next, a wedge resection of the underlying posterior lamella is performed or, alternatively, a lateral tarsal strip procedure is performed.

The traction sutures are tightened again with the artery clips exaggerating the anterior lamellar defect. Next, a template is taken of the defect using a piece of Steridrape and a gentian violet marker pen (Figure 5.37).

The template is transferred to the skin graft donor site and outlined with gentian violet (Figure 5.38a). The skin is incised with a No. 15 Bard Parker blade along the mark. The skin graft is then raised at one end with a skin hook while countertraction is applied. The graft is then peeled away using a sweeping action with the blade (Figure 5.38b). The donor site is closed with a continuous interlocking 6/0 nylon suture. If the wound is under tension, the margins are undermined and interrupted 4/0 nylon sutures are placed in a vertical mattress fashion.

The skin graft is placed over the tip of the surgeon's forefinger with the raw surface uppermost. Westcott scissors are used to remove all subcutaneous tissue meticulously until the rete pegs are visible (Figure 5.39).

The graft is then transferred to the lower eyelid and sutured into the defect using four 6/0 silk bolster sutures. Continuous 7/0 Vicryl sutures are placed in between the silk sutures (Figure 5.40a). The graft is then covered in topical antibiotic ointment, a piece of Vaseline gauze and a piece of sterile sponge shaped from the template. The bolster sutures are tied over the sponge (Figure 5.40b).

Tincture of benzoin is painted on the forehead. The lower lid traction sutures are fixated to the forehead with Steri-strips. A firm compressive dressing is applied and left undisturbed for a period of 7 days.

The patient is instructed on wound aftercare when the sutures are removed at 1 week. The patient commences massage to the skin graft 2 weeks after the surgery and continues this for at least 3 months (Figure 5.41).

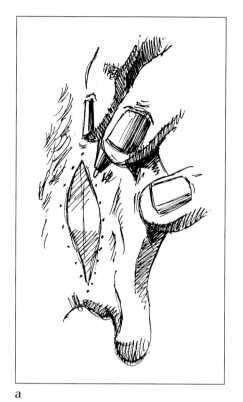 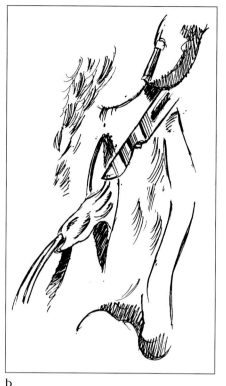

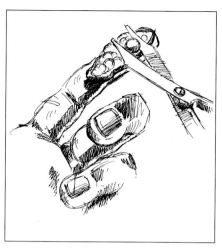

**Figure 5.39**
The skin graft is placed over the tip of the surgeon's forefinger with the raw surface uppermost. Westcott scissors are used to remove all subcutaneous tissue meticulously.

a        b

**Figure 5.38**
(a) The template has been transferred to the postauricular area and outlined with gentian violet. (b) The skin graft is harvested using a No. 15 Bard Parker blade.

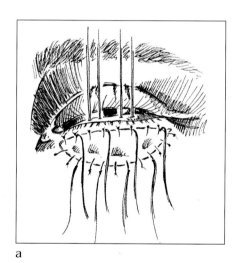 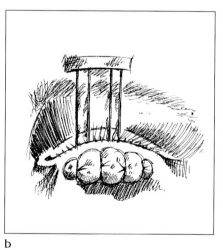

**Figure 5.40**
(a) The skin graft is anchored into place with interrupted 6/0 silk sutures, and interrupted 7/0 Vicryl sutures are placed in between. (b) The silk sutures are then tied over a sponge bolster.

a        b

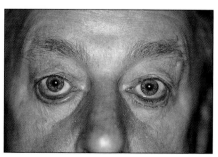 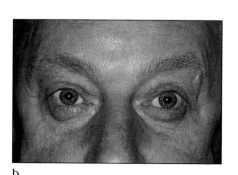

**Figure 5.41**
(a) A patient with a bilateral lower eyelid cicatricial ectropion. (b) The postoperative appearance 3 months following placement of lower eyelid skin grafts and lateral tarsal strips.

a        b

## *Mechanical ectropion*

The diagnosis of mechanical lower eyelid ectropion is made where a mass lesion or a mid-face ptosis is responsible for pushing or pulling the eyelid out of its normal position. The ectropion is managed by directing treatment at the underlying cause (Figure 5.42).

If a mid-face ptosis is causing the ectropion, as may be seen in a chronic facial palsy, the ptosis itself may be addressed in a number of ways, depending on the individual circumstances. Treatment may be by facial suspension techniques, e.g. fascia lata graft suspension, or by nerve substitution techniques, e.g. facial hypoglossal nerve anastomosis, cross facial nerve grafting, performed by plastic surgery or ENT colleagues. Alternatively, the cheek may be raised by a sub-orbicularis oculi fat (SOOF) lift or a subperiosteal mid-face lift procedure performed via a transconjunctival approach and combined with a lateral tarsal strip procedure (see Chapter 7, Facial Palsy).

In elderly patients, the mid-face ptosis can instead be accepted and the ectropion, whose aetiology may be multifactorial, may be addressed by means of a combination of eyelid procedures only, e.g. a medial spindle, a posterior approach retractor recession, a full-thickness skin graft and a lateral tarsal strip procedure (Figure 5.43).

## *Paralytic ectropion*

The surgical management of paralytic ectropion depends on the degree of ectropion, and on the additional aetiological factors that may be responsible for the ectropion, e.g. cicatricial changes from chronic epiphora, mechanical changes from a mid-face ptosis. A mild degree of paralytic ectropion in a patient with exposure keratopathy may benefit from a simple lateral tarsorrhaphy. A mild degree of ectropion alone may be managed with a lateral tarsal strip procedure. A chronic paralytic ectropion with medial canthal tendon laxity would be best managed with a medial canthal tendon resection procedure.

A mild degree of paralytic medial ectropion can be managed by means of a simple medial canthoplasty.

**Medial canthoplasty.** The eyelids are split medial to the puncta and anterior to the canaliculi using a Beaver micro-sharp

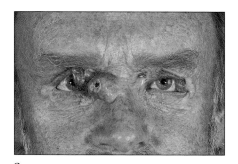
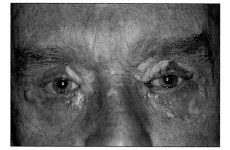

a                                    b

**Figure 5.42**
(a) A patient with a left lower eyelid mechanical ectropion from periocular xanthomata. (b) The postoperative appearance 3 months following excision of the xanthomata and placement of skin grafts. A left lower lid tarsal strip procedure has also been performed.

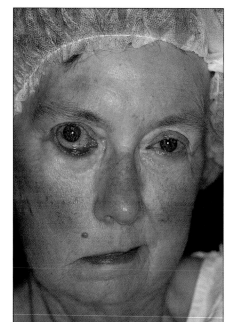
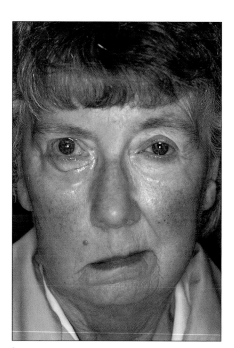

a                                    b

**Figure 5.43**
(a) A patient with a chronic right facial palsy and a right lower eyelid ectropion. The ectropion is due to a combination of factors. It is paralytic, involutional, cicatricial and mechanical. (b) The ectropion has been addressed by means of a posterior approach lower lid retractor recession, a lower eyelid skin graft and a lateral tarsal strip procedure and a medial spindle procedure. The mid-face ptosis has not been addressed.

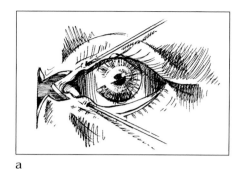

a

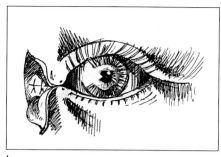

b

**Figure 5.44**
(a) The eyelids have been split medial to the puncta and anterior to the canaliculi. The skin has been undermined and a vertical relieving incision made inferiorly. (b) Two 7/0 Vicryl sutures have been passed though the pericanicular tissue and tied.

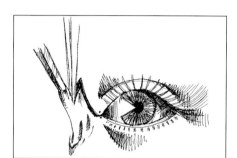

a

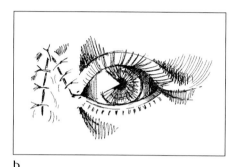

b

**Figure 5.45**
(a) The inferior skin flap is drawn medially and the dog ear removed. (b) The skin is closed with interrupted 7/0 Vicryl sutures.

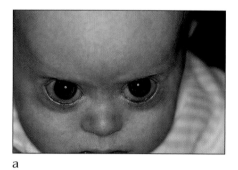

a

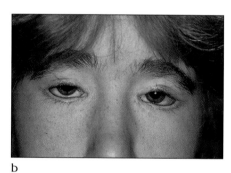

b

**Figure 5.46**
(a) An infant with a bilateral congenital lower eyelid ectropion due to a vertical skin shortening. The infant has Down syndrome. (b) A patient with a bilateral lateral cicatricial ectropion. The patient has a blepharophimosis syndrome. She had undergone medial canthal surgery and ptosis surgery elsewhere.

blade. The skin is undermined using blunt-tipped Westcott scissors. A vertical relieving incision is made inferiorly at the medial aspect of the inferior skin flap (Figure 5.44a). Two 7/0 Vicryl sutures are passed though the pericanicular tissue and tied (Figure 5.44b).

The inferior skin flap is drawn medially and the dog ear removed (Figure 5.45a). The skin is closed with interrupted 7/0 Vicryl sutures (Figure 5.45b)

## Congenital lower eyelid ectropion

The majority of patients with congenital ectropion of the lower eyelid have additional facial abnormalities, e.g. patients with Down syndrome (Figure 5.46a), blepharophimosis syndrome (Figure 5.46b), Möbius syndrome, lamellar ichthyosis (see Figure 5.7). The patient's ectropion is either cicatricial or paralytic in aetiology. The majority of such patients require a full-thickness skin graft. The cosmetic results of such surgery are poor in comparison to the results in adults.

# Further reading

1.  American Academy of Ophthalmology. *Basic and clinical science course: orbit, eyelids, and lacrimal system*, section 7. San Francisco: American Academy of Ophthalmology, 1998–99, pp. 138–48.

2.  Anderson RL, Gordy DD. The tarsal strip procedure. *Arch Ophthalmol* (1979) **97**:2192–6.

3.  Bosniak SL, Zilkha MC. Ectropion. In: Nesi FA, Lisman RD, Levine MR, eds, *Smith's ophthalmic, plastic and reconstructive surgery*, 2nd edn. St Louis: Mosby, 1987, pp. 290–307.

4.  Dutton JJ. *Atlas of clinical and surgical orbital anatomy*. Philadelphia: WB Saunders, 1994.

5.  Gilbard SM. Involutional and paralytic ectropion. In: Bosniak S, ed., *Principles and practice of ophthalmic plastic and reconstructive surgery*, Vol 1. Philadelphia: WB Saunders, 1996, pp. 422–37.

6.  Giola VM, Linberg JV, McCormick SA. The anatomy of the lateral canthal tendon. *Arch Ophthalmol* (1987) **105**:529–32.

7.  Jordan DR, Anderson RL. The lateral tarsal strip revisited: the enhanced tarsal strip. *Arch Ophthalmol* (1989) **107**:604–6.

8.  Nowinski TS, Anderson RL. The medial spindle procedure for involutional medial ectropion. *Arch Ophthalmol* (1985) **103**:1750–3.

9.  Tse DT. Ectropion repair. In: Levine MR, ed., *Manual of oculoplastic surgery*, 2nd edn. Boston: Butterworth-Heinemann, 1996, pp. 147–56.

# 6

# Trichiasis

## Introduction

Trichiasis refers to a condition in which aberrant eyelashes turn inwards against the globe in the absence of any eyelid malposition (Figure 6.1). It is frequently seen in association with chronic blepharoconjunctivitis or cicatrizing conjunctivitis, e.g. ocular cicatricial pemphigoid. In contrast, distichiasis refers to a condition in which accessory eyelashes arise from the lid margin in an area other than the normal ciliary line, e.g. from the meibomian gland orifices (Figure 6.2). If eyelashes abrade the cornea the patient will experience constant irritation, photophobia and lacrimation. Fluorescein staining of the cornea will occur. Constant corneal abrasion by ingrowing eyelashes can result in visual morbidity, e.g. this can lead to failure of a penetrating keratoplasty. In contrast, however, infants tend to tolerate corneal contact with soft lashes without such symptoms.

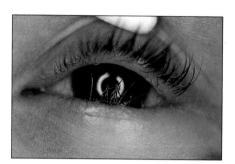

**Figure 6.1**
Trichiasis.

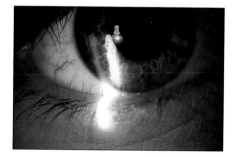

**Figure 6.2**
Distichiasis.

## Management

1. Epilation
2. Bandage contact lens
3. Electrolysis
4. Cryotherapy
5. Surgical excision

## *Bandage contact lens*

A temporary relief from symptoms can be obtained by the fitting of a bandage contact lens while definitive treatment is being arranged.

## *Epilation*

Epilation of eyelashes provides a temporary relief from symptoms, but the symptoms are often exacerbated as the eyelashes regrow. The eyelashes are initially short and stubby, creating more corneal damage. Epilation also prevents definitive treatment by electrolysis until the eyelashes have begun to regrow, which enables the surgeon to identify the offending eyelashes.

## *Electrolysis*

Electrolysis is an appropriate form of treatment if only a few eyelashes are present, particularly if these are located at various points in the eyelids. The Ellman Surgitron radiofrequency device is particularly suited for electrolysis provided the patient does not have a cardiac pacemaker (Figure 6.3). Alternatively, a

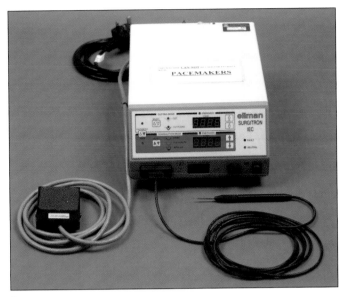

a

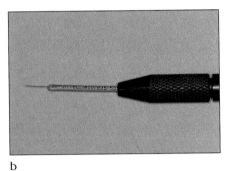

b

**Figure 6.3**
(a) The Ellman radiofrequency device. (b) The Ellman probe with electrolysis needle.

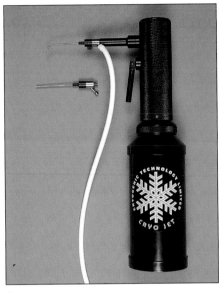

a

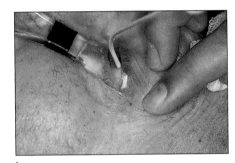

b

**Figure 6.4**
(a) A 'Cryojet' cryotherapy device which utilizes liquid nitrogen. A series of interchangable delivery heads are available. (b) The globe is protected with a plastic eyeguard when the cryotherapy is applied to the eyelids.

Colorado needle holder can be fitted with an electrolysis needle and used. The globe should be protected with a plastic eyeguard coated with a lubricant ointment. The electrolysis needle is inserted into the hair root under microscopic control and the current applied. The appearance of blanching or bubbles at the eyelid margin indicates that sufficient current has been applied. The eyelash should then drop out spontaneously or should be easily epilated without any resistance. The patient should be warned that some lashes may fail to respond to treatment and that a further treatment session a few weeks later may be required.

## Cryotherapy

Cryotherapy is an appropriate form of treatment for more extensive trichiasis or distichiasis. The application of liquid nitrogen to the affected area is the most effective method of delivering cryotherapy. The temperature at the level of the eyelash follicle should be monitored with a thermocouple. The globe must be protected with a plastic eyeguard lightly coated with a lubricant ointment on the surface in contact with the globe (Figure 6.4). The goal is to reduce the temperature to approximately −25°C which should destroy the lash follicle without

inducing tissue necrosis. A double freeze–thaw cycle is used. At this level of temperature, however, pigment cells in the skin are destroyed, leaving hypopigmentation.

Alternatively, a nitrous oxide cryotherapy unit can be used with a block probe (Figure 6.5), which allows a greater area of the eyelid to be treated with each application than a retinal cryotherapy probe. This can also be used in conjunction with a thermocouple. The probe is held against the lid margin in the affected area while the temperature is reduced. The application duration is usually approximately 30 seconds. A double freeze–thaw cycle is again used. With thin, atrophic eyelids, a shorter freeze time should be used to avoid the risk of inducing necrosis of the eyelid. Each area is frozen in a similar manner, using a freeze–thaw–refreeze cycle. The patient should be warned about the risk of recurrence and the likely requirement for repeated treatment.

## Surgical excision

A localized area of trichiasis in a patient with eyelid laxity may be more conveniently managed by a wedge excision and direct closure of the defect. Although it is feasible to expose and individually remove eyelash roots via an upper eyelid skin crease

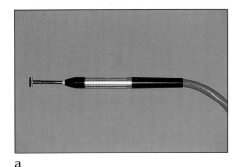
a

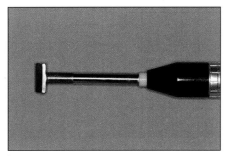
b

**Figure 6.5**
(a) An eyelid cryoprobe. (b) A close-up of the end of the cryoprobe.

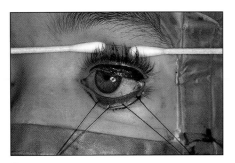
a

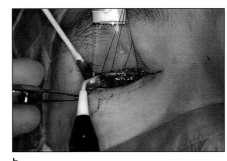
b

**Figure 6.6**
(a) The upper eyelid has been separated into anterior and posterior lamellae. (b) Cryotherapy is being applied to the posterior lamella of the lower eyelid.

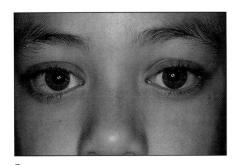
a

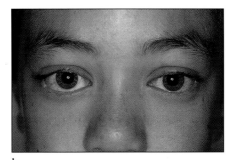
b

**Figure 6.7**
(a) A patient with distichiasis affecting the upper and lower eyelids bilaterally. (b) The patient following eyelid splitting and cryotherapy to the posterior lamellae. The upper eyelid lashes have mostly survived but there is extensive loss of eyelashes in the lower eyelids.

or lower eyelid subciliary incision, this is a tedious exercise and rarely required.

Distichiasis is managed by splitting the eyelids along the grey line with a micro-sharp blade and dividing the eyelids into anterior and posterior lamellae with blunt-tipped Westcott scissors (Figure 6.6a). Cryotherapy is then applied to the posterior lamella only (Figure 6.6b).

The posterior lamella is advanced 2 mm and the anterior lamella is sutured to the anterior surface of the posterior lamella in a recessed position to avoid any subsequent contracture and eyelid malposition. Although the goal of this approach is to avoid damage to the normal eyelashes, many of these rarely survive, particularly in the lower eyelids (Figure 6.7). It is important that the patient is suitably counselled about this beforehand.

# Further reading

1.  American Academy of Ophthalmology. *Basic and clinical science course: orbit, eyelids, and lacrimal system*, section 7. San Francisco: American Academy of Ophthalmology, 1998–99, pp. 155–6.
2.  Anderson RL, Harvey JT. Lid splitting and posterior lamella cryosurgery for congenital and acquired distichiasis. *Arch Ophthalmol* (1981) **99**:631–3.
3.  Anderson RL, Wood JR. Complications of cryosurgery. *Arch Ophthalmol* (1981) **90**:460–3.
4.  Bartley GB, Lowry JC. Argon laser treatment of trichiasis. *Am J Ophthalmol* (1992) **113**:71–4.
5.  Martin RT, Nunery WR, Tanenbaum M. Entropion, trichiasis and distichiasis. In: McCord CD, Tanenbaum M, Nunery WR, eds, *Oculoplastic surgery*, 3rd edn. New York: Raven Press, 1995, pp. 230–48.
6.  Rose GE, Collin JRO. Management of entropion and trichiasis. In: *American Academy of Ophthalmology Monographs, surgery of the eyelid, orbit, and lacrimal system*, Vol. 2, 1994, pp. 34–52.
7.  Sullivan JH, Beard C, Bullock JD. Cryosurgery for treatment of trichiasis. *Am J Ophthalmol* (1976) **82**:117–21.

# 7

# Facial palsy

## Introduction

The ophthalmologist may be the first clinician to see a patient who presents with an acute facial nerve palsy. Under such circumstances the ophthalmologist should make every effort to establish the underlying cause of the facial palsy and should ensure that the patient's cornea is adequately protected. Many patients presenting with a facial palsy are incorrectly labelled as 'Bell's palsy'. This is a diagnosis of exclusion. Approximately 10% of patients presenting with an acute facial palsy have a treatable lesion.

The ophthalmologist should be aware of:

1. The varied disorders which may cause a facial palsy (Table 7.1)
2. The detailed evaluation of the patient with a facial palsy
3. The various medical and surgical treatments available

A number of other disciplines may be involved in the care of the patient with a facial palsy, e.g. an ENT (ear, nose and throat)

**Table 7.1** The more common causes of facial palsy

- Bell's palsy
- Ramsay Hunt syndrome
- Otitis media
- Mastoiditis
- Cholesteatoma
- Trauma
- Acoustic neuroma surgery
- Sarcoidosis
- Parotid tumour
- Lymphoma
- Nasopharyngeal carcinoma
- Metastatic carcinoma
- Congenital

surgeon, a neurosurgeon, a neurologist, a plastic surgeon, a physician. *It is essential that effective communication exists between such clinicians for the optimal care of the patient. The ophthalmologist must be made aware of the prognosis for recovery of facial nerve function, e.g. following the removal of an acoustic neuroma, and of any plans for surgery by other colleagues, e.g. facial reanimation surgery.* The ophthalmologist should be involved in the care of any patient in whom a facial palsy may be anticipated postoperatively, e.g. acoustic neuroma surgery. In the early postoperative period following acoustic neuroma surgery, periorbital swelling can cause a patient with a complete facial palsy to have apparently normal eyelid closure. As the swelling subsides the patient develops severe lagophthalmos, which may be compounded by reduced corneal sensation and a poor Bell's phenomenon.

> The priority for any clinician involved in the management of a patient with a facial palsy is prevention of exposure keratopathy. It is much simpler to prevent corneal ulceration from exposure than it is to treat this once it has occurred (Figure 7.1).

A facial palsy can have a devastating effect on a patient. It is associated with a number of potential problems that need to be addressed on an individual basis:

1. Visual defects from corneal exposure or its medical and surgical management
2. Ocular pain or discomfort
3. Chronic lacrimation and epiphora from corneal exposure, paralytic ectropion, lacrimal pump failure
4. Cosmetic disfigurement
5. Difficulties with speech/drooling

These problems can affect a patient's ability to work, drive and to interact socially. Patients may lose self-esteem and become discouraged and depressed.

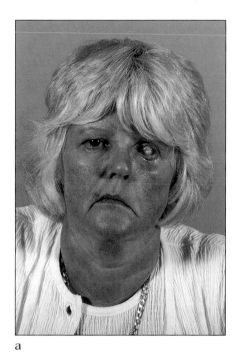

a

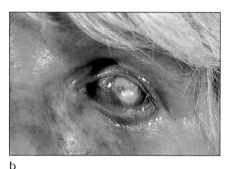

b

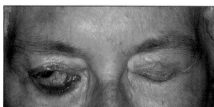

a

b

**Figure 7.1**
(a) A patient referred with a complete left lower motor neuron facial palsy and a painful left eye. (b) A close-up photograph of the patient's left eye. She had marked lagophthalmos and a dry eye. Her neglected exposure keratopathy had resulted in a secondary corneal abscess and endophthalmitis. The eye had to be eviscerated.

**Figure 7.2**
(a) A patient with a right lower motor neuron facial palsy demonstrating upper eyelid retraction, a brow ptosis and a lower eyelid ectropion. (b) The same patient demonstrating marked right lagophthalmos and a poor Bell's phenomenon.

# History and examination

A full history should be taken and a comprehensive examination performed to determine the cause of the facial palsy. Specific questions should be asked about the following:

1. Onset and duration of the palsy
2. Any prior trauma
3. Any past ENT history
4. Any symptoms of hearing loss or hyperacusis
5. Any symptoms of ear pain or discharge
6. Any symptoms of other cranial nerve dysfunction, e.g. diplopia, anosmia, difficulty swallowing, neurosensory facial deficits
7. Past medical history, e.g. diabetes, sarcoidosis, myasthenia
8. Any skin rashes

The patient's presenting ocular complaints should be noted.

The patient should be carefully observed during the history taking. An incomplete blink may be noted as well as any facial asymmetry or loss of the nasolabial fold or forehead creases. The patient should then be examined systematically:

1. The muscles of facial expression should be tested to determine if the patient has a facial nerve paresis or a complete paralysis. In a chronic palsy, signs of aberrant reinnervation should be looked for.

2. The degree of facial motor nerve palsy can be graded to assist in monitoring the return of facial nerve function. *In general, the temporal branches of the facial nerve are the most severely affected and the last to return.*

3. The frontalis muscle should be tested to differentiate an upper motor neuron (intact frontalis action) from a lower motor neuron lesion (impaired frontalis action).

4. The extent of passive and forced eyelid closure should be determined and the degree of lagophthalmos measured (Figure 7.2). The patient's reflex blink should be observed.

5. Any upper eyelid retraction is noted (Figure 7.2). (The upper eyelid retracts in chronic facial palsy due to the unopposed action of the levator muscle. In some patients there is a chronic shortening of the anterior lamella, which further aggravates lagophthalmos.)

6. *The corneal sensation is tested before the instillation of any topical anaesthetic agents and the sensation in the distribution of the trigeminal nerve is also tested.*

7. The tear film is examined and a Schirmer's test performed to determine tear production.

8. The cornea is examined on a slit lamp and fluorescein instilled (Figure 7.3). The dye disappearance can also be observed and compared with the fellow eye. The blink can also be observed.

9. The presence or absence of a Bell's phenomenon is determined (Figure 7.4).

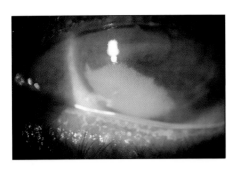

**Figure 7.3**
A patient with exposure keratopathy highlighted by the use of fluorescein.

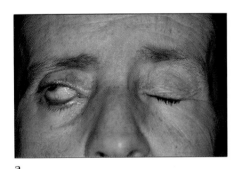

a

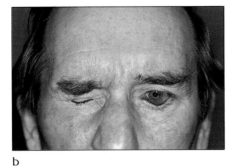

b

**Figure 7.4**
(a) A patient with lagophthalmos but a good Bell's phenomenon. (b) A patient with lagophthalmos and an absent Bell's phenomenon.

**Figure 7.5**
A patient with a left post-traumatic facial palsy. Her widened left palpebral aperture is due to both upper and lower eyelid retraction.

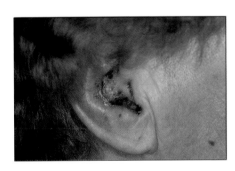

**Figure 7.6**
A patient with Ramsay Hunt syndrome.

10. The lower eyelid should be examined for any retraction or frank ectropion (Figures 7.2 and 7.5).
11. The ocular motility should be carefully tested. This is important as the cranial nerves subserving ocular motility lie in close anatomical proximity intracranially to the facial nerve nucleus and fascicles.
12. The patient's hearing should be tested and the ear examined for rashes, e.g. herpes zoster (Ramsay Hunt syndrome) (Figure 7.6).
13. The parotid glands should be palpated for masses.
14. The lacrimal glands should be palpated (these may be enlarged in sarcoidosis).
15. The submandibular and cervical lymph nodes should be palpated.
16. The oropharynx should be examined

Although the patient's visual acuity should be recorded, this can be inaccurate due to the presence of therapeutically applied ointments.

# General treatment considerations

The patients who are at high risk of exposure keratopathy and corneal ulceration should be identified early. The following are significant risk factors:

1. Absence of corneal sensation
2. Facial paralysis with severe lagophthalmos
3. An absent Bell's phenomenon
4. A dry eye

Patients may have more than one risk factor that compounds the problem further. *Loss of corneal sensation indicates a severely guarded prognosis for patients with facial palsy and demands urgent and aggressive treatment.*

Other factors must also be considered in determining the most appropriate medical or surgical treatment of an individual patient. These include the patient's age, general health and ability to comply with medical therapy regimens and frequent follow-up visits.

# Medical treatment

A number of relatively simple medical therapies can be applied particularly for a limited time in the patient who has a good prognosis for the recovery of facial nerve function and who has no risk factors for the development of exposure keratopathy.

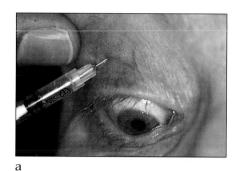

a

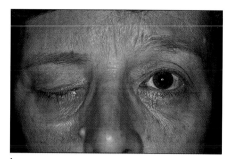

b

**Figure 7.7**
(a) The technique of botulinum toxin injection into the levator muscle. (b) A patient with a right facial palsy 3 days following an upper eyelid botulinum toxin injection. She had a complete right ptosis.

These include:

1. The use of frequent topical lubricants
2. The avoidance of ocular irritants
3. The use of spectacle side shields/moisture chamber goggles
4. Taping the eye closed at night
5. Upper eyelid botulinum toxin injections
6. The application of external eyelid weights
7. The use of eyelid adhesives

The most common ophthalmic treatment for facial palsy is the use of frequent lubricants. The use of ointment provides more efficient corneal protection than drops but with more blurring of vision. Patients should avoid ocular irritants, e.g. smoke, air conditioners.

Most patients do not tolerate moisture chamber goggles or plastic wrap occlusive dressings but spectacle side shields are relatively unobtrusive and well tolerated.

The upper eyelid can be taped closed over the eye at night but it is essential to ensure full closure to prevent further trauma to the cornea by the tape.

Botulinum toxin can be injected into the levator muscle to induce a ptosis for a patient with a temporary facial palsy (Figure 7.7). This is, however, expensive and commits the patient to monovision for a period of 8–12 weeks when spontaneous recovery occurs. The patient can develop problems with fusion and suffer diplopia. In addition, as the superior rectus can be weakened, the Bell's phenomenon may be adversely affected, creating more problems with exposure keratopathy during the recovery phase.

An external eyelid weight may be applied to the upper eyelid with a tissue adhesive. The weight is flesh coloured to make it less conspicuous. Such weights are useful for a temporary facial palsy but can also be used for a trial period before subjecting a patient to an upper eyelid gold weight implant.

Tissue adhesives are rarely tolerated for more than very short periods.

# Surgical treatment

Surgical treatment in the management of the patient with facial palsy has a number of indications:

1. The prevention or management of corneal exposure
2. The correction of lower eyelid ectropion
3. The management of brow ptosis

The surgical planning should take into consideration any plans for surgery by other clinicians, e.g. facial reanimation surgery.

# *The prevention or management of corneal exposure*

## Punctal occlusion

In patients with decreased tear production who cannot be managed adequately with topical lubricants alone, punctal occlusion is beneficial. This can be achieved temporarily with the use of silicone punctal plugs. If these are tolerated without secondary epiphora, surgical punctal occlusion can be performed under local anaesthesia. A simple disposable cautery device is used with a brief application to the puncta. This method does not prevent the reopening of the puncta at a later stage if necessary.

## Lateral tarsorrhaphy

A lateral tarsorrhaphy has been the time-honoured simple surgical method of providing adequate corneal protection in the management of the patient with a facial palsy.

### Advantages
1. Simple and quick to perform
2. Inexpensive
3. Reversible

### Disadvantages
1. Cosmetic disfigurement
2. Limitation of visual field
3. Complications, e.g. trichiasis

It is preferable to perform a more extensive tarsorrhaphy than is thought to be required as it is easier to partially open the tarsorrhaphy at a later date than to have to extend the tarsorrhaphy. In a patient with absent corneal sensation, who is at risk of a neurotrophic keratopathy, the lateral tarsorrhaphy should be very extensive and, unless the corneal sensation recovers, may have to be permanent.

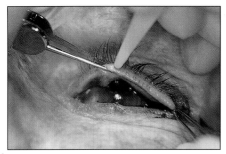

a

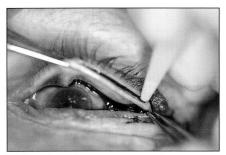

b

**Figure 7.8**
(a) The upper eyelid is being held taught with toothed forceps. (b) The positioning of the eyelid enables a linear incision to be made using a micro-sharp blade.

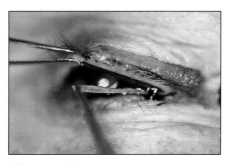

**Figure 7.9**
A strip of eyelid margin is excised from the posterior aspect of the eyelid margin.

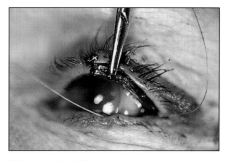

**Figure 7.10**
A 5/0 Vicryl suture is being passed horizontally through the tarsus, taking a partial-thickness bite.

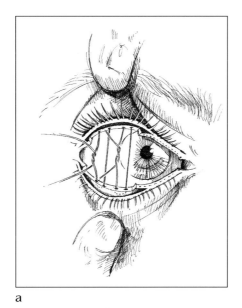

a

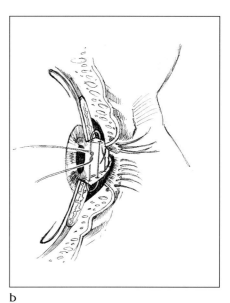

b

**Figure 7.11**
(a) The sutures are tied ensuring that the suture knots are away from the cornea. (b) A lateral view demonstrating the position of the sutures.

## Surgical technique

1. The upper and lower lids are injected with 2–3 ml of 0.5% bupivacaine and 1:200,000 units of adrenaline.
2. The eyelid is held taught centrally and laterally with toothed forceps (Figure 7.8a).
3. An incision 2–3 mm deep is made along the grey line of each eyelid using a Beaver micro-sharp blade (7530) mounted in a Beaver blade handle (Figure 7.8b).
4. Using the same blade, two incisions are made at 90 degrees to the grey line incision posteriorly. Next, using a 0.12 toothed forceps and a sharp-tipped Westcott scissors, a 0.5 mm strip of eyelid margin tissue is carefully removed posteriorly (Figure 7.9).
5. Two interrupted 5/0 Vicryl sutures on a 1/4-circle needle are passed horizontally through the tarsal plates of the upper and lower lids and tied with the knot placed anteriorly away from the cornea (Figures 7.10 and 7.11).
6. Interrupted 7/0 Vicryl sutures are placed through the anterior lips of the grey line incisions (Figure 7.12).

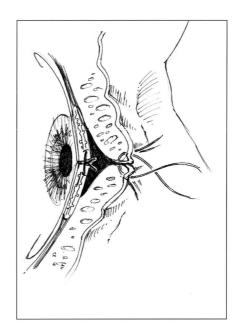

**Figure 7.12**
Interrupted 7/0 Vicryl sutures are placed through the anterior lips of the grey line incisions.

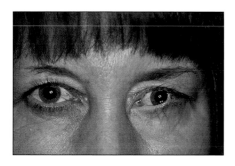

**Figure 7.13**
A healed lateral tarsorrhaphy.

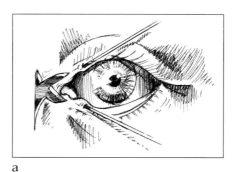

a                                                    b

**Figure 7.14**
(a) The eyelids have been split medial to the puncta and the skin undermined with Bowman probes protecting the canaliculi. An inferior relieving incision has been made. (b) Two 7/0 Vicryl sutures have been passed through the pericanalicular tissue and tied.

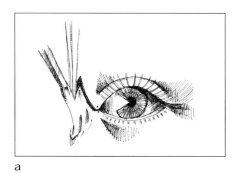

a                                                    b

**Figure 7.15**
(a) The inferior skin flap is drawn medially and the dog ear removed with scissors. (b) The wound is closed with interrupted 7/0 Vicryl sutures.

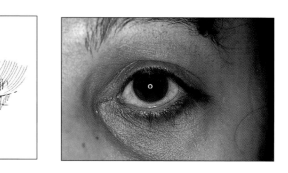

**Figure 7.16**
A patient who has undergone a medial canthoplasty and a small lateral tarsorrhaphy.

There is no requirement for any external bolsters. Topical antibiotic ointment is applied for 2 weeks. The eyelids fuse laterally (Figure 7.13). The tarsorrhaphy can be partially or completely reversed as required by simply dividing the eyelids with straight scissors.

## Medial canthoplasty

The eyelids are split medial to the puncta and anterior to the canaliculi using a Beaver micro-sharp blade (7530) (Figure 7.14a). The skin is undermined using blunt-tipped Westcott scissors (Figure 7.14a). A vertical relieving incision is made inferiorly at the medial aspect of the inferior skin flap (Figure 7.14a). Two 7/0 Vicryl sutures are passed though the pericanalicular tissue and tied (Figure 7.14b).

The inferior skin flap is drawn medially and the dog ear removed (Figure 7.15a). The skin is closed with interrupted 7/0 Vicryl sutures (Figure 7.15b).

A patient who has undergone a medial canthoplasty and a smal lateral tarsorrhaphy is shown in Figure 7.16.

## Upper lid retractor recession

A gentle recession of the upper eyelid retractors may benefit the patient with a chronic facial palsy with upper eyelid retraction

who has lagophthalmos but a moderate Bell's phenomenon, normal corneal sensation and normal tear production. Such patients may demonstrate exposure signs that affect only the inferior 1/3 of the cornea. The procedure is performed under local anaesthesia.

## Surgical technique

1.  The upper eyelid is everted and 0.5% bupivacaine and 1:200,000 units of adrenaline are injected subconjunctivally.
2.  A 4/0 silk traction suture is placed through the grey line of the upper eyelid.
3.  The upper eyelid is everted over a large Desmarres retractor.
4.  A conjunctival incision is made at the upper border of the tarsus with a No. 15 Bard Parker blade.
5.  The conjunctiva is undermined for 4–5 mm.
6.  The upper eyelid retractors are now gently incised with blunt-tipped Westcott scissors.
7.  The patient is placed into an upright sitting position and the eyelid height and contour inspected. The eyelid should be 1 mm lower than the fellow upper eyelid.
8.  The retractors are weakened further until the end point has been achieved.

No sutures are required. Postoperatively, topical antibiotic drops are prescribed. The patient is instructed to apply traction to the

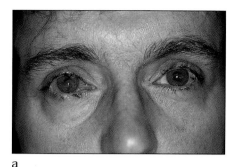
a

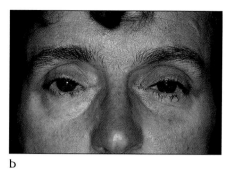
b

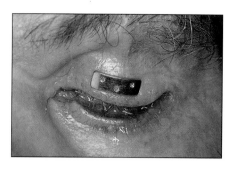

**Figure 7.17**
(a) A patient with a bilateral facial palsy and bilateral exposure keratopathy who has reduced corneal sensation. (b) The exposure keratopathy has resolved following a bilateral upper eyelid retractor recession and a bilateral medial canthoplasty.

**Figure 7.18**
A gold eyelid weight fixated to the upper eyelid with a small piece of adhesive tape. The patient is able to effect a passive closure of the eye.

eyelid lashes to maintain the desired eyelid height and contour as soon as the eyelid has started to rise (Figure 7.17).

# Gold weight insertion

Gold weight implantation is a simple and useful procedure for the patient with lagophthalmos but who has a good Bell's phenomenon, normal corneal sensation and normal tear production. It is particularly useful in the patient who has had a lateral tarsorrhaphy performed and is dissatisfied with the cosmetic appearance. The success of gold weight implantation depends on careful patient selection. It is not advisable to implant a gold weight into patients with very thin pale skin, with an atrophic orbicularis muscle and an upper lid sulcus defect. The weight is likely to be visible and obtrusive in such individuals. Patients should be carefully counselled preoperatively so that they understand the aims of the procedure and the disadvantages as well as the advantages. The procedure improves eyelid closure but it does not restore a normal reflex blink.

## Advantages
1. Simple surgical procedure
2. Reversible
3. Few complications

## Disadvantages
1. Eyelid closure may be impeded in the fully recumbent position
2. The gold weight may be visible
3. The gold weight may migrate or extrude
4. The patient may suffer an allergic reaction

**Preoperative evaluation**. It is relatively simple to determine the weight required for complete eyelid closure in the case of a patient who has not previously undergone any eyelid surgery. It is more difficult in the case of a patient with a lateral tarsorrhaphy that is to be opened at the time of placement of the weight. A weight is selected and fixated to the upper eyelid skin just below the skin crease with adhesive tape. The upper eyelid position and degree of closure are assessed (Figure 7.18).

The optimal weight is one that creates a minimal degree of ptosis but which permits complete eyelid closure. Generally, a 1.0 g or 1.2 g weight is used. Although the weights are available commercially, it is preferable to shape them to the contour of the patient's individual tarsus.

**Surgical technique.** The procedure is performed as follows:
1. A skin crease incision is marked at the desired level in the upper eyelid using gentian violet and a cocktail stick after cleansing the skin with an alcohol wipe.
2. A volume of 1–1.5 ml of 0.5% Marcain with 1:200,000 units of adrenaline is injected subcutaneously into the upper eyelid.
3. A 4/0 silk traction suture is placed through the grey line of the upper lid and fixated to the face drapes with an artery clip.
4. A 7 mm skin crease incision is made with a No. 15 Bard Parker blade (Figure 7.19).

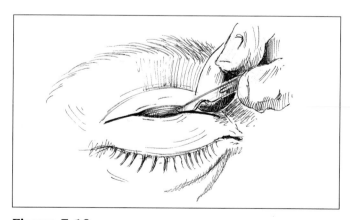

**Figure 7.19**
A small central incision is made. This reduces the risk of postoperative exposure of the implant. It also reduces the degree and duration of postoperative pretarsal oedema and minimizes postoperative sensory loss.

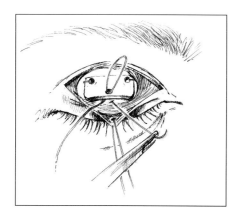

**Figure 7.20**
The gold weight can be fixated to the torsus using non-absorbable sutures passed through holes in the gold weight.

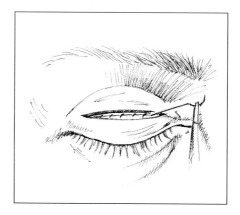

**Figure 7.21**
The orbicularis muscle is reapproximated before the skin is closed.

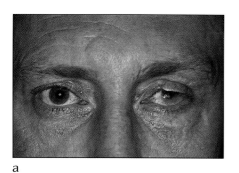

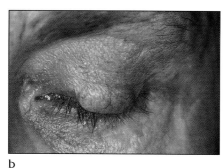

a                                          b

**Figure 7.22**
(a) A patient with a left upper eyelid gold weight which has migrated anteriorly. (b) A close-up photograph of the left upper eyelid demonstrating the abnormal position of the gold weight, which is clearly visible through the thinned and stretched upper eyelid skin.

5. The orbicularis muscle is grasped and opened with Westcott scissors down to the tarsal plate.
6. The glistening white tarsal plate is identified and a space opened medially, laterally and also inferiorly, taking care to avoid damaging the lash roots.
7. If the patient has significant eyelid retraction, the eyelid retractors may be gently recessed prior to insertion of the gold weight.
8. The gold weight is inserted into the space created. Some surgeons fixate the weight to the tarsus with nonabsorbable sutures (Figure 7.20). Care should be taken to avoid passing such sutures through the full thickness of the tarsus and to avoid causing any buckling of the tarsus.
9. The orbicularis muscle is closed over the weight with interrupted 7/0 Vicryl sutures (Figure 7.21).
10. The skin is closed with interrupted 7/0 Vicryl sutures.

**Complications.** Complications are usually minimal. A patient who is allergic to gold may develop an apparent chronic cellulitis that resolves when the weight is removed. Some upper lid swelling and intermittent redness around the weight does not necessitate removal in the absence of other symptoms or signs. A ptosis of 1–2 mm is common and usually resolves after removal of the gold weight. If the weight migrates or becomes exposed, elective removal of the weight is undertaken (Figure 7.22).

## Additional eyelid closure procedures

Most patients with lagophthalmos due to a facial palsy can be managed with the procedures described above. A number of other procedures have been described to effect closure of the eyelid:

1. Silicone rod cerclage
2. Palpebral spring implantation
3. Temporalis fascia transfer

The silicone rod cerclage consists of placing a rod of silicone around the upper and lower eyelids. When the upper eyelid opens, tension is placed on the silicone rod cerclage. When the patient relaxes the levator muscle, the stretched cerclage causes closure of the eyelid.

The palpebral spring consists of a piece of orthodontic wire fashioned into a spring and placed laterally in the upper eyelid. As the eyelid is opened, tension is placed on the wire. Once the levator muscle relaxes, the tension of the spring causes the eyelid to close.

With the temporalis fascia transfer, the force of closure is generated by a cerclage around the eyelid of a strip of temporalis fascia attached to the temporalis muscle. When the patient clenches the jaw, tension is placed on the eyelid, causing it to close.

Both the silicone rod cerclage and the palpebral spring procedures are technically more demanding than gold weight implantation and have a tendency to extrude. For this reason these procedures are not advocated by the author.

The temporalis fascia transfer relies on a conscious effort being made by the patient to clench the jaw in order to close the eyelid. The patient still experiences lagophthalmos at night as the patient's temporalis muscle relaxes. The temporalis fascia tends to loosen with time. This is not a procedure which is used by the author.

## The correction of lower eyelid ectropion

A patient with a mild degree of paralytic ectropion and lagophthalmos may benefit from a simple lateral tarsorrhaphy alone. The management of greater degrees of ectropion in a patient with a facial palsy depends on an evaluation of the aetiology of the ectropion, e.g. chronic epiphora may lead to cicatricial changes that may require a skin graft procedure (Figures 7.23 and 7.24). This is discussed in detail in Chapter 5 (Lower Eyelid Ectropion).

In patients who are poor candidates for a facial reanimation procedure, the mid-face ptosis may be addressed either with a static sling using autogenous fascia lata to pull the lip and face upward toward the zygomatic arch, or with a sub-orbicularis oculi fat (SOOF) or mid-face lift. These procedures help to eliminate the inferior traction of the sagging face from the lower eyelid.

In a fascia lata facial suspension, the fascial strips must be inserted from the muscles around the mouth and lip subcutaneously using a Wright's fascia lata needle. The strips are then fixated near the zygomatic arch and must be tightened as much as possible.

In an SOOF lift, the inferior orbital margin is approached via a lower eyelid transconjunctival incision combined with a lateral canthotomy and inferior cantholysis. The SOOF lateral to the infraorbital neurovascular bundle is raised down to the lower border of the maxilla. The SOOF is raised and reattached with nonabsorbable sutures to the arcus marginalis and to the superficial temporal fascia. In patients with a more severe mid-face ptosis, a subperiosteal mid-face lift may be performed. In such patients the advanced tissues are fixated using polypropylene sutures passed through drill holes in the bone of the inferior orbital margin.

## The management of brow ptosis

A unilateral brow ptosis may be severe enough to cause impairment of the superior visual field as well as a cosmetic deformity (Figure 7.25). It can cause a pseudo-blepharoptosis, and may lead to a secondary misdirection of the upper eyelid lashes with constant ocular irritation.

Although a number of different surgical approaches for the management of a brow ptosis complicating a facial palsy have been described, the preferred approaches are:

1.   A direct brow lift
2.   An endoscopic brow lift

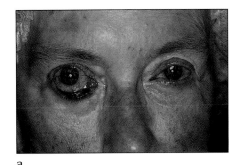 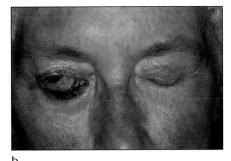

a                                         b

**Figure 7.23**
(a) A patient with a right facial palsy who has a severe lower eyelid ectropion. The ectropion is not only paralytic in aetiology but is also cicatricial (due to skin excoriation secondary to chronic epiphora) and mechanical (secondary to a mild mid-face ptosis). (b) The patient also has marked lagophthalmos.

**Figure 7.25**
A patient with a right lower motor neuron facial palsy. Her right brow ptosis is causing a marked restriction of her visual field.

**Figure 7.24**
(a) The same patient (as in Figure 7.23) following a lower eyelid full-thickness skin graft and lateral tarsal strip procedure. (b) Her lagophthalmos has also been improved with the placement of an upper eyelid gold weight.

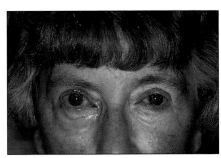 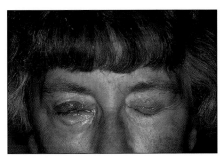

a                                         b

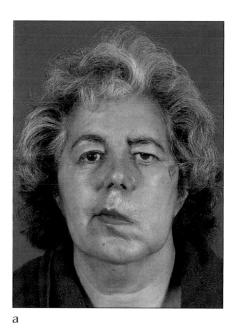

a

b

**Figure 7.26**
(a) A patient with a left facial palsy and a moderate left brow ptosis. (b) The appearance of the eyebrows at rest 2 weeks after a left direct brow lift.

## A direct brow lift

A direct brow lift is a simple but effective procedure to correct a unilateral brow ptosis (Figure 7.26). It can be combined, if necessary, with an upper lid blepharoplasty. If a blepharoplasty is deemed to be necessary, the brow lift should be performed first. The blepharoplasty should be conservative to avoid aggravating any lagophthalmos.

## Endoscopic brow lift

An endoscopic approach to the management of a unilateral brow ptosis has a number of advantages but also some disadvantages.

### Advantages
1.  Small incision scars hidden behind the hairline
2.  A reduced risk of postoperative sensory loss in the forehead
3.  A faster postoperative recovery

### Disadvantages
1.  Time consuming
2.  Expensive
3.  Higher recurrence rate

These surgical procedures are described in Chapter 22 (Eyebrow Ptosis).

# Aberrant reinnervation of the facial nerve

Aberrant reinnervation following recovery from a facial palsy is relatively common and patients should be warned about its possible occurrence. The degree of disability from aberrant reinnervation is variable. Some patients experience complete eyelid closure when using the perioral muscles. Such patients may be treated with botulinum toxin injections to the orbicularis oculi muscle, but such treatment inevitably leaves the patient with lagophthalmos and the need for frequent topical lubricants.

# Further reading

1.  Catalano PJ, Bergstein MJ, Biller HF. Comprehensive management of the eye in facial paralysis. *Arch Otolaryngol Head & Neck Surg* (1995) **121**:81–6.
2.  Leatherbarrow B, Collin JR. Eyelid surgery in facial palsy. *Eye* (1991) **5**:585–90.
3.  May M. *The facial nerve.* New York: Thieme Stratton, 1986.
4.  Wulc AE, Dryden RM, Khatchaturian T. Where is the gray line? *Arch Ophthalmol* (1987) **105**:1092–8.

# 8

# Eyelid tumours

## Introduction

Eyelid and periocular skin lesions are common in patients referred to ophthalmologists. The main goal in the evaluation of these lesions is to differentiate malignant from benign lesions. In general, the majority of malignant tumours affecting the eyelids and periocular area are slowly enlarging, destructive lesions that distort or frankly destroy eyelid anatomy. There are a number of subtle features that can help to differentiate malignant from benign eyelid tumours (Table 8.1). It can, however, be extremely difficult to make the correct diagnosis of an eyelid lesion without a biopsy. Some malignant lesions may appear innocuous (Figure 8.1a). Conversely, some benign lesions may appear extremely sinister (Figure 8.2a).

| **Table 8.1** Clinical signs suggestive of malignancy |
|---|
| • A localized loss of lashes<br>• Obliteration of the eyelid margin<br>• Pearly telangiectatic change<br>• Ulceration<br>• A new enlarging pigmented lesion<br>• An area of diffuse induration<br>• Irregular borders<br>• A scirrhous retracted area |

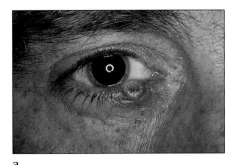

a

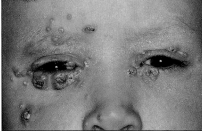

b

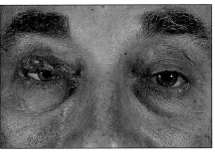

a

b

### Figure 8.1
(a) A lower eyelid squamous cell carcinoma referred as a suspected molluscum contagiosum. (b) Multiple eyelid molluscum contagiosum lesions. The skin lesions are usually multiple, dome-shaped, umbilicated papules. They are self-limiting in immunocompetent patients. An associated follicular conjunctivitis may occur. The lesions can be treated by incision and curettage, surgical excision, electrodessication and cryotherapy. Severe and aggressive involvement of the periocular region may occur in AIDS patients.

### Figure 8.2
(a) This patient was referred with a suspected upper eyelid squamous cell carcinoma. A biopsy proved the lesion to be a cryptococcus infection. (b) The patient following repair of an upper lid wedge incisional biopsy and a 6-week course of fluconazole.

Alternatively, the clinical pattern of some malignant eyelid tumours can simulate other tumour types, e.g. pigmented eyelid tumours are much more frequently basal cell carcinomas than melanomas (see Figure 8.16).

Early diagnosis can significantly reduce morbidity and, indeed, mortality associated with malignant eyelid tumours. However, *malignant eyelid tumours are diagnosed early only if a high degree of clinical suspicion is applied when examining all eyelid lesions.* The appropriate management of malignant eyelid tumours requires a thorough understanding of their clinical characteristics and their pathological behaviour.

Slit lamp examination can highlight these various features that help to differentiate benign from malignant tumours (Figure 8.3). A classification of malignant eyelid tumours is given in Table 8.2.

Most benign eyelid tumours can be readily diagnosed on the basis of their typical clinical appearance and behaviour (Figures 8.4–8.11).

**Table 8.2** Classification of malignant eyelid tumours

*Epithelial*
- Basal cell carcinoma
- Sebaceous gland carcinoma
- Squamous cell carcinoma
- Keratoacanthoma

*Non-epithelial*
- Lymphoma – mycosis fungoides
- Merkel cell tumour
- Kaposi's sarcoma
- Metastatic tumours
- Melanoma

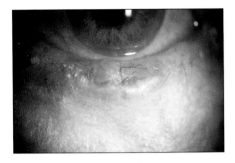

### Figure 8.3
Lower eyelid margin basal cell carcinoma demonstrating typical localized loss of eyelashes, pearly telangiectatic change and distortion of the eyelid margin.

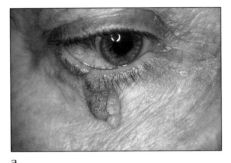

a

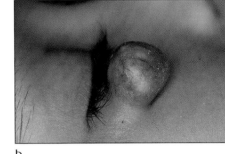

b

### Figure 8.4
(a) A lower lid seborrhoeic keratosis. These are common acquired lesions in middle-aged and elderly patients. On the eyelids they typically appear lobulated, papillary or pedunculated. The surface of the lesions has friable excrescences. These lesions are easily removed by simple shave excision, leaving a flat surface which re-epithelializes. (b) A lower eyelid pilomatrixoma (calcifying tumour of Malherbe) in a child. This tumour develops from hair matrix cells. The eyelid and eyebrow are sites of predilection for this tumour. The tumour is easily removed surgically.

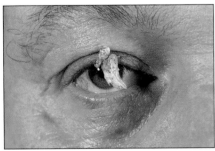

a

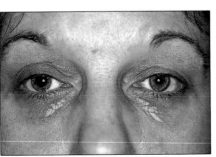

b

### Figure 8.5
(a) A verruca vulgaris lesion of the eyelid. These lesions appear as circumscribed elevated lesions with a hyperkeratotic, filiform surface. Treatment is by surgical excision. (b) A typical sebaceous cyst.

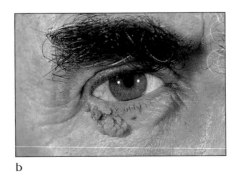

a

b

### Figure 8.6
(a) Typical xanthelasmata. These are easily treated by the topical application of trichloroacetic acid used very sparingly, taking care to protect the globes from inadvertent injury. (b) Inverted follicular keratosis. This lesion has a verrucous morphology. These lesions may also appear papillomatous or cystic.

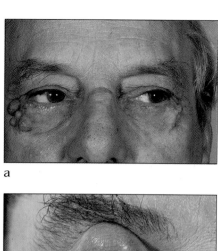

a

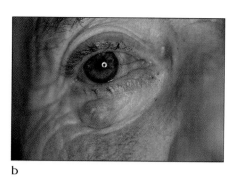

b

### Figure 8.7

(a) Syringomata of the right lower eyelid. These are typically multiple, flesh-coloured, soft, waxy nodular lesions predominantly affecting the lower eyelids. They may be removed surgically. (b) A lower eyelid varix. This appears as a dark blue cystic lesion in elderly patients.

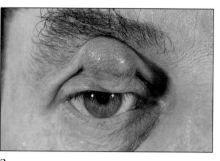

a

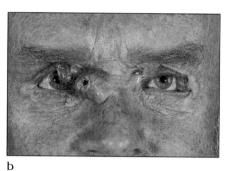

b

### Figure 8.8

(a) An eccrine spiradenoma. This is an uncommon lesion that occurs as a solitary, flesh-coloured nodule.
(b) Tuberous xanthomata. Xanthomata of the eyelids are commonly associated with hyperlipidaemia. The lesions are situated more deeply in the dermis than xanthelasmata.

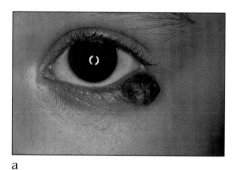

a

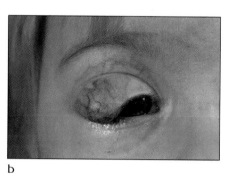

b

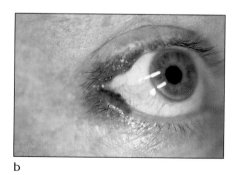

a

### Figure 8.9

(a) A pyogenic granuloma. The lesion appears as a pedunculated reddish lesion often with superficial ulceration. Treatment is by surgical excision. (b) An upper eyelid capillary haemangioma. This represents the most common benign periocular tumour of infancy. The tumour tends to grow rapidly during the first few months of life before undergoing spontaneous regression. The clinical appearance varies with the depth of the lesion. Although benign, the lesion may cause amblyopia from occlusion or secondary astigmatism. Lesions which threaten to cause astigmatism should be treated with intralesional steroid injections (triamcinolone and betamethasone). Surgical debulking or excision may be required for those which fail to respond to steroid injections.

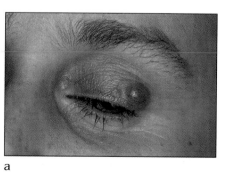

a

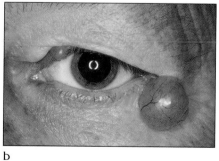

b

### Figure 8.10

(a) A typical meibomian cyst. (b) A cyst of Moll (apocrine hidrocystoma). These lesions are thin-walled and translucent, sometimes with a bluish tinge. They may be confused diagnostically with a cystic basal cell carcinoma.

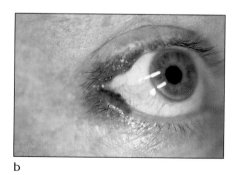

b

### Figure 8.11

(a) Multiple trichoepitheliomata. These lesions can be solitary or multiple. Multiple trichoepitheliomata tend to arise in younger patients and affect other areas of the face as well as the eyelids. They can be effectively treated with $CO_2$ laser application. (b) A 'kissing' compound naevus. This lesion occurs following the deposition of naevus cells in the eyelid fold while the eyelids are fused during embryogenesis.

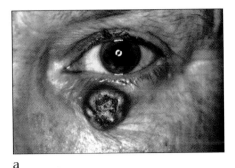
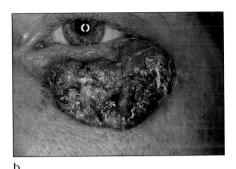

a                                          b

## Figure 8.12

(a) A small keratoacanthoma in a middle-aged patient. (b) A large keratoacanthoma in a young patient. Classically, the lesion commences as a small, flesh-coloured papule which rapidly develops into a dome-shaped nodule with a central keratin-filled crater and elevated, rolled margins. The lesion may increase in size quite rapidly. The lesion then tends to regress spontaneously over the course of 3–6 months. Although this lesion has long been regarded as a benign, self-limiting lesion that mimics a squamous cell carcinoma, it should be regarded as a low-grade squamous cell carcinoma and should be surgically excised while still small.

A number of lesions, however, cannot be easily and reliably differentiated from malignant eyelid lesion and require a biopsy, e.g. a keratoacanthoma (Figure 8.12). For small lesions an *excisional* biopsy serves two functions: diagnosis and treatment. For larger lesions an *incisional* biopsy is undertaken for diagnostic purposes. Shave biopsies should only be used for lesions in which characteristic histopathological changes are anticipated to be confined to the epidermis or superficial dermis, e.g. seborrhoeic keratosis.

It is important that biopsies are performed meticulously or errors in diagnosis will occur. *The tissue must be handled very carefully in order not to induce crush artefact.* The tissue sample should be of adequate size and depth and ideally should include adjacent normal eyelid tissue. This is of particular importance with regard to biopsies of suspected keratoacanthoma. If a sebaceous gland carcinoma is suspected it is important to alert the pathologist of this suspicion so that appropriate stains are utilized. Some biopsy material may need to be presented on filter paper because of the very small size of the samples, e.g. random conjunctival sac biopsies in cases of suspected diffuse sebaceous gland carcinoma.

*It is important to orientate tissue for the pathologist where biopsies are attempted excisional biopsies in case one or more edges are not clear of tumour involvement.* Sutures of various lengths can be employed as markers for this purpose. A tumour excision map should be enclosed with the pathology form to assist the pathologist. A classification of benign eyelid tumors is given in Table 8.3.

## Biopsy technique

A number of lesions cannot be easily and reliably differentiated from malignant eyelid lesion and require a biopsy. For small

---

**Table 8.3**  Classification of benign eyelid tumours

*Benign lesions of the epidermis*
- Achrocordon (skin tag)
- Seborrhoeic keratosis
- Inverted follicular keratosis
- Cutaneous horn

*Benign lesions of the dermis*
- Dermatofibroma
- Neurofibroma
- Capillary haemangioma
- Pyogenic granuloma
- Xanthelasma
- Xanthoma
- Juvenile xanthogranuloma

*Benign lesions of the adnexa*

*Tumours of sweat gland origin*
- Syringoma
- Eccrine spiradenoma

*Tumours of hair follicle origin*
- Trichofolliculoma
- Pilomatrixoma

*Tumours of sebaceous gland origin*
- Sebaceous gland hyperplasia
- Sebaceous adenoma

*Benign pigmentary lesions*
- Congenital naevus
- Junctional naevus
- Compound naevus
- Intradermal naevus
- Lentigo simplex
- Lentigo senilis

lesions an *excisional* biopsy serves two functions: diagnosis and treatment. For larger lesions an *incisional* biopsy is undertaken for diagnostic purposes. In general, shave biopsies should only be used for lesions in which characteristic histopathological changes are anticipated to be confined to the epidermis or superficial dermis, e.g. seborrhoeic keratosis. Exceptions to this rule include naevi that affect the eyelid margin. Although an intradermal naevus by definition extends into the dermis, it is reasonable to perform a shave biopsy as the visible portion of the lesion is removed without subjecting the patient to a more invasive procedure. This leaves a good cosmetic result, with an intact eyelid margin.

It is important that biopsies are performed meticulously or errors in diagnosis will occur. *The tissue must be handled very carefully in order not to induce crush artefact.* The tissue sample should be of adequate size and depth and ideally should include adjacent normal eyelid tissue. This is of particular importance with regard to biopsies of suspected keratoacanthoma. The periphery of the lesion should be selected for incisional biopsy. Material taken from an area of central ulceration may only yield necrotic material.

If a sebaceous gland carcinoma is suspected it is important to alert the pathologist of this suspicion so that appropriate stains are utilized. Some biopsy material may need to be presented on filter paper because of the very small size of the samples, e.g. random conjunctival sac biopsies in cases of suspected diffuse sebaceous gland carcinoma.

*It is important to orientate tissue for the pathologist where biopsies are attempted excisional biopsies in case one or more edges are not clear of tumour involvement.* Sutures of various lengths can be employed as markers for this purpose. A tumour excision map should be enclosed with the pathology form to assist the pathologist.

---

*Note*

1. All eyelid lesions that are removed should be submitted for histopathological examination and the patient informed of the result.
2. It is not acceptable to remove an eyelid or periocular malignant tumour without obtaining histological confirmation that the tumour margins are clear.
3. It is not acceptable to reconstruct an eyelid or periocular tumour excision defect (except by simple direct closure) before obtaining histological confirmation that the tumour margins are clear.

---

# Basal cell carcinoma

Basal cell carcinoma (BCCs) account for approximately 90–95% of all malignant eyelid tumours. Ultraviolet light exposure is an important aetiological factor in the development of eyelid epithelial malignancies. This tumour is prevalent in fair-skinned people. The effects of sun exposure are cumulative, as reflected in the increasing incidence of the tumour with advancing age. BCC may, however, occur in younger patients, particularly those with a tumour diathesis such as the basal cell naevus syndrome (Gorlin's syndrome). Patients with Gorlin's syndrome in the advanced stage are shown in Figure 8.13.

In descending order of frequency, BCCs involve the following locations (Figure 8.14):

- Lower eyelid
- Medial canthus
- Lateral canthus
- Upper eyelid

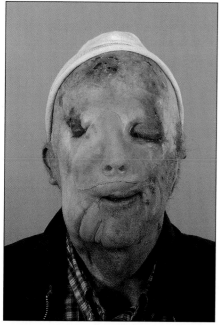

a

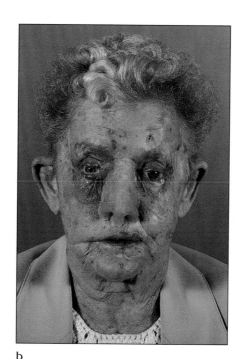

b

**Figure 8.13**
Patients with Gorlin's syndrome in the advanced stages of their disorder. Both patients are wearing prosthetic noses.

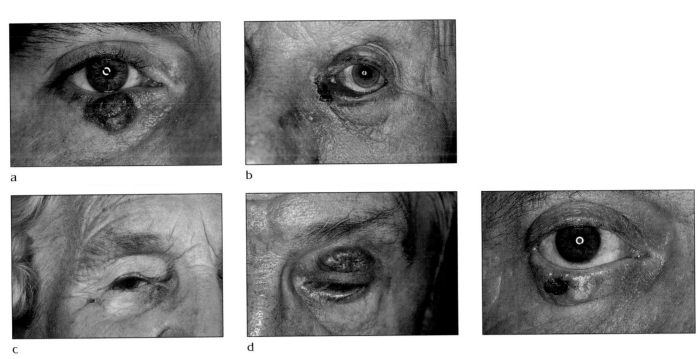

**Figure 8.14**
(a) Lower eyelid nodular basal cell carcinoma (BCC) in a young patient. (b) Medial canthal nodulo-ulcerative BCC in a patient presenting with a cicatricial ectropion. (c) Morphoeic lateral canthal BCC. (d) Upper eyelid nodular BCC.

**Figure 8.15**
Typical lower eyelid nodulo-ulcerative basal cell carcinoma.

BCCs have a variety of clinical appearances, reflecting the various histopathological patterns of the tumour. The tumour arises from undifferentiated cells in the basal layer of the epidermis. As these cells do not produce keratin, BCCs are not associated with hyperkeratosis in contrast to squamous cell carcinomas. The most common presentation is a nodular pattern. The epithelial proliferation produces a solid pearly lesion contiguous with the surface epithelium. The superficial nature of telangiectatic vessels may predispose these lesions to spontaneous bleeding. With prolonged growth, central umbilication and ulceration occurs. The typical presentation is of a chronic, indurated, non-tender, raised, pearly, telangiectatic, well-circumscribed lesion with an elevated surround and depressed crater-like centre (Figure 8.15).

## Clinical varieties

- Nodular
- Ulcerative
- Cystic
- Pigmented
- Morpheaform

The most commonly encountered morphological patterns of BCC are the nodular and ulcerative forms. Nodular BCCs may assume various clinical presentations, such as papilloma (secondary to increased keratin production), a naevus (secondary to pigmentation) and a cyst (due to central tumour necrosis). The variety of clinical presentations of BCC accounts for the high incidence of misdiagnosis. Clinical awareness of the various presentations of the tumour minimizes incorrect clinical diagnoses and management. The pigmented BCC is easily mistaken for an eyelid melanoma that is, in fact, very rare (Figure 8.16).

Occasionally, patients present with a lower eyelid ectropion that has occurred as a consequence of the cicatricial effects of a BCC (Figure 8.17a). The underlying BCC may be missed with a cursory examination (Figure 8.17b).

The morpheaform lesion has clinically indistinct margins and has a tendency to deep invasion, especially at the medial canthus. Orbital invasion by a BCC is manifest clinically as a fixed, non-mobile tumour and/or a 'frozen globe'. Although BCCs 'never' metastasize, approximately 130 cases of metastases have been described in the literature.

The most difficult BCCs to manage are:

- Morpheaform BCCs (Figure 8.18a)
- BCCs that are fixed to bone (Figure 8.18b)
- Medial canthal BCCs (Figure 8.18c)
- BCCs with orbital invasion (Figure 8.18d)
- Recurrent BCCs, especially following radiotherapy (Figure 8.18e)

## Sebaceous gland carcinoma

Sebaceous gland carcinomas (SGCs) are very rare, with a predilection for the periocular area. In addition, SGC of the eyelids has a tendency to produce widespread metastasis,

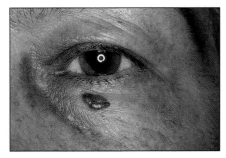

**Figure 8.16**
A pigmented lower lid basal cell carcinoma.

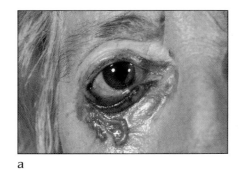

a

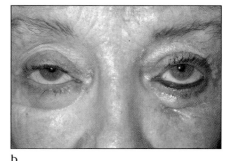

b

**Figure 8.17**
(a) An obvious basal cell carcinoma (BCC) with cicatricial lower eyelid ectropion. (b) A lower lid ectropion secondary to a BCC adherent to the inferior orbital margin. The presence of the BCC would be easily missed on a cursory examination.

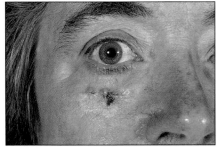

a

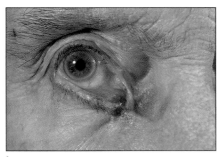

b

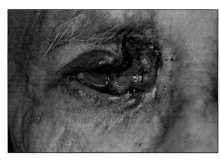

c

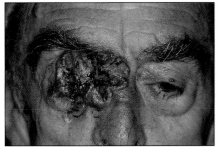

d

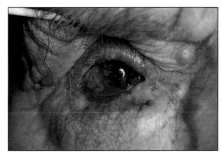

e

**Figure 8.18**
(a) Extensive right lower eyelid morpheaform basal cell carcinoma (BCC). (b) Right lower eyelid nodulo-ulcerative BCC fixed to the inferior orbital margin. (c) Extensive right medial canthal BCC with orbital invasion. (d) Neglected periocular BCC with orbital invasion. (e) Recurrence of lower eyelid BCC after previous radiotherapy.

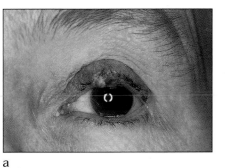

a

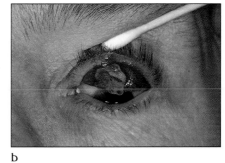

b

**Figure 8.19**
(a) Left upper eyelid sebaceous gland carcinoma masquerading as a recurrent chalazion. (b) Appearances on eversion of the upper eyelid.

whereas such tumours occurring elsewhere on the skin rarely metastasize. SGC occurs with increasing frequency with advancing age. The tumour has a predilection for the upper eyelid, but diffuse upper and lower eyelid involvement may occur in patients presenting with chronic blepharoconjunctivitis.

*This tumour is well recognized for its ability to masquerade as chronic blepharitis/blepharoconjunctivitis or recurrent chalazion ('masquerade syndrome')* (Figures 8.19 and 8.20). Recurrent chalazion or atypical solid chalazia should alert the ophthalmologist to the possibility of underlying sebaceous gland carcinoma.

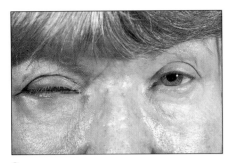
a

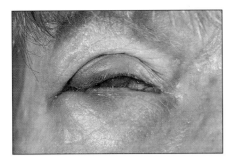
b

**Figure 8.20**
(a) Sebaceous gland carcinoma masquerading as chronic unilateral blepharoconjunctivitis in a patient with acne rosacea. (b) Close-up of same patient.

Histopathological features of SGC are characteristic and may be confirmed by lipid stains (oil red O) on fresh tissue specimens. Multicentric origin is a feature of some SGCs. Clinical presentation of chronic blepharoconjunctivitis has been correlated with the pathological features of pagetoid involvement of the surface epithelium.

*Despite the characteristic features, the tumour is frequently misdiagnosed.* The aggressive behaviour and significant morbidity and mortality associated with SGCs have traditionally been attributed to the misdiagnosed tumours. It is clear that early diagnosis and appropriate therapy significantly reduce the long-term morbidity and mortality associated with this tumour. An advanced neglected SGC is shown in Figure 8.21.

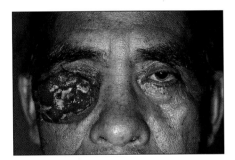

**Figure 8.21**
Advanced neglected sebaceous gland carcinoma.

## Clinical features

- Affects females more commonly than males
- More common in oriental patients
- Tends to occur in older patients
- Has a predilection for the upper eyelid
- Arises most commonly from the meibomian glands
- Has a lesser tendency to ulcerate
- Masquerades as recurrent chalazion or chronic blepharoconjunctivitis ('masquerade syndrome')
- May metastasize prior to establishing correct diagnosis
- High incidence of metastases
- Difficult delineation of tumour margins due to intraepithelial pagetoid spread and/or multicentric pattern
- May be misdiagnosed histologically, especially if lipid stains are not used on properly prepared tissue

## Poor prognostic factors

- Invasion – vascular, lymphatic, or orbital
- Diffuse involvement of both eyelids
- Multicentric origin
- Tumour diameter > 10 mm
- Symptoms present > 6 months

## Note

- In the pagetoid pattern there is often involvement of both eyelids as well as the conjunctiva
- Approximately 30% of SGCs recur
- Systemic extension occurs by contiguous growth, lymphatic spread, and haematogenous seeding
- The tumour spreads mainly to the orbit, the preauricular/submandibular nodes or parotid gland – less frequently to the cervical nodes, lung, pleura, liver, brain and skull.
- Some patients remain alive and well for long periods with regional node involvement – radical neck dissection for isolated cervical node disease is often indicated
- Mortality is approximately 10–20% mainly due to late diagnosis

## Diagnosis

*A high index of suspicion is required*

- Shave biopsy – may only show inflammation
- Full-thickness eyelid biopsy is required
- Random conjunctival biopsies should be performed
- Fat stains are required – alert the pathologist about the suspected diagnosis

# Squamous cell carcinoma

Squamous cell carcinoma (SCC) in the eyelids is similar to that occurring elsewhere on the skin, with low metastatic potential and low tumour-induced mortality. It represents approximately 1–2% of all malignant eyelid lesions. The tumours tend to spread to regional nodes but direct perineural invasion into the central nervous system is usually the cause of death in this group of patients. A patient with a periocular SCC who develops a cranial nerve palsy has neurotrophic spread until proven otherwise. The tumour occurs with increasing frequency with advancing age. Radiation therapy is a significant aetiological factor in the production of SCC.

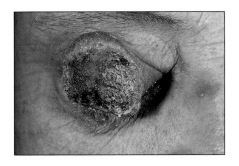

**Figure 8.22**
Right upper eyelid squamous cell carcinoma. The patient also has an upper eyelid xanthelasma.

## Clinical features

*There is no pathognomonic presentation.* These tumours tend to appear as thick, erythematous, elevated, lesions with indurated borders and with a scaly surface (Figures 8.22 and 8.23). *Cutaneous horn formation or extensive keratinization are the most consistent features.* When an SCC occurs at the eyelid margin the lashes are destroyed. Squamous cell carcinomas may be derived from actinic keratoses. With chronicity and cicatricial changes of the skin, secondary ectropion may occur. The clinical features of the tumour are an exaggeration of those found with actinic keratosis. The lesions of actinic keratosis occur in areas of actinic damage and appear as flesh-coloured, yellow/brown plaques, sometimes with erythema. As these areas have malignant potential, such patients should be closely monitored.

Benign tumours such as inverted follicular keratosis, and pseudoepitheliomatous hyperplasia simulate features of SCC. The common variable with these tumours is inflammation that stimulates epithelial proliferation. Clinically, rapid growth is characteristic of these benign lesions.

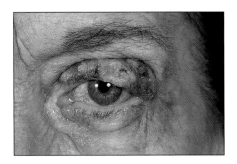

**Figure 8.23**
Left upper eyelid squamous cell carcinoma.

## Keratoacanthoma

Keratoacanthoma is an uncommon epithelial tumour usually occurring on the lower eyelid in patients over 50 years of age. Classically, the lesion commences as a small, flesh-coloured papule which rapidly develops into a dome-shaped nodule with a central keratin-filled crater and elevated, rolled margins (see Figure 8.12). The lesion may increase in size quite rapidly. The lesion then tends to regress spontaneously over the course of 3–6 months. Although this lesion has long been regarded as a benign, self-limiting lesion that mimics an SCC, it should be regarded as a low-grade SCC and should be surgically excised while still small.

## Pigmented eyelid lesions

Pigmented eyelid lesions can lead to diagnostic confusion as any common eyelid lesion can be pigmented, e.g. a BCC (see Figure 8.16). A pigmented eyelid lesion may not, therefore, be derived from abnormal pigment cells, e.g. a naevus or a melanoma. In addition, it should be borne in mind that an eyelid lesion which is derived from abnormal pigment cells may in fact be non-pigmented.

## Benign pigment cell lesions

### Naevi

Naevi have different clinical appearances in different age groups. A *congenital naevus* usually appears as a small flat oval or round light or dark brown macule, although it may range in size. It can contain hairs. This lesion has malignant potential (approximately 5% over the course of a patient's lifetime) and should be removed. A kissing naevus is an unusual form of congenital naevus (see Figure 8.11b).

Acceleration of a naevus during puberty leads to a brown flat *junctional naevus* that lies at the junction of the epidermis and dermis. A naevus that has become more raised and dome-shaped in early adulthood is a *compound naevus*. The naevus of older adults that becomes more raised and nodular in shape with a loss of pigment, becoming flesh coloured, is an *intradermal naevus*. These lesions are commonly seen at the eyelid margin.

### Lentigines

Lentigines are acquired macules varying from light to dark brown in appearance. There are three main varieties: *lentigo simplex, lentigo senilis* and *lentigo maligna* (Hutchinson's freckle). *Lentigo simplex* lesions appear as small, well-circumscribed macules which does not darken with exposure to sunlight. They are entirely benign. *Lentigo senilis* lesions appear as regular light to dark brown gradually enlarging macules appearing in patients usually over 50 years of age. They are seen in areas of the skin exposed to sunlight, particularly the face and arms. They are benign. In contrast, *lentigo maligna* lesions have malignant potential. These lesions have a variable degree of pigmentation with irregular borders. They tend to occur in the lateral cheek and temple regions, affecting patients usually over 50 years of age. As malignant transformation may affect up to 50% of such lesions, surgical excision at an early stage is warranted, although some clinicians follow a policy of close observation with biopsy in the event of a change in size, pigmentation or shape.

## Melanoma

Melanomas represent less than 1% of malignant eyelid tumours. Pigmented BCCs are 10 times more common than melanoma as a cause of pigmented eyelid tumours; however, 40% of eyelid melanomas are non-pigmented.

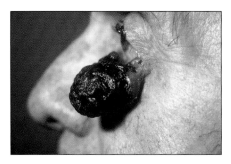

**Figure 8.24** Large left lower eyelid nodular melanoma.

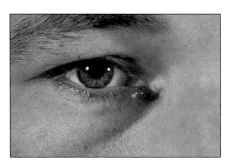

**Figure 8.25** A lower eyelid Kaposi's sarcoma in a patient with AIDS.

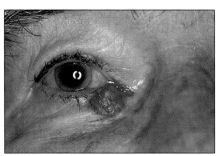

**Figure 8.26** Typical Merkel cell tumours.

a

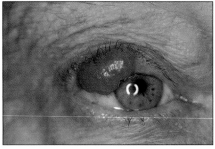

b

## Clinical features

These tumours tend to have irregular borders, variegated pigmentation often with inflammation, occasional bleeding and ulceration. Occasionally, the eyelid may be secondarily involved by a conjunctival melanoma.

## Classification

- Lentigo maligna melanoma
- Superficial spreading melanoma
- Nodular melanoma

Superficial spreading melanoma appears typically as a brown lesion with shades of red, white and blue – it is initially flat but becomes nodular with increase in vertical growth. Nodular melanoma appears as a nodule or plaque, is dark brown or black in colour but can be amelanotic. It shows little radial growth, but extensive vertical growth (Figure 8.24).

Two classic histological classifications are based on:

- Anatomical level of involvement (Clark)
- Tumour thickness (Breslow)

Tumour thickness is the most important predictor of prognosis. The average time to metastasis for cutaneous melanomas varies according to tumour thickness. The late onset of widespread disease is rare (cf. choroidal melanomas).

## Kaposi's sarcoma

Prior to 1981 most cases of Kaposi's sarcoma occurred in elderly Italian/Jewish men or African children. It very rarely involved periocular structures prior to acquired immune deficiency syndrome (AIDS) but is now a relatively common manifestation of AIDS (Figure 8.25).

## Clinical features

Lesions tend to be violaceous in colour. The conjunctiva may be diffusely involved and simulate inflammation.

## Rare eyelid malignancies

- Merkel cell tumour
- Lymphoid tumours – mycosis fungoides
- Metastatic eyelid tumours

Such rare eyelid tumours are usually only diagnosed on histological examination and do not tend to have pathognomonic clinical features. The Merkel cell tumour is highly malignant in its behaviour (Figure 8.26). It is thought to develop from precursor cells that give rise to keratinocytes. They tend to appear as raised dark red lesions close to the eyelid margin of elderly patients. It frequently invades lymphatic vessels and early spread to regional lymph nodes is common. Recurrences are also very common.

# Further reading

1. American Academy of Ophthalmology: *Basic and clinical science course: orbit, eyelids, and lacrimal system*, section 7. San Francisco: American Academy of Ophthalmology, 1998–99, pp. 167–87.
2. Conlon MR, Leatherbarrow B, Nerad JA. Benign eyelid tumors. In: Bosniak S, ed., *Principles and practice of ophthalmic plastic and reconstructive surgery*. Philadelphia: WB Saunders, 1996, pp. 323–41.
3. Doxanas MT. Malignant epithelial eyelid tumors. In: Bosniak S, ed., *Principles and practice of ophthalmic plastic and reconstructive surgery*. Philadelphia: WB Saunders, 1996, pp. 342–51.
4. Howard GR, Nerad JA, Carter KD, Whitaker DC. Clinical characteristics associated with orbital invasion of cutaneous basal cell and squamous cell tumors of the eyelid. *Am J Ophthalmol* (1992) **113**:123–33.
5. Kivela T, Tarkkanen A. The Merkel cell and associated neoplasms in the eyelids and periocular region. *Surv Ophthalmol* (1990) **35**:171–87.
6. Margo CE, Waltz K. Basal cell carcinoma of the eyelid and periocular skin. *Surv Ophthalmol* (1993) **38**:169–92.
7. McCord CD, ed. Management of eyelid neoplastic disease. In: *Eyelid surgery: principles and techniques*. Philadelphia: Lippincott-Raven, 1995, pp. 312–29.
8. Nerad JA, Whitaker DC. Periocular basal cell carcinoma in adults 35 years of age and younger. *Am J Ophthalmol* (1988) **106**:723–9.
9. Sacks EH, Lisman RD. Diagnosis and management of sebaceous gland carcinoma. In: Bosniak S, ed., *Principles and practice of ophthalmic plastic and reconstructive surgery*. Philadelphia: WB Saunders, 1996, pp. 190–5.
10. Tanenbaum M, Grove AS, McCord CD. Eyelid tumors: diagnosis and management. In: McCord CD, Tanenhaum M, Nunery WR, eds, *Oculoplastic surgery*, 3rd edn. New York: Raven Press, 1995, pp. 145–74.
11. Von Domarus H, Steven PJ. Metastatic basal cell carcinoma. Report of five cases and review of 170 cases in the literature. *J Am Acad Dermatol* (1984) **10**:1043–60.

# 9

# Management of malignant eyelid/periocular tumours

## Introduction

Many different treatment modalities have been advocated, by a variety of medical practitioners, for the management of malignant tumours in the periocular region.

> The management of all malignant eyelid tumours depends on:
>
> - Correct histological diagnosis
> - Assessment of tumour margins
> - Assessment of local and systemic tumour spread

The vast majority of malignant periocular tumours are non-melanoma cutaneous malignancies (basal and squamous cell carcinomas). The major considerations in selecting a treatment for these tumours are:

- The selected treatment modality must be capable of totally eradicating all tumour cells to which it is applied
- A mechanism must exist to ensure that the treatment is applied to all the existing tumour cells

Tumours of the eyelids and canthi often exhibit slender strands and shoots of cancer cells which can infiltrate the local tissues beyond the clinically apparent borders of the tumour. For this reason appropriate monitoring to ensure that the treatment modality reaches all of the tumour cells is essential. Numerous studies have demonstrated that clinical judgement of tumour margins is inadequate, significantly underestimating the area of microscopic tumour involvement. The introduction of frozen-section control to document adequacy of tumour excision marked a major advancement in the treatment of malignant eyelid tumours and now constitutes the standard of care. Any treatment modality that does not utilize microscopic monitoring of tumour margins must instead encompass a wider area of adjacent normal tissue in the hope that any microscopic extensions of tumour will fall within this area.

> The goals in the surgical management of malignant eyelid tumours are:
>
> - Complete eradication of the tumour
> - Minimal sacrifice of normal adjacent tissues
>
> These concepts are of the utmost importance in the surgical management of periocular malignancy because of the complex nature of the periocular tissues and the functional importance of the eyelids in ocular protection, in addition to the grave risks that are posed by tumour recurrence in this area.
>
> Mohs micrographic surgery represents the gold standard in the management of basal cell and squamous cell carcinomas.

In the periocular region, focal malignancy can be treated with:

- Surgery
- Irradiation
- Cryotherapy

> The choice of therapy depends on:
>
> - The size of the tumour
> - The location of the tumour
> - The type of tumour
> - The age and general health of the patient
> - The clinician's relative expertise

The choice of treatment is particularly important in:

- Diffuse tumours
- Tumour extension to bone/the orbit
- Patients with a cancer diathesis, e.g. the basal cell nevus syndrome
- Young patients

A comprehensive examination of the patient is important, with palpation of the regional lymph nodes and a whole body skin examination wherever possible. If orbital invasion is suspected from the clinical examination, e.g. restriction of ocular motility, it is appropriate to request thin-section, high-resolution computed tomography (CT) scans with bone windows. In selected cases, chest and abdominal CT is required with liver function tests to evaluate systemic spread. Such patients should be managed with the assistance of an oncologist. If systemic spread is found, palliation only may be preferable.

# Basal cell carcinoma

*Unfortunately, basal cell carcinomas have traditionally been regarded as relatively benign, rarely invasive tumours and as such have commonly been casually excised. This has been associated with a high incidence of recurrence, unnecessary morbidity, and occasionally avoidable mortality.* A dedicated approach to tumour eradication is clearly essential in the management of these patients:

- Surgery in conjunction with histological monitoring of tumour margins
- Irradiation
- Cryotherapy

The surgical management of basal cell carcinoma consists of surgical removal of the tumour, with monitoring of the excised margins, either by permanent or frozen section. A close working relationship with a pathologist offers a major advantage in the efficient delivery of such care. In the majority of cases the diagnosis is evident on clinical grounds alone. *Where the diagnosis is unclear, a biopsy should be performed before definitive treatment.* Although Mohs' micrographic surgery is now considered by many to represent the *gold standard* in the management of periocular basal cell carcinomas, this treatment modality is unavailable in many centres in this and other countries.

*Although it is reasonable to close small defects immediately, no defect should be formally reconstructed without definitive histopathological evidence of complete tumour clearance.* Exenteration is reserved for cases where orbital invasion has occurred and aggressive surgical management is appropriate for the individual patient.

> Note: Tumours which recur after radiation are often poorly controlled with other modalities

# Squamous cell carcinoma

The following treatment modalities are used for the management of squamous cell carcinoma:

- Surgery in conjunction with histological monitoring of tumour margins
- Radiation

The surgical management of squamous cell carcinoma consists of surgical removal of the tumour with monitoring of the excised margins, either by permanent or frozen section. It is appropriate to obtain a biopsy of a suspicious tumour before undertaking a definitive surgical procedure. *Great care should be taken to obtain a representative section of the tumour.* Shave biopsies do not allow determination of dermal invasion by the epithelial tumour. Benign tumours such as actinic keratosis, inverted follicular keratosis and pseudoepitheliomatous hyperplasia can be differentiated only by evaluation of dermal extension. As such, the pathologist is frequently forced to give a diagnosis of squamous cell carcinoma because inadequate tissue has been submitted for review. It is not unusual for a tumour that has been reported as squamous cell carcinoma to have resolved by the time definitive surgical resection can be scheduled for this reason.

# *Biopsy technique*

If the lesion is small, an excisional biopsy with direct closure of the defect should be performed. If the lesion is larger, an incisional biopsy should be performed. The specimen should be handled with care to avoid any crush artefact. If the lesion involves the eyelid margin, the biopsy should be full thickness. Wherever possible, the base of the lesion and adjacent normal tissue should be included. The specimen should be oriented and a tumour map recorded for the pathologist. 'Laissez-faire' is useful for healing of many biopsy sites.

As in the management of basal cell carcinoma, Mohs' surgery is the *gold standard*. Exenteration is reserved for cases where orbital invasion has occurred and aggressive surgical management is appropriate for the individual patient.

# Sebaceous gland carcinoma

The preferred management of sebaceous gland carcinoma consists of complete surgical extirpation of the tumour. With heightened appreciation of the clinical presentation of the tumour, early surgical excision significantly enhances the long-term prognosis. Numerous procedures for incision and drainage of suspected recurrent chalazia delay the appropriate diagnosis of sebaceous gland carcinoma.

Localized sebaceous gland carcinoma is managed by a permanent section biopsy to establish the diagnosis. A full-thickness block resection of the eyelid is required to establish the diagnosis in patients with diffuse thickening of the eyelid. An incisional biopsy is appropriate in the patient presenting with a solid mass. The tumour can arise from multifocal non-contiguous tumour origins. It is for this reason that it is not appropriate to subject this tumour to Mohs' micrographic surgery nor is intraoperative frozen-section control of the surgical margins appropriate.

Following confirmation of the diagnosis a wide resection of the affected eyelid is performed and the specimen sent for permanent section analysis. *Because of the possible multicentric origin of sebaceous gland carcinoma, it is important to perform random conjunctival sac biopsies which should be carefully mapped and recorded.* If the pathologist is able to confirm that the margins are clear and that the random biopsies do not contain tumour, the defect can be reconstructed.

Close postoperative observation is always crucial in the management of these patients to exclude recurrent disease. In patients with diffuse eyelid/conjunctival involvement or orbital extension, orbital exenteration is recommended.

Radiation therapy has a limited role in the management of sebaceous gland carcinoma. The tumour is radiosensitive and does respond to radiation therapy, but recurrences are inevitable. In addition, patients develop significant ocular complications such as keratitis, radiation retinopathy and severe pain. Radiation therapy is therefore considered a palliative procedure to reduce tumour size. It should not be viewed as a curative modality.

# Melanoma

## *Surgery*

The extent of tumour-free margins does not correlate with survival. It is therefore appropriate to take relatively small tissue margins to preserve eyelid function wherever possible. If the tumour has extended to Clark level IV or V or its thickness exceeds 1.5 mm, a referral for lymph node dissection should be considered.

## *Radiation*

Radiotherapy is rarely used in the management of eyelid melanoma. Doses sufficient to destroy the tumour will destroy the eye/ocular adnexae.

# Merkel cell tumour

Merkel cell tumour is a rare but highly malignant tumour. It should be managed by urgent aggressive surgical resection with wide margins. Postoperative radiotherapy should also be considered.

# Metastatic eyelid tumour

The management of metastatic eyelid tumours is the realm of the oncologist and usually involves chemotherapy and/or radiation therapy. Surgical excision can be considered if the tumour is localized and unresponsive to other modalities.

# Lymphoma

The management of eyelid lymphoma is also the realm of the oncologist.

# Kaposi's sarcoma

Local control is usually easily achieved with radiation.

# Irradiation

Historically, irradiation as a treatment modality for periocular cutaneous malignancies was very popular in the UK, and a number of studies reported better than 90% cure rates for periocular basal cell carcinomas. More recently, however, investigators have noted that basal cell carcinomas treated by irradiation recur at a higher rate and behave more aggressively than tumours treated by surgical excision.

The radiation dose used to treat patients varies, depending on the size of the lesion and the estimate of its depth. The treatments are usually fractionated over several weeks, depending on local protocols. The proponents of radiation therapy point to the lack of discomfort with radiation treatment and to the fact that no hospitalization or anaesthesia is required.

Although radiation therapy is no longer to be recommended as the treatment of choice for periocular cutaneous malignancies, there are occasionally patients who, for various reasons, cannot undergo surgical excision and reconstruction and for whom radiation may be useful. However, it is important to continue to look closely for evidence of recurrence well beyond the 5-year postoperative period routinely utilized for surgically managed cutaneous malignancies.

## *Disadvantages*

*It is now generally accepted that basal cell carcinomas recurring after radiation therapy are more difficult to diagnose, present at a more advanced stage, cause more extensive destruction, and are much more difficult to eradicate.* The greater extent of destruction may be explained by the presence of adjacent radiodermatitis, which may mask underlying tumour recurrence and allow the tumour to grow more extensively before it can be clinically detected

(Figure 9.1). The damaging effect of radiation on periocular tissues poses another drawback to its use.

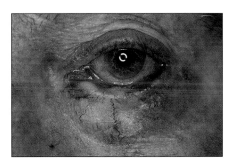

**Figure 9.1**
Lower eyelid scarring/telangiectasia with a cicatricial ectropion following irradiation of a basal cell carcinoma.

Note the potential complications associated with the use of irradiation for treatment of periocular malignancy:

- Skin necrosis
- Cicatricial ectropion
- Telangiectasia
- Epiphora
- Loss of eyelashes
- Keratitis
- Cataract
- Dry eye
- Keratinization of the palpebral conjunctiva

> Note:
> The most serious complications occur after treatment of large tumours of the upper eyelid even when the eye is shielded.

Although most surgeons would oppose the use of radiotherapy as the primary modality in treating periocular skin cancers, it is felt to be specifically contraindicated for lesions in the medial canthus, lesions greater than 1 cm and recurrent tumours.

Although a number of studies reported high success rates with radiation for periocular basal cell carcinomas, many of these studies did not include long-term follow-up. Investigators have now determined that it may take longer for a recurrence of a radiation-treated malignancy to become clinically apparent than for a surgically treated tumour. Recent studies with longer follow-up have reported a recurrence rate between 17% and 20%.

The radiation changes induced in surrounding tissue make it more difficult to track recurrent tumours micrographically and render subsequent reconstruction after excision more difficult. It has also been reported that radiation therapy may disturb the protective barrier offered by the periosteum and allow for greater likelihood of bony cancerous involvement with recurrences. A final concern with radiation therapy, which is not shared by other treatment modalities, is that the treatment itself may induce new tumour formation.

# Cryotherapy

Cryotherapy is an effective alternative therapy for small localized basal cell carcinomas, especially those located in the vicinity of the puncta/canaliculi which are relatively resistant to damage by the temperatures required to kill tumour cells. It is useful in debilitated patients who are unfit for surgery. It is a single session treatment (cf. radiotherapy). *A diagnostic biopsy should be performed prior to treatment.* The entire tumour must be frozen to −30°C. Liquid nitrogen is the most effective freezing agent. The globe and adjacent tissue must be adequately protected. A thermocouple should be used and a cycle of freeze–thaw, freeze thaw utilized.

## *Disadvantages*

There is an approximate 10% recurrence rate due to the inadvertent inclusion of morpheaform/diffuse tumours. There is a profound tissue reaction to cryotherapy with exudation and a prolonged period of healing.

Note the potential complications associated with the use of cryotherapy for treatment of periocular malignancy:

- Eyelid notching
- Ectropion
- Hypertrophic scarring
- Pseudoepitheliomatous hyperplasia
- Symblephara

Pseudoepitheliomatous hyperplasia is difficult to manage as it can mimic recurrent tumour.

# Mohs' micrographic surgery

Mohs' micrographic surgery is a refinement of frozen-section control of tumour margins that, by mapping tumour planes, allows a three-dimensional assessment of tumour margins rather than the two-dimensional analysis provided by routine frozen section. In this technique, the surgical removal of the tumour is performed by a dermatological surgeon with specialized training in tumour excision and mapping of margins.

The unique feature of Mohs' micrographic surgery is that it removes the skin cancer in a sequence of horizontal layers monitored by microscopic examination of horizontal sections through the undersurface of each layer. Careful mapping of residual cancer in each layer is possible, and subsequent horizontal layers are then excised in cancer-bearing areas until cancer-free histological layers are obtained at the base and on all sides of the skin cancer.

## *Advantages*

Mohs' micrographic excision has been shown to give the highest cure rate for most cutaneous malignancies occurring on various body surfaces. In addition to its high cure rate, the technique offers several other advantages. The Mohs' technique obviates the need to remove generous margins of clinically normal adjacent tissue by allowing precise layer-by-layer mapping of tumour cells. This is extremely important in the periocular regions because of the specialized nature of the periocular tissues and the challenges in creating ready substitutes that will obtain a satisfactory functional and cosmetic result.

Because routine frozen-section monitoring of periocular skin cancers in the operating theatre involves a significant loss of time while waiting for turnaround of results from the pathologist, Mohs' micrographic excision performed in the dermatologist's minor operating theatre allows for more efficient use of operating theatre time.

Although small lesions may be allowed to granulate, excision in the majority of periocular cases is followed by immediate or next day reconstruction, by a separate oculoplastic surgeon who has expertise in reconstructing periocular defects. Reconstruction can be scheduled immediately following Mohs' micrographic excision or on a subsequent day with better prediction of the operating theatre time required. Taking responsibility for tumour excision out of the hands of the reconstructing surgeon also assures that concern over the difficulties of reconstruction do not limit aggressive tissue removal where it is required.

Mohs' micrographic excision has been shown to provide the most effective treatment for non-melanoma cutaneous malignancies, i.e basal cell and squamous cell carcinomas. It is not suitable for the management of sebaceous gland carcinomas. However, it is particularly recommended for the following types of periocular cutaneous malignancy:

- Skin tumours arising in the medial canthal region, where, because of natural tissue planes, the risk of deeper invasion is greater and where the borders of involved tissue are more difficult to define
- Recurrent skin tumours
- Large primary skin tumours of long duration
- Morpheaform basal cell carcinomas
- Any tumours whose clinical borders are not obviously demarcated
- Tumours in young patients

## *Disadvantages*

Although Mohs' micrographic surgery allows for the most precise histological monitoring, some cancer cells may rarely be left behind and a 2–3% long-term recurrence rate has been reported for primary periocular skin cancers. Careful follow-up, searching for early signs of recurrence, remains important.

> Patients must be able to tolerate local anaesthesia for this procedure

For periocular tumours the surgical excision and surgical reconstruction are usually divided between two surgeons and often at two different physical sites. In addition, Mohs' micrographic surgeons are not available in many centres in this and other countries.

## Further reading

1. Abide JM, Nahai F, Bennett RG. The meaning of surgical margins. *Plast Reconstr Surg* (1984) **73**:492–6.

2. American Academy of Ophthalmology. *Basic and clinical science course: orbit, eyelids, and lacrimal system*, section 7. San Francisco: American Academy of Ophthalmology, 1998–99, pp. 167–87.

3. Anderson RL, Ceilley RI. Multispeciality approach to excision and reconstruction of eyelid tumours. *Ophthalmology* (1978) **85**:1150–63.

4. Carter KD, Nerad JA, Whitaker DC. Clinical factors influencing periocular surgical defects after Mohs' micrographic surgery. *Ophthal Plast Reconstr Surg* (1999) **15**:83–91.

5. De Potter P, Shields CL, Shields JA. Sebaceous gland carcinoma of the eyelids. *Int Ophthalmol Clin* (1993) **33**:5–9.

6. Inkster C, Ashworth J, Murdoch JR, Montgomery P, Telfer NR, Leatherbarrow B. Oculoplastic reconstruction following Mohs' surgery. *Eye* (1998) **12**:214–18.

7. Leshin B, Yeatts P, Anscher M, Montano G, Dutton JJ. Management of periocular basal cell carcinoma: Mohs' micrographic surgery versus radiotherapy. *Surv Ophthalmology* (1993) **38**:193–212.

8. Mohs FE. Micrographic surgery for the microscopically controlled excision of eyelid cancers. *Arch Ophthalmol* (1986) **104**:901–9.

9. Rivlin D, Moy RL. Mohs' surgery for periorbital malignancies. In: Bosniak S, ed., *Principles and practice of ophthalmic plastic and reconstructive surgery*, Vol. 2. Philadelphia: WB Saunders, 1996, pp. 352–5.

10. Sacks EH, Lisman RD: Diagnosis and management of sebaceous gland carcinoma. In: Bosniak S, ed., *Principles and practice of ophthalmic plastic and reconstructive surgery*, Philadelphia: WB Saunders, 1996, pp. 190–5.

11. Shriner DL, McCoy DK, Goldberg DJ, Wagner RF Jr. Mohs' micrographic surgery. *J Am Acad Dermatol* (1998) **39**:79–97.

12. Tanenbaum M, Grove AS, McCord CD. Eyelid tumors: diagnosis and management. In: McCord CD, Tanenhaum M, Nunery WR, eds, *Oculoplastic surgery*, 3rd edn. New York: Raven Press, 1995, pp. 145–74.

13. Telfer NR, Colver GB, Bowers PW. Guidelines for the management of basal cell carcinoma. British Association of Dermatologists. *Br J Dermatol* (1999) **141**:415–23.

# 10

# Eyelid reconstruction

## Introduction

The goals in eyelid reconstruction following eyelid tumour excision are preservation of normal eyelid function for the protection of the eye and restoration of good cosmesis. Of these goals, preservation of normal function is of the utmost importance and takes priority over the cosmetic result. Failure to maintain normal eyelid function, particularly following upper eyelid reconstruction, will have dire consequences for the comfort and visual performance of the patient. In general, it is technically easier to reconstruct eyelid defects following tumour excision surgery than following trauma.

## General principles

A number of surgical procedures can be utilized to reconstruct eyelid defects. In general, where less than 25% of the eyelid has been sacrificed, direct closure of the eyelid is possible. Where the eyelid tissues are very lax, direct closure may be possible for much larger defects occupying up to 50% of the eyelid. Where direct closure without undue tension on the wound is difficult, a simple lateral canthotomy and cantholysis of the appropriate limb of the lateral canthal tendon can effect a simple closure.

To reconstruct eyelid defects involving greater degrees of tissue loss, a number of different surgical procedures have been devised. The choice depends on:

- The extent of the eyelid defect
- The state of the remaining periocular tissues
- The visual status of the fellow eye
- The age and general health of the patient
- The surgeon's own expertise

In deciding which procedure is most suited to the individual patient's needs, one should aim to re-establish the following:

- A smooth mucosal surface to line the eyelid and protect the cornea
- An outer layer of skin and muscle
- Structural support between the two lamellae of skin and mucosa originally provided by the tarsal plate
- A smooth, nonabrasive eyelid margin free from keratin and trichiasis
- In the upper eyelid, normal vertical eyelid movement without significant ptosis or lagophthalmos
- Normal horizontal tension with normal medial and lateral canthal tendon positions
- Normal apposition of the eyelid to the globe
- A normal contour to the eyelid

Large eyelid defects generally require composite reconstruction in layers with a variety of tissues from either adjacent sources or from distant sites being used to replace both the anterior and posterior lamellae. It is essential that only one lamella should be reconstructed as a free graft. The other lamella should be reconstructed as a vascularized flap to provide an adequate blood supply to prevent necrosis.

## Lower eyelid reconstruction

Defects of the lower eyelid can be divided into those that involve the eyelid margin and those that do not.

## *Eyelid defects involving the eyelid margin*

### Small defects

An eyelid defect of 25% or less may be closed directly. In patients with marked eyelid laxity, even a defect occupying up to 50% of

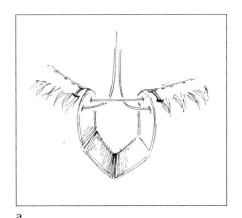
a

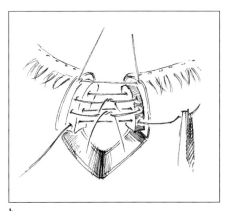
b

**Figure 10.1**
(a) Reapproximation of the eyelid margin is achieved with a single-armed 5/0 Vicryl suture passed symmetrically through the superior aspect of the tarsus on each side of the defect. (b) Once the eyelid margin is satisfactorily aligned, the initial suture is loosened and used to put the eyelid on gentle traction. The rest of the tarsus is reapproximated with interrupted 5/0 Vicryl sutures.

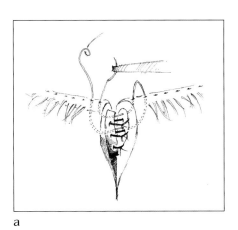
a

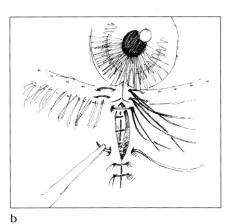
b

**Figure 10.2**
(a) Once the tarsal sutures have been placed, 6/0 silk sutures are placed along the lash line and along the line of the meibomian glands in a vertical mattress fashion. (b) The skin is closed with interrupted 7/0 Vicryl sutures.

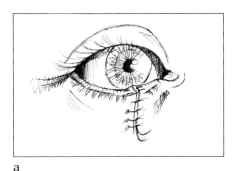
a

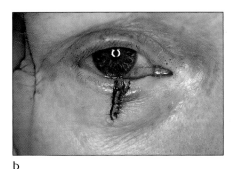
b

**Figure 10.3**
Direct closure of a lower eyelid defect completed with eversion of the eyelid margin wound. The silk sutures have been left long and have been incorporated into the skin closure sutures. The conjunctiva is left to heal spontaneously without suture closure. The skin sutures may be removed in 5–7 days but the eyelid margin sutures should be left in place for 14 days.

the eyelid may be closed directly. The two edges of the defect should be grasped and pulled together to judge the facility of closure. If there is no excess tension on the lid, the edges may be approximated directly. The lid margin is reapproximated with a single-armed 5/0 Vicryl suture on a 1/2-circle needle. This is passed through the most superior aspect of the tarsus, ensuring that the suture is anterior to the conjunctiva to avoid contact with the cornea (Figure 10.1).

This suture is tied with a single throw and the eyelid margin approximation checked. If this is unsatisfactory, the suture is replaced and the process repeated. Proper placement of this suture will avoid the complications of eyelid notching and trichiasis. Once the margin approximation is good, the suture is untied and the ends fixated to the head drape with a haemostat. This

elongates the wound, enabling further single-armed Vicryl sutures to be placed in the lower tarsus.

These sutures are tied. The uppermost Vicryl suture is then tied. Improper placement or tying of the suture or too great a degree of tension on the wound will result in dehiscence of the wound. Next, a 6/0 silk suture is passed in a vertical mattress fashion along the lash line and a second suture along the line of the meibomian glands (Figure 10.2).

These sutures are tied with sufficient tension to cause eversion of the edges of the eyelid margin wound. A small amount of pucker is desirable initially, to avoid late lid notching, as the lid heals and the wound contracts. The sutures are left long and incorporated into the skin closure sutures to prevent contact with the cornea (Figure 10.3).

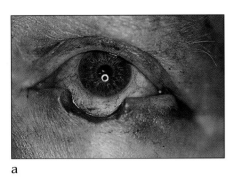

a

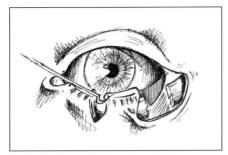

b

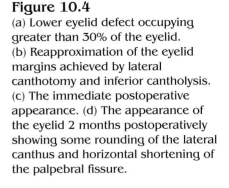

**Figure 10.4**
(a) Lower eyelid defect occupying greater than 30% of the eyelid.
(b) Reapproximation of the eyelid margins achieved by lateral canthotomy and inferior cantholysis.
(c) The immediate postoperative appearance. (d) The appearance of the eyelid 2 months postoperatively showing some rounding of the lateral canthus and horizontal shortening of the palpebral fissure.

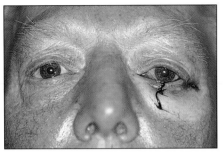

c

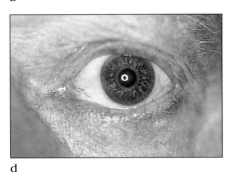

d

## Moderate defects

**Canthotomy and cantholysis.** Where an eyelid defect cannot be closed directly without undue tension on the wound, a lateral canthotomy and inferior cantholysis can be performed. The inferior cantholysis is performed by cutting the tissue between the conjunctiva and the skin close to the periosteum of the lateral orbital margin with the lateral lid margin drawn up and medially (Figure 10.4).

**Semicircular flap.** A semicircular flap (Tenzel flap) is useful for the reconstruction of defects up to 70% of the lower eyelid where some tarsus remains on either side of the defect, particularly where the patient's fellow eye has poor vision. Under these circumstances it is preferable to avoid a procedure which necessitates closure of the eye for a period of some weeks. A semicircular incision is made starting at the lateral canthus, curving superiorly to a level just below the brow and temporally for approximately 2 cm.

The flap is widely undermined to the depth of the superficial temporalis fascia, taking care not to damage the temporal branch of the facial nerve that crosses the mid-portion of the zygomatic arch. A lateral canthotomy and inferior cantholysis are then performed. The eyelid defect is closed as described above. The lateral canthus is suspended with a deep 5/0 Vicryl suture passed through the periosteum of the lateral orbital margin to prevent retraction of the flap (Figure 10.5). Any residual dog ear is removed and the lateral skin wound closed with simple interrupted sutures. The conjunctiva of the inferolateral fornix is gently mobilized and sutured to the edge of the flap with interrupted 8/0 Vicryl sutures.

## Large defects

**Upper lid tarsoconjunctival pedicle flap.** The upper lid tarsoconjunctival pedicle flap (Hughes flap) is an excellent technique for the reconstruction of relatively shallow defects

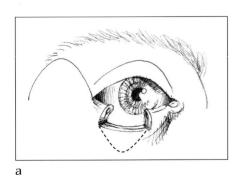

a

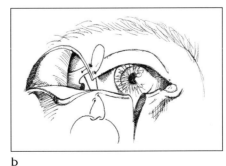

b

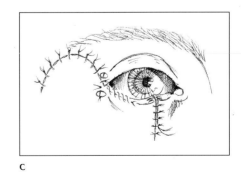

c

**Figure 10.5**
(a) Large defect of the lower eyelid. (b) Lateral canthotomy, inferior cantholysis with dissection of semicircular flap. The flap is suspended from the periosteum of the lateral orbital margin with a suture. (c) The final appearance following wound closure.

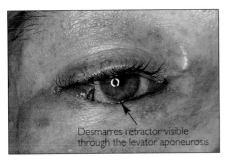

**Figure 10.6**
A lower eyelid defect suitable for reconstruction using a Hughes procedure.

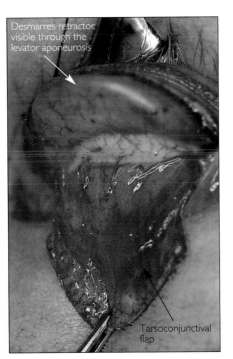

**Figure 10.7**
A tarsoconjunctival flap.

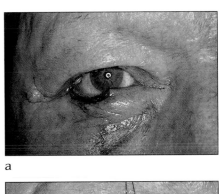

a

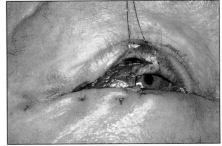

b

**Figure 10.8**
(a) Lateral lower eyelid defect.
(b) Lateral tarsoconjunctival flap with a skin–muscle advancement flap. The flap is held in the advanced position with two 5/0 Vicryl sutures that are anchored to the tarsus.

involving up to 100% of the eyelid (Figure 10.6). With defects extending horizontally beyond the eyelids, it can be combined with periosteal flaps from the canthi to recreate canthal tendons. *Great care, however, should be taken in the planning and construction of the flap in order not to compromise the function of the upper eyelid. It is essential that the patient can cope with occlusion of the eye for a period of 8–10 weeks.*

A 4/0 silk traction suture is passed through the grey line of the upper eyelid, which is everted over a Desmarres retractor. The size of the flap to be constructed is ascertained by pulling together the edges of the eyelid wound firmly and measuring the residual defect. A horizontal incision is made centrally through the tarsus 3.5 mm above the lid margin. It is important to leave a tarsal height of 3.5 mm below the incision in order to prevent an upper eyelid entropion and to prevent any compromise of the eyelid margin blood supply. The horizontal incision is completed with blunt-tipped Westcott scissors, and vertical relieving cuts are made at both ends of the tarsal incision. The tarsus and conjunctiva are dissected free from Müller's muscle and the levator aponeurosis up to the superior fornix. The tarsoconjunctival flap is mobilized into the lower lid defect (Figure 10.7).

The tarsus is sutured to the lower lid tarsus with interrupted 5/0 Vicryl sutures. The lower lid conjunctival edge is sutured to the inferior border of the mobilized tarsus with a continuous 7/0 Vicryl suture.

Sufficient skin to cover the anterior surface of the flap can be obtained either by harvesting a full-thickness skin graft or by advancing a myocutaneous flap from the cheek. This flap can be elevated by bluntly dissecting a skin and muscle flap inferiorly toward the orbital rim and incising the lid and cheek skin vertically. Relaxing triangles (Burow's triangles) may be excised on the inferior medial and lateral edges of the defect. The flap of skin and muscle is then advanced with sufficient undermining so that it will lie in place without tension. This flap is then sewn in place with its upper border at the appropriate level to produce the new lower lid margin. Two interrupted 5/0 Vicryl sutures are passed through the flap and anchored to the tarsus (Figure 10.8). The skin edge is sewn to the superior aspect of the tarsus using a continuous 7/0 Vicryl suture.

In the patient with relatively tight, non-elastic skin, such an advancement may eventually lead to eyelid retraction or an ectropion. In such cases, it is wiser to use a free full-thickness skin graft from the opposite upper lid, preauricular area, retroauricular area or from the upper inner arm area. The graft should not be taken from the upper lid of the same eye as the Hughes flap, as the resultant vertical shortening of both the anterior and the posterior lamellae may produce vertical contracture of the donor lid. If possible, a flap of orbicularis muscle can be advanced alone after dissecting it free from overlying skin. This will improve the vascular recipient bed for the skin graft. If a full-thickness skin graft has been utilized, an occlusive dressing is applied for 5–7 days. Skin sutures may be removed after 5–7 days. The patient is instructed to massage the area in an upward direction for a few minutes 3–4 times per day to keep the tissues supple and prevent undue contracture.

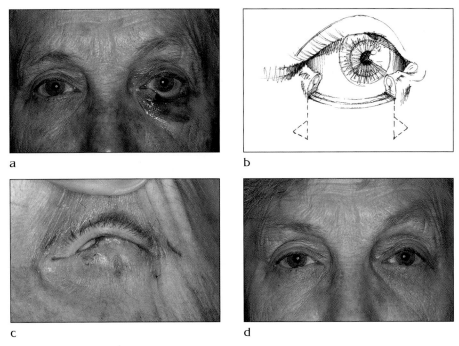

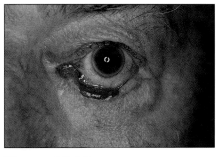

**Figure 10.10**
An unsatisfactory result from a Hughes procedure with a lower eyelid ectropion, retraction and an unsightly eyelid margin.

**Figure 10.9**
(a) Central shallow lower eyelid defect occupying greater than 50% of the eyelid. (b) Diagram showing position of Burow's triangles. (c) Upper eyelid raised showing the typical appearance of a skin–muscle advancement flap. (d) The appearance of the reconstructed eyelid 1 month after the second stage division of the flap. The upper eyelid shows some mild retraction.

The flap can be opened approximately 6–8 weeks (or longer if necessary) after surgery. This is done by inserting one blade of a pair of blunt-tipped Westcott scissors just above the desired level of the new lid border and cutting the flap open. It is unnecessary to angle the scissors to leave the conjunctival edge somewhat higher than the anterior edge. Traditionally, this provides some conjunctiva posteriorly to be draped forward and create a new mucocutaneous lid margin, but this leaves a reddened lid margin which is cosmetically poor. It is preferable to allow the lid margin simply to granulate, as the appearance is far better. The upper lid is then everted and the residual flap is excised flush to its attachment. If Müller's muscle has been left undisturbed in the original dissection of the flap, eyelid retraction is minimal and no formal attempt is needed to recess the upper lid retractors. The Hughes procedure provides excellent cosmetic and functional results for lower lid reconstruction (Figure 10.9).

## Complications
- Lower eyelid retraction
- Lower eyelid ectropion
- A reddened eyelid margin
- Upper eyelid retraction

These complications following the use of a Hughes procedure can be avoided if the basic principles outlined above are closely adhered to (Figure 10.10). The lower eyelid will retract if a skin–muscle advancement flap has been used where there is insufficient residual anterior lamella, if the flap has been divided too soon or if the patient has not applied sufficient postoperative massage.

An unsightly eyelid margin is avoided by performing a simple division of the flap without formal overlapping or suturing of the conjunctiva. Some upper eyelid retraction is inevitable but can be kept to a minimal degree either by excluding Müller's muscle from the flap where a skin graft is not required or by performing an upper lid retractor recession at the second stage division of the flap.

**Periosteal flap.** For the repair of lateral lid defects in which the tarsus and the lateral canthal tendon have been completely excised, a periosteal flap provides excellent support for the reconstruction. The periosteum should be elevated as a rectangular strip from the outer aspect of the lateral orbital rim at the mid-pupillary level to provide upward support. The flap should be 4–5 mm in height, and the length can be judged based on the size of the defect to be reconstructed. The hinged flap is elevated and folded medially and secured to the edge of the residual tarsus or to the inner aspect of a myocutaneous flap with 5/0 or 6/0 absorbable sutures.

Although the Hughes procedure is traditionally used for the reconstruction of shallow marginal defects of the lower eyelid, it can be used in conjunction with local periosteal flaps for a simplified reconstruction of more extensive defects of the lower lid (Figures 10.11–10.14). This avoids more invasive procedures and

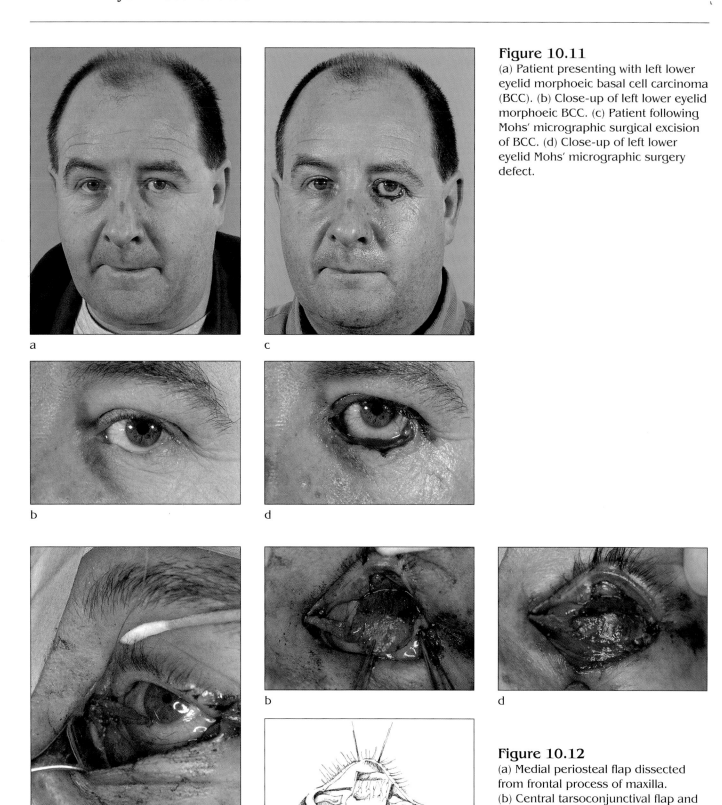

a

b

c

d

a

c

b

d

**Figure 10.11**
(a) Patient presenting with left lower eyelid morphoeic basal cell carcinoma (BCC). (b) Close-up of left lower eyelid morphoeic BCC. (c) Patient following Mohs' micrographic surgical excision of BCC. (d) Close-up of left lower eyelid Mohs' micrographic surgery defect.

**Figure 10.12**
(a) Medial periosteal flap dissected from frontal process of maxilla.
(b) Central tarsoconjunctival flap and medial and lateral periosteal flaps dissected. (c) Diagram demonstrating periosteal flap dissection. (d) Flaps sutured in place prior to skin–muscle advancement flap.

can still be performed under local anaesthesia. The term 'maximal Hughes procedure' has been coined for this reconstructive technique.

The Hughes procedure may be combined with other reconstructive techniques to achieve the best result for an individual patient (Figure 10.15).

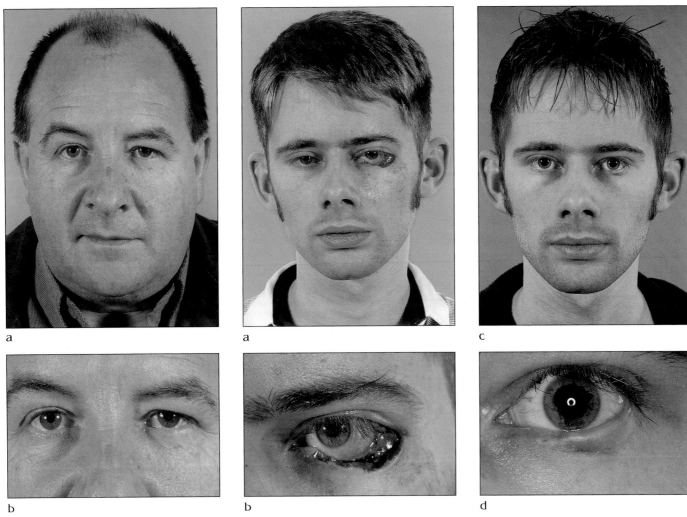

### Figure 10.13
Postoperative appearance of reconstructed eyelid following a 'maximal Hughes procedure'.

### Figure 10.14
(a) Young patient with extensive lower eyelid Mohs' micrographic surgery defect. (b) Close-up of defect. (c) Postoperative appearance following a 'maximal Hughes procedure' with a skin graft. (d) Close-up of reconstructed eyelid.

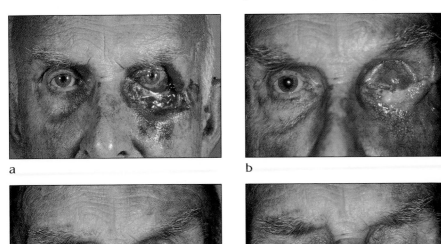

### Figure 10.15
(a) Extensive Mohs' micrographic surgery defect of lower eyelid and lateral part of upper eyelid. (b) Defects reconstructed with medial tarsoconjunctival flap, large periosteal flaps and a Fricke flap.
(c) Postoperative appearance following division of flaps. (d) Adequate closure of eyelids achieved.

**Free tarsoconjunctival graft.** Adequate tarsal support may be provided by harvesting a free tarsoconjunctival graft from either upper lid. The upper lid is everted as described above. The size of the graft needed is determined in a similar manner as well. Again, the tarsus is incised across the width of the lid, 3–4 mm above the lash line, to prevent upper lid instability and lash loss. The flap is elevated by blunt dissection in the pretarsal space, and vertical cuts are made to the tarsal base. The tarsus is then amputated at its base and grafted into the recipient lower lid, as described above. Because this graft is inherently avascular, it must be covered by a vascularized myocutaneous advancement flap.

This technique is useful in lower lid reconstruction for a monocular patient, because it does not occlude the visual axis. If the surgical defect extends to involve the canthal tendons, the free graft should be anchored to periosteal flaps.

**Mustard cheek rotation flap.** With the development and popularity of other reconstruction techniques and with the tissue-conserving advantages of Mohs' micrographic surgery, the Mustard rotational cheek flap is more rarely utilized than in the past. It is reserved for the reconstruction of very extensive deep eyelid defects usually involving more than 75% of the eyelid.

A large myocutaneous cheek flap is dissected and used in conjunction with an adequate mucosal lining posteriorly. The posterior lamellar tarsal substitute is usually a nasal septal cartilage graft or a hard palate graft. The important points in designing a cheek flap are summarized by Mustard as follows.

A deep inverted triangle must be excised below the defect to allow adequate rotation (Figure 10.16). The side of the triangle nearest the nose should be practically vertical. Failure to observe this point will result in pulling down the advancing flap because the centre of rotation of the leading edge is too far to the lateral side.

The outline of the flap should rise in a curve toward the tail of the eyebrow and hairline and should reach down as far as the lobule of the ear (Figure 10.16).

The flap must be adequately undermined from the lowest point of the incision in front of the ear across the whole cheek to within 1 cm below the apex of the excised triangle (Figure 10.17). Great care must be exercised to avoid damage to branches of the facial nerve.

Where necessary (in defects of three-quarters or more), a back cut should be made at the lowest point, 1 cm or more below the lobule of the ear. The deep tissue of the flap should be hitched up to the orbital rim, especially at the lateral canthus, to prevent the weight of the flap from pulling on the lid (Figure 10.18). A typical early result following this reconstructive procedure is shown in Figure 10.19.

---

Cheek flaps can be followed by many complications, including facial-nerve paralysis, haematoma, necrosis of the flap, ectropion, entropion, epiphora, sagging of the lower lid (Figure 10.20) and excessive facial scarring. It is very important to plan the design of the flap and to appreciate the plane of dissection to avoid inadvertent injury to the facial nerve, resulting in lagophthalmos. Meticulous attention to haemostasis is important, as is placement of a drain and a compressive dressing at the conclusion of surgery.

---

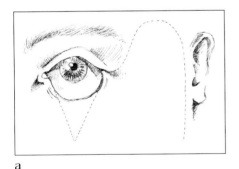
a

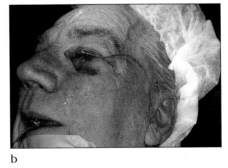
b

**Figure 10.16**
(a) A deep inverted V is excised to permit the flap to rotate adequately. (b) The Mustard cheek rotation flap is marked out.

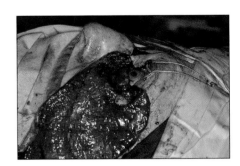

**Figure 10.17**
Mustard cheek rotation flap dissected.

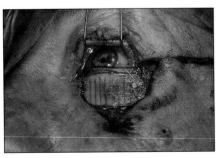
a

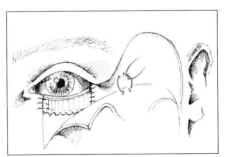
b

**Figure 10.18**
(a) A nasal septal cartilage graft scored vertically, creating an anterior convexity of the graft. A frill of nasal mucosa is left superiorly to create a mucocutaneous junction. (b) The deep tissue of the flap is hitched to the periosteum of the lateral orbital margin.

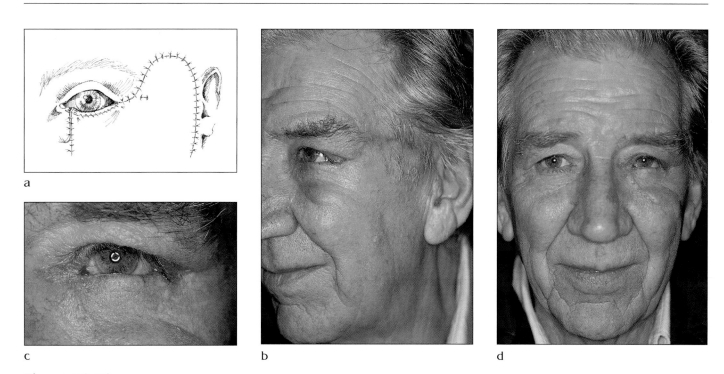

**Figure 10.19**
(a) A cheek rotation flap and posterior lamellar nasal septal cartilage flap completed. (b) A lateral view of a patient 1 week following surgery. (c) A close-up view of the reconstructed eyelid. (d) A full-face view of the same patient.

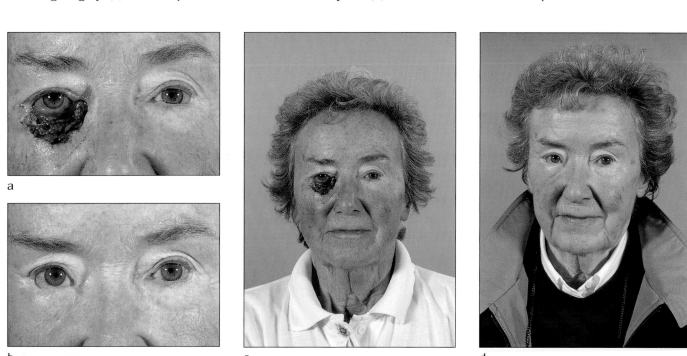

**Figure 10.20**
(a) An extensive right lower eyelid Mohs' micrographic surgery defect. (b) The patient 6 weeks following a Mustard flap reconstruction with nasal septal cartilage graft. The flap was not adequately hitched to the periosteum of the lateral orbital margin, with a resultant sagging of the flap laterally. (c) A full-face view of the same patient preoperatively. (d) A full-face view of the same patient postoperatively.

There are a number of alternative local periocular flaps which can be utilized for anterior lamellar replacement. It is important to respect a length–width ratio of approximately 4:1 where such flaps are not based on an axial blood supply to avoid necrosis. A particularly useful flap is the Fricke flap harvested from above the brow and based temporally (Figure 10.21). It provides good vertical support but requires a second stage revision. Other local flaps which are harvested from the lower lateral cheek area or

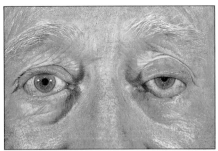

a

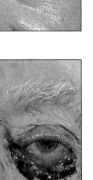

b

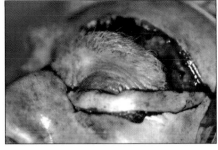

c

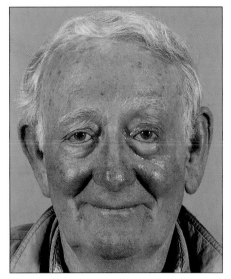

d

### Figure 10.21

(a) Left lower eyelid basal cell carcinoma. (b) Extensive left lower eyelid Mohs' micrographic surgery defect. (c) Fricke flap and hard palate mucosal graft reconstruction. (d) Final result 2 months postoperatively.

the nasojugal area have the disadvantage of secondary lymphoedema, which can take many months to resolve.

The Fricke flap can be expanded intraoperatively by 10–15% with the use of a Foley catheter. This is inserted into the forehead subcutaneously via a small incision temporally (Figure 10.22). Blunt dissection is used to create a pocket. The 14-gauge catheter is inflated and deflated at intervals of 10 min for approximately 30 min.

The Fricke flap also leaves the ipsilateral eyebrow elevated. A regime of postoperative massage lowers the eyebrow to a satisfactory level. A contralateral direct brow lift can be performed to improve symmetry if necessary.

A flap can be used from the upper eyelid where there is sufficient redundant tissue. Occasionally, the flap can be created as a 'bucket handle' based both temporally and nasally (a Tripier flap). It is essential, however, to ensure that the creation of such flaps does not cause lagophthalmos.

## *Eyelid defects not involving the eyelid margin*

If the lid border is spared and the tumour does not invade orbicularis or deeper tissues, a full-thickness section of lid does not have to be excised. If the lesion is small, the defect may be closed with direct approximation of the skin edges after undermining or with the use of a horizontal skin–muscle advancement (Figure 10.23). It is important to close the wound horizontally to avoid a postoperative ectropion.

In larger lesions where the adjacent skin is tight, a full-thickness skin graft may be necessary to prevent ectropion of the lower lid (Figure 10.24). If the lid is lax, this may have to be combined with a lateral tarsal strip procedure or a wedge resection in order to prevent a lower eyelid ectropion.

A piece of cellulose sponge can then be placed over the grafted area and secured with the suture ends that were left long.

This bolster and the sutures are removed in 7–10 days. Eyelid tissues are highly vascular and full-thickness skin grafts usually survive very well. Postoperative wound massage is mandatory to prevent undue contracture.

## Upper eyelid reconstruction

Reconstruction of upper eyelid tumour defects must be performed meticulously to avoid ocular surface complications. A number of surgical procedures can be utilized to reconstruct an upper lid defect and it is important to select the procedure best suited to the individual patient's needs.

Lagophthalmos following reconstruction may cause exposure keratopathy, particularly in the absence of a good Bell's phenomenon. The problem is compounded by loss of accessory lacrimal tissue. Lacrimal tissue should be preserved when dissecting in the lateral canthal, lateral levator and lateral anterior orbital areas. Poor eyelid closure is usually due either to adhesions, wound contracture or to a vertical skin shortage. It may also be caused by over-enthusiastic dissection of lateral periocular flaps, with damage to branches of the facial nerve.

When levator function is preserved following surgical defects of the eyelid, ptosis can usually be avoided or corrected. It is important to carefully identify the cut edges of the levator and to ensure that the levator is reattached to the reconstructed tarsal replacement with a suitable spacer if required.

## *Eyelid defects involving the eyelid margin*
### Small defects

As in the lower lid reconstruction, an eyelid defect of 25% or less may be closed directly, and in patients with marked eyelid laxity,

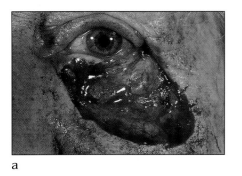
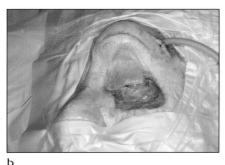
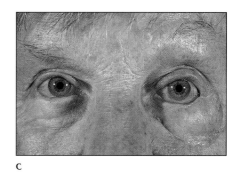

a                         b                         c

**Figure 10.22**
(a) Extensive lower eyelid/cheek Mohs' micrographic surgery defect. (b) Rapid intraoperative expansion of Fricke flap using Foley catheter. (c) Final result after reconstruction with expanded Fricke flap, lateral tarsoconjunctival flap and skin graft at inferior aspect of wound.

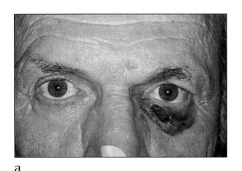
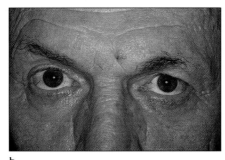

a                         b

**Figure 10.23**
(a) Small lower eyelid skin defect. (b) Appearance 2 weeks following horizontal skin–muscle advancement flap.

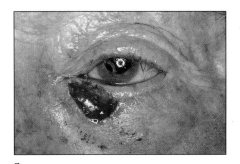
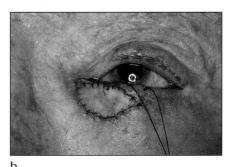

a                         b

**Figure 10.24**
(a) Moderate anterior lamellar defect. (b) Placement of full-thickness skin graft.

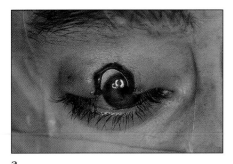
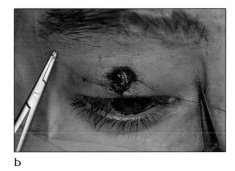
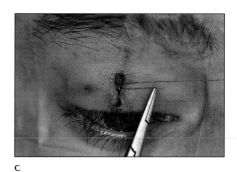

a                         b                         c

**Figure 10.25**
Direct closure of an upper eyelid wedge resection defect.

even a defect occupying up to 50% of the eyelid may be closed directly (Figure 10.25). The surgical procedure is as described above. It is important that the tarsal plate is aligned precisely and closed with 5/0 Vicryl sutures, ensuring that the bites are partial thickness to avoid the possibility of corneal abrasion. After closure of the tarsus, the eyelid margin is closed with interrupted 6/0 silk sutures placed at the grey line and lash margin. All eyelashes should be everted away from the cornea. The ends of the margin sutures are left long and sutured to the external skin tissue to avoid corneal irritation.

## Moderate defects

**Canthotomy and cantholysis.** Where an eyelid defect cannot be closed directly without undue tension on the wound, a lateral canthotomy and superior cantholysis can be performed. *It is very important that the cantholysis is performed meticulously to avoid any inadvertent damage to the levator aponeurosis or to the lacrimal gland.*

**Semicircular flap.** A lateral, inverted, semicircular flap may be combined with direct closure for full-thickness defects of up to two-thirds of the eyelid margin. An inverted semicircle is marked on the skin surface, beginning at the lateral canthus and extending laterally approximately 3 cm. The skin and orbicularis muscle are undermined under the entire flap, and a superior cantholysis performed. The lateral aspect of the eyelid may then be advanced medially to cover the defect (Figure 10.26).

The posterior surface of the advanced semicircular flap may be covered by a tarsoconjunctival advancement flap from the lateral aspect of the lower eyelid. A vertical, full-thickness, lower eyelid incision is made, and the tarsoconjunctival advancement flap is prepared by excising the lower eyelid skin tissue and lash margin from the flap. The tarsus and conjunctiva may then be advanced superiorly into the lateral aspect of the upper eyelid flap. The lower eyelid defect may be repaired primarily, anterior to the tarsoconjunctival flap. The lateral tarsoconjunctival flap may be released in 4–6 weeks.

As an alternative to semicircular skin advancement, the advanced lower lid tarsoconjunctival flap may be covered with full-thickness skin tissue rather than a rotated, inverted semicircle.

## Large defects

**Sliding tarsoconjunctival flap.** Horizontal advancement of an upper eyelid tarsoconjunctival flap is useful for full-thickness defects of up to two-thirds of the upper lid margin. The residual upper eyelid tarsus is bisected horizontally. The superior portion of the tarsus is advanced horizontally along with its levator and Müller's muscle attachments. The tarsoconjunctival advancement flap created is then sutured in a side-to-side fashion to the lower portion of the upper lid tarsus and to the lateral or medial canthal tendon. The lower portion of the upper lid tarsus remains attached to the orbicularis and skin tissue. After the horizontal tarsoconjunctival advancement, the external skin tissue is rebuilt by using full-thickness skin grafting or semicircular adjacent tissue advancement.

**Free tarsal graft.** A free tarsal graft may be harvested from the contralateral upper eyelid, leaving at least 3.5 cm of undisturbed tarsus above the eyelid margin to prevent instability of the eyelid (Figure 10.27). This must be covered by a local skin–muscle flap and is sewn edge to edge to the residual tarsus or to the local periosteal flaps (Figure 10.28).

**Cutler–Beard reconstruction (modified).** A Cutler–Beard reconstruction is useful for upper eyelid defects covering up to 100% of the eyelid margin. The upper lid defect is measured horizontally while gently drawing the edges of the wound together. A three-sided inverted U-shaped incision is marked on the lower eyelid, beginning 4–5 mm below the eyelid margin (Figure 10.29). The eyelid is everted over a

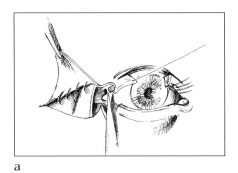
a

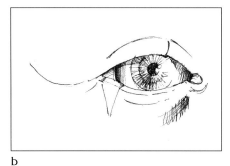
b

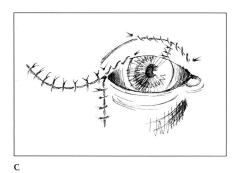
c

**Figure 10.26**
(a) A semicircular flap is undermined and a lateral canthotomy and superior cantholysis performed. (b) The posterior lamellar defect is reconstructed with a lower eyelid tarsoconjunctival flap. (c) The wounds are closed.

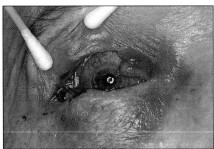
a

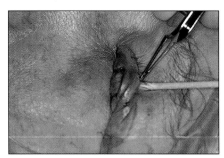
b

**Figure 10.27**
(a) Extensive Mohs' micrographic surgery defect of upper eyelid. (b) Free tarsal graft harvested from contralateral upper eyelid.

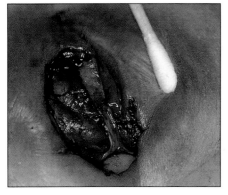

a

**Figure 10.28**
(a) Periosteal flap dissected and attached to free tarsal graft.
(b) Preoperative appearance of patient with large right upper eyelid squamous cell carcinoma.
(c) Postoperative appearance after use of upper eyelid skin–muscle advancement flap.

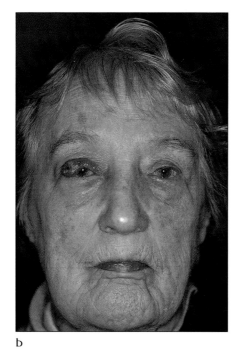

b

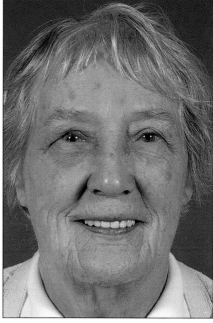

c

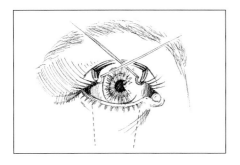

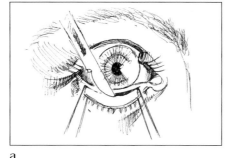

a

b

**Figure 10.29**
The edges of the upper eyelid defect are gently drawn together before the defect is measured.

**Figure 10.30**
(a) A horizontal incision is made through the conjunctiva just below the tarsus.
(b) The conjunctival flap is mobilized into the upper eyelid defect. Two 4/0 silk traction sutures identify the cut edge of the levator aponeurosis. The conjunctival flap is sutured to the cut edge of the upper eyelid conjunctiva.

Desmarres retractor and a conjunctival incision is made below the tarsus (Figure 10.30a). A conjunctival flap is fashioned and dissected into the inferior fornix and onto the globe. The flap is advanced into the upper eyelid defect and sewn edge to edge with the remaining upper fornix conjunctiva using 7/0 Vicryl with care being taken to avoid corneal irritation. The cornea is now protected (Figure 10.30b).

An incision is made through the lower eyelid horizontally below the tarsus and extended inferiorly to create a skin–muscle advancement flap (Figure 10.31). The lower lid skin–muscle flap is then advanced to the upper lid to cover an auricular cartilage graft, used to replace the tarsus (Figure 10.32).

Tarsal support to the upper eyelid is replaced by placing an autogenous auricular cartilage graft, which has been suitably shaped, anterior to the conjunctival flap (Figure 10.32). The edges are sewn horizontally to either tarsal remnants or to

periosteal flaps. The edge of the levator aponeurosis is sutured to the anterior surface of the superior one-third of the cartilage graft. If the levator aponeurosis has been resected it may be necessary to interpose a 'spacer', e.g. a piece of temporalis fascia. The lower lid tissue is advanced posteriorly to the remaining lower lid tarsal and lid margin bridge (Figure 10.33).

The bridge flap is left intact for at least 8 weeks prior to separation. When the bridge flap is separated, a full-thickness incision should be made through the flap at a position inferior to the lower lid bridge margin. The conjunctiva and skin are then sutured directly in the newly separated upper eyelid tissue (Figure 10.34). The inferior margins of the lower lid bridge are freshened and reanastomosed to the remaining lower lid skin and conjunctival layers. It is common for the lower lid to become very lax and to require a wedge resection at the second stage.

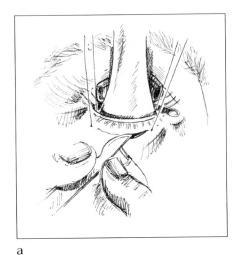

a

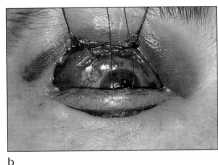

b

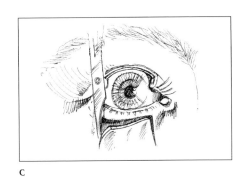

c

### Figure 10.31
(a) A horizontal incision is made through the eyelid 4–5 mm below the eyelid margin to match the dimension of the upper eyelid defect. (b) The incision here is shown before the conjunctival flap has been dissected. (c) Two parallel vertical incisions are made to create a skin–muscle advancement flap.

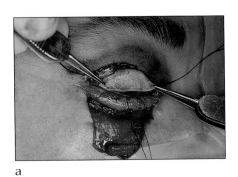

a

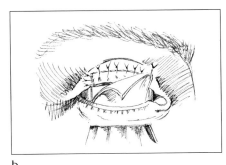

b

### Figure 10.32
(a) An auricular cartilage graft is used to reconstruct the upper eyelid tarsal plate. (b) The cartilage graft is sutured to the tarsal remnants or periosteal flaps and to the remaining levator aponeurosis.

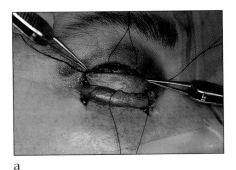

a

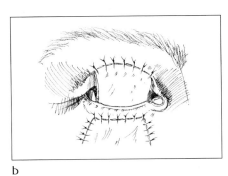

b

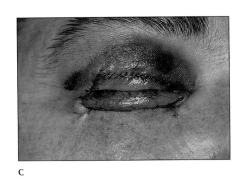

c

### Figure 10.33
(a) The skin–muscle flap is advanced under the lower lid margin. (b) The skin edges are closed with interrupted 7/0 Vicryl sutures. (c) The appearance of the reconstructed eyelid at the completion of the first stage of surgery.

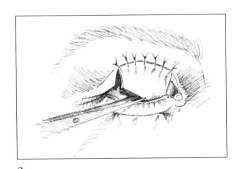

a

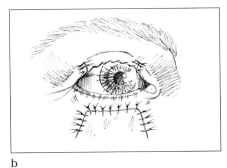

b

### Figure 10.34
(a) The flap is divided with blunt-tipped Westcott scissors, leaving a frill of conjunctiva. (b) The lower eyelid defect is refashioned and closed.

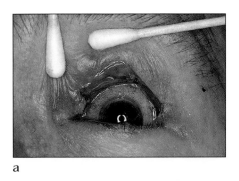

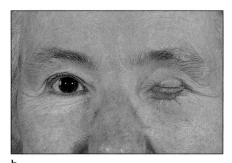

a                                    b

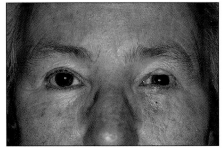

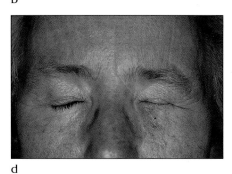

c                                    d

**Figure 10.35**
(a) Extensive upper eyelid defect.
(b) Postoperative appearances 6
weeks following Cutler–Beard
reconstruction. (c) Appearance of
upper eyelid reconstruction 4 weeks
following division of flaps and a
wedge resection of lower eyelid.
(d) Satisfactory passive closure
of the reconstructed upper eyelid.

## Complications

It is extremely important to ensure that sutures are kept away from the cornea. It is very difficult to assess a complaint of a foreign body sensation following the reconstruction. Exposed suture ends abrading the cornea can lead to severe corneal morbidity.

The skin of the upper eyelid may slide anteriorly, bringing fine skin hairs into contact with the cornea. This can be managed either with the application of cryotherapy or with a skin resection at the lid margin, leaving the area to granulate.

A typical result following a Cutler–Beard reconstruction of an upper eyelid defect is shown in Figure 10.35. The use of a labial mucous membrane graft in conjunction with a Cutler–Beard procedure for the reconstruction of a more extensive upper eyelid and conjunctival defect is demonstrated in Figure 10.36.

**Full-thickness composite graft.** A full-thickness en bloc section of tissue from the other upper eyelid may be transplanted into defects of the upper eyelid margin (Figure 10.37). The resection of the normal eyelid should be performed below the lid crease and should be done only when the remaining normal eyelid can be easily closed with direct closure. The lashes of the transplanted lid rarely survive. The overlying skin and orbicularis are removed and a rotation/advancement flap fashioned to cover the graft.

**Rotation of the lower lid.** Rotation and inversion of the lower lid margin and tarsus into an upper lid defect provides good lid function as well as lashes for the upper eyelid. This procedure is best used, however, for large upper lid defects and it necessitates complete reconstruction of the lower eyelid margin, utilizing a lateral Mustardé cheek flap reconstruction combined with a hard palate or nasal chondromucosal graft for the reconstruction of the lower eyelid tarsus and conjunctiva. This technique is particularly useful for reconstruction of upper eyelid colobomata.

The lower lid margin needed for upper lid reconstruction is outlined laterally, and a horizontal full-thickness incision is made inferiorly in the lower eyelid flap. The lateral aspect of the lower eyelid is then advanced medially through the use of a lateral Mustardé flap. The lower eyelid margin is then inverted and sutured into the upper lid defect. The lower lid rotation is closed medially, and the lateral aspect of the new lower lid margin is backed with a nasal chondromucosal composite graft or a hard palate graft. The bridge adjoining the upper and lower lids is separated after 6–8 weeks. Although some surgeons use this technique with success, it is cumbersome and requires both lower eyelid construction and lateral facial advancement.

## *Eyelid defects not involving the eyelid margin*

If a small skin defect can be closed directly, this should be performed horizontally, leaving a vertical scar in order to prevent vertical contracture of the wound and secondary lagophthalmos or eyelid retraction. If horizontal closure of the tissue is not possible, a full-thickness skin graft may be placed over the defect to prevent lagophthalmos.

## Full-thickness loss of upper and lower lids

Reconstruction of the upper eyelid becomes much more of a challenge when additional periocular tissue and part of the lower eyelid have been lost. The type of reconstruction will then depend very much on the age and general health of the patient and the visual status of the fellow eye. Frequently, concerns

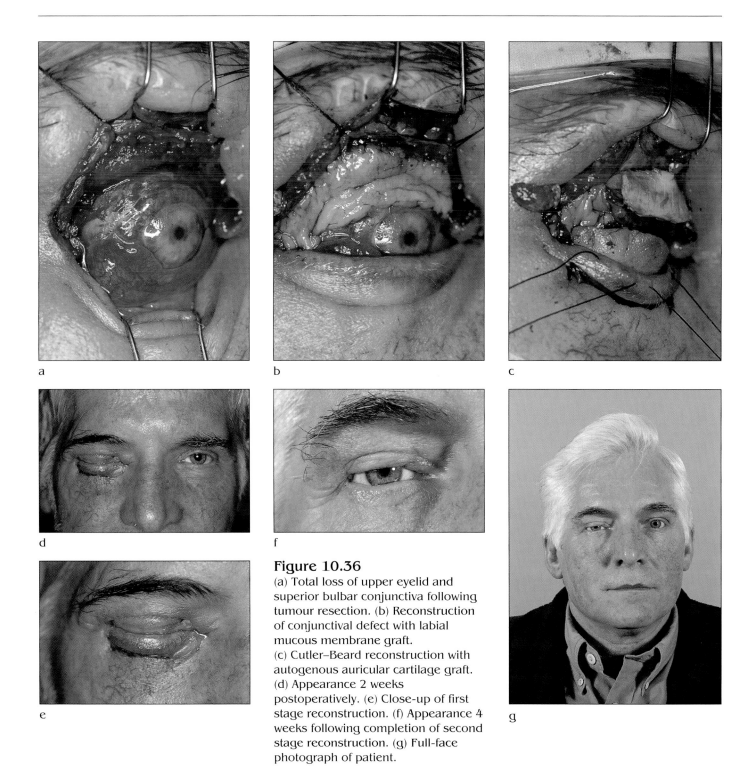

a

b

c

d

f

e

g

**Figure 10.36**
(a) Total loss of upper eyelid and superior bulbar conjunctiva following tumour resection. (b) Reconstruction of conjunctival defect with labial mucous membrane graft.
(c) Cutler–Beard reconstruction with autogenous auricular cartilage graft. (d) Appearance 2 weeks postoperatively. (e) Close-up of first stage reconstruction. (f) Appearance 4 weeks following completion of second stage reconstruction. (g) Full-face photograph of patient.

about cosmesis will have to be sacrificed to concerns about adequate corneal protection.

When a full-thickness defect includes the entire upper and lower eyelids, the goal of reconstruction becomes preservation of the globe by complete coverage with mucous membrane and skin tissue. Usually, sufficient conjunctiva is available on the bulbar surface to allow undermining and reflection over the corneal surface. The reflected bulbar conjunctiva inferiorly is sutured to the reflected conjunctiva superiorly. This can then be covered with a full-thickness skin graft or a rotation flap from the lateral face or mid-forehead. After maturation of the tissue, a small opening can be made to permit central corneal vision. Because the upper and lower eyelids are immobile, only a small palpebral fissure should be created to minimize the risk of lagophthalmos and exposure.

If available bulbar conjunctiva is insufficient to cover the globe, full-thickness buccal mucous membrane may be grafted to the posterior surface of the lateral cheek or midline forehead flap to provide a mucosal lining for the globe.

When ample conjunctiva with a good blood supply is available, the reflected mucosal covering may be adequate to support full-thickness skin grafting externally as an alternative to larger flap rotations.

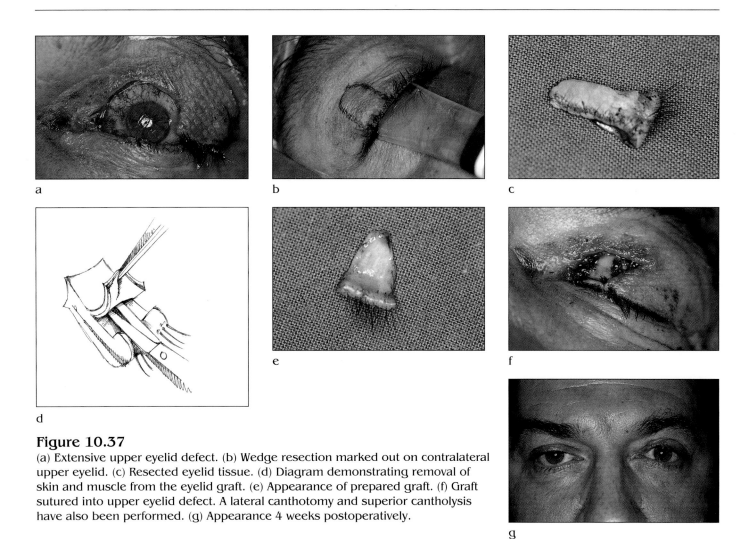

**Figure 10.37**
(a) Extensive upper eyelid defect. (b) Wedge resection marked out on contralateral upper eyelid. (c) Resected eyelid tissue. (d) Diagram demonstrating removal of skin and muscle from the eyelid graft. (e) Appearance of prepared graft. (f) Graft sutured into upper eyelid defect. A lateral canthotomy and superior cantholysis have also been performed. (g) Appearance 4 weeks postoperatively.

# Medial canthal reconstruction

The medial canthal region is a unique area that represents the convergence of skin units of differing texture, thickness and contour. The unique contour of the medial canthal region is dependent on the interrelationship of the eyelids, brow, cheek, nose and glabellar regions. This can present difficulties in the reconstruction of surgical defects in this region.

Medial canthal tumour defects can be closed by a variety of methods depending on their size, location, depth, patient age and patient preference. Spectacle wear by the patient should also be taken into account. The methods include:

1.  Laissez-faire
2.  Full-thickness skin grafting
3.  A variety of local flaps, e.g. a glabellar flap, a bilobed flap, a rhomboid flap and a median forehead flap
4.  Epicranial flap combined with full-thickness skin grafting

If the lacrimal drainage system has been sacrificed, it is not formally reconstructed at the time of reconstruction of a medial canthal tumour defect. The patient may in fact remain symptom-free. If postoperative epiphora is problematic, a conjunctivo-dacryocystorhinostomy (CDCR) with placement of a Lester Jones tube may be undertaken. It is preferable to ensure that the patient has been free from any signs of recurrence of the tumour for a period of at least 3 years before disturbing the local perios-teum, an important tumour barrier.

## *Laissez-faire*

Laissez-faire can yield excellent results in the medial canthal region. This is particularly useful for small defects and defects in elderly or medically unfit patients. It can, however, lead to unsatis-factory scarring and unpredictable results in younger patients. An unsatisfactory result for an elderly patient is shown in Figure 10.38.

## *Full-thickness skin grafting*

Full-thickness skin grafting generally yields very good results in the medial canthus provided the defect is not too deep. Deep defects exposing bone require a local flap. Skin grafting takes longer to perform than a local flap unless an assistant is available to harvest the graft and close the donor site. Patients with thick

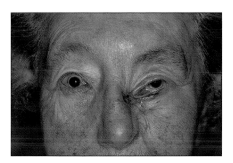

**Figure 10.38**
A very unsatisfactory result from laissez-faire in an elderly patient who refused medial canthal reconstruction following a Mohs' micrographic surgical excision of a basal cell carcinoma.

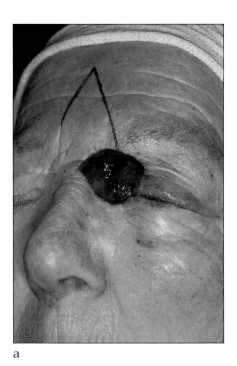

a

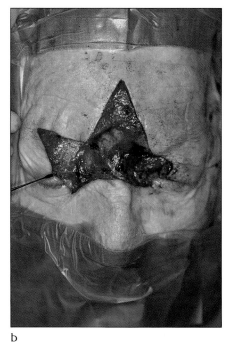

b

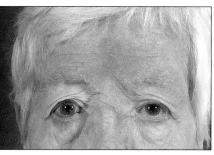

c

**Figure 10.39**
(a) Glabellar flap marked out.
(b) Glabellar flap dissected.
(c) Postoperative appearance after 2 weeks.

sebaceous skin are prone to 'pin cushioning' of the graft, which will require massage and patience before a satisfactory result is achieved after a period of many months.

## Local flap

A local flap procedure is relatively quick to perform but such a flap may hide tumour recurrence. As with any formal reconstructive technique other than direct closure, it should only be used after ensuring complete tumour excision by histological monitoring of all the margins of the excised tissue.

## Glabellar flap

The glabellar flap is a time-honoured local flap used for medial canthal reconstruction. The glabellar flap is a V–Y flap which allows the transposition of skin from the glabellar region into a defect. The ideal defect for this flap does not extend laterally below the brow or too far below the medial canthus into the skin of the cheek. It is rounded, so that width and height of the defect are approximately the same.

A number of factors predispose to unsatisfactory results with the glabellar flap, including a large and irregular medial canthal defect; a defect extending across the nose; a defect extending laterally under the brow; young patients; tight facial skin; a very deep medial canthus; a very oval defect oriented vertically and extending well below the lower eyelid; or patients with a continuous brow.

The outline of the flap begins with the location of the apex of the V within the glabellar region. The first arm of the V arises directly from the defect and passes superomedially towards the apex across the medial brow. The second arm arises from the apex at an angle to the first arm and passes inferiorly. The V of the flap thus has two arms, and once the flap has been raised, it has three borders: an inferior, a lateral and a superior border.

Once the flap is raised, there is a very large defect continuous with the original defect (Figure 10.39). Closure commences vertically to create a V–Y pattern, and this may be facilitated by undermining tissue margins. Deep 5/0 Vicryl sutures are placed to reduce the tension on the cutaneous closure, which is performed with either a 6/0 nylon or 7/0 Vicryl suture. Once the vertical closure is complete, the original defect is closed with the flap. Some redundant tissue at the apex of the flap is excised as required.

Dissection should be deep to include the subdermal plexus but not into procerus or corrugator supercilii. A superficial dissection risks flap necrosis but provides a thinner flap. The deep

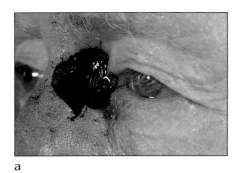 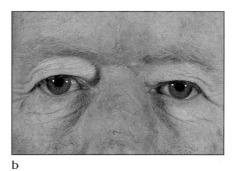 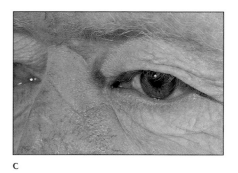

a                         b                         c

## Figure 10.40
(a) An irregular Mohs' micrographic surgery medial canthal defect. (b) Postoperative appearances 6 weeks following a glabellar flap reconstruction. (c) A side view of the reconstruction.

surface of the flap is anchored to the periosteum to reform the concave contour of the medial canthus. The nasal skin is closed with 6/0 nylon vertical mattress sutures and the lid skin is closed with 7/0 Vicryl sutures. A dental roll wrapped in paraffin gauze is applied under a firm pressure bandage. These measures help prevent haematomas and aid in reforming the concave contour of the medial canthus. After at least 4 days the dressing is removed and the sutures removed. Topical antibiotic ointment is applied for 1 week. Digital massage over the flap begins at suture removal and continues for at least 2 months. A typical early result of a glabellar flap reconstruction is shown in Figure 10.40.

## Rhomboid flap

The defect is conceptualized as a rhomboid shape with its long axis vertical. The rhomboid consists of two equilateral triangles placed base to base (Figure 10.41). For medial canthal defects there are two possible rhomboid flaps. These are constructed as follows. A line of the same length as the bases of the triangles is drawn horizontally across the nose from the base of the triangles. Two vertically oriented lines from the tip of the horizontal line are drawn at an angle of 60 degrees (Figure 10.41a). These lines are the same length and parallel to the side of the rhomboid. The upper flap is used because of the greater laxity of the upper nasal skin. The resultant scar is also more easily hidden. The flap is oriented parallel to the lines of maximal extensibility (LME), allowing the donor site and defect to be closed with the minimum tension (Figures 10.41b,c). The LME are perpendicular to the horizontally oriented relaxed skin tension lines (RSTL) on the bridge of the nose. The scar from closure of the flap's donor site is hidden in an RSTL. Despite three sections of the scar being oriented almost perpendicular to the RSTL (Figure 10.41d), in most cases this becomes insignificant after several weeks (Figure 10.42).

The deep surface of the flap is anchored to the periosteum to reform the concave contour of the medial canthus. The nasal skin is closed with 6/0 nylon vertical mattress sutures and the lid skin is closed with 7/0 Vicryl sutures. A dental roll wrapped in paraffin gauze is applied under a firm pressure bandage. These measures help prevent haematomas and aid in reforming the concave

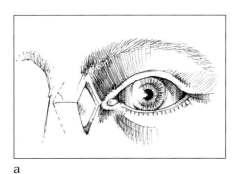 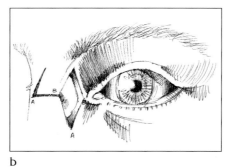

a                         b

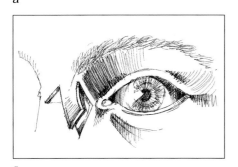 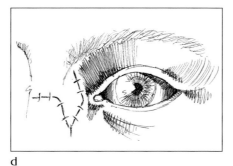

c                         d

## Figure 10.41
(a) The rhomboid flap is marked out, selecting either a superior or inferior flap. (b) The incisions are made. (c) The flap is undermined and transposed. (d) The wounds are closed.

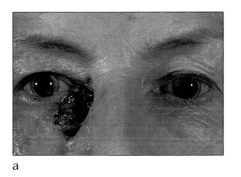

a

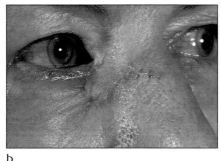

b

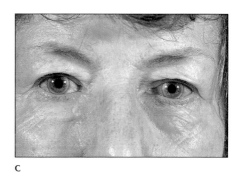

c

## Figure 10.42
(a) Right medial canthal Mohs micrographic surgery defect. (b) Postoperative appearance of medial canthal defect 2 weeks after reconstruction with a rhomboid flap. (c) Patient 6 months after rhomboid flap reconstruction.

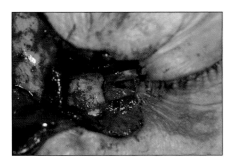

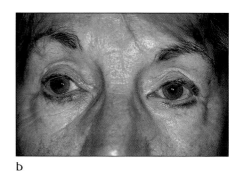

a

b

## Figure 10.43
Periosteal flaps dissected from the nasal bone can be used to reconstruct a medial canthal tendon.

## Figure 10.44
(a) Right lower eyelid Mohs' micrographic surgery defect. (b) Postoperative result following reconstruction using a medial periosteal flap and a small medial rhomboid flap combined with a small skin graft harvested from the ipsilateral upper eyelid.

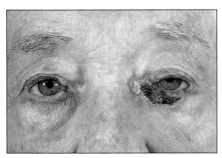

a

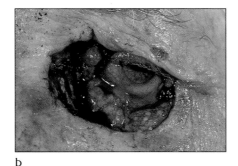

b

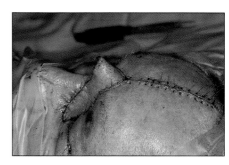

## Figure 10.46
Median forehead flap reconstruction of medial canthal defect.

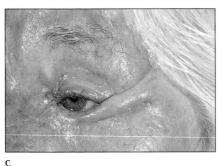

c

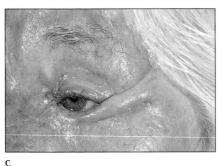

d

## Figure 10.45
(a) Large left lower eyelid and medial canthal basal cell carcinoma. (b) Extensive Mohs' micrographic surgery defect. (c) Defects reconstructed with a rhomboid flap, hard palate graft and Fricke flap. Appearance 4 weeks postoperatively.
(d) Appearance 4 weeks following division of the Fricke flap.

contour of the medial canthus. After at least 4 days the dressing is removed and the sutures removed. Topical antibiotic ointment is applied for 1 week. Digital massage over the flap begins at suture removal and continues for at least 2 months.

Defects involving the areas above and below the medial palpebral ligament can be closed by rhomboid flaps from the adjoining glabellar and nasal tissues, respectively. In closing inferiorly placed defects, the flap can be extended inferiorly by lengthening the vertical incision. In closing defects which extend laterally into the upper or lower lid, the lateral lid skin can be undermined and pulled medially to meet the rhomboid flap. The orientation of the defect parallel to the LME minimizes distortion on surrounding tissues. When the medial palpebral ligament has been excised, periosteal flaps can be used to reattach the cut ends of the tarsal plates (Figure 10.43). A periosteal flap will pull the lids medially and helps reduce the size of the defect (Figure 10.44).

The rhomboid flap is extremely versatile. Reconstructing a medial canthal defect with a rhomboid flap enables a close skin match and potentially better cosmesis. A rhomboid flap is quicker to perform than a glabellar flap, is less invasive and has much shorter suture lines, which heal with less obvious scars in many cases. It can be combined with other medial canthal and periocular reconstructive procedures (Figure 10.45).

## Median forehead flap

This flap requires two stages. It is cosmetically disfiguring and rarely required (Figure 10.46). The alternative of an epicranial flap with a full-thickness skin graft is much preferred for the reconstruction of extensive deep medial defects.

## *Epicranial flap with full-thickness skin graft*

In this procedure an epicranial flap is dissected from the forehead region. The flap is based on the supraorbital vessels on the contralateral side. A central vertical forehead incision is made down to and through the galea and between the frontalis muscle bellies (Figure 10.47b). The epicranial flap is measured to fit the

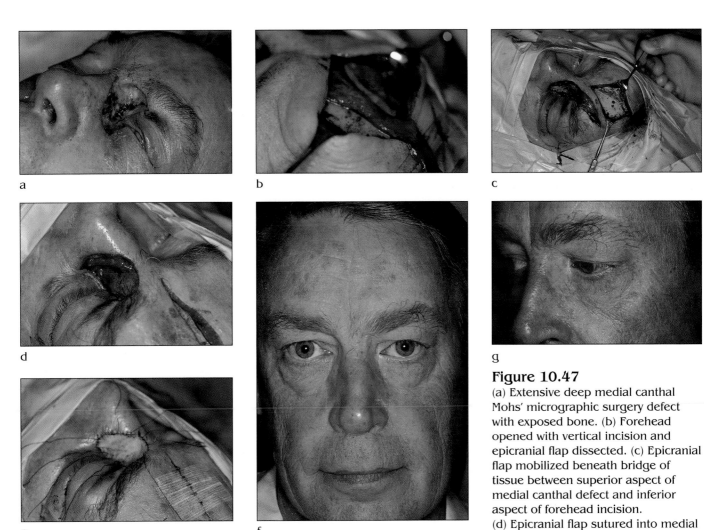

a

b

c

d

e

f

g

**Figure 10.47**
(a) Extensive deep medial canthal Mohs' micrographic surgery defect with exposed bone. (b) Forehead opened with vertical incision and epicranial flap dissected. (c) Epicranial flap mobilized beneath bridge of tissue between superior aspect of medial canthal defect and inferior aspect of forehead incision.
(d) Epicranial flap sutured into medial canthal defect. (e) Skin graft placed over epicranial flap. (f and g) Appearance of reconstructed medial canthus 9 months postoperatively.

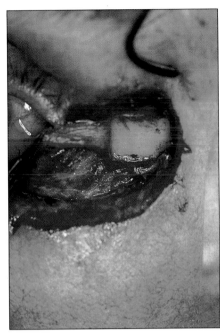

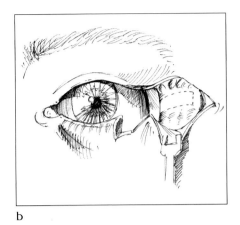

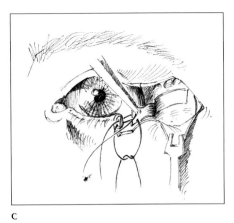

**Figure 10.48**
(a) A periosteal flap. (b) A diagram demonstrating the position of the periosteal flap. (c) The flap is mobilized and sutured to the tarsus, recreating a lateral canthal tendon.

defect before it is dissected. It is then turned and passed beneath the bridge of tissue between the medial canthal defect and the inferior aspect of the forehead incision (Figure 10.47c). The flap is sutured into the medial canthal defect to provide bulk to the medial canthus and to provide a blood supply to a full-thickness skin graft, which is sutured into place over the flap (Figure 10.47e). The forehead wound is closed easily as it is not under tension. This procedure avoids placing a thick tissue flap over a site which has the potential for tumour recurrence and it does not affect the position of the eyebrows.

## Lateral canthal reconstruction

Skin defects at the lateral canthus can be reconstructed with full-thickness skin grafts or with a variety of local flaps. The rhomboid flap is particularly versatile at the lateral canthus.

In reconstructing lateral canthal defects it is important to note that the attachment of the lateral canthal tendon to the lateral orbital tubercle lies posterior to the lateral orbital margin. Attachment of eyelid tissue to the periosteum lying over the lateral orbital rim results in an anteriorly displaced lateral canthal angle.

Periosteal flaps can be raised at the lateral canthus to reconstruct a lateral canthal tendon (Figure 10.48). A short flap may be raised by incising the periosteum horizontally. If a longer flap is required, this can be raised from the malar eminence and rotated to lie horizontally. The flap should be dissected into the internal aspect of the lateral orbital wall to mimic the anatomical arrangement of the lateral canthal tendon.

The periosteal flap may be split to form both superior and inferior lateral canthal tendon crura. The conjunctiva can be sutured to the edge of the periosteal flaps.

## Further reading

1. American Academy of Ophthalmology. *Basic and clinical science course: orbit, eyelids, and lacrimal system*, section 7. San Francisco: American Academy of Ophthalmology, 1998–99, pp. 167–91.
2. Anderson RL, Gordy DD. The tarsal strip procedure. *Arch Ophthalmol* (1979) **97**:2192–6.
3. Bartley GB, Putterman AM. A minor modification of the Hughes' operation for lower eyelid reconstruction. *Am J Ophthalmol* (1995) **119**:96–7.
4. Bullock JD, Koss N, Flagg SV. Rhomboid flap in ophthalmic plastic surgery. *Arch Ophthalmol* (1973) **90**:203–5.
5. Cohen MS, Shorr N. Eyelid reconstruction with hard palate mucosa grafts. *Ophthal Plast Reconstr Surg* (1992) **8**:183–95.
6. Collin JRO. Eyelid reconstruction and tumour management. In: Collin JRO, ed. *Manual of systematic eyelid surgery*, 2nd edn. London: Churchill Livingstone, 1989, p. 93.
7. Cutler NL, Beard C. A method for partial and total upper lid reconstruction. *Am J Ophthalmol* (1955) **39**:1.
8. Dailey RA, Habrich D. Medial canthal reconstruction. In: Bosniak S, ed., *Principles and practice of ophthalmic plastic and reconstructive surgery*, Vol. 2. Philadelphia: WB Saunders, 1996, pp. 387–200.
9. Dryden RM, Wulc AE. The preauricular skin graft in eyelid reconstruction. *Arch Ophthalmol* (1985) **103**:1579–81.
10. Foster JA, Scheiner AJ, Wulc AE, Wallace IB, Greenbaum SS. Intraoperative tissue expansion in eyelid reconstruction. *Ophthalmology* (1998) **105**:170–5.
11. Giola VM, Linberg JV, McCormick SA. The anatomy of the lateral canthal tendon. *Arch Ophthalmol* (1987) **105**:529–32.
12. Hewes EH, Sullivan JH, Beard C. Lower eyelid reconstruction by tarsal transposition. *Am J Ophthalmol* (1976) **81**:512–14.
13. Hughes WL. *Reconstructive surgery of the eyelids*. 2nd edn. St Louis: CV Mosby, 1954.
14. Jackson IT, ed. *Local flaps in bead and neck reconstruction*. St Louis: CV Mosby, 1985.

15.  Jordan D: Reconstruction of the upper eyelid. In: Bosniak S, ed., *Principles and practice of ophthalmic plastic and reconstructive surgery*, Vol. 2. Philadelphia: WB Saunders, 1996, pp. 356–86.

16.  Leone CR. Periosteal flap for lower eyelid reconstruction. *Am J Ophthalmol*. (1992) **114**:513–14.

17.  Limberg AA. *Mathematical principles of local plastic procedures on the surface of the human body*. Leningrad: Megriz, 1946.

18.  Lowry JC, Bartley GB, Garrity JA. The role of second-intention healing in periocular reconstruction. *Ophthal Plast Reconstr Surg* (1997) **13**:174–88.

19.  Maloof AJ, Leatherbarrow B. The glabellar flap dissected. *Eye* (2000) **14**:597–605.

20.  McCord CD. System of repair of full-thickness eyelid defects. In: McCord CD, Tanenbaum M, Nunery WR, eds, *Oculoplastic surgery*, 3rd edn. New York: Raven Press, 1995, pp. 85–97.

21.  McCord CD, Nunery WR, Tanenbaum M. Reconstruction of the lower eyelid and outer canthus. In: McCord CD, Tanenbaum M, Nunery WR, eds, *Oculoplastic surgery*, 3rd edn. New York: Raven Press, 1995, pp. 119–44.

22.  Mustardé JC. *Repair and reconstruction in the orbital region*. Edinburgh: Livingstone, 1966.

23.  Ng SG, Inkster CF, Leatherbarrow B. The rhomboid flap in medial canthal reconstruction. *Br J Ophthalmol* (2001) **85**:556–9.

24.  Patrinely JR, Marines HM, Anderson RL. Skin flaps in periorbital reconstruction. *Surv Ophthalmol* (1987) **31**:249–61.

25.  Putterman AM. Viable composite grafting in eyelid reconstruction: a new method of upper and lower lid reconstruction. *Am J Ophthalmol* (1978) **85**:237–41.

26.  Rohrich RJ, Zbar RI. The evolution of the Hughes tarsoconjunctival flap for the lower eyelid reconstruction. *Plast Reconstr Surg* (1999) **104**:518–22; quiz 523; discussion 524–6.

27.  Shotton FT. Optimal closure of medial canthal defects with rhomboid flaps: "rules of thumb" for flap and rhomboid defect orientations. *Ophthalmic Surg* (1983) **14**:46–52.

28.  Sullivan TJ, Bray LC. The bilobed flap in medial canthal reconstruction. *Aust NZ J Ophthalmol* (1995) **23**:42–8.

29.  Tenzel RR, Stewart WB. Eyelid reconstruction by the semicircle flap technique. *Ophthalmology* (1978) **85**:1164–9.

30.  Tucker SM, Linberg JV. Vascular anatomy of the eyelids. *Ophthalmology* (1994) **101**:1118–21.

31.  Weinstein GS, Anderson RL, Tse DT, Kersten RC. The use of a periosteal strip for eyelid reconstruction. *Arch Ophthalmol* (1985) **103**:357–9.

32.  Werner MS, Olson JJ, Putterman AM. Composite grafting for eyelid reconstruction. *Am J Ophthalmol* (1993) **116**:11–16.

33.  Wesley RE, McCord CD. Reconstruction of the upper eyelid and medial canthus. In: McCord CD, Tanenbaum M, Nunery WR, eds, *Oculoplastic surgery*, 3rd edn. New York: Raven Press, 1995, pp. 99–117.

# 11

# Management of eyelid trauma

## Introduction

All ophthalmologists, regardless of the type of practice they have, may be called upon to assist in the management of patients who have sustained acute eyelid or orbital trauma. A systematic approach to the evaluation and management of such patients by the ophthalmologist is essential and will:

- Maximize the results of primary treatment
- Minimize the need for secondary reconstruction
- Lessen the exposure of the ophthalmologist to medicolegal risks

When called upon to manage a patient who has sustained acute eyelid or orbital trauma it is useful to apply a set of cardinal principles (Table 11.1).

**Table 11.1** Cardinal principles

- Examine and treat the patient for *all* injuries
- Maintain a high index of suspicion for undetected injury
- Determine the priority for repair
- The results of primary repair are superior to secondary repair
- Delay major reconstruction if the necessary expertise is not available
- Delay the repair until operating conditions are optimal
- Document all injuries very carefully
- Remove dirt and debris
- Reposition tissues to their correct anatomical alignment
- Do not discard or excise tissue unnecessarily

Most patients who suffer acute eyelid or orbital trauma present to a general Accident and Emergency (A&E) department. There, initial triage and stabilization begin. Although the diagnosis of associated injuries is usually made independent of the ophthalmologist's examination, a certain redundancy in evaluation is necessary for trauma to be treated appropriately and expeditiously. *It is imperative that the patient is examined thoroughly so that additional injuries are not overlooked.* The ophthalmologist should assist other specialists in determining the priority for repair of the patient's injuries.

- Examine and treat the patient for *all* injuries

## History

## *Mechanism of injury*

Even before seeing the patient, the ophthalmologist can anticipate the types of injuries that are likeliest to be encountered from a knowledge of the mechanism of injury. An accurate history is essential, but in many instances, the history may be inaccurate: e.g. self-inflicted trauma, a child whose injury was not witnessed. *Apparently trivial eyelid trauma may be associated with serious sight-threatening or even life-threatening injury which will go undetected unless a high index of suspicion is maintained during the patient's evaluation.* The examination of such patients should be performed very delicately and meticulously to exclude associated trauma to the globe (Figure 11.1).

NB: *Lacerations of the eyelid have an underlying perforating injury of the globe, or even a penetrating injury of the brain, until proven otherwise* (Figure 11.2).

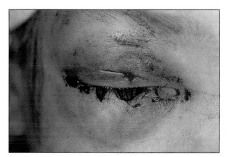

a

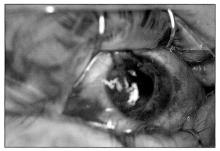

b

**Figure 11.1**
(a) Patient presenting with apparently trivial upper eyelid laceration.
(b) Careful examination of the globe revealed a penetrating eye injury with an iris prolapse.

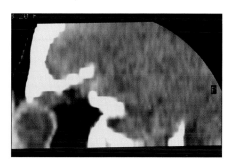

**Figure 11.2**
Sagittal computed tomography (CT) scan of a patient with apparently trivial upper eyelid injury but who developed a frontal lobe abscess 3 days following her fall onto a rose bush. She had sustained a fracture of the roof of her orbit and a penetrating injury of her brain. She had no other symptoms on presentation.

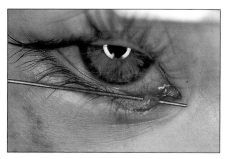

**Figure 11.3**
Right lower eyelid laceration involving the inferior canaliculus.

NB: *Lacerations of the medial canthal area involve the lacrimal drainage apparatus until proven otherwise* (Figure 11.3).

- Maintain a high index of suspicion for undetected injury

Traumatic injuries occur after contact with sharp or blunt objects, toxic substances, or sources of thermal or electromagnetic energy. Combination injuries may be present, such as those seen in road traffic accidents.

## *Sharp trauma*

Sharp trauma tends to produce a clean wound of the eyelids without actual tissue loss. Sharp trauma can be associated with ocular injury, injury to extraocular muscles or other orbital structures, or, through penetration of the orbital walls, craniocerebral or upper respiratory tract injuries. The ophthalmologist must maintain a high index of suspicion for undetected injury and for retained foreign bodies, e.g. in young children whose injury has not been witnessed (Figure 11.4).

## *Blunt trauma*

Abrasions, irregular lacerations and partial avulsions are commoner with blunt trauma than with sharp trauma. Associated neurological injury (intracranial or cervical), facial fractures, orbital wall blowout fractures, concussive ocular injury or globe rupture must be ruled out. A computed tomography (CT) scan examination should be performed whenever there is clinical evidence of orbital trauma or of an intraorbital foreign body.

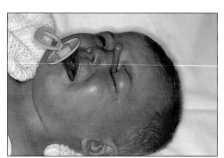

a

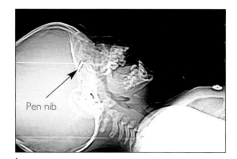

Pen nib

b

**Figure 11.4**
This infant was unsupervised playing with a pen when he fell. The pen nib was embedded in the body of the sphenoid with no other intracranial or ophthalmic injury. It was removed and the infant made a full recovery. Had the infant pulled the pen out the only visible sign of injury would have been a minor medial canthal wound.

# *Bites*

Eyelid injuries caused by bites pose unique problems. The injuries themselves can be a combination of sharp and blunt trauma, causing lacerations and tearing-type injuries and, rarely, actual tissue loss. In addition, *all bite wounds should be considered contaminated and preventive measures need to be taken against possible infection.*

Most periorbital bites are caused by domestic dogs (Figure 11.5). Facial and eyelid bites from other animals are extremely rare. Periorbital human bites are also rare but potentially serious.

# Patient evaluation

Eyelid trauma is highly visible and, in most cases, alarming in appearance to the patient. Anxiety about the possibility of loss of vision and disfigurement is high and must be managed tactfully. Patients who are under the influence of drugs or alcohol are often particularly difficult to evaluate satisfactorily. Steps should be taken to prevent further inadvertent injury.

It should be borne in mind that legal actions often result from the injury, and possibly from the treatment, if the results are unsatisfactory.

# *Systemic considerations*

*Determine the priority for repair.* The ophthalmologist may be working alone in the case of a patient who has sustained an eyelid laceration and a penetrating eye injury or he/she may be part of a multidisciplinary team managing a severely traumatized patient, e.g. following a road traffic accident. After life-threatening associated injuries have been ruled out, acute sight-threatening conditions must be assessed. The patient's injuries must be dealt with in their order of importance and severity. It is obvious to an ophthalmologist that repair of a penetrating injury takes precedence over repair of eyelid lacerations. It may not be obvious to another team, however, that the immediate management of a sight-threatening orbital haematoma takes precedence over visually dramatic facial lacerations once haemostasis has been obtained (Figure 11.6). The evaluation of the unconscious patient is particularly difficult. The ophthalmologist plays a very important role in such a situation where the proper evaluation of a relative afferent pupil defect cannot be delegated to other clinicians.

- Determine the priority for repair

Resuscitation, if needed, and stabilization of vital signs are the initial goals for the treatment of any trauma patient. *It must be borne in mind that any patient who has sustained trauma has the potential of developing shock during the evaluation process as a result of occult serious or life-threatening injury* (see Figure 11.2). Periodic monitoring of vital signs during the examination process is therefore prudent.

Once the patient is stabilized, the presence of life-threatening associated injury must be ruled out. Understanding the mechanism of injury is most helpful in this regard, e.g. an eyelid injury from a screwdriver in a child may be associated with a serious central nervous system (CNS) injury.

All patients with significant eyelid trauma should receive a complete ophthalmic examination, but the order and venue for the examination (in the Emergency Department or the Operating Room) are dictated by the severity of associated ocular injury. It is important to ensure that all steps have been taken to exclude possible associated trauma (e.g. CNS injury in a patient with an upper lid puncture wound) by CT scanning, before the patient is anaesthetized. It is highly unsatisfactory to discover other injuries,

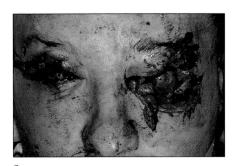
a
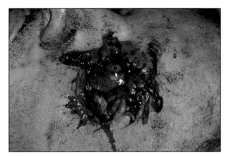
b

**Figure 11.5**
Severe dog bite injury with tissue loss.

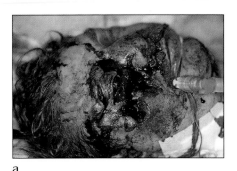
a
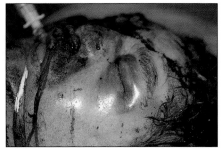
b

**Figure 11.6**
A patient who has sustained severe blunt facial trauma. (a) The right globe is damaged beyond repair. (b) The left orbit has an expanding orbital haematoma whose management takes precedence over his other facial injuries once haemostasis has been obtained and his airway protected.

which require the expertise of other specialists/operating facilities that are located elsewhere, once the patient is anaesthetized.

In patients with animal bites it is important to establish whether or not the patient is immunocompromised and, in particular, whether or not a prior splenectomy has been performed, so that increased risk of possible post-traumatic infection with unusual organisms can be assessed. The management of any secondary infection in this situation should be undertaken with the assistance of a microbiologist. The patient's tetanus immunization status should be investigated and tetanus toxoid given where appropriate. The risk of contracting rabies in the UK is extremely low, but must be borne in mind when managing such injuries in other countries.

## Evaluation of eyelid injuries

It is convenient to divide eyelid injuries into the following categories:

- Marginal injuries
- Extramarginal injuries
- Avulsion injuries
- Injuries involving tissue loss

## Marginal injuries

Most full-thickness marginal lid lacerations are easily identified. It is easy, however, to overlook medial canthal injuries, particularly when dried coagulum obscures the area in a child. Relatively minor trauma, even to the lateral aspect of the eyelids, can result in rupture of the attachment of the medial canthal tendon to the tarsus, an area of anatomical weakness, with resulting disruption of the canalicular system. This is particularly true of dog bites, injuries from hooks, and even finger-poking injuries. *All marginal trauma to the medial canthal region should be assumed to have damaged the canalicular system, unless proved otherwise* (see Figure 11.3). Assessing the lacrimal system may be difficult in a child with injury to the medial canthus and, in some situations, the patient must be anaesthetized for the examination. Failure to identify and repair a canalicular laceration primarily will have long-term consequences for the patient (Figure 11.7).

- The results of primary repair are superior to secondary repair

## Extramarginal injuries

In most instances, extramarginal lid lacerations tend to follow the relaxed skin tension lines (RSTLs) and are oriented parallel to the free margin of the eyelid (see Figure 11.1). All such lacerations should be considered to be associated with possible underlying injury to the eye, the orbit, or contiguous structures such as the cranial cavity. Depending on the mechanism of injury and the clinical findings, appropriate imaging studies should be undertaken to evaluate the extent of associated orbital trauma and to rule out the presence of retained foreign bodies. The wound should be gently explored to measure its depth. The presence of fat in the wound indicates that the wound has at least breached the orbital septum (Figure 11.8).

*In the upper lid it is important not to confuse fat with the lacrimal gland.* The fat may be cleaned and gently reposited. It is not necessary to attempt a repair of the orbital septum. If the fat has been exposed for a long period of time, it may be difficult to reposit it. If it is removed, it should be very carefully cross-clamped with a curved haemostat, first taking care not to apply any traction to the fat. The fat should then be cauterized carefully and the haemostat gently released but immediately reclamped in the event of any bleeding. In general, the fat should be left alone to prevent postoperative eyelid asymmetry.

Tissue loss is sometimes seen with extramarginal lacerations, particularly in lacerations from a broken windshield, which produce a characteristic series of partial and sometimes full-thickness linear gouges together with irregular lacerations and abrasions. It may also be seen with some animal bites (see Figure 11.5).

Extramarginal lacerations of the upper eyelid may involve the levator aponeurosis or levator muscle. Any laceration of these structures should be explored and repaired as soon as possible. In an adult it is helpful if the repair can be undertaken under local anaesthesia so that the height and contour of the lid can be adjusted appropriately.

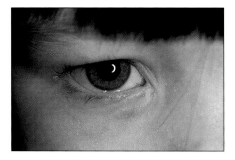

**Figure 11.7**
Lower lid marginal laceration, which involved the inferior canaliculus. The canalicular injury was not recognized. The small laceration was managed with Steri-strips. The patient now has constant epiphora and will require a conjunctivodacryorhinostomy (CDCR) with a Lester Jones tube.

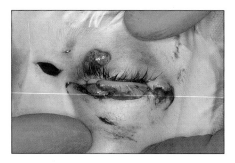

**Figure 11.8**
A dog bite injury with several eyelid puncture wounds with orbital fat prolapse and a lower lid marginal laceration.

## Avulsion injuries

Full-thickness marginal lacerations of the eyelids of the medial canthal region can also be associated with tangential extensions of the lacerations at the level of the eyelid creases and distal borders of the tarsi (Figure 11.9). Disruption of the orbicularis muscle allows retraction of the cut edges, and gives the appearance of tissue loss. This is, however, very rarely the case.

## Injuries involving tissue loss

Although tissue loss in the periocular region is rare, it is important to recognize, as a formal reconstruction may be required. This requires particular oculoplastic expertise (see Figure 11.5). Attempts to undertake such work in inexperienced hands may seriously compromise the result.

- Delay major reconstruction if the necessary expertise is not available

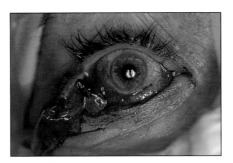

**Figure 11.9**
A lower eyelid avulsion injury with typical tangential extension of the laceration at the level of the eyelid crease.

should be carried out, and a suitable protective dressing should be applied until surgery can be performed. This is particularly important with respect to bite wounds.

- Delay the repair until operating conditions are optimal

## Management decisions

After the nature and extent of the injuries have been appropriately evaluated, management decisions can be made. The repair of eyelid injuries may be delayed for up to 72 hours if the operating conditions are not optimal. It is preferable, however, to repair such injuries as soon as possible after trauma for the following reasons:

1. Decontamination of the wounds is far more effective the earlier it is performed
2. Post-traumatic tissue oedema increases during the first 24 hours after injury
3. The surgical repair becomes more difficult to perform after the first 24 hours

If the ophthalmologist has doubts regarding the suitability of the facilities in the A&E Department or the patient's cooperation, the surgical repair should be undertaken in the operating theatre. If a formal repair of a lacrimal drainage system damage is contemplated, it is preferable to undertake such surgery under general anaesthesia. If the surgical repair must be delayed, e.g. because of potential anesthetic problems, decontamination of the wounds

## *Medicolegal considerations*

> *Documentation*
> Accurate and detailed documentation is essential. Many injuries will result in civil or criminal legal proceedings.

An accurate detailed legible history must be recorded and signed. It is particularly important to record any eyewitness statements and to record the names of anyone who administered any first aid. In the case of road traffic accidents it is important to record who was driving the vehicle. A record of the patient's vision is mandatory, unless this could not be recorded. A detailed description of the ocular and physical examination findings with drawings should be recorded.

Photographic documentation of the nature and extent of the injuries is particularly helpful and should always be considered (Figure 11.10). Photographic documentation offers significant advantages over drawings:

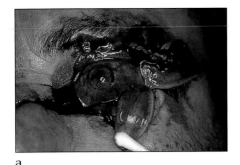

a

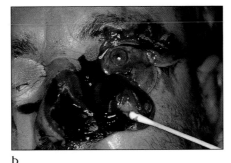

b

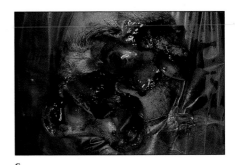

c

**Figure 11.10**
(a–c) Severe facial trauma caused by a relative of the patient. The photographs were used in legal proceedings.

1. Photographs provide objective documentation of the patient's preoperative appearance
2. Objective documentation may be useful in supporting claims filed with solicitors, insurance companies or the Criminal Injury Compensation Board
3. The photographs can illustrate the ophthalmologist's testimony should it be required in the future

• Document all injuries very carefully

## Remove dirt and debris

Tetanus prophylaxis must be considered in all patients. Patients with clean wounds who have been immunized within the last 10 years do not require tetanus toxoid injections. This criterion is reduced to 5 years for wounds with devitalized tissue or for contaminated wounds. Patients with clean wounds who have not been immunized should be treated with tetanus toxoid. Patients with contaminated wounds or devitalized tissue should also receive tetanus immune globulin.

# Surgical management

## *Wound decontamination*

In is essential that all wounds are thoroughly cleaned and all foreign bodies removed before any surgical repair is undertaken. Wounds should be carefully explored and a high degree of suspicion maintained that retained foreign material is present, depending on the circumstances of the injury (see Figure 11.2). Failure to remove particulate matter, as seen following explosions or contact from road surfaces in road traffic accidents, will lead to a traumatic tattoo that will prove extremely difficult to remove at a secondary procedure.

The role of prophylactic antibiotic administration in the treatment of traumatic eyelid and facial wounds remains controversial and is no substitute for meticulous wound decontamination. Grossly contaminated wounds, wounds associated with significant tissue devitalization, wounds involving the orbit, and animal/human bites certainly warrant antibiotic therapy, which should be started as soon as possible in consultation with a microbiologist (Figure 11.11).

# *Sequence of periocular laceration repair*

It is important to approach the repair of periocular wounds in a systematic fashion. Many periocular wounds are simple and straightforward to repair but some are complex lacerations with associated damage to the lacrimal drainage system, the globe and the bony orbital walls (Figure 11.12).

# *Lacrimal drainage system wounds*

After the wound has been decontaminated, it should be repaired in methodical fashion. Canalicular lacerations should be repaired meticulously. In the past, many surgeons have advocated a very conservative approach to the management of

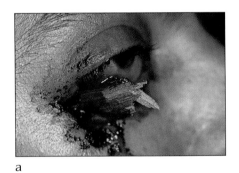

a

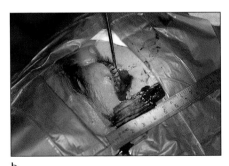

b

**Figure 11.11**
(a) A wooden foreign body removed under general anaesthesia. (b) Careful orbital wound exploration was essential to ensure no residual foreign bodies were left *in situ*.

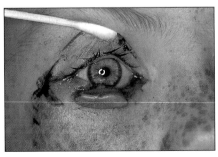

a

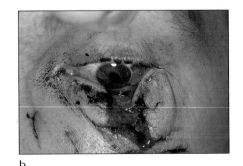

b

**Figure 11.12**
(a) This patient has sustained a lower lid avulsion injury in addition to a lateral marginal laceration. It is preferable to repair the avulsion injury and the inferior canalicular laceration before proceeding with a repair of the lateral marginal laceration. (b) This patient has a severe lower lid marginal laceration and a penetrating eye injury with iris prolapse. The globe must be repaired first followed by a meticulous eyelid repair, taking care to avoid undue pressure on the globe

canalicular lacerations for fear of causing iatrogenic damage not only to the affected canaliculus but also to the uninvolved canaliculus or to the common canaliculus. It is mandatory to avoid such iatrogenic trauma, which was particularly seen with the use of the pigtail probe, for which reason it has fallen into disrepute. The technique of passing bicanalicular silicone stents is much simpler than using a pigtail probe. *In the hands of a skilled and experienced surgeon bicanalicular silicone intubation causes little if any iatrogenic trauma and offers significant advantages over monocanalicular intubation:*

- When tightened, the silicone loop aids in the anatomical realignment of the eyelid, although the loop must be loosened once the sutures are in place to avoid any cheese-wiring of the puncta and canaliculi.
- Patients more readily tolerate the loop of silicone at the medial canthus for long periods than monocanalicular stents, which also tend to occlude the puncta and cause secondary epiphora.

It is therefore reasonable for the skilled and experienced surgeon to attempt a repair of a lacerated superior canaliculus when the inferior canaliculus is intact. If the surgeon is inexperienced, however, the priorities are to avoid iatrogenic trauma and to achieve a good anatomical alignment of the eyelid. Under these circumstances, the use of a monocanalicular stent is preferable. When both canaliculi have been severed, it is mandatory to attempt a repair.

Numerous methods have been described to assist in the identification of the proximal end of a lacerated canaliculus.

These are very rarely required, as the proximal end of the lacerated canaliculus can almost always be readily identified using the operating microscope. It is more difficult to locate following an avulsion injury when good retraction of the surrounding oedematous tissues is essential using cotton-tipped applicators. The lighter colour of the canaliculus is contrasted with the surrounding orbicularis muscle (Figure 11.13).

At induction of anaesthesia the nose should be packed with small neurosurgical patties moistened with a vasoconstrictor, e.g. 5% cocaine solution. These should be placed under and around the inferior turbinate. Shrinkage of the mucosa of the inferior turbinate will permit much easier retrieval of the silicone stent from the nose without bleeding.

It is essential to insert good-quality silicone stents atraumatically. The author's first choice is the Crawford silicone stent. This is reinforced with a white thread within the silicone and has a fine flexible wire introducer with a small olive tip (Figure 11.14). It is essential to check the attachment of the silicone to the introducer. This should be rounded and smooth, permitting easy passage through the canaliculi. Some stents have a flattened attachment that causes trauma to the canaliculi. These stents should be avoided.

This is easily retrieved from beneath the inferior turbinate, either with the use of a nasal endoscope and a hook retriever or with a Tse–Anderson grooved director placed under the inferior turbinate and used by 'feel'. This is a modified Quickert grooved director with a tip designed to catch the olive tip of the wire introducer (Figure 11.15). A similar device, the Anderson Hwang grooved director, is now available from Altomed Limited.

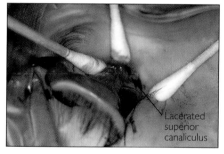

**Figure 11.13**
A patient with an upper eyelid avulsion injury. The lighter colour of the lacerated superior canaliculus is contrasted with the surrounding orbicularis muscle.

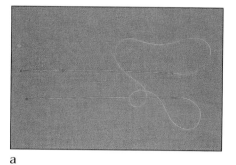

a                                                    b

**Figure 11.14**
(a) A Crawford silicone stent. (b) The olive tip of the stent introducer.

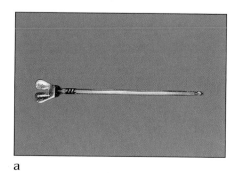

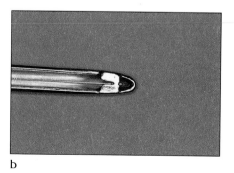

a                                                    b

**Figure 11.15**
(a) A Tse–Anderson grooved director. (b) The modified tip of the grooved director.

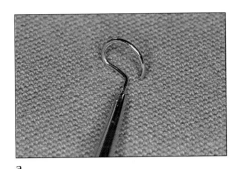

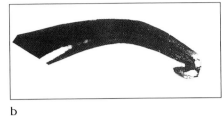

b

**Figure 11.16**
(a) A pigtail probe with a barbed tip.
(b) A diagram of the pigtail probe with a barbed tip.

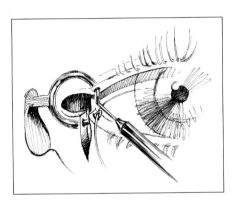

a

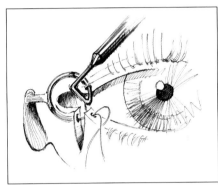

b

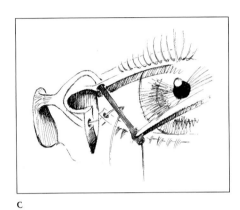

c

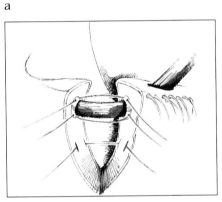

d

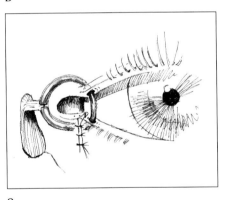

e

**Figure 11.17**
(a) A pigtail probe has been passed via the superior canaliculus and a 6/0 nylon suture threaded through the eye of the probe. (b) The probe is rotated back and the suture withdrawn through the superior canaliculus. (c) Silicone tubing is threaded over the suture. (d) 8/0 Vicryl sutures are placed through the substantia propria of the canaliculus. (e) The tubing is cut to size and the central nylon suture tied and the knot rotated into the lacrimal sac.

It is essential that an attempt be made to pass the stent via the lacerated canaliculus first. Only if this manoeuvre is successful should the stent then be passed via the uninvolved canaliculus. The stent is left in place and removed after 9–12 months in the absence of any problems. If the central thread has been denuded and used to tie the knot, retrieval via the canaliculi is easy and less uncomfortable for the patient.

If the stents cannot be passed into the nose successfully, e.g. there is an associated nasal fracture, the pigtail probe can be used. This requires more skill and care and does not offer the advantage of assisting the anatomical realignment of the eyelid in contrast to bicanalicular intubation. The pigtail probe is passed via the uninvolved canaliculus. A single attempt should be made to gently rotate the probe into position. If this is difficult, or any resistance is encountered, the attempt should be abandoned.

It is important to select a pigtail probe of appropriate size. A common error is to assume that one size fits all because only a single size is available. The probe should be smooth, with a small

eye at the tip through which a 6/0 nylon suture is passed. No probe should be used which has a barb at the tip. This causes severe trauma to the canaliculi and its use is largely responsible for the pigtail probe falling into disrepute (Figure 11.16).

Once the nylon has been retrieved and the probe removed, a fine silicone tube is passed over the suture. A Crawford stent is ideal. This is cut and the central thread removed, leaving a hollow tube. The tubing is then trimmed to size, taking great care not to cut the suture. The suture is then tied and cut and the knot rotated into the lacrimal sac (Figure 11.17).

This procedure is ideally suited to minor lacerations (Figure 11.18).

With more major lacerations or avulsion injuries of the lower eyelid, the medial canthal ligament should be reconstructed with a permanent suture (e.g. 5/0 Ethibond) after the silicone tubing has been placed but not yet tied. It is essential to ensure that the suture is initially placed through the posterior lacrimal crest. This requires good assistance and retraction of the tissues. The posterior lacrimal crest is approached by dissection between the caruncle and the plica semilunaris. The crest can be felt with a Freer periosteal elevator. The use of a 1/2–circle needle is essential to facilitate good fixation to the posterior lacrimal crest and easier retrieval of the needle. Failure to attach the avulsed lid to this position will lead to antero-positioning of the lower lid, poor cosmesis and epiphora (Figure 11.19).

The Ethibond suture is passed through the tarsus, taking care not to damage the canaliculus further, and is then tied with a slip knot to ensure correct anatomical placement of the eyelid, but then loosened so that a microsurgical repair of the canaliculus itself can proceed. When possible, the canaliculus should be repaired with three equally spaced 8/0 Vicryl sutures placed through the substantia propria of the canaliculus. These sutures should be left untied until all three are placed.

The silicone tubing can then be gently tightened and the Ethibond posterior fixation suture tied. This action takes all tension off of the 8/0 sutures, which can then be tied blindly and cut. The orbicularis muscle is repaired with the remaining Vicryl suture. The lid margin is sutured with two interrupted 6/0 Vicryl sutures placed in a vertical mattress fashion, again taking care not to damage the canaliculus or the stent. Finally, the stent is loosened so that there is no tension on it and then tied in the nose (Figure 11.20).

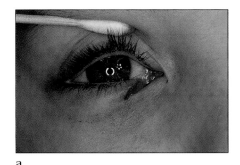
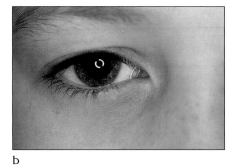

a    b

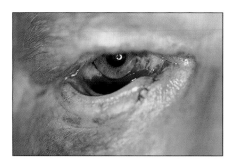

### Figure 11.18
(a) Minor lower lid marginal laceration involving the inferior canaliculus.
(b) Canalicular laceration repaired using a pigtail probe. The nylon suture is visible in the silicone stent.

### Figure 11.19
(a) Lower lid ectropion following lower lid avulsion injury. No attempt has been made to repair the medial canthal tendon.

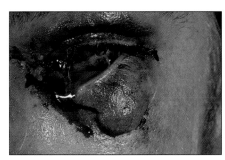

a

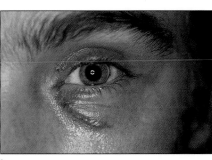

b

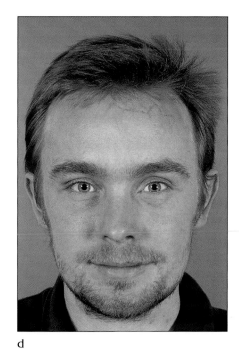

c                                    d

### Figure 11.20
(a) Severe left lower eyelid avulsion injury with secondary eyelid oedema and bruising. (b) One week following repair with bicanalicular silicone intubation. (c) Severe left lower eyelid avulsion injury with secondary eyelid oedema and bruising. (d) Eight weeks following repair with bicanalicular silicone intubation.

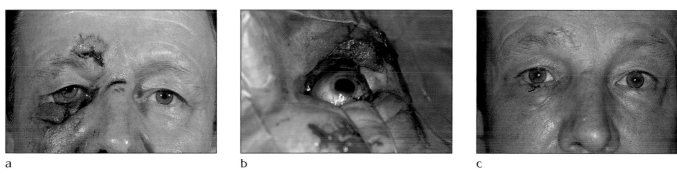

a                        b                        c

### Figure 11.21

(a) Severe right lower eyelid avulsion injury combined with marginal laceration. (b) Small pedicle of attachment with dusky appearance to avulsed eyelid tissue. (c) Result of anatomical realignment 2 weeks later prior to lid margin suture removal.

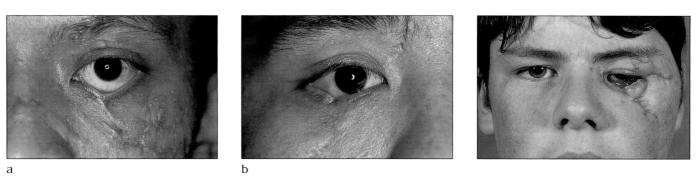

a                        b

### Figure 11.22

(a) Lower eyelid retraction with severe cutaneous and deep scar formation.
(b) Central lower eyelid notch with retraction.

### Figure 11.23

Severe periocular scarring and left lower lid wound breakdown.

## *Marginal injuries*

Marginal injuries can be difficult to repair because of secondary eyelid bruising and swelling as well as irregularity of the wound (Figure 11.21). Although it is reasonable to debride shredded devitalized tissue, this should be kept to a minimum. The blood supply to the periorbital area is excellent and tissue, which may appear non-viable, will usually survive even if replaced as a free graft.

* Reposition tissues to their correct anatomical alignment

The goals in the repair of marginal lacerations are:

* Meticulous anatomical alignment of the eyelid margin
* Avoidance of secondary trichiasis and eyelid notching
* Restoration of the structural integrity of the tarsus
* Avoidance of any eyelid retraction or lagophthalmos
* A limitation of cutaneous and deep scar formation

Failure to observe basic principles of eyelid repair and postoperative wound management will result in failure to achieve these goals and poor results (Figures 11.22 and 11.23). Secondary surgery will not achieve as good a result.

Figure 11.23 illustrates the reconstructive problems caused by a poor attempt at a primary repair.

* The results of primary repair are superior to secondary repair

The principles involved in the repair of eyelid marginal lacerations are very similar to those involved in the closure of wedge defects of the eyelid. It is rarely the case that tissue is missing from the eyelid. Depending on the age of the patient, it may be possible to convert a wound to a standard wedge excision by segmental excision of the involved area. If, however, the extent of the tissue loss is too great, a formal reconstruction will be required.

After the eyelid margin and tarsus have been repaired, any horizontal defects of the eyelid retractors should be repaired before the orbicularis and skin are closed as separate layers (Figure 11.24). Failure to repair defects of the eyelid, retractors

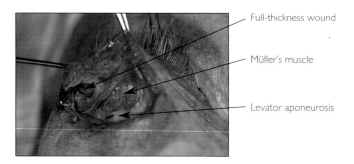

Full-thickness wound

Müller's muscle

Levator aponeurosis

### Figure 11.24

An upper eyelid extramarginal laceration with a full-thickness hole laterally and a lacerated levator aponeurosis. The skin wound was extended to effect a repair of the levator aponeurosis.

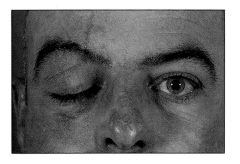

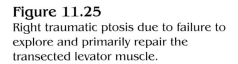

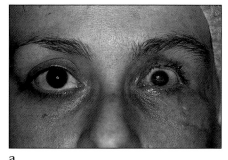

a

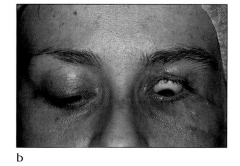

b

**Figure 11.25**
Right traumatic ptosis due to failure to explore and primarily repair the transected levator muscle.

**Figure 11.26**
(a) Left upper eyelid retraction, phthisis bulbi and periorbital severe cutaneous and deep scar formation following a road traffic accident. (b) Severe lag on downgaze due to overzealous debridement of upper lid tissues which appeared to be devitalized.

may result in a severe ptosis that is much more difficult to correct secondarily (Figure 11.25). Following windscreen injuries, multiple flaps and puncture wounds may be present and it may be a very difficult task to ascertain the correct anatomical location for the tissues. This task is made even more difficult by the possibility of tissue loss.

# *Extramarginal injuries*

It is to be re-emphasized that extramarginal lacerations are associated with more serious underlying injuries until proved otherwise.

The goals in the repair of extramarginal lacerations are:

- Meticulous anatomical alignment of the eyelid tissues
- Avoidance of any eyelid retraction or lagophthalmos (Figure 11.26)
- A limitation of cutaneous and deep scar formation

In the upper lid, if the lacerations extend to the eyebrow, it is preferable to realign the eyebrow first. Suturing of the orbicularis muscle with 5/0 Vicryl aids in the alignment of irregular skin flaps and removes the tension from the skin sutures. The minimal number of sutures should be placed in order to limit deep scarring. The sutures should not strangulate tissue. As in all repairs, slight eversion of the skin edges minimizes the chances of depressed scars.

- Do not discard or excise tissue unnecessarily

# *Eyelid injuries with associated severe penetrating globe injury*

*The decision to repair a severely traumatized eye with no prospect of useful vision may compromise the patient's outcome if this decision prevents the adequate primary repair of associated complex eyelid*

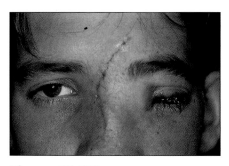

**Figure 11.27**
This patient suffered a severe left globe rupture and a comminuted nasoethmoidal fracture. A maxillofacial surgeon undertook the repair of the nasoethmoidal fracture after the severe globe rupture had been repaired. The maxillofacial surgeon was unable to effect a satisfactory repair of the fractures for fear of damaging the globe. The globe had no visual prospects and was enucleated the next day.

*lacerations and orbital fractures* (Figure 11.27). This may save the patient from numerous further operative procedures. This can be extremely difficult *and any decision to proceed with a primary enucleation must be made at the most senior level.* It is particularly important when the ophthalmic surgeon is operating as part of a multidisciplinary team. Good communication with other members of the team is vital. Detailed postoperative documentation is also imperative.

# *Postoperative care*

Measures should be taken to prevent excessive postoperative eyelid oedema, which can adversely affect the outcome. These are:

- Elevation of the patient's head
- Prolonged application of a pressure dressing
- Ice packs

For most injuries the pressure dressing can be removed the following day. Prolonged application of a pressure dressing should be avoided in young children, to avoid occlusion amblyopia. The eyelid can instead be protected with a clear Cartella shield.

In the case of severe eyelid avulsion injuries where the wound is under tension (see Figure 11.20), the tarsal fixation suture should be supported by a pressure dressing, which is applied with the tape fixed to the cheek area and then drawn up to the forehead. This holds tension off the wound until the wound has had a chance to heal and also reduces the chances of further postoperative oedema, which can cause the sutures to give way (see Figure 11.23). Such a dressing should be further supported with the use of a head bandage and can be maintained in place for up to 1 week.

Ideally, sutures should be removed in wounds not under tension on the fourth or fifth day after surgery, and Steri-strips used to support the wound for a few days more. This is not necessary, however, where dissolvable sutures have been used. Eyelid margin sutures should be left in place for 2 weeks.

> The patient should be advised on postoperative wound massage. Massage after placement of ointment prevents wound contracture and softens the resultant scar. Massage should be performed regularly and for months after the surgery. Compliance with such aftercare can prevent the need for further surgical intervention.

# Secondary repair

Although the aim of a good primary repair of eyelid injuries is to avoid the necessity for any secondary reconstructive surgery, such secondary intervention is occasionally necessary for a variety of reasons:

- Severe aesthetic deformity (see Figure 11.23)
- Lagophthalmos with exposure keratopathy (see Figure 11.26)
- Mechanical keratitis from eyelid malposition/trichiasis
- Lower lid retraction/ectropion (see Figure 11.22)

- An overlooked foreign body
- Tattooing of the wound
- An overlooked injury to the canalicular system (see Figure 11.7)
- A deformity of the medial or lateral canthi (see Figure 11.23)
- Ptosis (see Figure 11.25)
- Conjunctival scarring with restriction of ocular motility

The timing of the secondary intervention depends on the degree of urgency of the problem and can be categorized as early, intermediate or late: e.g. lagophthalmos with exposure keratopathy which cannot be managed conservatively.

If the opportunity arises to reintervene early where there has been a failure to apply the basic principles discussed earlier, the wound can be simply recreated and repaired appropriately. An alternative strategy may need to be employed, however, for an eyelid that is shortened by loss of tissue or scar formation. A superior result may be achieved by a reconstruction with a full-thickness skin graft combined with an orbicularis muscle advancement undertaken as an aesthetic procedure (Figure 11.28).

The management of a ptosis following trauma can be a challenge. It can be very difficult to differentiate a mechanical ptosis from eyelid swelling and haematoma from a neurogenic ptosis or from a myogenic/aponeurotic ptosis following a direct laceration to the levator muscle or its aponeurosis. The ptosis may in fact have a mixed aetiology. If it is known that the levator muscle or its aponeurosis has been transected, it is preferable to reintervene early and repair the laceration with the patient under local anaesthesia. The presence of eyelid swelling and haematoma, however, may make this impractical. Alternatively, it is reasonable to delay reintervention for some months unless there is a risk of amblyopia in an infant. The ptosis and levator function may improve spontaneously. The ptosis can then be re-evaluated and the ptosis managed according to basic principles.

If the opportunity for an early reintervention for canalicular lacerations has been missed the secondary reconstruction can be particularly difficult and may fail to achieve freedom from epiphora without a conjunctivo dacryocystorhinostomy (CDCR) and a Lester Jones tube.

Late reintervention for scar revisions is indicated once the scars have matured and the wounds have been extensively massaged.

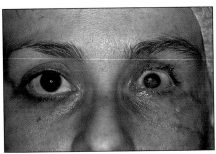

a

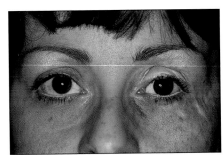

b

**Figure 11.28**
(a) Left upper eyelid retraction, phthisis bulbi and periorbital severe cutaneous and deep scar formation following a road traffic accident.
(b) Result after a full thickness postauricular skin graft combined with an orbicularis muscle advancement and fitting of a cosmetic shell.

# Burns

Burns can be classified as:

- Thermal
- Chemical
- Electrical
- Radiational

This section will deal only with thermal burns.

Patients who have sustained thermal burns to the eyelids are often critically ill. The majority of such patients are managed in a specialist burns unit. Severe burns are rarely confined to the eyelids and periocular region (Figure 11.29).

Fortunately, the eye is rarely affected acutely by facial burns because of the protective mechanisms afforded by reflex eyelid closure and the Bell's phenomenon.

Burns are classified as:

- First degree
- Second degree
- Third degree

A first-degree burn only involves the epidermis and is characterized by erythema typically seen in a mild sunburn. A second-degree (partial thickness) burn involves the epidermis and superficial layers of the adjacent dermis. Regeneration of the skin occurs from remaining epithelial elements. This degree of burn is characterized by pain, erythema, blistering and weeping, as typically seen following $CO_2$ laser resurfacing (Figure 11.30).

A third-degree burn (full thickness) involves total and irreversible destruction of both the epidermis and dermis. Such a burn is painless and is characterized by the absence of oedema, with the area affected by the burn appearing hard and inelastic (see Figure 11.29).

## *Management*

The immediate management of thermal burns of the eyelids is conservative. The goals are:

- To prevent infection
- To prevent secondary corneal complication

First-degree burns usually require no further treatment. Second- and third-degree burns should be cleaned and any foreign material removed. *If the burned tissue is extensive enough to cause destruction resulting in corneal exposure, it is imperative to protect the eye with a combination of topical lubricants and antibiotics. If corneal protection cannot be achieved satisfactorily a temporary suture tarsorrhaphy may be necessary.*

Once cicatricial changes begin in the eyelids with ectropion and lagophthalmos, there is often a rapid deterioration of the ocular surface. More aggressive treatment may be necessary to prevent irreversible ocular morbidity (Figure 11.31). Although

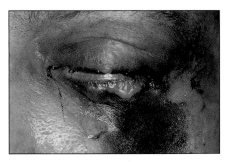

**Figure 11.29**
Self-inflicted third-degree burn of lower eyelid, lateral aspect of upper eyelid and cheek in a schizophrenic patient caused by direct contact with a cigarette lighter flame.

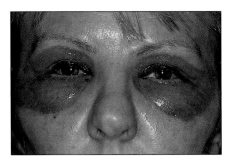

**Figure 11.30**
$CO_2$ resurfacing burns.

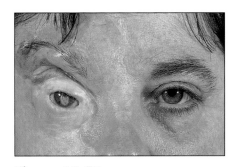

**Figure 11.31**
Corneal scarring in spite of extensive periocular skin grafting combined with a lateral tarsorrhaphy and a medial canthoplasty.

skin grafting is usually delayed until cicatricial changes stabilize, the use of early full-thickness skin may be necessary to reduce ocular morbidity.

The late management of thermal eyelid burns involves excision of the scar with the use of full-thickness skin grafts. The recipient lid should be placed on maximum stretch with the use of eyelid margin silk sutures in order to increase the area to be grafted. This allows for postoperative skin graft contraction, which should be minimized by a strict protocol of postoperative massage.

# Further reading

1.  American Academy of Ophthalmology. *Basic and clinical science course: orbit, eyelids and lacrimal system*, section 7. San Francisco: American Academy of Ophthalmology, 1998–99, pp. 101–9, 138–41.

2.  Gonnering RS. Eyelid trauma. In: Bosniak S, ed., *Principles and practice of ophthalmic plastic and reconstructive surgery*, Vol. 1. Philadelphia: WB Saunders, 1996, pp. 452–64.

3.  Grossman MD, Berlin AJ. Management of acute adnexal trauma. In: Stewart WB, ed., *Surgery of the eyelids, orbit and lacrimal system*, *Vol. 1. Ophthalmology monographs 8*. San Francisco: American Academy of Ophthalmology, 1993, pp. 170–85.

4.  Jordan DR, Nerad JA, Tse DT. The pigtail probe revisited. *Ophthalmology* (1990) **97**:512–19.

5.  Kulwin DR. Thermal, chemical and radiation burns. In: Stewart WB, ed., *Surgery of the eyelids, orbit and lacrimal system. Vol. 1, Ophthalmology monographs 8*. San Francisco: American Academy of Ophthalmology, 1993, pp. 186–97.

6.  Mustarde JC. *Repair and reconstruction in the orbital region*. Edinburgh: Livingstone, 1966.

7.  Shore JW, Rubin PA, Bilyk JR. Repair of telecanthus by anterior fixation of cantilevered miniplates. *Ophthalmology* (1992) **99**:1133–8.

# 12

# Orbital wall blowout fractures

## Introduction

The term 'pure orbital blowout fracture' is used to describe a fracture of the orbital floor, the medial orbital wall or both, with an intact bony orbital margin. The term 'impure orbital blowout fracture' is used when such fractures occur in conjunction with a fracture of the orbital rim, e.g. as part of a zygomatic complex fracture. The most common site for a blowout fracture to occur is in the posteromedial aspect of the orbital floor medial to the infraorbital neurovascular bundle where the maxillary bone is very thin. As the lamina papyracea is also very thin, the medial orbital wall is also prone to fracture, either in isolation or in association with a fracture of the orbital floor or other facial bones.

## Aetiology

There are two mechanisms thought to be responsible for pure orbital wall blowout fractures:

1. The backward displacement of the globe caused by a blunt non-penetrating object, e.g. a tennis ball, which raises the intraorbital pressure sufficiently to fracture the postero-medial orbital floor and/or the lamina papyracea of the ethmoid.
2. A transient deformation of the orbital rim transmits the force of injury directly to the orbital wall.

These fractures may occur following any blunt trauma to the periorbital region, e.g. following a blow with a fist (Figure 12.1). The weak areas of the orbital walls provide some means of protection to the globe and orbital tissues, permitting these to expand into the maxillary antrum and/or ethmoid sinus rather than being compressed against the other more rigid areas of the orbit. Although a rupture of the globe can complicate such fractures, this occurrence is rare. Conversely, *any patient who has*

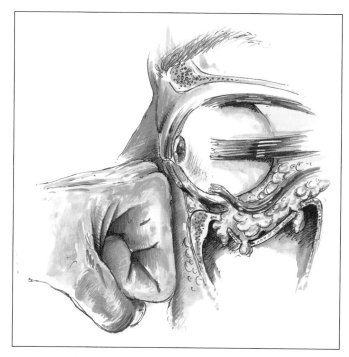

**Figure 12.1**
Production of an orbital floor blowout fracture with a prolapse of orbital fat into the maxillary antrum.

*suffered blunt trauma sufficient to cause a ruptured globe has an orbital wall blowout fracture until proven otherwise.* Such a fracture is commonly overlooked.

## Diagnosis

A high index of suspicion should be maintained for the presence of a blowout fracture in any patient who has sustained blunt periorbital trauma. The patient's clinical signs will depend on the timing of the examination in relation to the traumatic episode. A patient presenting some months after the traumatic event may have enophthalmos as the only physical sign.

## Clinical signs

1.  Eyelid ecchymosis/haematoma
2.  Subcutaneous emphysema
3.  Neurosensory loss in the distribution of the infraorbital nerve
4.  Limitation of ocular motility
5.  Enophthalmos/proptosis/hypoglobus
6.  Upper eyelid sulcus deformity
7.  Pseudoptosis

## Eyelid ecchymosis/haematoma

Although eyelid ecchymosis, haematoma or oedema are usually present when the patient is seen soon after trauma has occurred, these signs may be absent as seen in the 'white eyed blowout fracture'.

## Subcutaneous emphysema

A blowout fracture communicates with an air-filled sinus. Air may escape into the orbit and/or eyelids, particularly in medial orbital wall blowout fractures. Subcutaneous emphysema may result in palpable crepitus. Patients should be urged not to blow their nose or to hold the nose when sneezing, or emphysema may be greatly exacerbated. Very rarely, air forced into the orbit can cause severe proptosis, and an orbital compartment syndrome with a compromise of the blood supply to the optic nerve or globe (Figure 12.2).

## Neurosensory loss in the distribution of the infraorbital nerve

Dysfunction of the infraorbital nerve is almost pathognomonic of an orbital floor blowout fracture. The patient is usually aware of altered sensation in the ipsilateral cheek, upper teeth or tip of the nose. This occurs because the fracture extends along the infraorbital groove or canal, injuring the infraorbital nerve. Not all patients with an orbital floor blowout fracture, however, experience such sensory defects. These annoying sensory defects tend to resolve spontaneously with time but may be exacerbated by surgical intervention for the fracture. Very rarely, persistent pain in the distribution of the infraorbital nerve may be an indication for surgical decompression of the nerve, which may be compressed by bone fragments.

## Limitation of ocular motility

The patient with an orbital floor blowout fracture may have vertical diplopia due to a variety of different mechanisms.

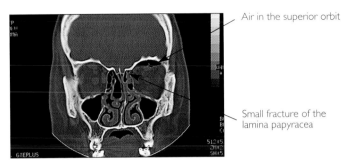

Air in the superior orbit

Small fracture of the lamina papyracea

**Figure 12.2**
This patient sustained a small medial orbital wall blowout fracture complicated by air forced into the orbit under pressure when the patient sneezed.

Horizontal diplopia in the presence of a medial orbital wall blowout fracture is less commonly seen. The mechanisms which may be responsible for limitation of ocular motility are:

1.  Entrapment of connective tissue septa or an extraocular muscle within the fracture
2.  Haematoma and/or oedema in the orbital fat adjacent to the fracture
3.  Haematoma or contusion of an extraocular muscle(s)
4.  Palsy of an extraocular muscle(s) due to neuronal damage
5.  Volkmann's ischaemic contracture of an entrapped extraocular muscle

## Enophthalmos/proptosis/hypoglobus

Enophthalmos is produced by an enlarged orbital volume and varies from insignificant to cosmetically disfiguring depending on the degree of orbital bony expansion. Fat atrophy contributes little if anything to the enophthalmos. It may be masked by orbital haematoma/oedema/air which may even cause proptosis in the first few days following trauma. Proptosis, however, may be associated with a 'blow-in' fracture where the fragmented bones of the orbital floor are displaced upwards into the orbit. Enophthalmos is always significant in the presence of combined fractures of the orbital floor and medial orbital wall. Hypoglobus is seen in the presence of extensive orbital floor blowout fractures. In some patients, the maxillary antrum extends laterally for some distance beyond the infraorbital neurovascular bundle, with the ensuing orbital floor defect occupying almost the whole of the orbital floor. Very rarely, the globe may come to lie within the maxillary antrum or even within the ethmoid sinus (Figures 12.3 and 12.4).

## Upper eyelid sulcus deformity/pseudoptosis

Enophthalmos results in decreased support of the upper eyelid, which leads to a secondary pseudoptosis and an upper eyelid sulcus deformity (Figure 12.5).

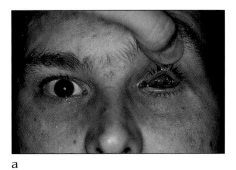

a

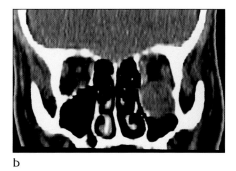

b

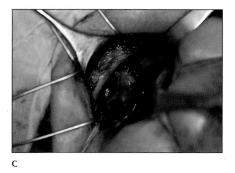

c

**Figure 12.3**
(a) This patient was referred for the management of an apparent anophthalmic socket. (b) Coronal CT scan of the patient demonstrating an extensive orbital floor blowout fracture with the globe prolapsed into the maxillary antrum. (c) The position of the globe below the inferior orbital margin seen intraoperatively.

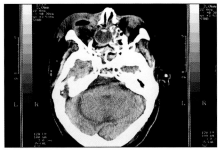

**Figure 12.4**
An extensive medial orbital wall and orbital floor blowout fracture with the globe prolapsed into the ethmoid sinus and nasal cavity.

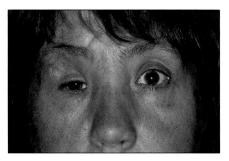

**Figure 12.5**
A patient demonstrating enophthalmos, ptosis and an upper lid sulcus deformity following extensive orbital floor and medial wall blowout fractures.

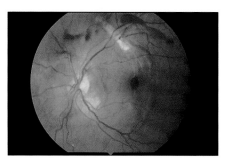

**Figure 12.6**
Choroidal rupture, macular haemorrhage and widespread retinal haemorrhages following blunt ocular trauma.

# Clinical evaluation

Any patient who has sustained blunt orbital trauma should undergo a complete ophthalmic examination to exclude associated ocular injuries (Table 12.1 and Figure 12.6). The incidence of ocular injuries has been reported as 14–30%. *The possibility of a globe rupture must always be considered and excluded before a forced duction test is performed.*

Any proptosis or enophthalmos should be measured using an Hertel exophthalmometer. Any vertical displacement of the globe should also be measured and recorded. The eyelids and periorbital tissues should be palpated for subcutaneous emphysema and for any orbital rim fractures. The malar eminences should be palpated and any depression noted (Figure 12.7).

The patient should be asked to open and close his/her mouth to ensure there is no associated pain or trismus. Such signs and symptoms are suggestive of a zygomatic complex fracture. A record of the extent of any infraorbital sensory loss should be made.

A full orthoptic assessment should be performed with prism measurements in nine positions of gaze, a Hess chart, a monocular and binocular visual field assessment, a forced duction test and an active force-generation test. Prior to the performance of a forced duction test, a cotton-tipped applicator is soaked in topical anaesthetic drops and held against the limbus for a few minutes. The patient should be recumbent. Fine-toothed forceps are then used to grasp the conjunctiva and Tenon's capsule just by the limbus. The patient is then asked to look in the direction of restriction of movement of the eye while the examiner attempts to move the globe in the same direction (Figure 12.8). The results of this test need to be interpreted with caution. If the examiner is unable to move the globe normally, this implies entrapment of the inferior orbital septa, but a positive forced duction test can also be caused by extraocular muscle/orbital haematoma and oedema. A strongly positive forced duction test, in a patient with evidence of

**Table 12.1** Ocular injuries complicating blowout fractures

| | |
|---|---|
| Globe rupture | Lens subluxation |
| Retinal tears | Traumatic cataract |
| Retinal dialysis | Choroidal rupture |
| Vitreous haemorrhage | Commotio retinae |
| Angle recession | Macular scarring |
| Hyphaema | Traumatic mydriasis |

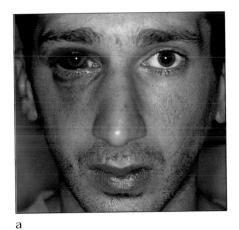

a

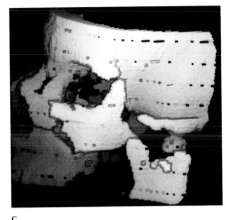

c

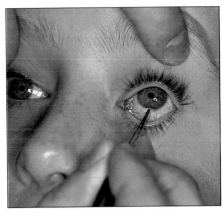

**Figure 12.8**
A forced duction test.

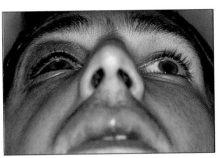

b

**Figure 12.7**
(a) Patient with a right zygomatic complex fracture showing a depression over the right malar eminence. (b) The abnormality is better appreciated from below. (c) This three-dimensional CT scan reconstruction demonstrates why the patient is experiencing trismus.

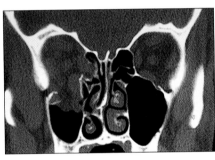

**Figure 12.9**
Coronal, axial and sagittal CT scan views demonstrating the extent of the orbital floor and medial wall fractures and the relationship of the inferior rectus and medial rectus muscles to the fractures.

**Figure 12.10**
This patient sustained an orbital floor blowout fracture following accidental blunt trauma. She represented to the A&E Department 2 days later with a severe orbital cellulitis and a blind eye.

a blowout fracture on a computed tomography (CT) scan, does suggest tissue entrapment as the cause of ocular restriction. An active force generation test is useful in differentiating extraocular muscle paralysis from tissue entrapment. A patient with tissue entrapment will usually experience pain on attempted globe movement in the direction of restriction.

If a patient has symptoms and signs suggestive of an orbital wall blowout fracture, a CT scan should be performed in an axial plane with coronal and sagittal reconstructions (Figure 12.9). Images available in three planes are extremely valuable in assessing the full extent of the injury. A plain skull X-ray is of little use in the evaluation of a blowout fracture. CT demonstrates the relationship of the soft tissues to the fracture sites, permits an evaluation of any secondary effects of trauma – e.g. retrobulbar

haemorrhage, intraoptic nerve sheath haematoma, subperiosteal haematoma – and can demonstrate any complications of trauma, e.g. orbital cellulitis, orbital or subperiosteal abscess and retained orbital foreign bodies.

## Management

Patients should be urged not to blow their nose or to hold the nose when sneezing. The role of antibiotic prophylaxis is controversial. If the CT scan shows evidence of chronic sinusitis, antibiotics should be prescribed to prevent a secondary orbital cellulitis (Figure 12.10).

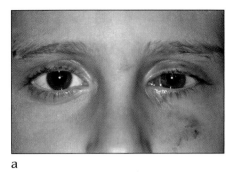
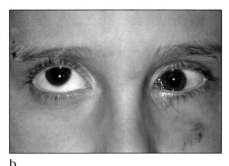
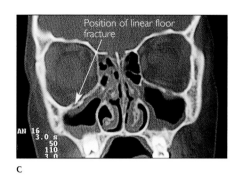

a                                       b                                       c

## Figure 12.11

(a) Boy presenting with diplopia on upgaze 2 days following blunt trauma to the left orbit. (b) Marked limitation of upgaze. A forced duction test was markedly positive. Early surgical release of the entrapped tissue is indicated. (c) Coronal CT scan of same patient. The radiographic images may be misleading in the absence of any obvious bony displacement.

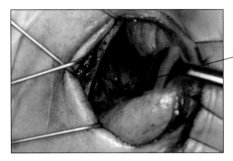

Linear 'trapdoor' fracture of the orbital floor after release of entrapped orbital contents

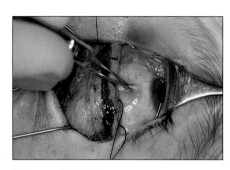

## Figure 12.12

The same patient as in Figure 12.12 demonstrating a linear fracture of the orbital floor in which orbital tissue was entrapped. The tissue was released with full recovery of ocular motility. No orbital floor implant was required.

## Figure 12.13

The forced duction test is repeated after release of the entrapped orbital tissue.

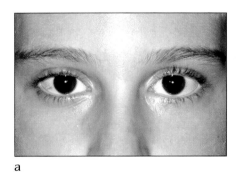
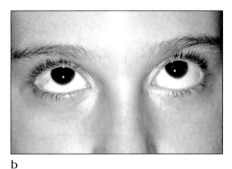

## Figure 12.14

(a) The same patient as in Figures 12.11–12.13 12 months following release of the entrapped orbital tissue. (b) The limitation of upgaze has completely resolved.

a                                       b

A number of different specialities compete for the treatment of patients with a blowout fracture, and opinions differ concerning the indications for surgery, the timing of surgery, the surgical approach and the use of orbital implant materials.

Although there are guidelines which can be used to advise the patient about surgical intervention, each patient should be managed as an individual. In general, the indications for the surgical repair of a blowout fracture are:

1.  Unresolving soft tissue entrapment with disabling diplopia
2.  Enophthalmos greater than 2 mm
3.  CT scan evidence of a large fracture

Patients with diplopia are observed for a period of approximately 2 weeks. If the diplopia resolves with a small fracture evident on CT,

no surgical intervention is required. There is an important exception to this. *Young patients with marked tissue entrapment and a linear fracture on CT (a 'trapdoor' fracture) are at risk of developing an ischaemic contracture unless the tissue entrapment is released very early* (Figures 12.11–12.14). *This is an indication for very early surgery.*

It is reasonable to defer operative decisions on the basis of the degree of enophthalmos for 2–3 weeks to determine with the patient whether or not the enophthalmos is cosmetically significant. This allows orbital oedema and haematoma to resolve, which in turn makes the surgery somewhat easier to perform. Extensive defects, particularly involving both the orbital floor and medial wall, suggest a high chance of progressive unsightly enophthalmos and support the decision for surgical intervention. *The patient must be fully informed of the risks and potential complications of such surgery.*

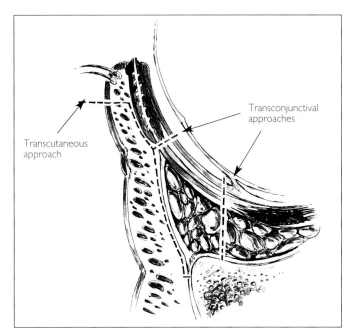

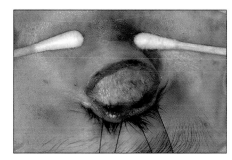

**Figure 12.16**
The surgeon's view of the dissection of a lower eyelid skin–muscle flap with the orbital septum maintained intact.

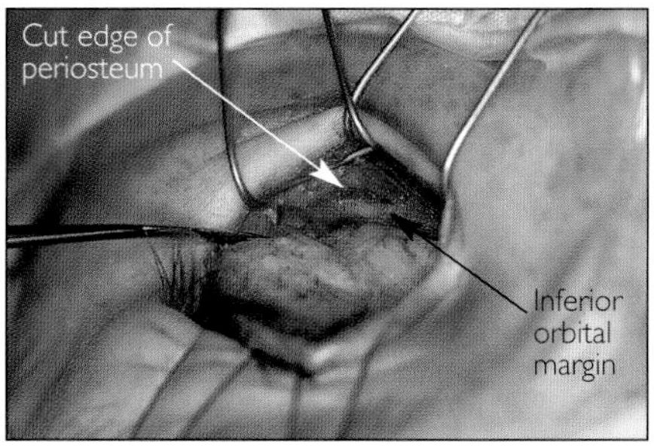

**Figure 12.17**
Periosteum of inferior orbital margin exposed.

**Figure 12.15**
Surgical approaches to the orbital floor.

# Surgical management

The surgical approach is the same whether the surgery is performed early after trauma (within 2 weeks) or is delayed. It is essential to use a headlight. *A forced duction test should be performed under general anaesthesia before surgery is commenced, and should be repeated once all the entrapped tissue has been freed from the fracture and again after placement of the orbital implant.* An orbital floor blowout fracture is usually approached via a lower eyelid incision. There is very rarely an indication for a Caldwell–Luc approach in which an opening is made into the maxillary sinus in the area of the superior gingiva. A medial wall fracture can also be repaired via the same lower eyelid incision. Alternatively, a transcaruncular approach can be used.

The lower eyelid incision can be made through the skin or through the conjunctiva (Figure 12.15). The author's preferred approach is transcutaneous. The scar, if the wound is properly constructed, closed and cared for postoperatively, is barely visible (see Figure 12.14).

## *Transcutaneous approach*

A variety of skin incisions can be utilized to gain access to the orbit. The subciliary incision is preferred by the author. An incision placed directly over the inferior orbital margin should be avoided as this is cosmetically unsatisfactory and is associated with postoperative eyelid lymphoedema.

Two 4/0 silk sutures are placed through the grey line of the lower eyelid and fixated to the head drapes. This places the lower eyelid tissues under tension to assist with the dissection through the tissue planes but it also permits the complete protection of the eye from the surgical instruments. The skin is incised with a Colorado needle just below the lashes and the orbicularis muscle incised down to the orbital septum. The avascular plane between the orbicularis muscle and the orbital septum is dissected and the orbital septum maintained intact to prevent any prolapse of fat and to prevent postoperative eyelid retraction (Figure 12.16).

The inferior orbital margin is exposed and the periosteum opened 2 mm below the inferior orbital margin. This is then elevated with a Freer periosteal dissector and the periorbita is elevated (Figure 12.17).

The majority of orbital floor fractures involve the posteromedial aspect of the floor, which is adjacent to the inferior orbital groove and the infraorbital canal. The infraorbital nerve is at risk from injury during the dissection as are the infraorbital artery and vein. Great care must be taken with the dissection to avoid damage to these vascular structures. Thermocautery should be used sparingly to avoid damage to the infraorbital nerve. All margins of the fracture should be exposed and prolapsing structures repositioned in the orbit. Overly aggressive dissection posteriorly risks damage to the optic nerve and other orbital apical structures. *It is useful to use a piece of Supramid with a Sewell retractor to keep prolapsing orbital fat from the surgical field during posterior dissection.*

Once the prolapsing orbital contents have been lifted out of the fracture site, an implant is placed over the fracture site ensuring that all margins are covered and that no tissue is allowed to herniate from the orbit again. The implant should be of an adequate size and shape to fulfil this objective (Figure 12.18).

It is very important to avoid the use of an unnecessarily large implant, to avoid compression of orbital apical structures. Likewise, it is important not to place the implant too far posteriorly in the orbit. The posterior margin of the fracture should be

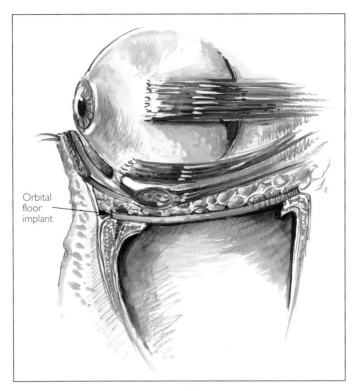

**Figure 12.18**
An orbital implant placed over margins of orbital floor blowout fracture. No fixation of the implant should normally be required.

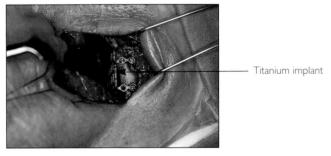

**Figure 12.19**
Titanium orbital implant fixated with screws to the inferior orbital margin and cantilevered back to the posterior margin of the fracture.

adequately exposed; this helps to support the implant, preventing it from prolapsing into the maxillary antrum. Fixation of an implant is usually unnecessary. If the fracture is so large that there is no posterior support, the implant should then be cantilevered over the fracture with microplates, which are fixated below the inferior orbital margin with screws (Figure 12.19).

Alternatively, channeled Medpor can be used in a very similar fashion (Figure 12.20). One or two linear microplates are inserted into the channels within the implant, with two or three holes left exposed anteriorly. This area is screwed to the inferior orbital margin. This implant is easy to fashion to the appropriate size and shape with scissors. It is very well tolerated. It is very rarely necessary to resort to autogenous bone grafting for the management of these fractures.

The edges of the periosteum are identified and closed with interrupted 5/0 Vicryl sutures, taking care to ensure that the orbital septum is not inadvertently included in the closure, which causes retraction of the lower eyelid. The skin edges are then reapproximated using a continuous 7/0 Vicryl suture. A compressive dressing is applied for 1 hour and then removed, and the patient's visual acuity and pupil reactions are checked. These are checked hourly for the first 12 hours postoperatively. Ice packs are then applied. Postoperative eyelid massage is commenced the day after surgery to prevent wound contracture and any eyelid retraction. Prophylactic broad-spectrum antibiotics are prescribed for 7 days postoperatively. The patient must be instructed not to blow the nose for 6 weeks postoperatively.

## *Transconjunctival approach*

This approach utilizes an incision through the conjunctiva of the inferior fornix combined with a lateral canthotomy and an inferior cantholysis. The eyelid is thereby detached from the lateral orbital rim. The conjunctiva and inferior retractors can be dissected free and lifted superiorly with traction sutures to provide corneal protection (Figure 12.21). The septum is again maintained intact to prevent postoperative lower eyelid retraction. The dissection then proceeds as described above. At the conclusion of surgery, the lateral canthal tendon is reattached after the conjunctiva and inferior retractors are reapproximated.

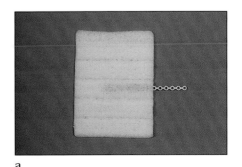
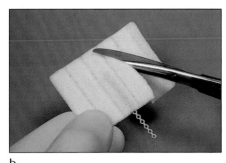
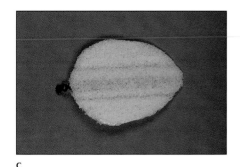

a      b      c

**Figure 12.20**
(a) A channeled Medpor implant. (b) The implant is cut to the appropriate size and shape using a template (usually a sheet of Supramid). (c) The implant ready for insertion to cover a large orbital floor fracture.

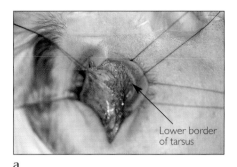

Lower border of tarsus

a

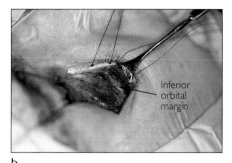

Inferior orbital margin

b

**Figure 12.21**
(a) Lateral canthotomy and inferior cantholysis with conjunctiva and inferior retractors lifted to protect the globe. (b) Inferior orbital margin exposed.

## Orbital implant materials

A variety of autogenous and synthetic materials have been used to cover an orbital wall blowout fracture, including silicone, Teflon, Supramid, Gelfilm, hydroxyapatite, methylmethacrylate, titanium, autogenous cartilage and autogenous bone. Autogenous bone can be harvested from the iliac crest or from the outer table of the skull. This entails a lengthier operation, a longer inpatient stay and risks donor site morbidity and complications. The author's preference is porous polyethylene (Medpor), which is easy to cut and shape to the precise dimensions required (see Figure 12.20). It lends good support for the majority of fractures and becomes ingrown by fibrovascular tissue. For larger fractures, channeled Medpor or a titanium microplate is preferred to lend greater support for the orbital contents, particularly when there is a large orbital floor fracture combined with a large medial wall fracture.

## Delayed treatment of diplopia

Long-term motility problems are quite rare in all types of orbital wall blowout fracture, with the exception of the linear 'trapdoor' fracture in the young. Spontaneous improvement in motility with resolution of diplopia is more common over a period of weeks to months whether a surgical repair of the fracture has been undertaken or not. There may be residual diplopia even after a successful repair of the fracture if there has been extraocular muscle or neuronal damage. Diplopia can, however, occur in the presence of normal extraocular muscles but with a large fracture and a markedly displaced globe. This is due to a change in the line of muscle pull. Such patients have clinically significant enophthalmos and the decision to proceed with a surgical repair is made on this basis.

A period of 4–6 months should be permitted to allow the diplopia to resolve or stabilize. Temporary relief can be provided with Fresnel prisms, which can be easily changed as alterations in the pattern of motility defect occur. Diplopia that does not resolve may not require any treatment if the patient is not disadvantaged by it. Alternatively, a permanent prism may be considered or strabismus surgery may be required.

In general, the goals of strabismus surgery following an orbital wall blowout fracture are to either enhance the action of the underacting muscles or weaken the action of the secondarily overacting muscles. The inverse Knapp procedure involves the transposition of the medial and lateral recti to the inferior rectus insertion to enhance the degree of depression of the affected

eye. This has been combined with recession of the inferior rectus, where this muscle shows contracture. A forced duction test must be performed before making a decision to recess this muscle. The risk of anterior segment ischaemia must also be taken into consideration. Surgery on other extraocular muscles may also be required to improve the field of binocular single vision. Patients must be counselled carefully prior to this surgery to ensure that they have realistic expectations.

## Complications of orbital wall blowout fracture surgery

### Blindness

Postoperative blindness is a rare complication. Nevertheless, the risk of this complication should be discussed with patients preoperatively and the risk weighed against the potential benefits of a surgical repair. It may be caused by:

1. *Intraoperative damage to the globe and/or optic nerve*
2. *Postoperative orbital haemorrhage*
3. *Compression of the optic nerve by misplacement of the orbital implant*

Every precaution should be taken to prevent its occurrence:

1. *A ruptured globe must be excluded before a patient undergoes an orbital wall blowout fracture repair*
2. *Meticulous haemostasis must be obtained before closure of the skin incision*
3. *The patient's vision must be monitored on recovery from general anaesthesia and at regular intervals thereafter for at least 12 hours*
4. *Great care must be taken to ensure that the orbital implant is of the correct size and shape and is not forced into the orbit beyond the posterior limit of the fracture*

### Diplopia

It is important to warn patients that it is not uncommon for diplopia to be worse in the first few weeks following surgery as a consequence of iatrogenic trauma from the surgical dissection to free entrapped orbital contents. It is important, however, to ensure that further inadvertent tissue entrapment has not been caused by misplacement of the orbital implant. For this reason the forced duction test must be repeated after placement of the orbital implant.

# Lower lid retraction

Lower eyelid retraction may be caused by:

1.  Incorrect closure of the periosteum over the infraorbital margin with inadvertent incorporation of the orbital septum in the sutures
2.  Adhesions of the orbital septum to the infraorbital margin (Figure 12.22)

Careful identification of the periosteal edges will avoid incorrect wound closure. Adhesions can be avoided by ensuring a meticulous dissection between the orbicularis oculi and the orbital septum, preventing any haematoma, and by early and prolonged postoperative eyelid massage.

The surgical correction of postoperative lower lid retraction is difficult. This is managed via a conjunctival incision at the lower border of the tarsus, a recession of the conjunctiva, the lower lid retractors and a dissection of all adhesions to the inferior orbital rim. A spacer, e.g. hard palate, is then interposed between the lower lid retractors and the lower border of the tarsus. In cases where there are extensive adhesions to the inferior orbital margin with a loss of preaponeurotic fat, a small dermis fat graft is placed over the rim to prevent further adhesions (Figure 12.23).

# Lower lid entropion

A lower lid entropion may occur after contracture of the wound following a transconjunctival approach to an orbital floor fracture. It is managed in a similar manner to lower lid retraction.

# Implant extrusion

Extrusion of an orbital implant may occur early or late after surgery for a blowout fracture. It may be seen many years after surgery. It may occur for a number of reasons:

1.  Infection
2.  The use of an oversized implant
3.  Inadequate closure of the periosteum along the inferior orbital margin

# Infection

Although an infection must be treated with systemic antibiotics, the implant will usually require removal. Late problems with sinusitis may occur.

# Infraorbital sensory loss

Patients should be warned about the potential for sensory loss in the distribution of the infraorbital nerve. Great care should be taken not to cause unnecessary intraoperative trauma to the

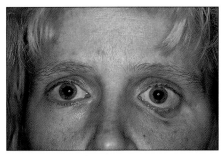

**Figure 12.22**
Left lower eyelid retraction following an orbital floor blowout fracture repair via a subciliary approach.

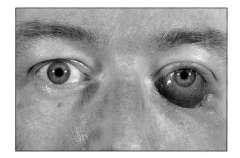

a

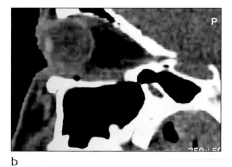

b

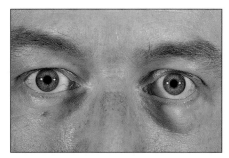

c

**Figure 12.23**
(a) Severe lower eyelid contracture and chemosis following infection of an orbital floor silastic implant. (b) CT scan demonstrating position of lower eyelid. (c) Result following removal of implant and insertion of dermis fat graft to prevent adhesion of lower eyelid to inferior orbital margin.

nerve and to remove any bone fragments which impinge on the nerve. Identification of the nerve may be difficult in the late management of large orbital floor fractures.

## *Undercorrection of enophthalmos*

Residual enophthalmos is usually the result of failure to reposition all prolapsed orbital tissues with placement of the orbital implant over the whole of the fracture, or of failure to treat any additional medial wall fracture. Although post-traumatic orbital fat atrophy can occur, this is usually overstated and the real cause of residual enophthalmos overlooked.

## *Proptosis/hyperglobus*

Proptosis or hyperglobus may occur from the use of oversized orbital implants, e.g. autogenous bone grafts. Care should be taken during surgery to avoid this complication by comparing the intraoperative position of the globe with that of the fellow globe in unilateral cases.

## *Lower lid lymphoedema*

Lower lid lymphoedema is usually seen following the use of a skin incision directly over the inferior orbital margin. Such an incision leaves an unsightly scar, predisposes the patient to implant extrusion and should be avoided unless there is a laceration in this location.

## *Chemosis*

Postoperative chemosis is more commonly seen following a transconjunctival approach to the repair of an orbital wall blowout fracture. It is rarely severe and usually resolves with the use of topical lubricants.

## Further reading

1.  Berkowitz RA, Putterman AM, Patel DB. Prolapse of the globe into the maxillary sinus after orbital floor fracture. *Am J Ophthalmol* (1981) **91**:253–7.
2.  Dutton GN, Al-Qurainy I, Stassen LFA, Titterington DM, Moos KF, El-Attar A. Ophthalmic consequences of mid-facial trauma. *Eye* (1992) **6**:86–9.
3.  Dutton JJ. *Atlas of clinical and surgical orbital anatomy.* Philadelphia: WB Saunders, 1994.
4.  Jordan DR, White GL, Anderson RL, Thiese SM. Orbital emphysema: a potentially blinding complication following orbital fractures. *Ann Emerg Med* (1988) **17**:853–5.
5.  Jordan DR, Allen LH, White J, Harvery J, Pashby R, Esmaeli B. Intervention within days for some orbital floor fractures: the white-eyed blowout. *Ophthal Plast Reconstr Surg* (1998) **14**:379–90.
6.  Koornneef L. Orbital septa: anatomy and functions. *Ophthalmology* (1979) **86**:876–80.
7.  Lyon DB, Newman SA. Evidence of direct damage to extraocular muscles as a cause of diplopia following orbital trauma. *Ophthal Plast Reconstr Surg* (1989) **5**:81–91.
8.  McGurk M, Whitehouse RW, Taylor PM, Swinson B. Orbital volume measured by a low-dose CT scanning technique. *Dentomaxillofac Radiol* (1992) **21**:70–2.
9.  Putterman AM, Stevens T, Urist MJ. Nonsurgical management of blowout fractures of the orbital floor. *Am J Ophthalmol* (1974) **77**:232–9.
10. Putterman AM. Management of orbital fractures: the conservative approach. *Surv Ophthalmol* (1991) **92**:523–8.
11. Rubin PA, Bilyk JR, Shore JW. Orbital reconstruction using porous polyethylene sheets. *Ophthalmology* (1994) **101**:1697–708.
12. Smith B, Regan WF. Blow-out fractures of the orbit. Mechanism and correction of internal orbital fracture. *Am J Ophthalmol* (1957) **11**:733–9.
13. Smith B, Lisman RD, Simonton J, Della Rocca R. Volkmann's contracture of the extraocular muscles following blowout fracture. *Plast Reconstr Surg* (1984) **74**:200–9.
14. Westfall CT, Shore JW. Isolated fractures of the orbital floor: risk of infection and the role of antibiotic prophylaxis. *Ophthalmic Surg* (1991): **22**: 409–11.

# 13

# Zygomatic complex fractures

## Introduction

A zygomatic complex fracture refers to a displacement of the zygoma and is often referred to as a tripod or tripartite fracture. This usually involves three areas of dislocation: the area of the frontozygomatic suture, the zygomaticomaxillary suture and the zygomatic arch (Figures 13.1 and 13.2).

## Aetiology

Zygomatic fractures usually occur following direct blunt trauma to the cheek.

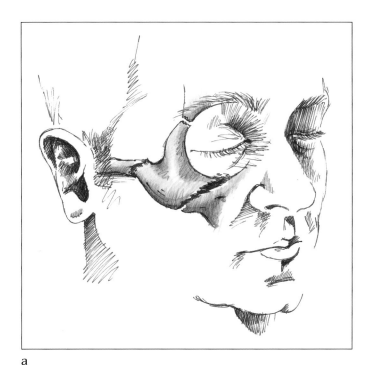

a

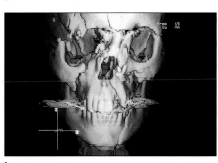

b

**Figure 13.1**
(a) Right zygomatic complex fracture demonstrating the areas of dislocation of the zygomatic bone. (b) A three-dimensional CT scan reconstruction demonstrating a marked displacement of the right zygoma.

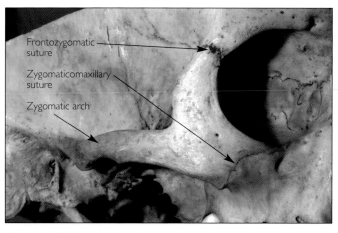

**Figure 13.2**
A lateral view of a skull demonstrating the potentially weak areas of the zygoma.

# Diagnosis

The presence of a zygomatic complex fracture should be suspected in any patient who has sustained blunt trauma to the cheek. The patient should be observed from below, looking for malar flattening. This may, however, be masked by oedema. The patient should be asked to open the mouth, looking for trismus (Figure 13.3). The orbital margin should be carefully palpated for gaps, steps and areas of tenderness. A neurosensory examination of the area should be performed, as hypoaesthesia or anaesthesia of the lower eyelid and cheek may be present. Imaging should be performed if there is a clinical suspicion of such a fracture.

# Clinical signs

Flattening of the cheek is usually noted (Figure 13.4).

Palpation of the inferior orbital margin may reveal gaps or steps. *The signs and symptoms of such a fracture depend on the degree of displacement of the zygoma and the direction of the displacement.* The lower eyelid may be dragged inferiorly, the lateral canthus may be displaced inferiorly, or there may be a bulge in the lateral cheek area (Figure 13.5).

There is usually an associated orbital floor fracture with enophthalmos but rarely signs of soft tissue entrapment. The fracture may be associated with other fractures, e.g. inferior orbital rim fractures.

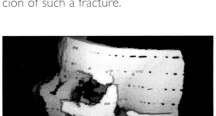

**Figure 13.3**
A three-dimensional CT scan reconstruction demonstrating a depressed zygomatic arch. This impinges on the coronoid process of the mandible and the adjacent temporalis muscle, causing both limitation of mouth opening and pain.

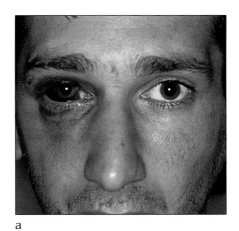
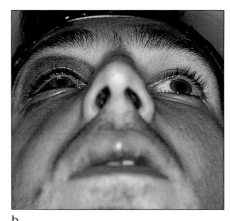

a                                  b

**Figure 13.4**
(a) A patient with a right zygomatic complex fracture demonstrating flattening of the right malar eminence. (b) This is best seen from below.

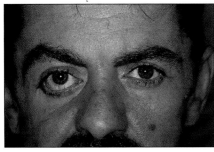

a

**Figure 13.5**
(a) Patient with a right zygomatic complex fracture with lower eyelid retraction, malar flattening and inferior displacement of the lateral canthus. (b) Diagram demonstrating zygomatic bone hinged at the frontozygomatic suture line. The attachment of the orbital septum to the inferior orbital margin causes lower eyelid retraction.

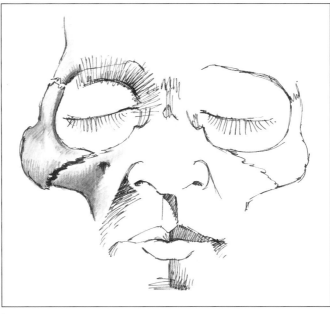

b

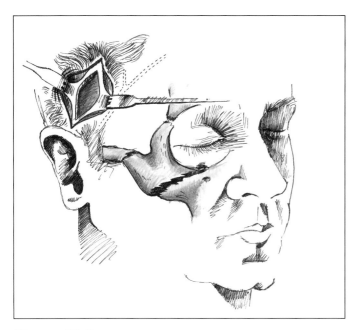

**Figure 13.6**
Incision for Gillies temporal approach for the management of a zygomatic complex fracture.

# Management

If the fracture is very minor, with no significant displacement of the zygoma, the patient should be managed conservatively. No surgery is indicated.

There are two basic surgical approaches for the management of a zygomatic complex fracture:

1.  Gillies temporal approach
2.  Direct approach

## *Gillies temporal approach*

This approach is used where the fractures are regular, recent and the displaced bone fragment is impacted on adjacent bone. A 5 cm incision is made approximately 2–3 cm behind the hairline over the temporal fossa, avoiding the superficial temporal vessels. The deep temporalis fascia is located and incised, exposing the underlying temporalis muscle (Figure 13.6).

Blunt dissection is performed in the plane between the temporalis fascia and the temporalis muscle. A Kilner elevator is then inserted and the blade manipulated under the zygoma (Figure 13.7). The instrument is then used to disimpact the bone fragment. This approach has the advantage of being relatively simple and fast but it does not permit an inspection of any associated orbital floor fracture.

## *Direct approach*

This approach is used if there is a marked degree of displacement of the zygoma or if the bone fragments are comminuted. Compression plates are used to gain stability at two fracture sites, usually the frontozygomatic and zygomaticomaxillary suture line areas. The frontozygomatic area is exposed by a direct incision in the lateral brow area (Figure 13.8). The zygomaticomaxillary area is exposed either by a subciliary transcutaneous incision or by a transconjunctival incision (Figure 13.9).

Three examples of the outcome following these surgical approaches are shown in Figures 13.8 and 13.9.

The bone fragments are manipulated into the correct position using an elevator inserted via the brow incision. The orbital floor can be inspected at the same time, any herniated orbital contents replaced and an orbital floor implant placed.

Two examples of the outcome following the use of these surgical approaches are given in Figures 13.10–13.13.

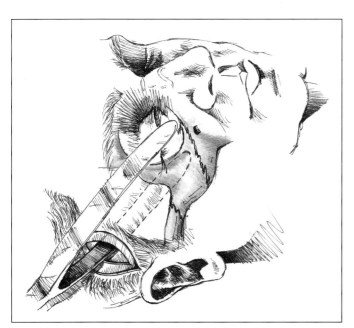

a

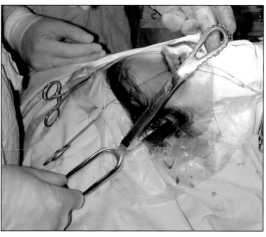

b

**Figure 13.7**
(a) Diagram demonstrating Kilner elevator blade inserted under zygoma. (b) Intraoperative photograph of patient undergoing Gillies approach repair of zygomatic fracture.

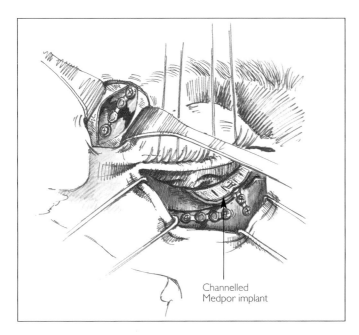

**Figure 13.8**
Incisions for the direct approach to the management of a zygomatic complex fracture.

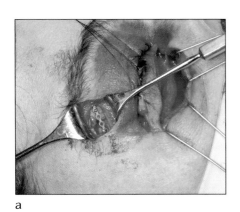

a

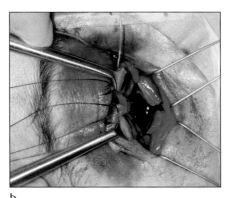

b

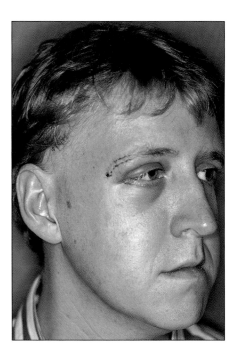

**Figure 13.9**
(a) The frontozygomatic fracture has been stabilized with a microplate. A transcutaneous approach to the inferior orbital margin has been used, as there was a large inferior eyelid laceration. A lateral canthotomy and inferior cantholysis had been performed for the urgent management of an orbital haematoma with compressive optic neuropathy. (b) The inferior orbital margin has comminuted fractures. These were reduced and fixated with microplates. A large orbital floor fracture is also visible. This was repaired with a channelled Medpor implant.

**Figure 13.10**
A patient who has undergone both a direct approach and a Gillies temporal approach to the repair of a right zygomatic complex fracture with a large orbital floor fracture. Incisions are seen in the temporal area, over the lateral aspect of the brow and in the lower eyelid.

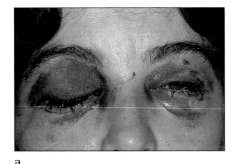

a

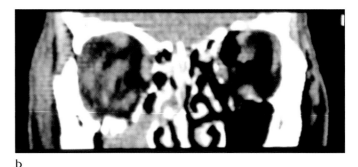

b

**Figure 13.11**
(a) Female patient following assault with a hammer. (b) Coronal CT scan demonstrating right zygomatic complex fracture and comminuted inferior orbital rim fractures. This patient's bony repairs are demonstrated in Figures 13.7 and 13.9.

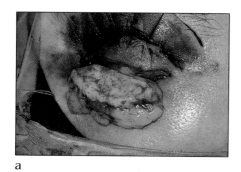
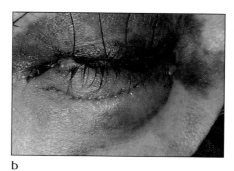

a

b

**Figure 13.12**
(a) A dermis fat graft was placed over the orbital rim to prevent adhesions and eyelid retraction or hollowing.
(b) The appearance at the completion of surgery.

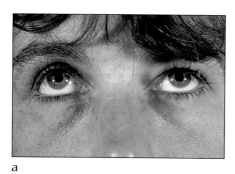
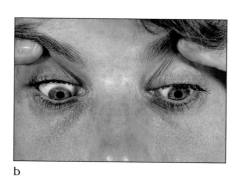

a

b

**Figure 13.13**
The appearance of the patient shown in Figures 13.11 and 13.12 at 3 months postoperatively.

# Further reading

1.  Aguilar EA. The reevaluation of the indications for orbital rim fixation and orbital floor exploration in zygomatic complex fractures. *Arch Otolaryngol Head Neck Surg* (1989) **115**:1025.
2.  Manson PN. Analysis of treatment for isolated zygomaticomaxillary complex fractures. Discussion. *J Oral Maxillofac Surg* (1996) **54**:400–1.

# 14

# Other orbital fractures

## Midfacial fractures

The site and extent of midfacial fractures depends on the type of impact and its direction and degree of severity. It is useful to have an understanding of the Le Fort classification of these fractures although pure Le Fort fractures are rarely encountered in clinical practice: they are often quite asymmetric.

## *Le Fort classification*

1. A Le Fort I fracture is a transverse fracture through the lower part of the maxilla above the teeth. The orbit is not involved (Figure 14.1).

2. A Le Fort II fracture has a pyramidal configuration involving the nasal, lacrimal and maxillary bones. The fracture lines extend through the frontal processes of the maxilla, through the lacrimal bones, the floor of the orbits, the area of the zygomaticomaxillary suture lines and involve the pterygoid plates (Figure 14.2). Orbital wall blowout fractures may be present and the lacrimal drainage system may be involved.

3. A Le Fort III fracture represents a true craniofacial dysfunction in which the entire facial skeleton is detached from the skull base and suspended only by soft tissues. This fracture involves the medial and lateral orbital walls and orbital floor. The fracture lines extend through the superior aspect of the nasal bones, the frontomaxillary suture area, through the ethmoid sinuses and medial orbital walls, below the optic canal to the inferior orbital fissures, and through the frontozygomatic suture areas (Figure 14.3).

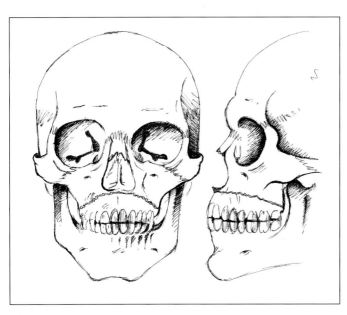

**Figure 14.1**
Le Fort I fracture.

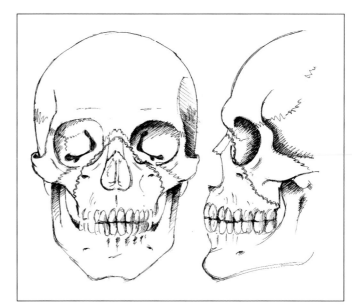

**Figure 14.2**
Le Fort II fracture.

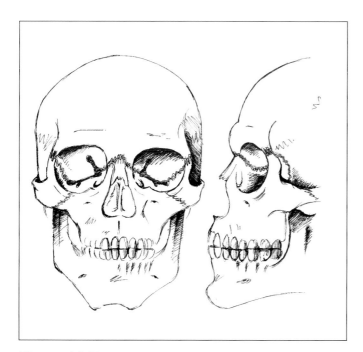

**Figure 14.3**
Le Fort III fracture.

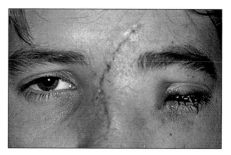

**Figure 14.4**
This patient suffered a severe comminuted nasoethmoidal fracture. A severe globe rupture necessitated enucleation. The failure to reduce the fractures adequately at the initial surgical repair will inevitably result in a severe secondary facial deformity.

# Naso-orbital fractures

Naso-orbital fractures comprise one of the most common patterns of fracture affecting the facial skeleton. They are most commonly the result of a severe impact across the bridge of the nose, e.g. in a motor vehicle accident in which an unrestrained passenger's face strikes the dashboard. The nasal bones are fractured and depressed. The medial canthal tendons are displaced laterally, leading to telecanthus. There are usually medial orbital wall blowout fractures. Damage to the cribriform plate may result in cerebrospinal fluid (CSF) rhinorrhoea. A severe epistaxis may result from laceration or avulsion of the anterior ethmoid arteries. Clinically, the patient usually presents with a flattened bridge of the nose and swollen medial canthal areas (Figure 14.4). Dacryostenosis is a common complication, requiring a dacryocystorhinostomy (DCR). Management of these injuries involves early surgical reduction of the fractures with the use of mini- and microplates. These fractures, along with mid-facial fractures, are best managed by a multidisciplinary team.

# Orbital roof fractures

Orbital roof fractures (Figure 14.5) may also involve the brain, cribriform plate and the frontal sinuses. They are usually caused by severe blunt trauma or occasionally by penetrating injuries. It is important to bear in mind the possibility of such an injury in children who may present with only a minor periocular laceration after falling on a pointed object. These fractures can lead to serious complications, e.g intracranial haemorrhage, brain contusion or laceration, infection, CSF rhinorrhoea, caroticocavernous fistula, pneumocephalus and traumatic optic neuropathy.

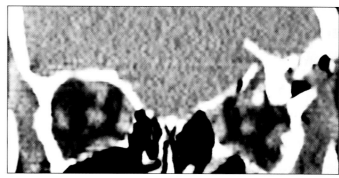

**Figure 14.5**
Severe left orbital roof fracture in a patient who fell 15 feet from a ladder.

Damage to the trochlea may result in diplopia. The patients may also experience painful limitation of upgaze due to inferior displacement of bone fragments. Ptosis may result from direct trauma to the levator muscle or to the oculomotor nerve.

The brain often sustains a concussion injury and may even be lacerated if there is a comminuted fracture. The supraorbital margin may be depressed with a palpable step-like deformity. The management of these fractures should be undertaken in close cooperation with a neurosurgeon.

# Further reading

1.    Greenwald MJ, Boston D, Pensler JM, Radkowski MA. Orbital roof fractures in childhood. *Ophthalmology* (1989) **96**:491–7.
2.    Markowitz BL, Manson PN. Panfacial fractures: organization and treatment. *Clin Plast Surg* (1989) **16**:105–14.
3.    Markowitz BL, Manson PN, Sargent L, *et al*. Management of the medial canthal tendon in nasoethmoid orbital fractures: the importance of the central fragment in classification and treatment. *Plast Reconstr Surg* (1991) **87**:843–53.

# 15

# Traumatic optic neuropathy

## Introduction

Injuries to the optic nerve are rare and may result from a variety of mechanisms:

- Direct injury to the optic nerve – penetrating orbital trauma (Figure 15.1), missiles, partial or complete avulsion (Figure 15.2), intraoptic nerve sheath haematoma (Figure 15.3)
- Indirect injury to the optic nerve – optic canal fracture with contusion of the optic nerve/oedema within the optic canal following a blow to the supraorbital area, expanding intra-orbital haematoma (Figure 15.4)

## Applied anatomy
### *The optic nerve*

The optic nerve runs from the optic chiasm to the globe. The length of the optic nerve is approximately 45–50 mm. It is divided into four parts:

- Intraocular (1 mm)
- Intraorbital (30 mm)
- Intracanalicular (5 mm)
- Intracranial 10 mm)

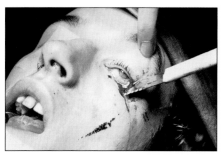

**Figure 15.1**
Direct optic nerve trauma from a knife.

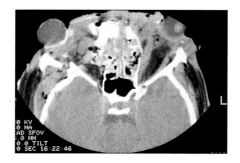

**Figure 15.2**
Severe orbital trauma following a motor vehicle accident with complete avulsion of both optic nerves.

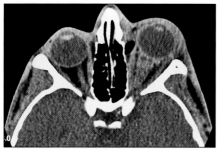

a

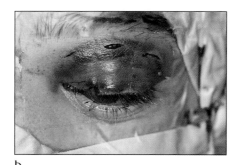

b

**Figure 15.3**
(a) Left intraoptic nerve sheath haematoma. (b) The same patient referred after inappropriate blind stabs had been made in the upper eyelid in a vain attempt to drain an orbital haematoma.

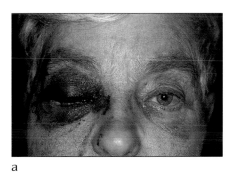

a

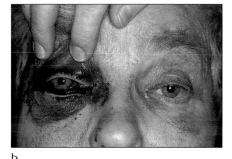

b

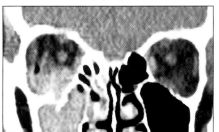

c

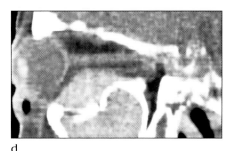

d

**Figure 15.4**
Complete visual loss occurred in this patient 30 min following blunt trauma to the right orbit due to the secondary development of a large subperiosteal haematoma. (a) Periorbital haematoma. (b) Proptosis and hyperglobus. (c) Coronal CT scan demonstrating orbital floor fracture and inferior orbital haematoma. (d) Sagittal CT scan demonstrating proptosis, orbital floor fracture and a subperiosteal haematoma extending to the orbital apex.

The nerve normally has an S-shaped configuration in the orbit. In contrast, the nerve is straightened in patients with proptosis. Dura, arachnoid and pia mater surround the nerve from the optic canal to the globe. The subarachnoid space is continued to the globe and is filled with cerebrospinal fluid. The space is enlarged just posterior to the globe in a bulbous part of the nerve. This is the site where an optic nerve sheath fenestration is performed for patients with benign intracranial hypertension. The central retinal artery enters the optic nerve in a variable position, usually on the inferomedial aspect approximately 10 mm posterior to the globe.

The intracanalicular part of the optic nerve is immobile as the dural sheath is fused to the periosteum of the optic canal. The anatomical arrangement of the nerve in this location leaves the nerve vulnerable to damage from blunt head trauma, which can lead to shearing of the pial vessels supplying the nerve. The intracanalicular nerve is also vulnerable to oedema.

The intracranial part of the nerve extends from the chiasm to the optic canal. The dura mater of the anterior cranial fossa has to be opened to gain access to the nerve in this location. This part of the nerve is closely related to the frontal lobe, the anterior cerebral, anterior communicating, middle cerebral, and internal carotid arteries and the cavernous sinus.

## The optic canal

The canal has a superomedial course as it exits the orbit. Its intra-orbital ostium is located in the lesser wing of the sphenoid in the medial orbital wall and has an oval shape, with its greatest dimension orientated vertically. The optic canal exits intracranially just medial to the anterior clinoid process. The intracranial ostium is also oval, but with its greatest dimension orientated horizontally. Along its entire intracanalicular length the optic nerve is strongly tethered to the very rigid adjacent structures. The annulus of Zinn

forms a tight stricture around the optic nerve as it enters the canal. Within the optic canal, the dural sheath is tightly adherent to the periosteum. As the optic nerve exits intracranially, it is restrained superiorly by a dural fold. The intracranial optic nerve continues its superomedial course to the optic chiasm. To expose the intracranial portion of the optic nerve, the dura must be opened.

For purposes of surgical anatomy, the optic canal may be considered as a triangle:

- The medial wall of the canal abuts the posterior ethmoid sinus and the sphenoid sinus
- The lateral wall of the canal is formed by the bone of the optic strut which separates it from the superior orbital fissure
- The roof lies adjacent to the cranial vault

When assessing a computed tomography (CT) scan, it is helpful to recall that the anterior clinoid process lies just lateral to the optic canal, a constant feature on axial and coronal images. The superior orbital fissure can be confused with the optic canal on CT scans. A number of findings assist in distinguishing these:

- The superior orbital fissure lies at a different level to the optic canal on axial images
- The superior orbital fissure lies on the same level as the cavernous sinus – the lateral wall of the cavernous sinus is usually visible on CT
- The optic canal typically lies at the same level as the superior rectus muscle

## Patient evaluation

Evaluation of the patient may be difficult, especially if the patient is unconscious. It is essential to monitor optic nerve function and pupillary reactions. It is important to establish the time of onset of visual loss. Immediate visual loss following trauma is associated with a very poor prognosis. This is usually due to severe direct penetrating trauma, severe intracanalicular contusion or optic nerve avulsion. A secondary visual loss is usually due to a circulatory disturbance subsequent to the initial trauma. This can occur from continued bleeding into the intraconal, extraconal or subperiosteal spaces.

It is important to exclude other causes of visual loss, e.g. a posterior globe rupture. High-resolution CT scanning examination of the orbits, paranasal sinuses, optic canals and brain should be performed. Plain skull X-rays have no role in the evaluation of the patient with traumatic optic neuropathy. It is imperative, however, that an urgent surgical decompression, if indicated, is not delayed by any imaging studies.

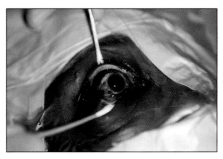

**Figure 15.5**
Lateral canthotomy and inferior cantholysis performed by the bedside prior to a formal exploration of a displaced lateral orbital wall fracture.

## Management

The treatment for posterior indirect traumatic optic neuropathy is determined on an individual basis. In the absence of contraindication to the use of corticosteroids, immediate treatment with high-dose intravenous methylprednisolone may be commenced if the patient has presented within the first 8 hours following trauma; this may be continued for 72 hours. If there has been an improvement in visual function, oral steroids may be continued and gradually tapered. If the patient is evaluated beyond 8 hours from injury, no steroids are indicated. Optic canal decompression may be considered on an individual basis, but the results overall are poor.

Haemorrhage and oedema in the orbit following trauma can cause increased pressure within the orbit, with the risk of vascular compromise. An acute rise in intraorbital pressure can compress the optic nerve at the orbital apex or can result in a closure of the central retinal artery. Under these circumstances an immediate lateral canthotomy and inferior cantholysis should be performed for decompression of the anterior orbit and for the relief of secondarily elevated intraocular pressure (Figure 15.5). Intravenous acetazolamide should be given in addition to topical therapy to lower intraocular pressure.

A formal orbital decompression may have to be performed in selected cases. An orbital haemorrhage cannot be drained through a needle, and blind stabs into the orbit in the vain hope of draining blood should *never* be considered. In contrast, needle aspiration of entrapped air within the orbit may be undertaken with extreme care if visual function is compromised.

## Further reading

1.  Bilyk JR, Joseph MP. Traumatic optic neuropathy. *Semin Ophthalmol* (1994) **9**:200–11.
2.  Goodall KL, Brahma A, Bates A, Leatherbarrow B. Lateral canthotomy and inferior cantholysis: an effective method of urgent orbital decompression for sight-threatening acute retrobulbar haemorrhage. *Injury* (1999) **30**:485–90.
3.  Miller NR. The management of traumatic optic neuropathy. Editorial. *Arch Ophthalmol* 1990;**108**:1086–7.
4.  Newton TH, Bilaniuk LT. *Radiology of the eye and orbit*. New York: Raven, 1990.
5.  Steinsapir KD, Goldberg RA. Traumatic optic neuropathy. *Surv Ophthalmol* (1994) **38**:487–518.

# 16

# Orbital disorders

## Introduction

This chapter deals with the evaluation of patients presenting with an orbital disorder. Such patients pose a potential diagnostic challenge and are encountered by most ophthalmic surgeons relatively infrequently. While it is tempting to save time in the evaluation of such a patient by routinely ordering orbital imaging, this should only be done where specifically indicated after a careful clinical evaluation of the patient. Likewise, the surgeon who is referred a patient who has already undergone orbital imaging may be tempted to examine the scans before seeing the patient. This is a bad habit which should be avoided, as it can cloud the surgeon's mind and lead to short cuts that adversely affect patient management. The scans taken may not have imaged the appropriate area satisfactorily.

The presentation and management of a number of specific orbital disorders are discussed. The disorders which have been selected are those more commonly encountered and which can be considered as very important in clinical practice.

## Evaluation of orbital disease

The surgeon should approach the patient presenting with an orbital disorder with the basic clinical patterns of orbital disease in mind:

1. Thyroid-related orbitopathy
2. Neoplastic disorder
3. Inflammatory disorder
4. Vascular disorder
5. Structural disorder
6. Degeneration/deposition

Although the patient's disorder may occasionally fall into more than one category, this framework allows the surgeon to proceed with the evaluation of the patient in a stepwise and logical manner.

*Thyroid-related orbitopathy is the most frequently encountered orbital disorder. It is the most common cause of unilateral or bilateral proptosis in an adult. It should always be considered in the differential diagnosis of a patient presenting with proptosis or orbital inflammatory signs (Figure 16.1). Although its classic presentation*

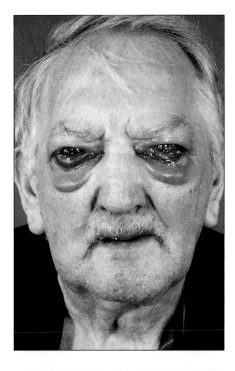

**Figure 16.1** Patient presenting with a rapidly progressive bilateral orbital inflammation and visual loss. He had 'malignant' thyroid eye disease with severe compressive optic neuropathy.

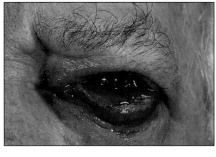

is easily recognized, it can have a variable and asymmetric presentation, making it difficult to diagnose.

Tumours may be primary or secondary, benign or malignant. They may spread to the orbit from the globe or from the paranasal sinuses. Cavernous haemangioma is the most commonly encountered benign orbital tumour. Lacrimal gland tumours represent a small but significant proportion of orbital disease. Lymphomas and metastatic tumours are the most commonly encountered malignant tumours in adults. *In a child a history of rapidly progressive proptosis demands the urgent exclusion of rhabdomyosarcoma as the cause.*

Many orbital disorders have inflammation as their pattern of presentation. The inflammatory process may be acute, subacute or chronic. Acute inflammation is typified by orbital cellulitis. Subacute inflammation may be seen with nonspecific orbital inflammatory syndrome, whereas a chronic inflammatory process is seen with idiopathic sclerosing inflammatory syndrome, or Wegener's granulomatosis. It is important to bear in mind that some tumours may present with signs of orbital inflammation which may respond to treatment with steroids. Such masquerade syndromes are important to exclude by means of a biopsy.

Vascular lesions which may be encountered include high- and low-flow arteriovenous fistulas, orbital varices and lymphangiomas. These lesions may mimic other orbital disorders, e.g. a low-flow arteriovenous shunt can mimic the appearance of thyroid eye disease.

Structural disorders may be congenital – e.g. dermoid cysts, sphenoid wing hypoplasia in neurofibromatosis, encephalocele, microphthalmia with orbital cyst – or acquired, e.g. orbital wall blowout fracture, silent sinus syndrome.

Degenerations and depositions are rarer disorders. Examples include amyloidosis, scleroderma and hemifacial atrophy.

The functional effect of the pathophysiological orbital process on the patient should also be considered. The patient may have a number of functional deficits:

- Visual disturbance
- Ocular motility restriction with diplopia
- Pain
- Neurosensory loss

It is important to be aware that orbital disease occurring in childhood has little overlap with that occurring in adulthood, although the approach to patient evaluation is very similar. Orbital cellulitis is the most commonly encountered orbital disorder of childhood. Malignant tumours, e.g. *rhabdomyosarcoma and neuroblastoma, are very rare but rhabdomyosarcoma must be considered in any child presenting with a rapidly progressive proptosis.* Choristomas, e.g. dermoid cysts, and hamartomas, e.g. capillary haemangiomas, are more commonly encountered orbital lesions. In contrast to adulthood, thyroid eye disease is rarely encountered in childhood.

# History

The history should be recorded in detail. It is important to listen carefully to the patient. Specific questions should be asked:

- What is the time course of the disorder? Acute, subacute or chronic
- Have there been any visual symptoms? Visual disturbance, gaze-evoked amaurosis
- Has there been any pain?
- Has the patient experienced diplopia?
- Has the patient experienced any periorbital neurosensory loss?
- Has there been a history of trauma?
- Is the patient aware of any bruits?
- Are the symptoms aggravated by any specific manoeuvre, e.g. coughing, straining, nose blowing?

The history may suggest a specific diagnosis. A sudden dramatic proptosis with conjunctival prolapse in a child with a recent upper respiratory tract infection may have bled into a lymphangioma. Gaze-evoked amaurosis may be associated with an orbital apical tumour. Pain associated with a short history of a mass in the region of the lacrimal gland suggests a diagnosis of a malignant lesion in contrast to a long history of a gradual painless mass in the region of the lacrimal gland suggestive of a benign pleomorphic adenoma. Periorbital neurosensory loss in the absence of trauma suggests a malignant lesion. A history of 'tinnitus' described by the patient may indicate an arteriovenous shunt. Proptosis provoked by straining may suggest orbital varices. A history of spontaneous unilateral periorbital bruising in an adult may suggest amyloidosis. Spontaneous bilateral bruising in a child may suggest a diagnosis of neuroblastoma. A history of acquired enophthalmos in a female patient with a past history of breast carcinoma suggests a scirrhous orbital metastasis.

A full past ophthalmic, medical and surgical history should be taken. A multitude of systemic disorders can affect the orbit. Unless prompted, the patient may omit details of a previous thyroid disorder, ear, nose and throat (ENT) disorder or treatment for a previous malignancy e.g. breast carcinoma.

Old photographs may be helpful in evaluating the patient. It is always helpful to suggest that these are brought to any consultation.

# Examination

The patient should undergo a full ocular examination, a specific orbital examination, and, where indicated, a full general physical examination. A careful examination of the globe and ocular adnexa may provide important clues to the underlying diagnosis, e.g. dilated episcleral vessels may suggest an arteriovenous shunt (Figure 16.2); opticociliary shunt vessels may suggest an optic nerve sheath meningioma (Figure 16.3); a 'salmon patch' lesion beneath the upper eyelid may indicate the presence of an orbital lymphoma (Figure 16.4); eversion of the upper eyelid may reveal a waxy yellow infiltrate with tortuous vessels suggesting an amyloid lesion – an S-shaped deformity of upper eyelid may suggest a plexiform neurofibroma (Figure 16.5).

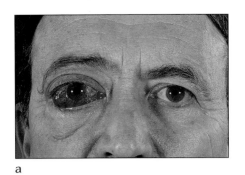

a

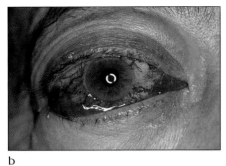

b

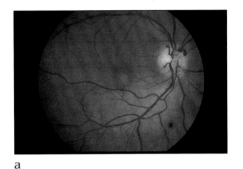

a

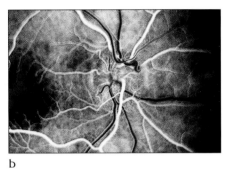

b

**Figure 16.2**
Patient with an acquired right arteriovenous malformation.

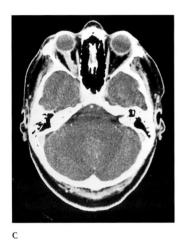

c

**Figure 16.3**
(a) Opticociliary shunt vessels on optic disc in a patient with an optic nerve sheath meningioma. (b) Fluorescein angiogram of the same patient. (c) Axial CT scan of the same patient demonstrating an optic nerve sheath meningioma.

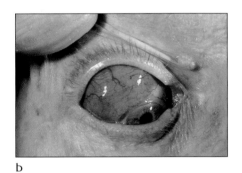

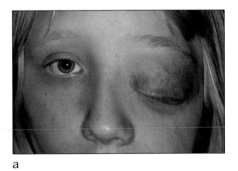

a

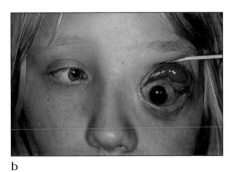

b

**Figure 16.4**
(a) Patient referred with acquired right ptosis. (b) Raising the upper eyelid revealed a large 'salmon patch' lesion. Biopsy confirmed the diagnosis of orbital lymphoma.

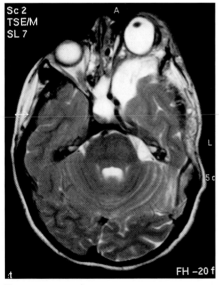

c

**Figure 16.5**
(a) Patient with type 1 neurofibromatosis with an S-shaped deformity of the upper eyelid. (b) Raising the upper eyelid revealed a displaced grossly buphthalmic pulsating globe. The upper eyelid is deformed due to the presence of an extensive plexiform neurofibroma. (c) An axial MRI scan demonstrating absence of the greater wing of the sphenoid with herniated intracranial contents and neurofibroma in the orbit.

## *Specific orbital examination*
### 1. Proptosis/enophthalmos should be assessed and measured using an exophthalmometer

As a general rule, any asymmetry greater than 2 mm is considered pathological. Pseudoproptosis (unilateral and bilateral) from high myopia should be excluded (Figure 16.6). It should be noted if the proptosis is axial or nonaxial. Axial proptosis usually suggests the presence of an intraconal mass. Nonaxial proptosis indicates an extraconal lesion. The globe is pushed in the opposite direction to the orbital mass lesion, e.g. a frontoethmoidal mucocoele causes an inferolateral displacement of the globe (Figure 16.7).

Unilateral proptosis can have a multitude of specific causes but bilateral proptosis, in general, has a more well-defined differential diagnosis. In general, the most common causes of bilateral proptosis include:

- Thyroid orbitopathy (Figure 16.8)
- Nonspecific orbital inflammatory syndrome
- Lymphomas
- Leukaemias
- Myeloma (Figure 16.9)
- Metastatic lesions
- Congenital craniofacial disorders (Figure 16.10)
- Arteriovenous shunts

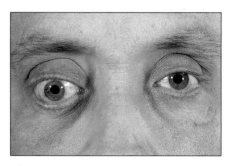

**Figure 16.6**
Pseudoproptosis from axial myopia. This patient has a 'heavy eyeball syndrome'.

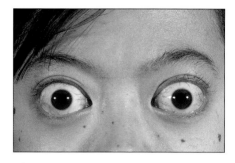

**Figure 16.8**
A 12-year-old boy of Chinese descent with bilateral proptosis due to thyroid eye disease. His proptosis is exaggerated by the presence of axial myopia and shallow orbits.

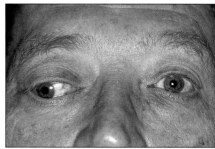

a

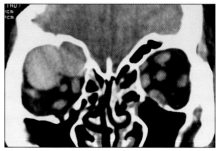

b

**Figure 16.7**
(a) Patient presenting with a right nonaxial proptosis. (b) Coronal CT scan demonstrating right frontal sinus mucocoele.

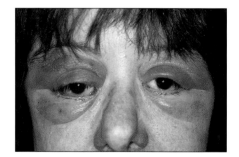

a

b

**Figure 16.9**
(a) Patient with multiple myeloma with nonaxial proptosis and orbital inflammatory signs. (b) Coronal CT scan demonstrating bilateral orbit masses.

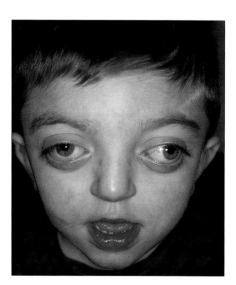

**Figure 16.10**
Crouzon's syndrome.

Enophthalmos may be subtle, presenting as a pseudoptosis or due to cosmetic asymmetry from the development of an upper lid sulcus. The causes are numerous and include:

- Orbital wall blowout fracture
- Silent sinus syndrome (Figure 16.11)
- Metastatic carcinoma (Figure 16.12)
- Parry–Romberg syndrome (Figure 16.13)
- Linear scleroderma
- Lipodystrophy
- Orbital irradiation

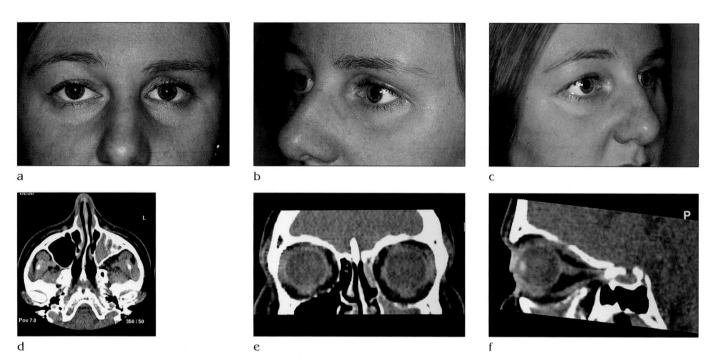

a                                    b                                    c

d                                    e                                    f

## Figure 16.11
(a–c) Patient presenting with a history of a gradual left enophthalmos. (d–f) Axial, coronal and sagittal CT scans of patient demonstrating appearances of a 'silent sinus syndrome'. The left maxillary antrum is small and opacified, the orbital floor is bowed inferiorly and the orbital volume is secondarily increased compared with the right side.

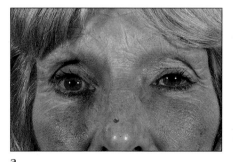

a

## Figure 16.12
(a) Patient presenting with a right upper eyelid sulcus deformity. She had 3 mm of enophthalmos. (b) An axial CT scan demonstrated a right cicatrizing orbital mass and enophthalmos. She was found to have carcinoma of the breast. The orbital mass was a metastatic deposit.

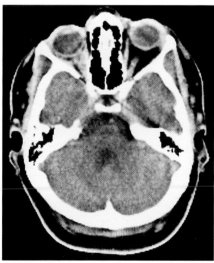

b

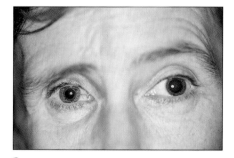

a

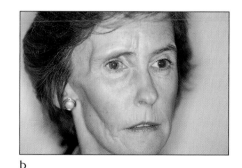

b

## Figure 16.13
Patient with Parry–Romberg syndrome.

## 2. The resistance to retropulsion should be assessed

A solid orbital tumour will cause marked resistance to retropulsion. This assessment of orbital compliance can help to determine the approach to orbital decompression in a patient with thyroid eye disease.

## 3. The orbital margins and eyelids should be palpated

An orbital mass may be palpable. Its characteristics should be noted: e.g. smooth or irregular, soft or hard, mobile or fixed, tender or nontender. A cystic mass may transilluminate. A clinical diagnosis may be suggested from these findings, e.g. a small firm, smooth, fixed, nontender lesion in the superotemporal quadrant of the orbit which has gradually increased in size in an infant suggests a dermoid cyst. A smooth inferior orbital mass in an infant with microphthalmia and a coloboma suggests microphthalmia with orbital cyst, a developmental anomaly. A fullness in the adjacent temple may suggest the presence of a sphenoid wing meningioma.

## 4. The patient should be observed for spontaneous ocular pulsations

The orbit should be palpated for thrills and auscultated for bruits.

## 5. The patient should be asked to perform a Valsalva manoeuvre

The effect on the globe position or a surface vascular lesion is observed at the same time (Figure 16.14).

## 6. The intraocular pressure should be recorded in upgaze as well as in the primary position

A rise in intraocular pressure may be seen in patients with restrictive myopathy, e.g. thyroid eye disease.

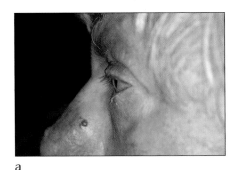

a

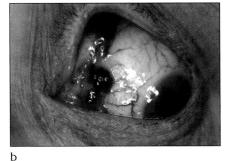

b

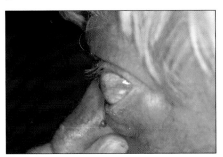

c

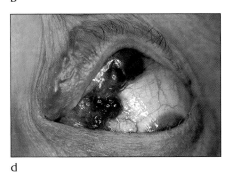

d

**Figure 16.14**
(a) Patient with left orbital venous anomaly. (b) Lesion visible on elevating left upper eyelid. (c) Patient performing Valsalva manoeuvre with immediate proptosis. (d) Lesion increasing in size on performing Valsalva manoeuvre.

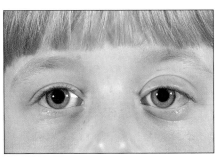

a

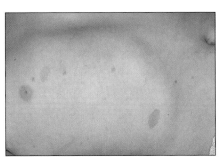

b

**Figure 16.15**
(a) A patient presenting with a left axial proptosis. (b) A general physical examination revealed multiple café au lait spots. The patient had neurofibromatosis and an optic nerve glioma.

# General physical examination

## 1. The patient's skin and oropharynx should be assessed

The presence of cutaneous or intraoral vascular lesions may suggest an orbital lymphangioma (see Figure 16.53b). The presence of café au lait spots suggests neurofibromatosis (Figure 16.15).

## 2. The regional and distant lymph nodes should be palpated

The presence of a generalized lymphadenopathy suggests a systemic lymphoproliferative disorder.

## 3. Cranial nerve examination

A cranial nerve examination should be performed, including an assessment of periorbital and corneal sensation.

## 4. Examination of chest and abdomen

An examination of the patient's chest and abdomen is important wherever there is the possibility of a systemic malignancy, e.g. undiagnosed breast carcinoma.

# Laboratory investigations

A number of laboratory investigations may assist in establishing the diagnosis of an orbital disorder, particularly where the disorder is a manifestation of a systemic disease. These include:

- Chest X-ray: sarcoidosis, bronchial carcinoma, Wegener's granulomatosis
- Thyroid function tests/thyroid antibodies: Graves' disease
- Angiotensin-converting enzyme: sarcoidosis
- Antinuclear cytoplasmic antibody (c-ANCA): Wegener's granulomatosis
- Renal function tests: Wegener's granulomatosis
- Immunology screen: systemic lupus erythematosus (SLE)

# Orbital imaging

Orbital imaging has become a cornerstone of orbital diagnosis and surgical planning. As orbital imaging technology continues to improve, the orbital surgeon has been able to refine preoperative differential diagnoses based on the imaging findings. Good communication between the surgeon and the radiologist is essential in obtaining appropriate studies. The better defined the differential diagnosis following a good history and clinical examination, the more appropriate the imaging will be. The selection of the appropriate type of scan, the area to be scanned and whether to use contrast media are crucial in obtaining the required information. Misinterpretation of images can result when the necessary information required could not be provided by the actual type of scan performed; consequently, it is essential that the surgeon reviews the scans and discusses them with the radiologist to ensure that the appropriate studies have been performed.

The imaging modalities available for the assessment of the patient with an orbital disorder are:

1.  Ultrasonography (USG)
2.  Computed tomography (CT)
3.  Magnetic resonance imaging (MRI)
4.  Magnetic resonance angiography (MRA)
5.  Arteriography

# Ultrasonography

Ultrasonography has a number of potential advantages:

1.  It is relatively cheap
2.  It can be repeated at regular intervals
3.  It provides dynamic information
4.  It has good resolution in the area of the optic nerve and sclera
5.  Colour-flow Doppler USG demonstrates vascular flow very well

These advantages can be exploited in the assessment of selected orbital disorders, e.g. it can be used to assist in the differentiation of posterior scleritis from other orbital inflammatory syndromes.

It has a number of disadvantages:

1.  It requires a skilled and experienced operator
2.  It may be difficult for the surgeon to interpret the findings
3.  The modality has poor resolution in the posterior orbit

For these reasons orbital USG has been largely replaced by CT and MRI, except in highly selected situations.

# Computed tomography

Computed tomography is the single most useful orbital imaging modality. It is relatively inexpensive, faster and easier to obtain than MRI in most centres. The scans can provide good resolution and soft tissue contrast and superior assessment of bone. It is ideal as an imaging modality to assess orbital trauma and lesions affecting bone. It does expose the patient to ionizing radiation and this should be borne in mind when ordering repeated CT imaging. Its major limitation is the loss of resolution at the orbital apex where soft tissue is enveloped by bone.

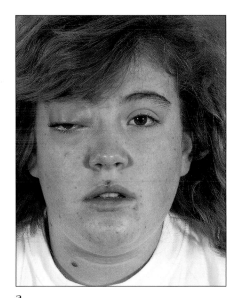

a

**Figure 16.16**
(a) Patient presenting with an acute
right orbital cellulitis. She had
experienced no previous symptoms.
(b–c) Axial CT scans demonstrating
orbitoethmoidal mass. (d–e) Coronal
and axial CT scans – bone windows.
The true extent of the bony mass is
clarified. The lesion proved to be a
benign fibro-osseous tumour which
had obstructed the sinus ostea,
leading to a sinusitis and a secondary
orbital cellulitis.

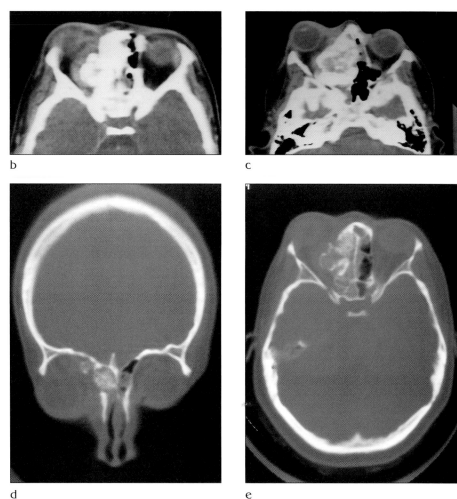

A single film does not have enough range of grey scale to display all the data from a scan. The data can be split and displayed on different films as soft tissue and bone windows. Bone windows should be requested wherever a bone lesion is suspected (Figure 16.16).

Spiral CT can produce volume data sets in the axial plane. These data sets can then be retrospectively reconstructed into thin sections in any other required plane, which minimizes the radiation dose in the acquisition of multiplanar images. It also overcomes problems of patient positioning in the scanner, as axial images are obtained in the supine position. Reconstruction is of most value in the coronal plane, which allows more detailed assessment of the inferior and superior recti and also the orbital floor. Spiral technology provides rapid image acquisition and therefore reduces problems with movement artefact. This is particularly useful when scanning younger patients.

Computed tomography can detect very small intraorbital metallic foreign bodies. Larger nonmetallic foreign bodies such as glass, some plastic materials and dry wood may also be visible on CT. With multiplanar imaging, CT can also accurately localize foreign bodies.

Computed tomography is sufficient for the assessment of tumours of the lacrimal gland. In this situation, the important factors to be assessed are the effects of the lesion on the adjacent orbital bone as well as the size, shape and consistency of the lesion.

A benign pleomorphic adenoma tends to be smooth and regular in outline, homogenous and causes indentation and remodelling of the lacrimal fossa. In contrast, a lacrimal gland carcinoma is irregular, with areas of enhancement and non-enhancement with contrast, and may cause irregular bone destruction (Figure 16.17).

The injection of intravenous contrast media can provide more information about orbital inflammatory lesions and tumours, e.g. the intraorbital and intracranial soft tissue extension of a sphenoid wing meningioma is better seen after the use of contrast. In many cases, however, it is unnecessary, given the wide range of intrinsic tissue contrast provided by various intraorbital structures against the hypodense background of orbital fat. The use of iodinated contrast media may, however, be contraindicated: e.g. renal dysfunction, a history of allergy to iodine-containing contrast media. An acute anaphylactic reaction can be potentially life threatening. The newer low-osmolar contrast media have an extremely low complication rate.

## Magnetic resonance imaging

Although MRI technology is continuing to improve, it is still more expensive than CT and more uncomfortable and claustrophobic for the patient. Magnetic resonance imaging is adversely affected by

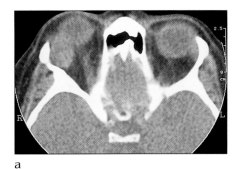
a

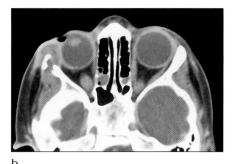
b

**Figure 16.17**
(a) Axial CT scan demonstrating pleomorphic adenoma of lacrimal gland with local remodelling of bone of lacrimal fossa. (b) Axial CT scan demonstrating bony destruction from adenoid cystic carcinoma of lacrimal gland.

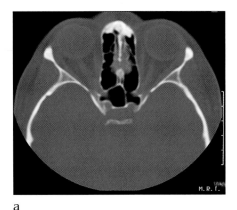
a

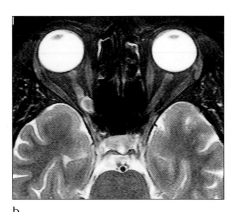
b

**Figure 16.18**
(a) An axial CT scan demonstrating ill-defined orbital apical lesion in a patient presenting with a visual field defect. (b) An axial MRI scan clearly demonstrating the presence of an orbital apical lesion which was compressing the optic nerve. This proved to be a small cavernous haemangioma.

patient movement: it does not, however, expose the patient to ionizing radiation, and has the advantage of allowing scans to be performed in any plane without the need to reposition the patient. Magnetic resonance imaging provides excellent soft tissue detail but, because bone is not differentiated from air, it is not a useful imaging modality for the evaluation of orbital fractures or lesions of bone. Magnetic resonance imaging is the preferred modality for imaging the intracanalicular and intracranial portions of the optic nerve. It is less sensitive for the detection of calcification.

For optic nerve tumours and orbital apex lesions, both CT and MRI may provide complementary information (Figure 16.18).

An MRI image is generated based on the movement of protons in tissues when a patient is placed into the magnetic field of a scanner and then subjected to a series of radiowave pulses. The radiowave pulses are varied by the radiologist to generate T1- and T2-weighted scans. A T1-weighted scan is recognized by the dark appearance of the vitreous in contrast to the very bright appearance of the vitreous on a T2-weighted scan (see Figure 16.20). T1-weighted scans provide the best anatomical detail. Fluid creates a bright signal on T2-weighted scans. A 'fluid void' is seen in areas of high vascular flow where the protons are moving too rapidly to be imaged. Cortical bone appears as a dark area on MRI scans, as the protons are too tightly bound to generate a signal.

The use of surface coil techniques can improve resolution in the orbit, but these are more sensitive to patient movement. A number of fat suppression techniques can be used to suppress the bright signal from orbital fat on T1-weighted images that can interfere with the signal from adjacent extraocular muscles and the optic nerve. The use of these techniques is essential in post-contrast imaging to prevent enhancing lesions from becoming 'lost' against the background of orbital fat. The use of intravenous gadolinium as a contrast medium in combination with fat suppression is particularly useful in the evaluation of optic nerve sheath meningiomas.

There are a number of contraindications to the use of MRI:

- Iron-containing intraocular foreign bodies
- Cochlear implants
- Intracranial vascular clips
- Cardiac pacemakers
- Older styles of prosthetic cardiac valves
- Claustrophobia

If an intraorbital foreign body is suspected, a plain X-ray of the orbit should be performed initially to ensure that an MRI scan is safe to perform.

## *Magnetic resonance angiography*

Magnetic resonance angiography permits noninvasive angiographic studies without the use of intravenous contrast media and spares the patient the dangers of exposure to ionizing radiation. It may provide adequate information to guide diagnosis and management for some orbital vascular lesions. It is, however, subject to a number of artefacts. It does not have the same resolution as catheter angiography and is not sensitive to slow blood flow. It cannot, therefore, exclude the presence of a low-flow dural fistula.

## Arteriography

Arteriography can be regarded as the gold standard to diagnose and characterize certain orbital vascular lesions, e.g. arteriovenous fistulae. It is not without its risks and potential complications. Interventional radiologists can also treat many of these lesions by the placement of intralesional coils via transarterial or transvenous routes. Occasionally, the orbital surgeon can assist such procedures by placement of a cannula into the superior ophthalmic vein. Such procedures do, however, carry risks.

## Review of images

The images should be reviewed in a systematic fashion. The basic preliminary data provided on the scan should be examined:

- The patient's name
- The date of the scan
- The technique performed
- Contrast or noncontrast
- Right–left orientation

The scout film should be examined. This shows the slices as sectioned by the computer (Figure 16.19), which assists in orientation of the plane of scanning performed. The images should be examined systematically, comparing both sides for any asymmetry. It is important to look for any rotation of the head that can lead to misleading asymmetries of no diagnostic significance. The bone structures are examined first, followed by the soft tissues. Interpretation of the images requires practice and experience. It is extremely helpful to review the images with the radiologist.

A number of lesions can be categorized according to their imaging characteristics, e.g. cystic lesions (dermoid cysts, mucocoeles, lymphangiomas, parasitic cysts), isolated lesions

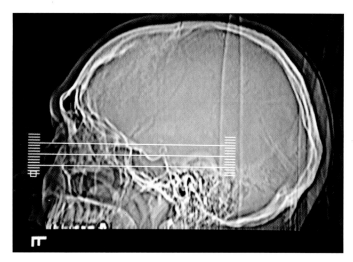

**Figure 16.19**
A scout film.

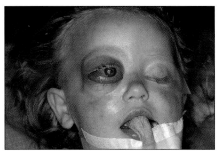

a

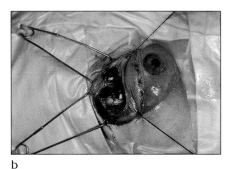

b

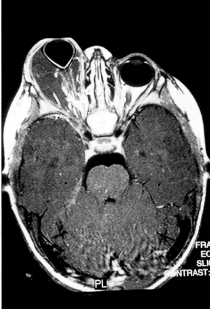

c

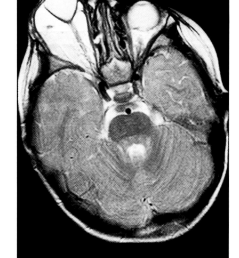

d

**Figure 16.20**
(a) An infant presenting with an acute proptosis following an upper respiratory tract infection. (b) The appearance at surgical exploration confirms the presence of a lymphangioma. (c) Axial T1-weighted MRI scan demonstrating extreme proptosis with tenting of the posterior pole of the globe with an extensive orbital mass. (d) The cystic nature of the lesion is demonstrated on the axial T2-weighted MRI scan with a fluid level visible.

(cavernous haemangioma, schwannoma), hyperostotic lesions (sphenoid wing meningioma, metastatic prostatic carcinoma), lesions with calcification (varices, optic nerve sheath meningioma). This can aid in the differential diagnosis (Figures 16.20–16.22).

Extraocular muscle enlargement, for example, suggests a number of potential differential diagnoses:

- Thyroid orbitopathy (Figure 16.23)
- Myositis (Figure 16.24)
- Metastases (Figure 16.25)
- Lymphoma
- Arteriovenous shunts
- Amyloidosis

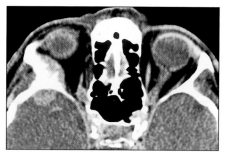

**Figure 16.21**
An axial CT scan with contrast demonstrating a right sphenoid wing meningioma. Marked hyperostosis of the zygoma and greater wing of sphenoid is clearly seen.

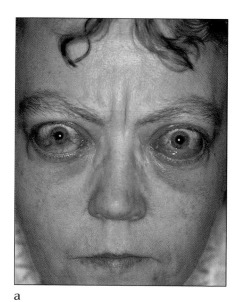

a

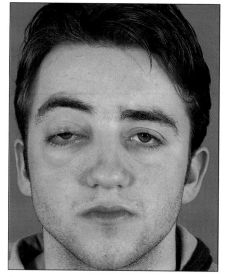

a

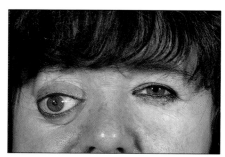

a

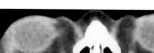

b

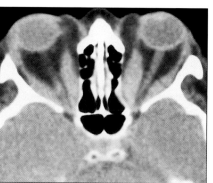

b

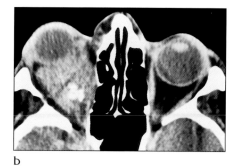

b

**Figure 16.22**
(a) This patient presented with an unrelated visual problem affecting the left eye. Her right nonaxial proptosis was long-standing. (b) An axial CT scan demonstrated orbital calcification within her orbital mass. This was a congenital venous anomaly.

**Figure 16.23**
(a) This patient with bilateral proptosis and known thyrotoxicosis presented with a rapidly progressive visual loss. (b) An axial CT scan demonstrates marked enlargement of the horizontal recti muscle bellies with sparing of the tendons of insertion on the globe. The medial recti are particularly enlarged, with secondary remodelling of the posterior lamina papyracea. The optic nerves are stretched and the orbital apices are crowded. Swelling of the orbital fat compartment also contributes to the marked proptosis. The findings are typical of dysthyroid orbitopathy with compressive optic neuropathy.

**Figure 16.24**
(a) This patient presented with an acute painful ophthalmoplegia. He has unilateral orbital inflammatory signs. (b) An axial CT scan demonstrates enlargement of the right medial rectus muscle. In contrast to the patient with thyroid eye disease, the tendon of insertion is not spared. This patient had acute orbital myositis, which rapidly responded to a short course of systemic steroid treatment.

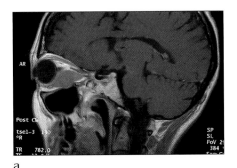 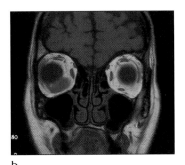

a                                    b

**Figure 16.25**
Sagittal and coronal MRI scans demonstrating a mass within the inferior rectus muscle. The patient had a small intestine carcinoid tumour with metastases.

# Orbital biopsy

Direct communication with the pathologist prior to surgery is extremely useful. Advice should be sought about any special handling of the tissue and the use of special fixatives. A fresh specimen may be required for certain immunohistochemical studies. Previous biopsy material obtained elsewhere may need to be reviewed by the pathologist and may aid in making a diagnosis.

An orbital biopsy may be incisional or excisional or may be obtained by fine-needle aspiration. An open incisional biopsy is performed with the intention of obtaining a diagnostic tissue sample with as little damage to adjacent structures as possible. It is very important to be aware of situations where this would be inappropriate, e.g. a pleomorphic adenoma of the lacrimal gland. In this situation, a complete extirpative excisional biopsy should be performed. An incisional biopsy requires careful preoperative planning and experience. It is essential to ensure that a representative sample is obtained which is sufficient for the pathologist to be able to examine. This can be difficult in situations where normal orbital anatomy is obscured by oedema and haemorrhage.

Fine-needle aspiration biopsy is appropriate for some situations but requires the services of a skilled and experienced cytopathologist. The tissue obtained may, however, be misleading: e.g. a mistaken diagnosis of nonspecific orbital inflammatory disease may be made from small samples of a lesion which is due to the presence of a parasite. Such misdiagnosis can have grave repercussions for the patient.

The biopsy material obtained must be handled carefully to avoid crush artefact. All forms accompanying the specimen must provide the pathologist with all relevant information.

# Selected orbital disorders

A comprehensive discussion of all orbital disorders is beyond the scope of this text. A number of disorders have been selected which represent either common or very important orbital problems.

# *Orbital inflammation*

A significant proportion of orbital disorders present with a picture of acute/subacute inflammation. The disorders most commonly encountered are:

- Acute thyroid orbitopathy
- Orbital cellulitis
- Nonspecific orbital inflammatory syndrome

Rarer causes are haemorrhage into a pre-existent lesion, e.g. a lymphangioma, a fulminant malignant tumour, and specific orbital inflammations, e.g. a systemic vasculitis.

# Acute thyroid orbitopathy

Thyroid orbitopathy is the most common orbital inflammatory disease, accounting for approximately 50% of cases seen. This disorder, in view of its unique character, has been addressed separately in Chapter 18.

# Orbital cellulitis

Microbial orbital cellulitis is a true ophthalmic emergency, requiring hospital admission. It is potentially sight and life threatening. The ophthalmic surgeon must play an active role in the diagnosis and be responsible for monitoring visual function.

**Aetiology.** The commonest cause is sinusitis. Children frequently present with a history of a recent upper respiratory tract infection. The locus of disease is usually ethmoidal and maxillary in children, in contrast to adults, who typically have disease in the frontoethmoidal complex. Many such adults have a previous history of polyps, allergy or trauma. Additional causes include contiguous spread from infections of the eyelid or face, e.g. dacryocystitis and dacryoadenitis, panophthalmitis, metastatic infection, foreign bodies, trauma, infected orbital implants and dental abscesses. Occasionally, orbital cellulitis can complicate surgery, e.g. retinal reattachment surgery. General medical conditions may predispose some patients to infection, e.g. diabetes mellitus.

The organisms responsible for microbial orbital cellulitis secondary to sinusitis are:

- Staphylococcal species
- Streptococci
- *Haemophilus influenzae*
- Diphtheroids
- *Escherichia coli*
- Pseudomonas species
- Polymicrobial aerobes and anaerobes

*Haemophilus influenza* is more common in children, whereas anaerobes are more frequently seen in adults. In debilitated or immunocompromised patients the possibility of fungal infection, in particular mucormycosis, should be considered.

**Clinical features.** The presentation and progress vary, depending on the virulence of the organism(s) responsible for the infection. Preseptal cellulitis is typified by eyelid oedema and erythema with a white eye and no orbital signs (Figure 16.26). *It should not, however, be regarded as benign but as stage 1 orbital cellulitis.*

Orbital cellulitis is typified by:

- Malaise
- Pyrexia
- Eyelid oedema and erythema
- Chemosis (Figure 16.27)
- Axial proptosis
- Restriction of ocular motility
- Increased intraocular pressure

As the condition worsens, the retinal veins may become engorged and the patient may develop optic disc oedema. The development of nonaxial proptosis should raise the suspicion that the patient has developed a subperiosteal abscess (Figure 16.28). The patient may then develop a reduction in visual acuity and a relative afferent pupil defect. The progression to a frank intraorbital abscess is heralded by increased proptosis, increased chemosis, ophthalmoplegia, increased malaise and spiking of the patient's temperature. The development of cavernous sinus thrombosis is heralded by severe headache, delirium, bilateral orbital signs, cranial nerve palsies, neurosensory loss, optic disc oedema and dusky discoloration of the eyelids.

**Diagnosis.** The diagnosis is made on the history and clinical examination findings. The patient should undergo a CT scan of the orbit and paranasal sinuses to determine the underlying cause and to exclude the development of complications such as an orbital abscess. In children it is important to exclude the possibility of a foreign body within the orbit or within the nasal passages. A CT scan demonstrates the location and extent of the inflammatory process and can be repeated if the clinical situation worsens. If the intraconal space is predominantly involved in the absence of associated sinus disease, an intraorbital foreign body should be suspected.

A subperiosteal abscess usually occurs adjacent to sinus disease. It is most commonly seen medially, secondary to ethmoiditis, and occasionally superomedially, secondary to a frontal sinusitis. As the abscess increases in size the periorbita, which is loosely attached to the orbital bones except at suture lines, bows away from the orbital walls, assuming a convex configuration (Figure 16.29).

Small subperiosteal abscesses in children may respond to antibiotic treatment alone. Subperiosteal abscesses in adults

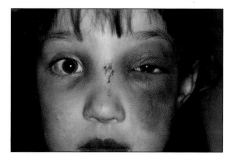

**Figure 16.26**
Child with an acute preseptal cellulitis.

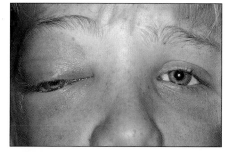

a

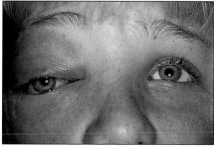

b

**Figure 16.28**
(a) A 13-year-old boy with orbital cellulitis and a nonaxial proptosis. (b) He has marked limitation of upgaze. A subperiosteal abscess should be suspected.

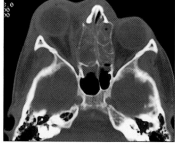

a

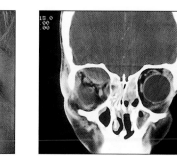

b

**Figure 16.29**
(a) An axial CT scan demonstrates a small medial subperiosteal abscess and extensive ethmoiditis. (b) The coronal CT scan demonstrates a large subperiosteal abscess along the roof of the orbit responsible for the globe displacement seen in Figure 16.28. The attachment of the periorbita at the frontoethmoidal suture line is visible.

**Figure 16.27**
A 12-year-old boy with a rapidly progressive severe orbital cellulitis secondary to acute ethmoiditis.

require prompt drainage. Undue delay in such management can result in severe morbidity. A frank intraorbital abscess may be identified as a poorly defined mass with variable enhancement with intravenous contrast.

Immunocompromised patients may have minimal signs of orbital inflammation as they are unable to mount an adequate white cell response. Such patients may also show less aggressive CT scan signs.

**Management.** The patient should be admitted to hospital and treatment commenced without delay. There has been a tendency in the past to regard preseptal cellulitis as relatively benign and a separate entity to orbital cellulitis. Preseptal cellulitis should, however, be regarded as a potentially serious infection. Spread into the orbit with serious consequences can occur.

It is essential that the patient is monitored very frequently during the first 24–48 hours following admission. The following should be assessed:

- Visual acuity
- Pupil reactions
- Changes in proptosis
- Nonaxial displacement of the globe
- Intraocular pressure
- Conjunctival chemosis
- Eyelid closure
- Ocular motility
- Fundus appearance
- Central nervous system (CNS) function

The assessment of visual acuity and pupil reactions in a fractious child with severe eyelid oedema can be extremely difficult. Under these circumstances the assessment of the other parameters assumes an even greater importance.

With increasing orbital oedema, the conjunctiva may prolapse. This must be lubricated frequently to prevent drying and ulceration. Occasionally, a lower eyelid Frost suture is required, but care should be taken to ensure that this does not abrade the cornea.

The patient's condition can deteriorate very rapidly. Repeated imaging studies are required if the clinical signs worsen. Facilities for surgical management should be available and prepared to accept the patient at short notice.

In patients with eyelid disease, wounds or foreign bodies, swabs should be taken of any discharging wound. Where sinusitis is the underlying cause, swabs should be taken from the nasopharynx and blood cultures taken. Specimens should be placed in both aerobic and anaerobic culture media and submitted without delay. Blood should also be drawn for a full blood count, glucose and biochemistry screen. An intravenous line should be inserted and intravenous antibiotics commenced. Antibiotics are commenced on an empirical basis initially (Table 16.1) and altered according to bacteriology results. The antibiotics to be used should be discussed with a local infectious diseases specialist. Antibiotic treatment should be continued until all signs of infection have completely subsided.

Nasal decongestants and adequate analgesia should be provided. If sinusitis is present, an ENT surgeon should be consulted. A decision may be taken to wash out the sinuses, which also provides an opportunity to obtain sinus aspirates for culture. If the clinical signs deteriorate in spite of appropriate medical treatment, surgical intervention may be required urgently to drain a subperiosteal/orbital abscess.

Abscesses should be drained via an external skin incision, which is usually carried out by a Lynch incision in the medial canthus (Figure 16.30).

The sinuses should be irrigated with an appropriate antibiotic solution and a drain inserted, which should be left in place for a few days. Attention should also be paid to adequate treatment of

---

**Table 16.1** Initial antibiotic regimen for orbital cellulitis

| Clinical variety | Likely organisms | Recommended antibiotics |
|---|---|---|
| Preseptal | Gram positives<br>   *Staphylococcus*<br>   *Streptococcus* | Clindamycin and ciprofloxacin[a]<br>Clindamycin and rifampicin[b] |
| Sinusitis related | Gram positives<br>   *Staphylococcus*<br>   *Streptococcus*<br>   *Haemophilus*<br>Anaerobes rarely | Clindamycin and ciprofloxacin[a]<br>Clindamycin and rifampicin[b] |
| Trauma or foreign body related | Gram positives<br>Anaerobes more likely | Clindamycin and ciprofloxacin |

*Doses recommended:* for orbital cellulitis in adults maximal doses are recommended; in children, liaison with a paediatrician is advised.
[a]Clindamycin: the incidence of pseudomembranous colitis is no greater than with other broad-spectrum antibiotics. Clindamycin has the advantage of greater soft tissue penetration as well as excellent Gram-positive and anaerobic cover.
   Ciprofloxacin: this provides good Gram-positive cover (although less for streptococcal species), excellent Gram-negative cover and some anaerobic cover. It is well tolerated and considered safe in children.
   Empirically, this combination is very broad spectrum, offering excellent tissue penetration and can be used in all situations. Alternatives such as Augmentin (co-amoxiclav) and metronidazole offer a similar spectrum of cover but do not achieve as high soft tissue concentrations.
[b]Rifampicin is useful if Gram-positives are suspected, but it should never be used as a single therapy.

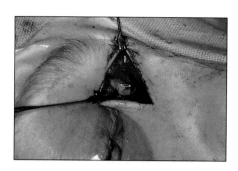

**Figure 16.30**
A subperiosteal abscess being drained via a Lynch incision.

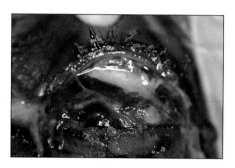

**Figure 16.31**
Patient with severe orbital cellulitis and orbital abscess formation.

the sinuses to re-establish appropriate drainage. This may be undertaken at a later stage. Occasionally, orbital abscesses may occur that require repeated drainage before response to antibiotic treatment is seen (Figure 16.31).

In rare circumstances where the intraorbital tension is very high in the absence of an abscess, a formal orbital decompression may have to be undertaken to prevent optic nerve/ocular ischaemia and exposure keratopathy.

**Complications**. The risk of serious complications following orbital cellulitis is greater in adults than children. Complications are more likely to follow inadequate or inappropriate treatment. The potential complications are:

- Exposure keratopathy
- Neurotrophic keratopathy
- Conjunctival ulceration
- Optic neuropathy
- Septic uveitis
- Panophthalmitis
- Blindness
- Death

## Nonspecific orbital inflammatory syndrome

A number of orbital inflammations currently elude specific diagnosis and are grouped under the term idiopathic or nonspecific orbital inflammatory syndrome. This syndrome was formerly known by the outdated term 'pseudotumour'. Patients tend to present with acute or subacute inflammation. Histologically, the syndrome is characterized by polymorphous infiltrations of inflammatory cells. The inflammation can vary in location, being either generalized or confined to a specific orbital structure, e.g. myositis. Orbital apical disease can lead to an orbital apex syndrome

with visual deterioration and cranial nerve palsies (Tolosa–Hunt syndrome). Patients usually respond to systemic corticosteroids or radiotherapy but a high index of suspicion for the possibility of an alternative pathological process – e.g. lacrimal gland carcinoma or lymphoproliferative disease – must be maintained. A biopsy may be required. Failure to perform a biopsy may delay appropriate treatment and lead to avoidable morbidity.

A specific variety of nonspecific orbital inflammatory syndrome is idiopathic sclerosing inflammation of the orbit. This entity has a characteristic pathological appearance with desmoplasia and considerable fibrosis; which results in an orbital mass lesion that slowly enlarges. Severe loss of function and a significant cosmetic deformity may occur, and early and aggressive treatment with a combination of corticosteroids, radiotherapy and cytotoxic drug therapy is required. Surgical debulking may be required. Advanced disease may even require an exenteration.

## Orbital tumours

A multitude of benign and malignant tumours can occur in the orbit. This section describes those which are commonly encountered.

## Cavernous haemangioma

Cavernous haemangiomas are the most common benign orbital tumours of adults. They typically affect patients between the ages of 30 and 70 years. They are usually intraconal and cause slowly progressive proptosis. They may cause choroidal folds. Those tumours located at the orbital apex can cause compressive optic neuropathy. Gaze-evoked amaurosis may occur. Many asymptomatic cavernous haemangiomas are picked up as incidental finding on head scans performed for unrelated indications.

Histologically, the lesions consist of large endothelial-lined channels with abundant loosely arranged smooth muscle fibres in the vascular wall. The lesions are surrounded by a fine capsule.

The lesions have very low-flow characteristics in contrast to infantile capillary haemangiomas.

A scan ultrasonography shows medium reflectivity and medium acoustic attentuation. The capsule demonstrates a high reflective spike (Figure 16.32a). B scan ultrasonography demonstrates a well-circumscribed usually regular mass, which is homogenous (Figure 16.32b). A CT scan typically demonstrates a well-defined, round or oval mass with a smooth outline that enhances with contrast (Figure 16.32c). More than one tumour is occasionally present.

The management is surgical removal for the majority of these tumours. This carries the risk of significant visual morbidity, however, where the tumour is located at the orbital apex. In this location the alternative management is endoscopic orbital apical decompression. At surgery the lesion has a typical slightly nodular appearance with a plum colour and vascular channels on its surface (Figure 16.33). It is usually easily separated from adjacent structures by careful blunt dissection. Delivery of the tumour may be aided by the use of a cryoprobe.

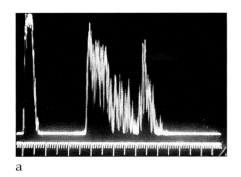
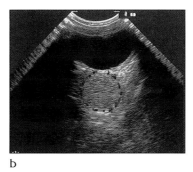
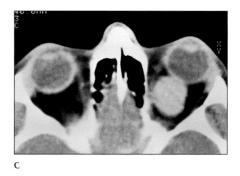

a b c

## Figure 16.32
(a) A scan echography of a cavernous haemangioma showing a high reflective initial spike from the capsule, medium internal reflectivity, medium acoustic attenuation and a second high spike from the capsule. (b) B scan echography of a cavernous haemangioma showing a relatively homogenous mass. (c) An axial CT scan demonstrating a well-defined, oval intraconal mass enhancing with contrast.

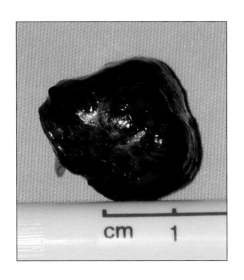

## Figure 16.33
A typical cavernous haemangioma.

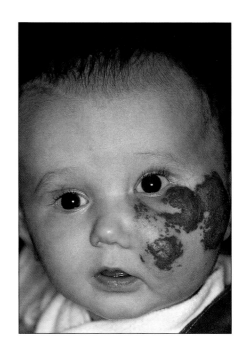

## Figure 16.34
Extensive capillary haemangioma.

Other benign orbital tumours which may mimic a cavernous haemangioma include the schwannoma, fibrous histiocytoma and solitary fibrous tumour.

## Capillary haemangioma

Capillary haemangiomas represent the most common ocular adnexal tumours of childhood (Figure 16.34). These vascular hamartomas typically appear during the perinatal period, enlarge rapidly over the next few months, remain stable for a period of several months, and then begin to involute spontaneously. Resolution of the lesion usually begins in the second year of life and is complete in 60% of cases by 4 years of age and in 76% of cases by 7 years of age. No treatment is therefore advocated unless the lesion threatens to cause amblyopia. The lesion can cause amblyopia by ocular occlusion or by inducing marked astigmatism. In this case, treatment is necessary and usually involves the administration of local or systemic corticosteroids (Figure 16.35).

Intralesional corticosteroid injections are preferred to avoid the numerous side effects associated with oral corticosteroids. A 50:50 mixture of triamcinolone (40 mg/ml) and betamethasone

(6 mg/ml) is used; 1–2 ml is injected within the substance of the haemangioma. A 27-gauge needle should be used and aspiration should be carried out prior to injection in the attempt to avoid intravascular injection. Use of a 10-cc syringe reduces the hydraulic pressure and thus the likelihood of flow reversal if inadvertent intravascular injection should occur.

The response to the corticosteroid injections is usually evident within 1–3 days, and the most marked involution occurs in the first 1–2 weeks. Gradual but slow involution may continue for 6–8 weeks. If the response to the first injection is inadequate, a second injection can be given approximately 8 weeks later. The mechanism of action of intralesional steroid injection is not fully understood, but corticosteroids are thought to produce intralesional vascular constriction, facilitating capillary closure with resultant local tissue hypoxia.

Although safer than systemic steroid administration, intralesional corticosteroid injection has also been associated with complications. These include visible subcutaneous deposits, fat atrophy,

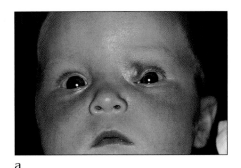

a

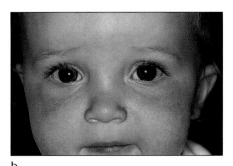

b

## Figure 16.35

(a) A small upper eyelid capillary haemangioma in an infant causing 5 dioptres of astigmatism. (b) The same patient 6 months after a local steroid injection with complete resolution of the haemangioma and the astigmatism.

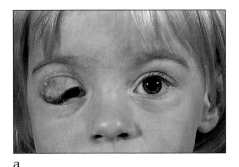

a

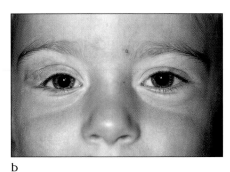

b

## Figure 16.36

(a) A right upper eyelid capillary haemangioma unresponsive to steroid injections. (b) The appearance 2 months following a debulking of the lesion, wedge excision and levator advancement.

eyelid skin necrosis, inadvertent intravascular injection with central retinal artery occlusion, adrenal suppression and growth retardation. Computed tomography should be performed prior to injection into deep orbital tumours for guidance. In such cases, however, oral steroids should be considered (prednisone, 1–2 mg/kg/day). Such treatment should be undertaken in conjunction with a paediatrician and the parents must be fully counselled about all the potential side effects of systemic steroid use.

The lesion may enlarge noticeably after the injection because of the bulk of medication and, rarely, haemorrhage, but mild pressure over the area assures haemostasis. The retinal vessels should be examined during and after the injection for possible compromise of the central retinal artery.

If the haemangioma is very large and requires an unacceptably high dose of corticosteroid, the injection should be limited to the most critical area, such as the upper lid when ptosis is obstructing the visual axis.

Surgical excision is occasionally effective for small, relatively localized adnexal haemangiomas that are unresponsive to pharmacological therapy and are causing amblyopia, and for the removal of remnants after regression. Occasionally, larger eyelid lesions can be safely removed surgically, but such surgery requires skill and experience (Figure 16.36). The Colorado needle is particularly useful in ensuring that such surgery is relatively bloodless.

Treatment with interferon alpha-2a has been generally reserved for life- or sight-threatening corticosteroid-resistant haemangiomas. The response to interferon therapy may be slow and often not rapid enough to alleviate impending amblyopia. Since daily injections for weeks or months may be required and the effect of interferon therapy is often mild, this treatment has enjoyed limited popularity for orbital lesions. Side effects are common and patients must be closely monitored during treatment.

# Optic nerve sheath meningioma

This tumour typically affects middle-aged adults. The tumour arises from the optic nerve meningeal sheath, leading to optic nerve compression usually before noticeable proptosis occurs. Patients usually present with slowly progressive painless visual loss. Unilateral optic disc oedema, optic disc atrophy and opticociliary shunt vessels may be seen (Figure 16.3a,b). These shunt vessels represent a dilatation of pre-existing venous channels occurring in response to obstruction of venous blood flow by a mass compressing the intraorbital portion of the optic nerve.

A CT scan may demonstrate subtle enlargement of the optic nerve. Occasionally an exophytic tumour may be present and may present a diagnostic challenge that requires a biopsy. Calcification may be seen very occasionally. A 'tram-track' sign is sometimes seen on an axial CT scan, where parallel radiodense lines are seen along the optic nerve sheath (see Figure 16.3c). A radiodense ring is seen on a coronal scan. This sign is diagnostic of an optic nerve sheath meningioma.

An MRI scan is performed to delineate the posterior extent of the lesion. A lesion confined to the optic canal can present a diagnostic challenge. Although benign, this lesion in patients under the age of 40 may behave more aggressively and may require surgical excision. Cystic forms of the tumour may spread into the orbit, making surgical excision extremely difficult. Stereotactic radiotherapy may be considered for patients who demonstrate growth of the lesion in order to preserve useful visual function for a longer period of time. Surgical excision is usually performed in younger patients who demonstrate active growth that threatens to extend intracranially. It may also be performed for patients with disfiguring proptosis and a blind eye. Such surgery requires a transcranial approach, with removal of the nerve from the chiasm to the globe.

## Sphenoid wing meningioma

A sphenoid wing meningioma is more commonly encountered than an optic nerve sheath meningioma. The growth of hyperostotic bone into the orbit usually causes a slowly progressive painless proptosis with inferior displacement of the globe. The degree of proptosis can become marked before visual loss from optic nerve compression occurs. Temporal 'fullness' is seen as the hyperostotic bone extends into the temporal fossa. The hyperostotic bone is readily seen on a CT scan but the full extent of the associated soft tissue lesion requires the use of an intravenous contrast agent (see Figure 16.21).

The tumour can be debulked but cannot be removed completely. Radiotherapy is occasionally used, but the tumour is not very radiosensitive. Recurrences are common and repeated surgery is required over the course of the patient's life.

## Optic nerve glioma

An optic nerve glioma, in contrast to an optic nerve sheath meningioma, is an intrinsic optic nerve tumour originating from the optic nerve tissue. It is usually seen initially in children under the age of 10 years. In contrast to an optic nerve sheath meningioma, which causes compression of the optic nerve and gradual loss of visual function, vision is usually reasonably well preserved in children with an optic nerve glioma. The lesion is considered to be a hamartoma rather than a true tumour. Patients tend to develop a very slowly progressive painless axial proptosis. Mucinous degeneration of the lesion can rarely lead to a more rapid progression.

Most optic nerve gliomas are unilateral. Approximately 25% of patients have neurofibromatosis. Bilateral optic nerve glioma is diagnostic of neurofibromatosis.

A CT scan usually shows fusiform enlargement of the optic nerve, although eccentric enlargement of the nerve may also be seen. In contrast to an optic nerve meningioma, there is an absence of calcification. An MRI scan should be performed to assess the posterior extent of the lesion. The optic chiasm may be affected in up to 50% of patients. Other intracranial areas can be affected and may be associated with a poor prognosis.

An incisional biopsy may be performed in those cases where the clinical diagnosis is uncertain or if the proptosis suddenly progresses. For most patients observation with serial MRI scans is appropriate. Surgical excision of the lesion is usually only required in patients with unsightly proptosis and blind eyes. For most patients this requires a transcranial approach.

## Lacrimal gland tumours

The major steps in the management of lesions of the lacrimal gland consist of accurate clinical and investigative categorization into neoplastic, inflammatory and structural processes. These processes may be intrinsic or extrinsic (Table 16.2).

The structural lesions – e.g. inclusion cysts, dermoid cysts and dermolipomas – are not usually difficult to differentiate from the other processes (Figures 16.37 and 16.38).

**Table 16.2** Space-occupying lesions of the lacrimal fossa

| Category | Intrinsic | Extrinsic |
|---|---|---|
| Neoplastic | Epithelial tumour/lymphoma | Myeloma |
| Inflammatory | Sarcoidosis | Granuloma |
| Structural | Dacryocoele | Dermoid cyst |

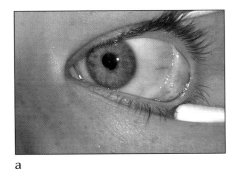 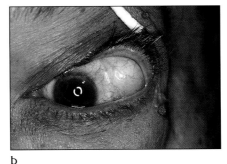 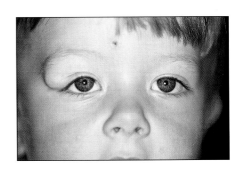

a                                         b

**Figure 16.37**
(a) A typical dermolipoma. The visible portion represents the 'tip of the iceberg'. The lesion typically extends deep into the orbit. Attempted surgical excision risks damage to the lacrimal ductules, resulting in a dry eye; the lateral rectus muscle, resulting in diplopia; the levator aponeurosis, resulting in ptosis; and the conjunctiva, with scarring and a restriction of ocular motility. (b) The typical appearance of a prolapse of orbital fat through a dehiscence in Tenon's capsule. This appearance should be differentiated from a prolapsed lacrimal gland, whose appearance is much paler.

**Figure 16.38**
A typical external angular dermoid cyst.

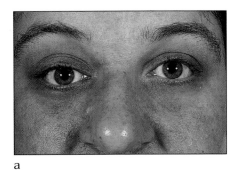
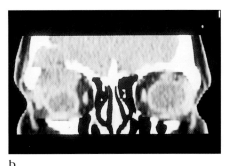
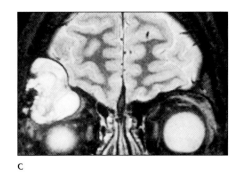

a                              b                              c

## Figure 16.39

(a) A patient who presented with a palpable mass in the region of the right lacrimal gland and a right hypoglobus. (b) A coronal CT scan demonstrating a lesion within the right frontal bone extending into the orbit responsible for the patient's hypoglobus. (c) A coronal MRI scan of the same lesion. The patient's prior history of blunt trauma to the area suggested the diagnosis of a cholesterol granuloma. This was confirmed histologically after surgical removal.

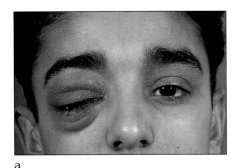
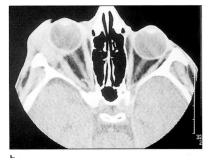

a                              b

### Figure 16.40

(a) A 15-year-old patient with a chronic orbital inflammatory mass. (b) Axial CT scan demonstrating mass in the region of the right lacrimal gland. A biopsy confirmed the diagnosis of an idiopathic sclerosing inflammation of the orbit.

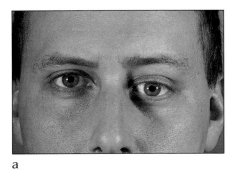
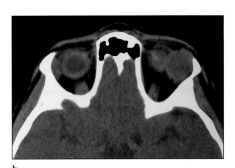

a                              b

### Figure 16.41

(a) Patient presenting with a 2-year history of a gradual painless nonaxial proptosis. (b) Axial CT scan demonstrating a well-defined mass in the left lacrimal fossa with pressure erosion of the adjacent bone. The preoperative diagnosis of a pleomorphic adenoma was confirmed histologically.

The inflammatory lesions (Figure 16.39), particularly those with a subacute or chronic course and imaging characteristics which suggest a non-destructive localized infiltration, should be subjected to an incisional biopsy (Figure 16.40). The management is based on the histological findings.

It has been generally held that approximately 50% of all intrinsic neoplastic lesions of the lacrimal gland are epithelial tumours and 50% lymphomas. Of the epithelial tumours, 50% are pleomorphic adenomas and 50% are carcinomas. Of the carcinomas, 50% are adenoid cystic carcinomas, with the remainder divided between mixed tumours and other carcinomas. Although useful as an aide-memoire, these figures have been challenged.

The main goal in the management of epithelial tumours of the lacrimal gland is the differentiation between pleomorphic adenoma (benign mixed cell tumour) and carcinomas. This can,

however, be far from straightforward. In general, pleomorphic adenoma is characterized by a long history and an absence of pain. It tends to occur between the ages of 20 and 50 years. An orbital CT scan usually demonstrates a well-defined, regular, homogenous mass that causes pressure erosion of the bone of the lacrimal fossa (Figure 16.41b).

In contrast, the carcinomas have a short history and are associated with pain in approximately 30% of cases. Adenoid cystic carcinoma has a peak incidence in the fourth decade. An orbital CT scan may show an irregular lesion with infiltration of adjacent structures, destruction of bone and calcification (Figure 16.42), although these features tend to absent in younger patients (Figure 16.43).

*The major goal is to identify the characteristic clinical and investigative features of the pleomorphic adenoma in order to ensure that complete en bloc surgical removal is the initial management and that*

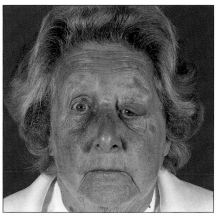

a

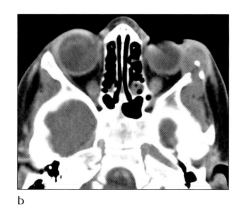

b

**Figure 16.42**
(a) Elderly patient presenting with a rapidly progressive nonaxial proptosis with pain. (b) An axial CT scan demonstrating a mass in the region of the lacrimal fossa with destruction of adjacent bone. A transeptal biopsy confirmed the diagnosis of adenoid cystic carcinoma of the lacrimal gland.

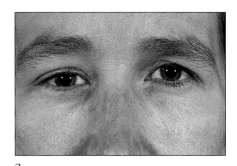

a

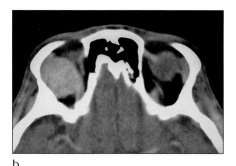

b

**Figure 16.43**
(a) A 40-year-old patient presenting with a 4-month history of a palpable mass in the region of the right lacrimal gland. (b) An axial CT scan showed a large but well-defined mass without any adjacent bony erosion or destruction. The lesion proved to be an adenoid cystic carcinoma.

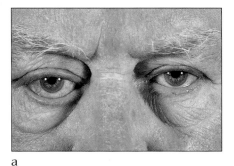

a

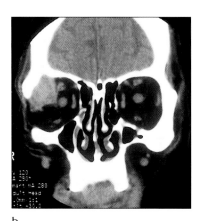

b

**Figure 16.44**
(a) A 66-year-old patient presenting with a 4-month history of a painless nonaxial proptosis. (b) A coronal CT scan demonstrated remodelling of the bone of the lacrimal fossa and a large irregular mass. The lesion was removed en bloc via a lateral orbitotomy. It proved to be a pleomorphic adenoma with malignant transformation affecting only the central core of the tumour.

*incisional biopsy is avoided.* This can be difficult in some patients who do not present with textbook symptoms and signs (Figure 16.44). Surgical intervention for diagnostic purposes in all other lesions involving the lacrimal fossa (with the exception of well-defined, noninfiltrative lesions, e.g. dermoid cysts) should be incisional biopsy.

The prognosis following appropriate management of a pleomorphic adenoma is excellent. There is, however, a high recurrence rate following incomplete excision or incisional biopsy. Recurrence following incomplete excision may be delayed for many years and may be associated with malignant transformation.

The prognosis for adenoid cystic carcinoma is very poor. The tendency to perineural invasion, which may extend centimetres beyond the apparent margins of the solid mass, is a dominant factor in the prognosis. The clinical course is one of painful local and regional recurrence followed by systemic spread. The median disease-free survival is 3 years and overall median survival is approximately 10 years.

When preoperative evaluation indicates a malignant tumour of the lacrimal gland, the recommended therapy is surgical with an initial transeptal diagnostic biopsy followed by exenteration, or en bloc resection, and radiotherapy. The role of radiotherapy is controversial.

## Lymphoid lesions

Lymphoid lesions of the orbit represent a large proportion of orbital tumours presenting in adulthood. Lymphomas form the largest group of lymphoproliferative disorders seen in the orbit. They usually affect patients over the age of 50 years. Typically, they occur in the anterior, superior or lateral aspects of the orbit extraconally and may be associated with a subconjunctival 'salmon patch' lesion (Figure 16.45). A gradual onset with slow painless progression is typical.

On CT scan examination they tend to mould themselves to the shape of the globe and to the adjacent orbital bone. They may involve the lacrimal gland. They tend to have a similar density on CT to that of the extraocular muscles (Figure 16.46).

Approximately 75% of orbital lymphomas are unilateral and 25% bilateral; approximately 50–60% of orbital lymphomas present as isolated orbital lesions; 40–50% have evidence of systemic disease on presentation. Of those patients who present with isolated orbital disease, approximately 15% subsequently develop systemic disease.

Obtaining an adequate safe biopsy is the key to management of orbital lymphoma. The classification of the lesions continues to change but in general they are classified histologically as:

- Benign reactive lymphoid hyperplasia (benign)
- Lymphoma (malignant)
- Atypical lymphoid hyperplasia (indeterminate)

Two tissue samples should be submitted for histopathological assessment. One sample should be sent fixed in formalin for haematoxylin and eosin staining and the other sample should be sent fresh for immunohistochemical evaluation.

The patient is referred to an oncology team with expertise in lymphoma management for systemic investigations to stage the disease followed by radiotherapy and/or chemotherapy. The patients are usually subjected to chest and abdominal CT scanning and bone marrow aspiration. Lesions confined to the orbit are usually treated with orbital radiotherapy alone.

## Metastases

The pathophysiology of orbital metastases reflects the character of the primary tumour. A metastasis may present as a rapidly progressive mass with proptosis, infiltrative signs and bone destruction or may present with an insidious cicatrization of soft tissues. The patient may already have a known primary tumour or may have had previous treatment for a tumour many years previously. Occasionally, the primary tumour is occult.

Some tumours show a tendency to metastasize to particular orbital structures: e.g. breast carcinoma to extraocular muscle, prostatic carcinoma to bone. Some tumours present with unusual systemic features: e.g. carcinoid tumour presenting as an orbital mass and features of carcinoid syndrome from the release of 5-hydroxytryptamine (5-HT) (Figure 16.47).

The tumours which most frequently metastasize to the orbit are:

- Breast carcinoma
- Bronchial carcinoma

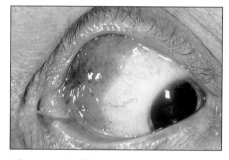

**Figure 16.45**
A typical 'salmon patch' lesion.

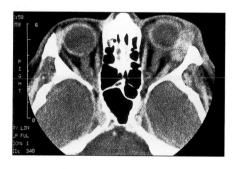

**Figure 16.46**
An axial CT scan demonstrating an orbital lymphoma moulding itself to adjacent structures.

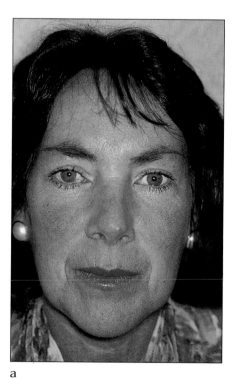
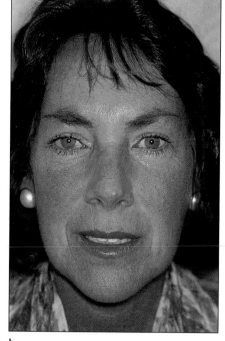

a                                    b

**Figure 16.47**
(a) Patient presenting with diplopia and a right proptosis. (b) The same patient 5 min later, experiencing symptoms of carcinoid syndrome from release of 5-HT. She had a small intestine carcinoid tumour with hepatic metastases and a metastasis to the right inferior rectus muscle (see Figure 16.25).

- Neuroblastoma
- Prostatic carcinoma
- Gastrointestinal tract carcinomas
- Renal carcinoma
- Melanoma
- Thyroid carcinoma
- Carcinoid tumour
- Ewing's sarcoma

Computed tomography scans show typically infiltrative masses which envelop the globe or encase the retrobulbar soft tissues. There may be extension into the paranasal sinuses or into the cranial cavity.

The role of the orbital surgeon is to perform a safe orbital biopsy. The patient should be referred to an oncology team for further investigations and appropriate management. The goal of management is usually palliative therapy, although long-term survival for some patients can be achieved.

## Rhabdomyosarcoma

Rhabdomyosarcoma is the most common primary malignant orbital tumour in children. Although it has been reported from birth to the seventh decade, the majority of cases occur before the age of 10 years. The most common presentation is a rapidly progressive proptosis with an inferolateral displacement of the globe. Associated inflammatory signs may lead to an initial misdiagnosis.

On CT scans, the tumour is often relatively well circumscribed but with associated destruction of bone (Figure 16.48). There may be extraorbital or intracranial extension.

The differential diagnosis of rhabdomyosarcoma is:

- Orbital cellulitis
- Neuroblastoma
- Chloroma

- Lymphangioma
- Capillary haemangioma
- Ruptured dermoid cyst
- Eosinophilic granuloma

Recognition of this tumour is extremely important. The tumour is lethal without urgent treatment. An urgent biopsy of the lesion should be performed. The patient is referred urgently to a paediatric oncology team for staging of the disease and treatment involving chemotherapy and radiotherapy. It is appropriate to consult the team prior to the performance of the orbital biopsy, as other tissue samples may be required under the same general anaesthetic, e.g. a bone marrow aspirate. The prognosis for survival is approximately 95% over 5 years.

## Secondary orbital tumours

The orbit may be invaded by benign or malignant tumours arising from adjacent structures, e.g. the paranasal sinuses, the globe and the eyelids.

Neglected eyelid tumours – e.g. squamous cell carcinomas, basal cell carcinomas, particularly morpheaform tumours occurring at the medial canthus – can invade the orbit and present with proptosis and diplopia. The ocular motility disturbance may be due to a mechanical restriction from the tumour mass itself or it may be paretic from cranial nerve involvement. Orbital exenteration may be required to effect a cure. Such surgery may need to be supplemented by radiotherapy in appropriate cases.

Extrascleral extension of a choroidal melanoma may present with proptosis, but this is rarely seen in Western societies (Figure 16.49). Small extensions are usually managed by a local resection of Tenon's capsule following enucleation. Exenteration is required only in more extreme cases.

Tumours of the paranasal sinuses may extend into the orbit and present with nonaxial proptosis. The direction of displacement of the globe reflects the location of the tumour and its

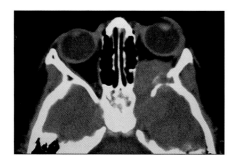

**Figure 16.48**
An axial CT scan of a child with a rhabdomyosarcoma involving the posterior orbit with local bone destruction and extension to the middle cranial fossa.

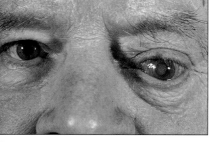
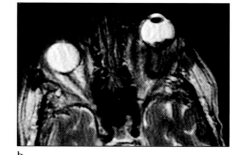

a

b

**Figure 16.49**
(a) Patient referred with a painful left nonaxial proptosis. He had a mature cataract and rubeotic glaucoma. The patient had a dark discoloration of his left upper eyelid. (b) An MRI scan demonstrated an intraocular lesion at the posterior pole and a large irregular intraorbital mass. The patient had a choroidal melanoma with massive extrascleral extension.

extension into the orbit. Such lesions should be referred to an ENT colleague for biopsy. The management of such tumours may require the skills of a multidisciplinary team and may involve the use of surgical resection, radiotherapy and chemotherapy.

## Vascular disorders

### Arteriovenous (a–v) shunts

Arteriovenous shunts may be congenital or acquired. They can follow trauma or occur spontaneously. They are classified haemodynamically as high flow or low flow. The high-flow shunts are usually post-traumatic caroticocavernous fistulas or a–v malformations, whereas the low-flow shunts are spontaneous dural a–v fistulas of the cavernous sinus region.

The clinical features of high-flow shunts are dramatic (Figure 16.50):

- Pulsatile proptosis
- Bruit
- Eyelid oedema
- Reduced visual acuity
- Chemosis/conjunctival prolapse
- Raised intraocular pressure secondary to raised episcleral venous pressure
- Retinal vascular dilatation
- Cranial nerve palsy

In contrast, the clinical features of low-flow shunts are far less dramatic and can lead to misdiagnosis (Figure 16.51):

- A red eye with episcleral venous dilation
- Mild proptosis
- Mildly raised intraocular pressure

This clinical presentation often leads to misdiagnoses of conjunctivitis, episcleritis, thyroid eye disease and glaucoma.

CT scan images demonstrate proptosis, enlargement of the superior ophthalmic vein (Figure 16.52) and enlargement of the extraocular muscles. Recognition of enlargement of the superior ophthalmic vein is important, as enlargement of the extraocular muscles in a patient with a red eye can reinforce the misdiagnosis of thyroid eye disease. Enlargement of the cavernous sinuses is an important radiological feature of a caroticocavernous fistula.

The diagnosis is confirmed by angiography. This also aids in planning treatment.

High-flow shunts usually require treatment, whereas low-flow shunts can be managed conservatively and the patient's visual status monitored as many low-flow shunts spontaneously resolve. Treatment of shunts requires the expertise of the interventional radiologist. Closure of shunts is usually achieved via the endovascular route, either arterial or venous, depending on the type of fistula and the haemodynamics. Embolic agents include balloons and coils for direct high-flow lesions and particles for low-flow fistulae. These techniques have significantly advanced the treatment of these lesions with relatively low complication rates. The associated risks of a cerebrovascular accident must, however, be taken into account.

## Varices

Orbital varices may be haemodynamically active or inactive. Active lesions have large connections with the systemic venous system and demonstrate enlargement in response to changes in venous pressure. Patients may present with intermittent proptosis and orbital pain aggravated by straining. Inactive lesions are more haemodynamically isolated and are characterized by stasis of blood, which can lead to thrombosis or occasionally haemorrhage.

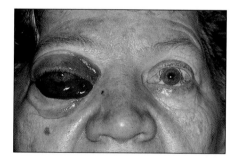

**Figure 16.50**
A caroticocavernous fistula.

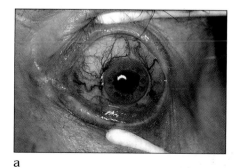

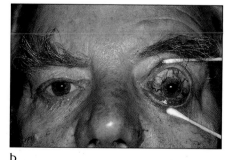

a        b

**Figure 16.51**
A patient with a low-flow arteriovenous shunt.

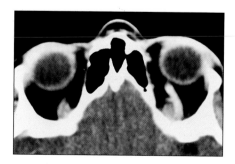

**Figure 16.52**
Enlargement of the superior ophthalmic vein.

Varices can be extremely difficult to manage. The indications for intervention are severe haemorrhage that causes pain and visual deterioration that is not amenable to conservative management, and severe cosmetic disfigurement. Lesions that are haemodynamically active must be approached with respect and caution (see Figure 16.14).

## Lymphangioma

Lymphangiomas are haemodynamically isolated thin-walled, endothelially lined vascular hamartomas. They are not affected by a Valsalva manoeuvre. They may be superficial and/or deep and tend to be diffuse. Superficial lesions may be confined to the conjunctiva and/or eyelid and may be amenable to resection if necessary. Deep lesions tend to present in infancy or early childhood as a gradually enlarging mass with decreased vision or as a sudden dramatic acute proptosis following a spontaneous haemorrhage into a previously unrecognized lesion. This typically occurs in the context of an upper respiratory tract infection. Deep orbital lesions which have a superficial component are readily diagnosed clinically. A deep lesion may present more of a diagnostic challenge. The patient may show other clues which assist in the diagnosis, e.g. intraoral vascular lesions (Figure 16.53).

Appearances on CT scans of deep lymphangiomas are typically low-density cystic masses in the intraconal and extraconal spaces. Contrast enhancement may occur around the lesions in approximately 50% of cases The lesions delineate extremely well on MRI (Figure 16.54).

Management should be conservative wherever possible. Surgery may be required if an acute haemorrhage has caused compressive optic neuropathy or exposure keratopathy which is not amenable to conservative management alone. Surgery should be conservative and aimed at removal of the major macrocysts, which raise intraorbital pressure, cause extreme proptosis or compress the optic nerve. Multiple surgical resections are associated with a poor final visual acuity.

Sclerosing agents have been advocated by some interventional radiologists for the management of some orbital lymphangiomas. It is essential to ensure that the lesion is haemodynamically isolated before such agents are used. The use of sclerosing agents represents an area of current controversy. Likewise, the use of systemic steroids for severe exacerbations is controversial.

## *Structural disorders*

### Dermoid cyst

A dermoid cyst is a choristoma which contains skin and skin appendages, i.e. hairs, keratin and sebaceous gland material. (An epidermoid cyst is very similar but does not contain skin appendages.) The lesion occurs in association with bony sutures, most commonly the frontozygomatic suture (Figure 16.55). It

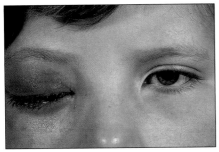

a

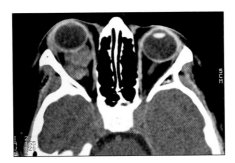

a

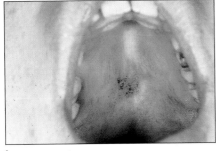

b

**Figure 16.53**
(a) A 10-year-old patient presenting with an acute right proptosis.
(b) Examination of the patient's hard palate revealed a vascular anomaly. The orbital lesion was a lymphangioma with an acute intralesional haemorrhage.

b

**Figure 16.54**
(a) Axial CT scan demonstrating appearances of orbital lymphangioma. (b) Axial T2 MRI scan of the same patient.

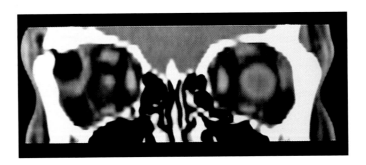

**Figure 16.55**
An intraorbital dermoid cyst related to the frontozygomatic suture.

usually presents in infancy as a smooth painless gradually enlarging cystic mass that lies outside the orbit (see Figure 16.37). It may be freely mobile or it may be fixed to the underlying bony suture. It may, however, present with a gradually progressive painless axial or nonaxial proptosis in a young adult if it arises from a deeper bony suture, e.g. the sphenozygomatic suture. Rarely, the lesion may rupture following minor trauma and present with an acute orbital inflammation.

Superficial freely mobile lesions are simple to remove and require no preoperative imaging. Superficial lesions at the lateral aspect of the eyebrow or superomedial orbit can be removed via an upper eyelid skin crease incision, avoiding a visible scar. Great care should be taken not to rupture the cyst during the surgical excision.

Lesions that are fixed to bone should be imaged with a CT scan. It is important to exclude the possibility of a 'dumb-bell' dermoid cyst, which extends through the lateral orbital bone into the orbit. The surgical approach can then be selected to adequately remove the lesion in its entirety. This may require a formal lateral orbitotomy. Failure to remove the entire lesion will lead to a recurrence, which will be more difficult to manage. A preoperative CT scan is certainly indicated for any lesion at the medial canthus. The differential diagnosis of a mass at the medial canthus includes an encephalocele, which should be excluded.

# Further reading

1. Bonavolonta G. Anterior, medial, lateral and combined surgical approaches to orbital tumor resection. In: Bosniak S, ed., *Principles and practice of ophthalmic plastic and reconstructive surgery*, Vol. 11. Philadelphia: WB Saunders, 1996, pp. 1060–9.
2. Bonavolonta G. Surgical approaches to the orbit. In: Bosniak S, ed., *Principles and practice of ophthalmic plastic and reconstructive surgery*, Vol. 11. Philadelphia: WB Saunders, 1996, pp. 1050–5.
3. Bosniak S. *Principles and practice of ophthalmic plastic and reconstructive surgery*. Philadelphia: WB Saunders, 1996, pp. 999–1006.
4. Char DH, Miller T, Kroll S. Orbital metastases: diagnosis and course. *Br J Ophthalmol* (1997) **81**:386–90.
5. Dutton J. *Atlas of clinical and surgical orbital anatomy*. Philadelphia: WB Saunders, 1994.
6. Haik BG, Karcioglu ZA, Gordon RA, Pechous BP. Capillary hemangioma (infantile periocular hemangioma). *Surv Ophthalmol* (1994) **38**:399–426.
7. Harris GJ. Orbital vascular malformations: a consensus statement on terminology and its clinical implications. Orbital Society. *Am J Ophthalmol* (1999) **127**:453–5.
8. Lacey B, Chang W, Rootman J. Nonthyroid causes of extraocular muscle disease. *Surv Ophthalmol* (1999) **44**:187–213.
9. McNab AA, Wright JE. Cavernous haemangiomas of the orbit. *Austral NZ J Ophthalmol* (1989) **17**:337–45.
10. McNab AA, Wright JE. Orbitofrontal cholesterol granuloma. *Ophthalmology* (1990) **97**:28–32.
11. McNab AA, Wright JE, Caswell AG. Clinical features and surgical management of dermolipomas. *Austral NZ J Ophthalmol* (1990) **18**:159–62.
12. McNab AA. Subconjunctival fat prolapse. *Austral NZ J Ophthalmol* (1999) **27**:33–6.
13. Rootman J, ed. *Diseases of the orbit*, Philadelphia: JB Lippincott, 1988.
14. Rootman J, Kao SC, Graeb DA. Multidisciplinary approaches to complicated vascular lesions of the orbit. *Ophthalmology* (1992) **99**:1440–6.
15. Rootman J, McCarthy M, White V, Harris G, Kennerdell J. Idiopathic sclerosing inflammation of the orbit. A distinct clinicopathologic entity. *Ophthalmology* (1994) **101**:570–84.
16. Rootman J. Why 'orbital pseudotumour' is no longer a useful concept. *Br J Ophthalmol* (1998) **82**:339–40.
17. Rose GE, Wright JE. Pleomorphic adenoma of the lacrimal gland. *Br J Ophthalmol* (1992) **76**:395–400.
18. Soparkar CN, Patrinely JR, Cuaycong MJ, et al. The silent sinus syndrome. A cause of spontaneous enophthalmos. *Ophthalmology* (1994) **101**:772–8.
19. Walker RS, Custer PL, Nerad JA. Surgical excision of periorbital capillary hemangiomas. *Ophthalmology* (1994) **101**:1333–40.
20. Wright JE, Stewart WB, Krohel GB. Factors affecting the survival of patients with lacrimal gland tumours. *Can J Ophthalmol* (1982) **17**:3–9.
21. Wright JE, Rose GE, Garner A. Primary malignant neoplasms of the lacrimal gland. *Br J Ophthalmol* (1992) **76**:400–7.

# 17

# Surgical approaches to the orbit

## Introduction

This chapter describes the surgical approaches used in the management of orbital lesions. The surgical approaches used to achieve a decompression of the orbit in the management of thyroid eye disease are described in Chapter 18. The surgical approaches used to manage orbital wall blowout fractures are described in Chapter 12.

It is important to ensure that the patient has been properly prepared for surgery before proceeding with an orbitotomy, particularly with regard to the management of hypertension and the use of antiplatelet and anticoagulant agents. Informed consent should be obtained ensuring that the patient understands the small risk of visual loss from intraoperative trauma to the optic nerve, or from postoperative intraorbital haemorrhage.

The anaesthetist should understand the surgical approach and the requirements for head position, nasal packing, the use of vasoconstrictive agents, hypotension, the potential risk of the oculocardiac reflex, the anticipated length of the surgical procedure and the requirements for postoperative pain medication.

It is essential that the patient's computed tomography/magnetic resonance imaging (CT/MRI) scans are available. These should be clearly visible on a viewing screen adjacent to the operating table. These should be reviewed before the orbitotomy is commenced and the correct side confirmed. The scans may need to be reviewed to confirm the location of the orbital lesion as the surgery proceeds, depending on the intraoperative findings.

The surgical plan should be coordinated with the nursing team to ensure that the appropriate surgical instrumentation is available. A potential change in the surgical approach depending on the intraoperative findings should be anticipated and the necessary instrumentation made available. It is also important to liaise with the pathologist prior to surgery and to complete pathology request forms prior to the commencement of surgery.

If a multidisciplinary team is involved in the surgical management of the patient, it is important to define the responsibilities of each member in advance. This also relates to the postoperative care of the patient.

## Selection of the surgical approach

The choice of surgical approach to an orbital lesion will depend on:

- The anatomical location of the lesion
- The size and extent of the lesion
- The suspected pathology
- The goal of the surgery

## *The anatomical location of the lesion*

Orbital tumours that lie anterior to the equator of the globe are most commonly approached via an anterior orbitotomy. Tumours located posterior to the equator of the globe require a more complex deep surgical approach, which is also influenced by the relationship of the tumour to the optic nerve. *A surgical approach should be selected which avoids crossing the optic nerve.*

## *The size and extent of the lesion*

Most orbital lesions can be managed adequately via a single orbitotomy approach. Some orbital lesions require a combination of orbitotomy approaches, e.g. a medial transconjunctival orbitotomy can be combined with a lateral orbitotomy which enables the globe to be retracted laterally. This can greatly improve safe surgical access to large or deep medial orbital lesions.

## The suspected pathology

The surgical approach is influenced by the aim of the operation. An incisional biopsy of a suspected lacrimal gland carcinoma should be performed via a trans-septal anterior orbitotomy. In contrast, a suspected pleomorphic adenoma of the lacrimal gland should not be subjected to an incisional biopsy but should be removed as an extirpative excisional biopsy via a lateral orbitotomy.

## The goal of the surgery

In the management of orbital tumours the goals of the surgery are usually to achieve as safely as possible an incisional biopsy, an excisional biopsy, debulking or decompression of the tumour. In general, infiltrative processes suggest a malignant lesion and require an incisional biopsy. Well-circumscribed lesions generally suggest a benign lesion that can be removed as an excisional biopsy, e.g. a cavernous haemangioma. Some benign orbital lesions may not be amenable to surgical excision but a debulking procedure may be beneficial, e.g. a plexiform neurofibroma. A small benign orbital apical tumour located medial to the optic nerve, causing compressive optic neuropathy, may be better managed by means of an endoscopic medial orbital wall decompression than by a much more invasive procedure, e.g. a transfrontal craniotomy.

## Applied anatomy
## The orbital walls

The orbit consists of four walls that angle posteriorly to form a pyramidal shape (Figure 17.1). The orbital rim is formed superiorly by the frontal bone, laterally by the zygomatic bone, medially by the frontal and maxillary bones and inferiorly by the zygomatic and maxillary bones. The orbital roof is concave and forms the floor of the anterior cranial fossa. In older patients portions of the bone of the orbital roof may be absorbed, leaving the periorbita in direct contact with the dura mater of the anterior cranial fossa. This should be borne in mind when assessing penetrating injuries of the orbit and when undertaking an exenteration. The concavity of the orbital roof is more exaggerated anterolaterally where the lacrimal gland is located within the lacrimal gland fossa. The orbital roof is separated from the lateral orbital wall by the superior orbital fissure (Figure 17.1).

The lateral orbital wall is relatively flat on the orbital side, but curved on its exterior surface to accommodate the temporalis muscle (Figures 17.1 and 17.2).

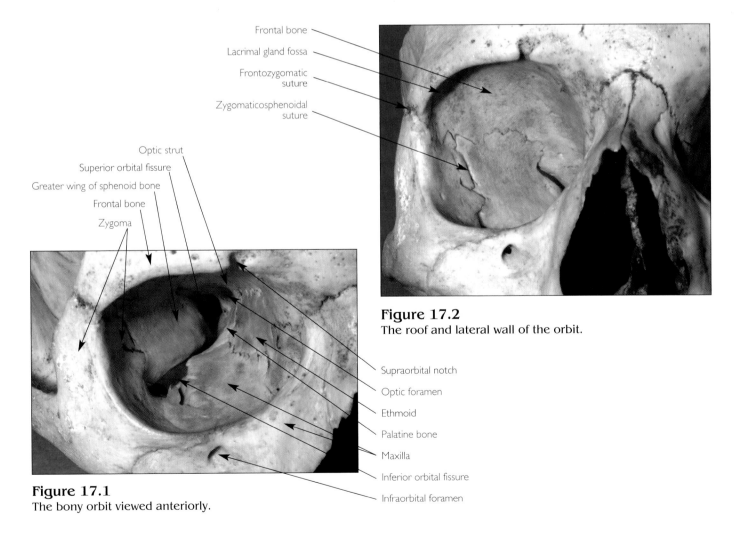

Frontal bone
Lacrimal gland fossa
Frontozygomatic suture
Zygomaticosphenoidal suture

Optic strut
Superior orbital fissure
Greater wing of sphenoid bone
Frontal bone
Zygoma

**Figure 17.2**
The roof and lateral wall of the orbit.

Supraorbital notch
Optic foramen
Ethmoid
Palatine bone
Maxilla
Inferior orbital fissure
Infraorbital foramen

**Figure 17.1**
The bony orbit viewed anteriorly.

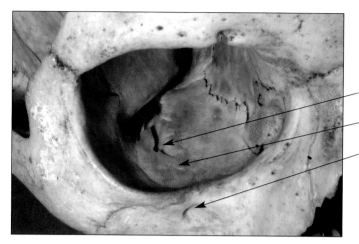

Infraorbital groove

Infraorbital canal

Infraorbital foramen

**Figure 17.3**
The floor of the orbit. The floor and the medial wall of the orbit are both convex.

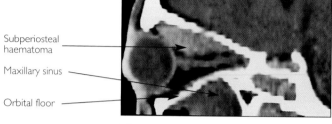

Subperiosteal haematoma

Maxillary sinus

Orbital floor

**Figure 17.5**
A sagittal CT scan of the orbit in a patient with a subperiosteal haematoma. The floor of the orbit is seen to slope upwards from the anterior orbital rim to the apex of the orbit.

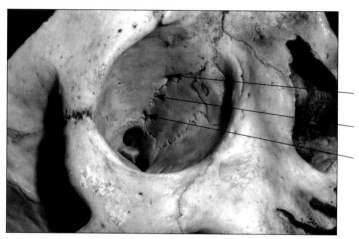

Anterior ethmoidal foramen

Frontoethmoidal suture line

Posterior ethmoidal foramen

**Figure 17.4**
The medial orbital wall.

The orbital floor forms the roof of the maxillary sinus and runs upward posteriorly to the orbital apex (Figures 17.3–17.5). The floor curves upwards medially to meet the medial orbital wall. The medial orbital wall is the lateral wall of the ethmoid sinus. The medial wall and the floor are both convex.

The medial wall and the roof of the orbit are separated by the frontoethmoidal suture line (see Figure 17.4). The anterior and posterior ethmoidal neurovascular bundles travel through the foramina in the suture line (Figure 17.4).

The bones of the orbital floor and medial wall are very thin. The medial wall of the orbit consists mainly of the very fine lamina papyracea. The infraorbital groove and canal separate the orbital floor into a thin medial portion and a thicker lateral portion. The thin bone of the medial orbital floor and the medial orbital wall is fractured in trauma.

The infraorbital groove runs anteriorly along the orbital floor from the inferior orbital fissure (see Figure 17.3). It usually acquires a bony roof midway along the orbital floor, forming the infraorbital canal. The canal leaves the orbit at the infraorbital foramen. The infraorbital neurovascular bundle travels in the infraorbital groove and through the infraorbital canal. The nerve is susceptible to injury from a blowout fracture and from any surgical manipulations performed along the orbital floor. A communicating branch of the infraorbital artery arises between the infraorbital groove and the infraorbital margin and passes through the periorbita into the orbit. This constant vessel is encountered when the periorbita is raised from the orbital floor and should be cauterized to prevent bleeding during an orbital floor dissection.

The anterior and posterior ethmoidal foramina lie along the frontoethmoidal suture line. The anterior ethmoidal foramen is situated approximately 25 mm posterior to the anterior lacrimal crest. The posterior ethmoidal foramen is located approximately 35 mm posterior to the anterior lacrimal crest. The optic foramen lies approximately 5–8 mm posterior to the posterior ethmoidal foramen. The ethmoidal neurovascular bundles form important surgical landmarks. They can be seen exiting the orbit within a sheath of periorbita. They should be carefully identified and cauterized before they are cut when performing an orbital exenteration. When performing a medial orbital wall decompression from the orbital approach, these neurovascular bundles

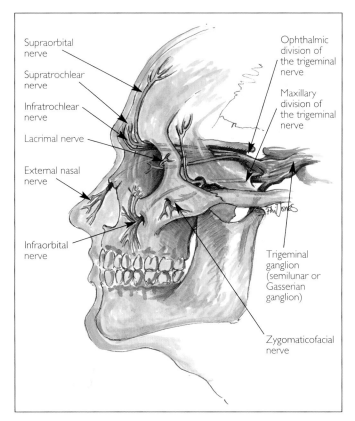

**Figure 17.6**
The course of the ophthalmic and maxillary divisions of the trigeminal nerve.

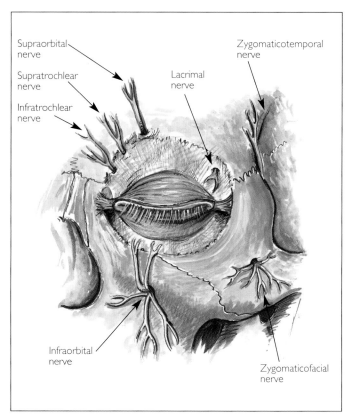

**Figure 17.7**
The location of the periorbital sensory nerves exiting the orbit.

should be avoided and the wall perforated and removed from below them.

The zygomaticotemporal and zygomaticofacial neurovascular bundles pass through the zygomaticotemporal and zygomaticofacial foramina in the lateral orbital wall (see Figures 17.6 and 17.7). The zygomaticotemporal and zygomaticofacial nerves are branches of the maxillary division of the trigeminal nerve. The nerves are severed during surgery on the lateral orbital wall, e.g. a lateral orbitotomy. This results in a small area of hypoaesthesia postoperatively over the zygoma and temple but this is usually insignificant in contrast to the sensory loss that follows damage to the infraorbital nerve. The zygomaticotemporal and zygomaticofacial arteries are branches of the lacrimal artery, which itself is a branch of the ophthalmic artery (see Figure 17.8). These vessels are encountered when the periorbita is raised from the lateral orbital wall. These vessels should be cauterized before they are severed.

## *The periorbita*

The periorbita covers all the bones of the internal orbit. Unlike the periosteum covering bones elsewhere, the periorbita is loosely adherent over the orbital walls, except at the orbital suture lines and along the orbital rims, where it is tightly adherent to the bone (Figure 17.9). The subperiosteal space is a potential

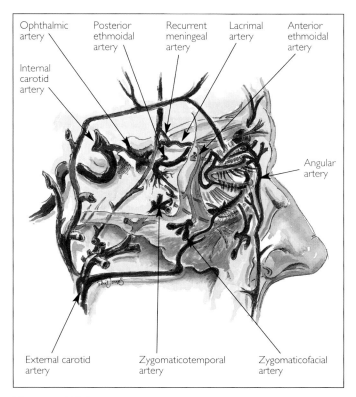

**Figure 17.8**
The relationship of the internal carotid and external carotid arterial systems in the orbital and periorbital regions.

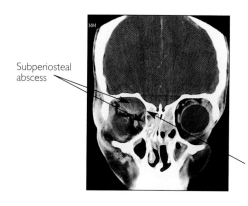

**Figure 17.9**
A coronal CT scan of a patient with ethmoiditis and a right subperiosteal orbital abscess.

Subperiosteal abscess

Periorbital attachment to the frontoethmoidal suture line

space that can be filled with blood (a subperiosteal haematoma) or pus (a subperiosteal abscess). The periorbita is lifted from the walls of the orbit in a characteristic dome-shaped fashion that is limited by the orbital suture lines (Figures 17.5 and 17.9).

The periorbita is dome-shaped over the roof and medial wall of the orbit, assuming a configuration limited by the attachment of the periorbita to the frontoethmoidal suture line.

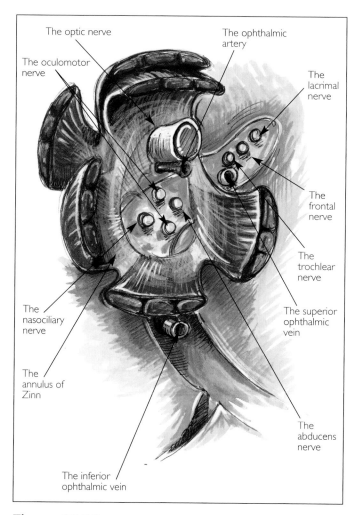

The optic nerve

The ophthalmic artery

The oculomotor nerve

The lacrimal nerve

The frontal nerve

The trochlear nerve

The superior ophthalmic vein

The nasociliary nerve

The annulus of Zinn

The abducens nerve

The inferior ophthalmic vein

**Figure 17.10**
An anterior view of the orbital apex. The separation of the superior orbital fissure into superior and inferior parts by the annulus of Zinn is demonstrated.

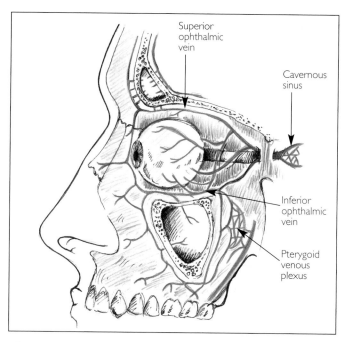

Superior ophthalmic vein

Cavernous sinus

Inferior ophthalmic vein

Pterygoid venous plexus

**Figure 17.11**
The orbital venous system.

## The orbital fissures

The superior orbital fissure is situated between the roof and lateral wall of the orbit and between the greater and lesser wings of the sphenoid bone. This fissure is divided into superior and inferior parts by the fibrous annulus of Zinn, from which the recti muscles take origin (Figure 17.10). The superior part of the fissure transmits the lacrimal, frontal and trochlear nerves, the superior ophthalmic vein and the anastomosis of the recurrent lacrimal and middle meningeal arteries, while the inferior part transmits the superior and inferior divisions of the oculomotor nerve, the nasociliary nerve, the abducens nerve and sympathetic nerves.

The inferior orbital fissure separates the lateral wall from the orbital floor (see Figure 17.1). The inferior orbital fissure connects the orbit to the infratemporal fossa and the ptery-gopalatine fossa. The inferior orbital venous system drains to the pterygoid venous plexus via this communication (see Figure 17.11). The fissure transmits the maxillary division of the trigeminal nerve, which becomes the infraorbital nerve.

## Surgical spaces of the orbit

Anatomically, the orbital spaces are divided into:

- Sub-Tenon's space
- Intraconal space
- Extraconal space
- Subperiosteal space

A good understanding of the surgical spaces of the orbit is essential in order to select the most appropriate surgical approach and to assist in navigation within the orbit during surgery (Figure 17.12).

## Extraconal space

The extraconal space contains the following:

- The lacrimal gland
- The oblique muscles
- The trochlea
- Orbital fat
- The superior ophthalmic vein
- Nerves and other vessels

The lacrimal gland is approached via an upper eyelid skin crease incision for an incisional biopsy for suspected lymphoma, non-specific orbital inflammatory syndrome or malignancy. A formal lateral orbitotomy with bone removal is required for the removal of a suspected lacrimal gland pleomorphic adenoma.

The extraconal fat includes the preaponeurotic fat that is important in the identification of the underlying eyelid retractors. Extraconal fat can be removed superiorly via an upper eyelid skin crease incision. Medial, lateral and inferior extraconal fat can be removed via transconjunctival incisions.

The anterior portion of the superior ophthalmic vein lies in the extraconal space. This can be accessed via an upper eyelid skin crease incision. In patients with arteriovenous shunts the vein is dilated and can provide alternative access for the insertion of platinum coils in conjunction with an interventional radiologist in selected cases.

## Intraconal space

The intraconal space lies within the recti and their intermuscular septa. The intraconal space contains the optic nerve, intraconal fat, nerves and vessels. Tumours of the optic nerve lie within this space.

The intraconal space may be accessed via a number of surgical approaches: e.g. in order to perform an optic nerve sheath fenestration, the optic nerve may be approached superomedially via an upper eyelid skin crease incision, medially via a conjunctival incision with disinsertion of the medial rectus muscle or laterally via a lateral orbitotomy, with or without bone removal. During a lateral orbitotomy approach with bone removal, the intraconal space is usually accessed by dissecting between the lacrimal gland and the lateral rectus muscle.

## Subperiosteal space

The subperiosteal space is a potential space that lies between the periorbita and the bony orbital walls. The periorbita has a loose attachment to the bone and can be easily separated from the bone except at the orbital sutures lines. This space is accessed surgically for the repair of orbital wall blowout fractures, for the drainage of subperiosteal abscesses or haematomas, for bony orbital decompression surgery or for the insertion of subperiosteal orbital implants in anophthalmic patients. This space can be accessed via a variety of transcutaneous or transconjunctival incisions.

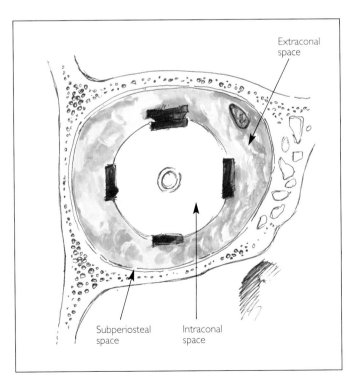

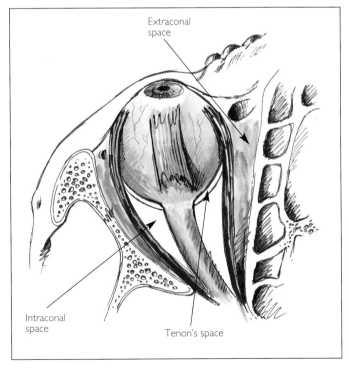

**Figure 17.12**
Surgical spaces of the orbit.

## Tenon's space

Tenon's space is a potential space situated between the globe and Tenon's capsule. It is not commonly involved in pathological processes. The space may be enlarged with fluid visible on echography in posterior scleritis or by infiltration by extraocular extension of intraocular tumours, e.g. choroidal melanoma.

## The optic nerve

The optic nerve runs from the optic chiasm to the globe. The length of the optic nerve is approximately 45–50 mm. It is divided into four parts:

- Intraocular (1 mm)
- Intraorbital (30 mm)
- Intracanalicular (5 mm)
- Intracranial 10 mm)

The nerve normally has an S-shaped configuration in the orbit. In contrast, the nerve is straightened in patients with proptosis. Dura, arachnoid and pia mater surround the nerve from the optic canal to the globe. The subarachnoid space is continued to the globe and is filled with cerebrospinal fluid. The space is enlarged just posterior to the globe in a bulbous part of the nerve. This is the site where an optic nerve sheath fenestration is performed for patients with benign intracranial hypertension. The central retinal artery enters the optic nerve in a variable position, usually on the inferomedial aspect approximately 10 mm posterior to the globe.

The intracanalicular part of the optic nerve is immobile as the dural sheath is fused to the periosteum of the optic canal. The anatomical arrangement of the nerve in this location leaves the nerve vulnerable to damage from blunt head trauma, which can lead to shearing of the pial vessels supplying the nerve. The intracanalicular nerve is also vulnerable to oedema.

The intracranial part of the nerve extends from the chiasm to the optic canal. The dura of the anterior cranial fossa has to be opened to gain access to the nerve in this location. This part of the nerve is closely related to the frontal lobe, the anterior cerebral, anterior communicating, middle cerebral, and internal carotid arteries and the cavernous sinus.

## The periorbital sensory innervation

The ophthalmic and maxillary divisions of the trigeminal nerve provide sensation to the periorbital area with considerable overlap of the branches of the sensory nerves (Figure 17.13). The ophthalmic and maxillary divisions of the trigeminal nerve arise from the semilunar ganglion, which lies in Meckel's cave over the apex of the petrous temporal bone, in the floor of the middle cranial fossa (Figures 17.6 and 17.14). They pass anteriorly in the lateral wall of the cavernous sinus.

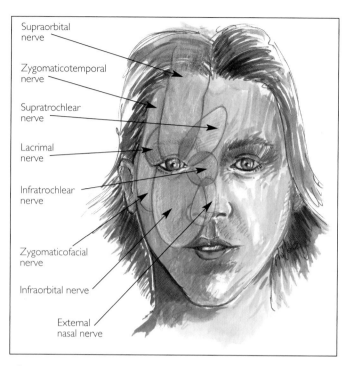

**Figure 17.13**
The overlap of the sensory innervation of the periocular region.

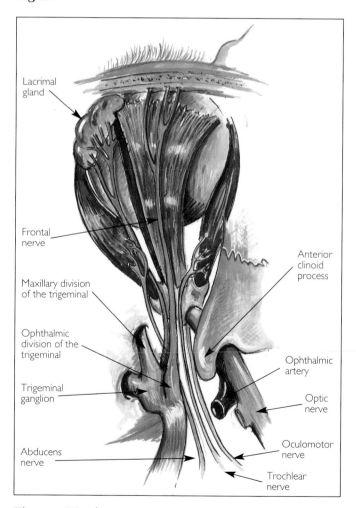

**Figure 17.14**
The orbital apical anatomy viewed from above.

# The ophthalmic division

The ophthalmic nerve divides into three main branches as it leaves the cavernous sinus:

- The lacrimal nerve
- The frontal nerve
- The nasociliary nerve

The arrangement of these nerves in the superior orbital fissure is illustrated in Figure 17.10. The largest branch is the frontal nerve. This travels forward from the orbital apex lying between the levator muscle and the periorbita (Figure 17.14). It is clearly visible when the periorbita is opened from above. It divides midway in the orbit into two branches:

- The supratrochlear nerve
- The supraorbital nerve

The supratrochlear nerve passes above the trochlea and supplies the lower part of the forehead and the medial aspect of the upper eyelid. The supraorbital nerve passes through the supraorbital foramen or notch and supplies the forehead to the vertex of the scalp, the upper eyelid and superior conjunctiva.

The nasociliary nerve innervates the globe. It crosses over the optic nerve from a lateral position after entering the orbit. It gives rise to a number of branches:

- The short ciliary nerves
- The long ciliary nerves
- The anterior ethmoidal nerve
- The posterior ethmoidal nerve

A small branch, the sensory root, runs along the lateral aspect of the optic nerve and enters the ciliary ganglion. The ciliary ganglion lies close to the apex of the orbit between the optic nerve and the lateral rectus muscle. The short ciliary nerves (5–20) then arise from the ciliary ganglion, and run with short ciliary arteries to the posterior aspect of the globe. They penetrate the sclera and provide sensory innervation to the cornea, the iris and the ciliary body. They also carry parasympathetic nerve fibres to the ciliary body and the sphincter pupillae.

The nasociliary nerve gives rise to the long ciliary nerves (2–3), which enter the sclera posteriorly and extend anteriorly along the medial and lateral aspects of the globe to provide sensory innervation to the cornea, iris and ciliary body. These nerves also carry sympathetic nerve fibres from the superior cervical ganglion to the dilator pupillae. After crossing the optic nerve, the posterior ethmoidal nerve is given off followed by the anterior ethmoidal nerve more anteriorly. This branch in turn gives rise to medial and lateral nasal branches and to the external nasal nerve. These branches provide sensory innervation to the nasal cavity and dorsum of the nose. After the anterior ethmoidal nerve has branched away, the nasociliary nerve continues as the infratrochlear nerve. This runs along the superior aspect of the medial rectus muscle and perforates through the orbital septum below the trochlea. It provides sensory innervation to the medial aspect of the skin of the eyelids, the lateral aspect of the nose, the lacrimal sac and the caruncular area. A regional nerve block permits good anaesthesia for an external dacryocystorhinostomy (DCR).

The lacrimal nerve runs along the lateral orbital wall above the lateral rectus muscle. As it runs to the lacrimal gland, it is joined by parasympathetic nerve fibres branching from the zygomaticotemporal nerve.

# The maxillary division

The maxillary division of the trigeminal nerve leaves the middle cranial fossa through the foramen rotundum and enters the pterygopalatine fossa. A number of branches arise in the pterygopalatine fossa:

- The zygomatic nerve
- The sphenopalatine nerves
- The posterior superior alveolar nerves

The zygomatic nerve enters the orbit through the inferior orbital fissure, runs along the lateral aspect of the orbit and divides into the zygomaticofacial and zygomaticotemporal nerves (see Figures 17.6 and 17.7).

The posterior superior alveolar nerves provide sensation to the upper molar teeth, the gingiva and the mucous membrane of the maxillary sinus.

The maxillary division enters the orbit through the central aspect of the inferior orbital fissure and continues forward as the infraorbital nerve through the infraorbital groove and infraorbital canal. In the canal it gives rise to:

- The middle superior alveolar nerve
- The anterior superior alveolar nerve
- The superior labial nerve

The middle superior alveolar nerve provides sensation to the upper premolar teeth. The anterior superior alveolar nerve supplies the upper incisor teeth and canines, and the mucous membrane of the maxillary sinus and of the inferior meatus of the nose. The superior labial nerve supplies the skin of the cheek and the skin and mucous membrane of the upper lip. These areas are affected by trauma to the infraorbital nerve following an orbital floor blowout fracture.

# The motor nerves to the extraocular muscles
## The oculomotor nerve

The oculomotor nerve provides motor innervation for:

- The levator muscle
- The superior rectus muscle
- The medial rectus muscle
- The inferior rectus muscle
- The inferior oblique muscle

It provides the pathway for parasympathetic nerve fibres to the ciliary muscle and the sphincter pupillae muscle.

The nerve leaves the lateral wall of the cavernous sinus and enters the orbit, where it divides into superior and inferior branches. It enters the orbit through the superior orbital fissure within the annulus of Zinn. The superior branch rises over the lateral aspect of the optic nerve and enters the undersurface of the superior rectus muscle at the junction of the posterior third with the anterior two-thirds. A branch of this nerve passes through or around the medial aspect of the superior rectus muscle to reach the levator muscle. The inferior branch gives rise to three further branches supplying the medial rectus, the inferior rectus and the inferior oblique muscles. The latter gives off a short root to the ciliary ganglion.

## The trochlear nerve

The trochlear nerve supplies the superior oblique muscle. The nerve enters the orbit through the superior orbital fissure outside the annulus of Zinn. It passes anteriorly and medially over the levator muscle and enters the superior oblique muscle on its outer aspect as three or four branches at the junction of the posterior third with the anterior two-thirds. The trochlear nerve is the only nerve that enters an extraocular muscle from the outer aspect. The other nerves enter the muscles from the conal surface.

## The abducens nerve

The abducens nerve supplies the lateral rectus muscle. The nerve enters the orbit within the annulus of Zinn. It enters the lateral rectus muscle on its conal surface at the junction of the posterior third with the anterior two-thirds.

## *The orbital vascular systems: arterial system*

The main orbital arteries arise from the ophthalmic artery. The terminal branches of the ophthalmic artery anastomose with terminal branches of the external carotid artery to form a rich arterial network of collateral circulation in the periocular region, making the tissues resistant to the effects of ischaemia and infection.

## Ophthalmic artery

The ophthalmic artery is the first branch of the internal carotid artery (see Figure 17.8). It is divided into intracranial, intracanalicular and intraorbital parts. The intracranial part lies below the optic nerve. The intracanalicular part lies below the optic nerve within its dural sheath. It enters the orbit inferolateral to the optic nerve and crosses either above or below the nerve, running towards the medial orbital wall.

The ophthalmic artery gives off a number of branches:

- Central retinal artery
- Medial and lateral posterior ciliary arteries
- Collateral branches to the optic nerve
- Multiple muscular arteries
- Lacrimal artery
- Supraorbital artery
- Supratrochlear artery
- Anterior and posterior ethmoidal arteries
- Infratrochlear artery
- Medial palpebral arteries

## Lacrimal artery

The lacrimal artery passes along the lateral orbital wall above the lateral rectus muscle. The branches from the lacrimal artery are:

- Recurrent meningeal artery
- Zygomatic
- Artery to the lacrimal gland
- Lateral palpebral artery

The zygomatic branches, the zygomaticotemporal and zygomaticofacial arteries, pass through foramina within the zygomatic bone and anastomose with anterior deep temporal and transverse facial arteries (Figures 17.8 and 17.15).

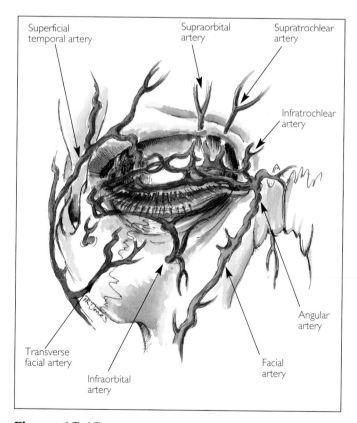

**Figure 17.15**
The arterial anatomy of the periorbital region viewed anteriorly.

## Supraorbital artery

The supraorbital artery branches from the ophthalmic artery as it crosses over the optic nerve. It runs along the medial border of the superior rectus and levator muscles. The artery exits the orbit through the supraorbital notch or foramen, supplying the forehead, brows and upper eyelid regions.

## Supratrochlear artery

The supratrochlear artery is one of the terminal branches of the ophthalmic artery. It supplies the medial aspect of the forehead and scalp and the superior medial canthal area.

## Infratrochlear artery

The infratrochlear artery is another of the terminal branches of the ophthalmic artery. It runs above the medial canthal tendon and anatomoses with the angular artery. It supplies the nasal bridge, scalp, medial forehead and medial canthal areas.

## Medial palpebral arteries

The medial palpebral arteries are also terminal branches of the ophthalmic artery and arise from the arteries lying just below the trochlea. They pass into the eyelids and anastomose with the lateral palpebral arterial branches.

## Ethmoidal arteries

The anterior and posterior ethmoidal arteries form important surgical landmarks. They exit the orbit via their respective ethmoidal foramina sheathed by periorbita. They form the superior limit of orbital bone removal in a medial orbital wall decompression. Inadvertent damage to these arteries can lead to brisk bleeding and the rapid development of a subperiosteal orbital haematoma.

## *The orbital vascular systems: the venous system*

Venous blood is drained from the orbit through three main systems:

- The cavernous sinus
- The pterygoid plexus
- The anterior venous system

The superior ophthalmic vein drains to the cavernous sinus. The inferior ophthalmic vein drains both to the superior ophthalmic vein and also to the pterygoid plexus (Figure 17.11). The venous system communicates anteriorly via the angular vein and its tributaries from the face and forehead.

## The superior ophthalmic vein

The superior ophthalmic vein is formed by the confluence of the supraorbital vein and the angular vein. It extends posteriorly from the medial aspect of the orbit to the medial border of the superior rectus muscle. It then runs below the superior rectus muscle and along its lateral margin to the superior orbital fissure and the cavernous sinus.

A supraorbital vein can be cannulated in order to pass a radiopaque dye to perform an orbital venogram. The supraorbital vein itself can be dissected and cannulated via an upper eyelid skin crease incision in order to embolize orbital vascular shunts if alternative endovascular routes are not feasible.

## The inferior ophthalmic vein

The inferior ophthalmic vein forms from a plexus of veins on the floor of the orbit. The vein runs posteriorly to communicate by a branch with the superior ophthalmic vein and by another smaller branch with the pterygoid plexus via the inferior orbital fissure.

## The central retinal vein

The central retinal vein exits from the optic nerve at a variable distance from the globe. It usually passes directly to the cavernous sinus.

# The principles of orbital surgery

The prerequisites for successful atraumatic orbital surgery are:

- A thorough knowledge of eyelid and orbital anatomy
- A thorough knowledge of orbital disorders
- A thorough understanding of imaging techniques
- Familiarity with the surgical approaches
- Familiarity with the required surgical instrumentation
- Proper illumination and magnification of the surgical field
- Adequate surgical exposure
- Meticulous surgical dissection
- Careful removal and presentation of biopsy specimens
- Good haemostasis

## *A thorough knowledge of eyelid and orbital anatomy*

It is essential to acquire a thorough knowledge of normal eyelid and orbital anatomy before undertaking surgical procedures in an orbit whose anatomy has been altered by a pathological process. A textbook of anatomy should be reviewed. It is wise to observe and assist at a variety of orbitotomy approaches. If possible, the opportunity to examine the orbital contents from above with the brain and orbital roof removed during a post-mortem examination should not be missed. This is particularly helpful prior to performing any surgery on the orbital apex.

## A thorough knowledge of orbital disorders

The evaluation of the patient with an orbital disorder is discussed in Chapter 16. This chapter deals with both common and important orbital disorders. A differential diagnosis based on a thorough history, a meticulous physical examination, imaging and laboratory investigations should enable a decision about appropriate management to be made. For the management of many orbital inflammatory, neoplastic or cystic lesions, a biopsy will be required. As a general rule, an incisional biopsy will be required for an orbital lesion that is suggestive of malignancy or inflammation (with the exception of myositis), whereas an excisional biopsy is indicated for the removal of a well-circumscribed or lesion suggestive of a benign process.

There are notable exceptions to this rule. A pleomorphic adenoma of the lacrimal gland may not always be well circumscribed. An incisional biopsy may predispose the patient to a malignant recurrence. An orbital lymphoma may appear well circumscribed, but an attempt at complete excision would be inappropriate.

## A thorough understanding of imaging techniques

Spending time with a neuroradiologist reviewing a variety of orbital CT and MRI images is an invaluable exercise.

## Familiarity with the surgical approaches

This can only be gained by experience. It is essential to observe and assist at a variety of surgical approaches to the orbit before undertaking this surgery.

## Familiarity with the required surgical instrumentation and equipment

This is also gained by experience. It is essential to understand the basic assembly of the drills and saws used in orbital surgery and the safety provisions for all members of the team. The handpiece should have a safe mode that is activated and deactivated by the surgeon (Figure 17.16). This avoids inadvertent activation of the drill/saw via a footswitch when using bipolar cautery. All members of the team should wear face guards to protect them from blood and bone fragments. Protection of the patient's globe from inadvertent injury by the instrumentation is the surgeon's responsibility.

A variety of burr sizes (both rose head and diamond) should be available. A variety of bone rongeurs are also required (Figure 17.17).

A microplating system and Medpor blocks and sheets are occasionally required to reconstruct complex bony orbitotomies, especially where additional bone has been burred away to gain improved access to the orbit. A variety of orbital retractors should be available in different sizes (Sewall, Wright's and malleable ribbon retractors). The retractors have different purposes and must be used appropriately. Sewall retractors have a sturdy handle that enables the assistant to apply traction with a hand (Figure 17.18). These are used during subperiosteal dissection in orbital decompression procedures or orbital blowout fracture repairs. These retractors are particularly efficient if used with a sheet of Supramid that prevents the prolapse of fat around the edges of the retractor. This makes dissection of all margins of a large orbital floor blowout fracture much simpler.

It is essential to appreciate the pressure on the globe that can be generated with these retractors. This is particularly important if the globe's integrity has been compromised (previous penetrating keratoplasty, penetrating injury repair, peripheral corneal gutter, staphyloma, etc.). Traction on the retractors should be released at regular intervals during surgery.

Wright's retractors have more delicate handles, and blades that are more appropriate for the retraction of fat around orbital tumours (Figure 17.19). These are held with the fingers, in contrast to the Sewall retractors. Malleable ribbon retractors are particularly useful for protecting the globe and surrounding tissues when using the drill and saw.

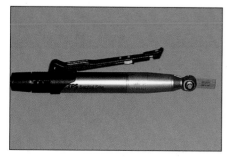

**Figure 17.16**
Stryker saw with finger switch.

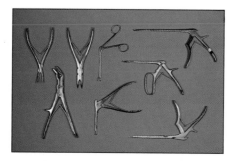

**Figure 17.17**
A variety of bone rongeurs used in orbital surgery.

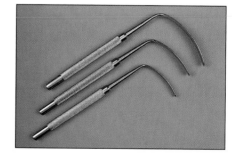

**Figure 17.18**
Sewall retractors.

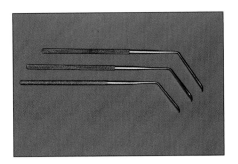

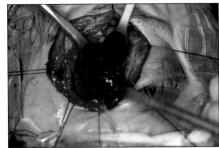

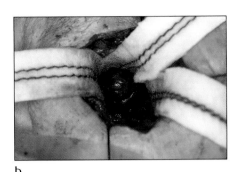

a                                              b

**Figure 17.19**
Wright's retractors.

**Figure 17.20**
(a) An orbital cavernous haemangioma is carefully exposed using Wright's retractors to hold back the orbital fat. (b) Neurosurgical cottonoids are used to aid the maintenance of a surgical field free of blood and fat.

# Proper illumination and magnification of the surgical field

A comfortable fibreoptic headlight provides excellent illumination of the orbital structures during most orbitotomy procedures. This should be used in conjunction with surgical loupes that provide a comfortable working distance, good magnification, a satisfactory depth of focus and an adequate field of view. It may be necessary for some orbital dissections to resort to the use of the operating microscope. This allows the surgical assistant and observers (via a TV monitor) to see precisely the same deeper orbital structures as the surgeon.

# Adequate surgical exposure

The surgical incision should be of an adequate length. Although incisions are generally selected to achieve the best postoperative cosmetic result possible, the main consideration is safe adequate surgical access. As the dissection proceeds into the deeper aspects of the orbit, the dimensions of the wound should be the same or even larger. Traction sutures should be carefully placed at strategic positions. These can be supplemented with self-retaining Jaffe retractors.

# Meticulous surgical dissection

Surgical dissection within the orbit requires a delicate patient approach. Lesions can often be palpated with the tip of the little finger, which can greatly assist orientation. This can be done at regular intervals if the lesion cannot be easily identified. Gentle blunt dissection should be undertaken using Wright's retractors in a hand-over-hand dissection technique. Once the surface of the lesion has been exposed, a Freer elevator can be used to gently separate the tissues and fat from the lesion with further blunt dissection. As the plane of dissection proceeds, the retrac-

tors can be repositioned (see Figure 17.20a). The dissection can be further facilitated by the placement of neurosurgical cottonoids, moistened with saline, into the wound (see Figure 17.20b). The retractors are then placed over these to prevent the prolapse of orbital fat into the surgical field. This also enables the efficient use of suction with a Baron suction tip, which is applied against the cottonoid to prevent the suction tip from engaging orbital fat.

Where required, careful dissection with blunt-tipped Westcott scissors can be used. The assistant should apply countertraction with the orbital retractors, as the surgeon manoeuvres the lesion away from the retractors with a cotton-tipped applicator, retractor or a combined Freer/suction elevator using the non-dominant hand. The tissues are gently dissected from the mass with the scissors in the dominant hand. For deep orbital dissection, blunt-tipped Yasargil neurosurgical scissors (curved or straight) may be used. Occasionally, a cryoprobe may assist the dissection by allowing the lesion to be gently pulled in different directions.

# Careful removal and presentation of biopsy specimens

The management of many undiagnosed orbital lesions requires an orbitotomy procedure with an incisional biopsy to obtain an accurate diagnosis. It is essential to ensure that the pathologist is presented with tissue samples that are:

- Of adequate size
- Representative of the entire lesion
- Undamaged by cautery or surgical instruments
- Appropriately stored

It may be necessary to provide more than one tissue sample, depending on the appearance of the lesion. Great care should be taken to ensure that the tissue samples are not damaged. It is preferable to use a right-angled 66 Beaver blade to obtain biopsies from a solid lesion. Small cup biopsy forceps are more appropriate for lesions that are friable. Very occasionally it is helpful to request a frozen section analysis of tissue samples taken from a small orbital lesion. The pathologist can confirm that adequate material has been obtained. No management decisions, however, should ever be based on the frozen section analysis of orbital biopsies. If frozen section analysis may be required, it is important to communicate this to the pathologist in advance. The pathology requisition forms should be completed prior to the commencement of surgery and should provide appropriate clinical information about the patient. The tissue samples should be quickly placed into the appropriate transport container to prevent desiccation. If fresh tissue samples are required by the pathologist, it is essential to communicate with the pathologist in advance and to ensure rapid transportation.

It is not appropriate to undertake fine-needle aspiration biopsies of orbital lesions on a routine basis. It can, however, be advantageous to perform an open approach fine-needle aspiration biopsy for deep orbital lesions from which it would be difficult and potentially dangerous to attempt to obtain a standard incisional biopsy. The surface of the lesion is carefully exposed. An 18–gauge needle (green) is attached to a 5 ml syringe. The needle is placed into the lesion and moved back and forth, while withdrawing on the plunger. The needle is carefully capped and the needle and syringe are sent to the cytopathologist.

## Good haemostasis

Good haemostasis is an extremely important prerequisite for successful orbital surgery. The fundamental principles underlying the successful achievement of good haemostasis are outlined in Chapter 1, Basic Principles. For orbital dissections, some points require emphasis:

- Only bipolar cautery should be used within the orbit
- Insulated bayonet bipolar forceps with delicate tips should be used
- The minimum power required should be used
- The minimum amount of cautery required should be used

It is essential that tissue to be submitted for histopathological examination is not damaged by cautery.

Gelfoam soaked with thrombin can be applied to the orbital wound during surgery and following removal of the orbital lesion to assist in haemostasis when there is generalized oozing without an identifiable source amenable to bipolar cautery.

For some orbital procedures a safe degree of hypotension is advantageous. The anaesthetist should be asked to restore a normal level of blood pressure following removal of an orbital lesion to ensure that intraoperative haemostasis is adequate before the orbit is closed. It is inevitable that the patient's venous pressure will rise on extubation. It is reasonable to apply a compressive dressing at the completion of surgery to tamponade the orbit and to remove this is in the recovery room as soon as the patient is awake and cooperative. The anaesthetist should be warned about this, so that the anaesthetic is not reversed too soon.

# The orbitotomy approaches

The surgical approaches which are most commonly used to gain access to the orbital spaces are:

- Anterior orbitotomy
    transcutaneous
    transconjunctival
    eyelid split
- Medial orbitotomy
    transcutaneous (Lynch incision)
    transconjunctival
    transcaruncular
    endoscopic
- Lateral orbitotomy
- Combined orbitotomies
- Transfrontal orbitotomy

## Anterior orbitotomy

An anterior orbitotomy is used for the incisional or excisional biopsy of anterior orbital lesions, for the biopsy of more posteriorly placed orbital lesions and for the drainage of haematomas/abscesses (Figure 17.21). An upper eyelid skin crease trans-septal approach is used particularly for superior lesions, whereas a transconjunctival approach may be preferred for inferior lesions, as this avoids a visible cutaneous scar. A lower eyelid transconjunctival approach can be combined with a lateral canthotomy and inferior cantholysis to provide improved exposure of the inferior and lateral orbit. The conjunctival incision can be extended into a transcaruncular incision to gain further access to the medial orbit.

Both approaches can also be used to gain access to the subperiosteal space as well as to the extraconal space, e.g. for the management of an orbital wall blowout fracture or for bony orbital decompression. *It is important, however, not to disturb the periosteum when performing a biopsy on potentially malignant orbital lesions, as the periosteum is an important barrier to tumour spread and an important surgical excision margin.* For the excision of more posteriorly placed lesions this approach may be combined with a lateral orbitotomy. Large superomedial orbital lesions may be approached by an upper eyelid split technique, where the upper eyelid is split vertically just lateral to the superior punctum (Figure 17.22).

### Trans-cutaneous anterior orbitotomy

1. A skin crease incision in the upper lid, or a subciliary or a skin crease incision in the lower lid is marked with a cocktail stick dipped in a gentian violet marker. Incisions over the inferior orbital margin should be avoided, as this leaves an unsightly scar and is associated with persistent postoperative lower eyelid lymphoedema. A large superior lesion which is palpable beneath the skin may be more easily approached by means of a skin incision placed directly over the lesion,

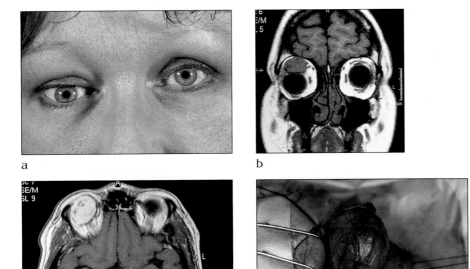

a

b

c

d

**Figure 17.21**

(a) A 40-year-old female patient who presented with a history of a gradual inferior displacement of the right globe. (b) A coronal MRI scan demonstrating a well-defined homogenous superior extraconal mass. (c) An axial MRI scan demonstrating that the lesion is anteriorly placed in the orbit. (d) The lesion was excised via an upper eyelid skin crease incision. A histopathological examination confirmed the lesion to be a solitary fibrous tumour.

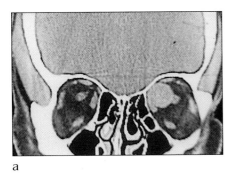

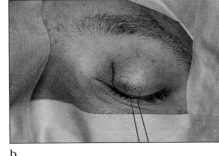

a

b

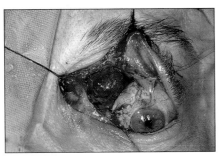

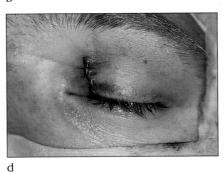

c

d

**Figure 17.22**

(a) A coronal CT scan demonstrating a superonasal orbital mass. (b) A vertical lid split incision has been marked nasal to the superior punctum extending into the superior fornix. (c) A cavernous haemangioma was exposed and an excision biopsy performed. (d) The eyelid split is carefully repaired.

although this will leave a visible scar. This is not of concern with suspected orbital malignancies. A superior subperiosteal abscess should be approached via a sub-brow incision, taking great care not to disturb the supraorbital and supratrochlear neurovascular bundles.

2. 0.5% Marcain with 1:200,000 units of adrenaline is injected subcutaneously.

3. A grey line traction suture is placed and fixated to the drapes with a curved artery clip.

4. The skin and orbicularis are incised with a Colorado needle.

5. The orbital septum is opened and a Jaffe eyelid retractor is placed.

6. The lesion is dissected and removed or biopsied and haemostasis obtained.

7. The orbital septum is not repaired.

8. The skin is closed with a continuous 7/0 Vicryl suture.

9. Topical antibiotic is applied to the wound.

10. A pressure dressing is applied and removed in the recovery room after approximately 45 min to begin monitoring of vision.

# Lower eyelid transconjunctival anterior orbitotomy

1. Subconjunctival injections of local anaesthetic solution containing adrenaline are avoided because of the effects on the pupil. The injections are instead given just beneath the skin in the lower eyelid and at the lateral canthus.
2. A lateral canthotomy and inferior cantholysis are performed (if required) with a Colorado needle.
3. Two 4/0 silk traction sutures are placed through the grey line of the lower eyelid and the lid everted over a Desmarres retractor.
4. A corneal protector is placed.
5. A conjunctival incision is made at the inferior border of the tarsus with a Colorado needle and extended through the lower eyelid retractors to approach the inferior orbital rim preseptally (Figure 17.23). An alternative is to make an incision in the inferior fornix. This provides rapid access to an anterior inferior orbital lesion but is a poor approach to the subperiosteal space, as it allows the prolapse of orbital fat into the surgical field.
6. The plane between the orbicularis muscle and the orbital septum is dissected to the inferior orbital margin (Figure 17.23).
7. 4/0 silk traction sutures are placed through the edges of the conjunctiva and inferior retractors and attached to the head drape with curved artery clips in order to protect the cornea.
8. Jaffe eyelid retractors are placed over the edge of the tarsus to assist retraction.
9. The orbital septum or the periorbita is opened, depending on the location of the lesion.
10. The lesion is exposed with the aid of Wright's retractors and removed or biopsied.
11. Haemostasis is obtained.
12. The conjunctiva is closed with interrupted 7/0 Vicryl sutures and the lateral canthotomy is repaired with a double-armed 5/0 Ethibond suture on a 1/2–circle needle passed from the tarsus to the lateral orbital periosteum. The skin is closed with interrupted 7/0 Vicryl sutures.
13. Topical antibiotic is applied to the wound.
14. A pressure dressing is applied and removed after approximately 45 min to begin monitoring of vision.

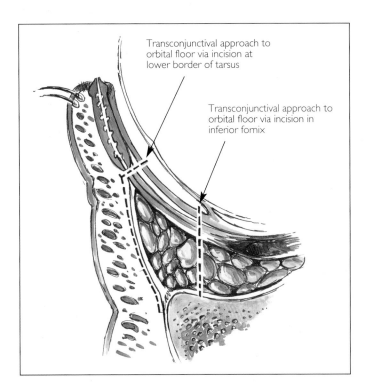

**Figure 17.23**
Surgical approaches to the orbit via lower eyelid conjunctival incisions.

## Eyelid split anterior orbitotomy

1. 0.5% marcain with 1:200,000 units of adrenaline is injected into the medial aspect of the upper eyelid.
2. The eyelid margin is incised 3–4 mm lateral to the superior punctum with a No. 15 Bard Parker blade. The incision is extended to the superior fornix with straight scissors.
3. The lesion is exposed with the aid of Wright's retractors and removed or biopsied.
4. The eyelid is repaired in layers.

# *Medial orbitotomy*

A medial orbitotomy via a skin incision (Lynch incision) can be used to approach the medial subperiosteal space, e.g. for the drainage of a subperiosteal abscess (Figure 17.24).

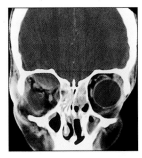 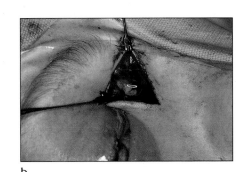

**Figure 17.24**
(a) A coronal CT scan demonstrating a large superior orbital subperiosteal abscess and a smaller medial wall subperiosteal abscess in a patient with an ethmoid sinusitis. The configuration of the subperiosteal abscess is determined by the attachment of the periorbita at the frontoethmoidal suture line. (b) A Lynch incision has been made in the same patient to drain the abscess.

a                          b

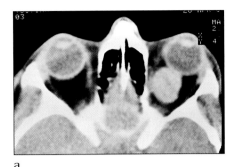

a

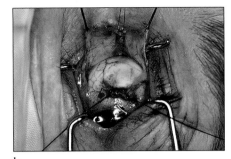

b

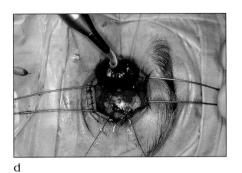

d

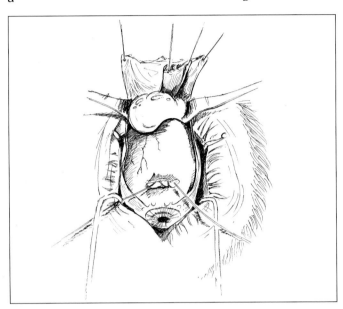

c

## Figure 17.25

(a) An axial CT scan demonstrating a medial intraconal orbital mass. (b) The medial rectus muscle has been sutured, detached from its insertion and drawn medially. Traction sutures have been placed through the medial rectus stump and the globe rotated laterally. Traction sutures have also been placed through the conjunctiva and anterior Tenon's fascia after radial relieving incisions have been made. (c) Wright's retractors are used to gently expose the lesion, which is then gently dissected free. (d) A cryotherapy probe insulated to the tip is being used to assist delivery of the lesion, a cavernous haemangioma.

A transconjunctival approach is used, often in conjunction with disinsertion of the medial rectus muscle, to remove intraconal lesions medial to the optic nerve or to perform an optic nerve fenestration procedure (Figure 17.25). A lateral orbitotomy can be combined with the medial orbitotomy to provide improved exposure.

A transcaruncular incision can be used to perform a medial orbital wall decompression for thyroid eye disease, to drain a medial subperiosteal haematoma or to repair a medial orbital wall blowout fracture. It can be used for the drainage of a sub-periosteal abscess, but it is a more uncomfortable location for a postoperative drain.

An endoscopic approach can be used for access to the posterior aspect of the medial orbit for the decompression of benign apical tumours or for an incisional biopsy in selected cases.

## Lynch incision medial orbitotomy

1. A curvilinear incision is marked within the medial canthus, midway between the medial commissure and the bridge of the nose (see Figure 17.24b).
2. 0.5% Marcain with 1:200,000 units of adrenaline is injected subcutaneously.
3. A skin incision is made with a Colorado needle.

4. The medial canthal vessels are retracted and the orbicularis muscle fibres spread apart to expose the periosteum on the lateral wall of the nose.
5. 4/0 silk traction sutures are inserted.
6. The periosteum is incised along the full length of the wound and elevated from the medial orbital wall along with the medial canthal tendon. A stump of the tendon is left on the nasal bone for reattachment of the tendon.
7. Greater exposure requires the careful cauterization and division of the anterior ethmoidal vessels.
8. Care must be taken in the region of the trochlea.
9. The wound is closed in layers and the medial canthal tendon is sutured back to its insertion using 5/0 Vicryl sutures.

## Transconjunctival medial orbitotomy

1. Subconjunctival injections of local anaesthetic solution containing adrenaline are avoided because of the effects on the pupil.
2. A medial 180-degree peritomy is performed with blunt-tipped Westcott scissors. Radial relieving incisions are made.
3. 4/0 silk traction sutures are placed through the conjunctiva edges.

4. The medial rectus muscle is hooked and interlocking 5/0 Vicryl sutures are placed behind the insertion, leaving a stump for the placement of 4/0 silk traction sutures.
5. The medial rectus muscle is disinserted and drawn medially.
6. The globe is drawn laterally with the traction sutures (Figure 17.25b).
7. Wright's retractors are used to aid exposure of the lesion.
8. The lesion is removed or biopsied.
9. Haemostasis is obtained.
10. The medial rectus muscle is reattached to its insertion on the globe and the conjunctiva is closed with 7/0 Vicryl sutures.

## Transcaruncular medial orbitotomy

1. Subconjunctival injections of local anaesthetic solution containing adrenaline are avoided because of the effects on the pupil.
2. An incision is made between the caruncle and the plica using blunt-tipped Westcott scissors (Figure 17.26a).
3. Blunt dissection with Stevens scissors is used to expose the medial orbital wall posterior to the posterior lacrimal crest.
4. 4/0 silk traction sutures are placed to improve exposure.
5. The periorbita is incised and elevated using a Freer periosteal elevator.
6. Wright's retractors or a narrow Sewall retractor are used to gain exposure of the posterior aspects of the medial wall (Figure 17.26b).

7. The conjunctiva is closed with interrupted 7/0 Vicryl sutures at the completion of surgery.

## *Lateral orbitotomy*

The lateral orbitotomy provides a good approach to the intraconal space and to lesions lateral to the optic nerve. It can be combined with other approaches to allow the globe to be moved laterally to facilitate improved surgical exposure. It can also be used as part of an orbital decompression procedure. The lateral orbital wall can be approached by means of different surgical incisions:

1. The Berke–Reese approach
2. The Stallard–Wright approach
3. An upper eyelid skin crease approach
4. A bicoronal flap approach

The Stallard–Wright approach is the approach of choice of the author (Figure 17.27).

The Berke–Reese approach leaves a less satisfactory scar and disturbs the lateral canthus. The upper eyelid skin crease approach can help to camouflage the scar but may leave the patient with a mechanical ptosis for some weeks due to pretarsal oedema (Figure 17.28).

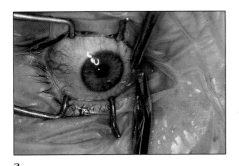

a

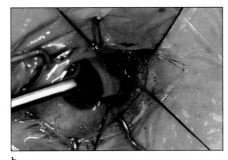

b

**Figure 17.26**
(a) An incision is made between the caruncle and the plica semilunaris.
(b) A Sewall retractor has been inserted into the wound to assist in exposing the medial orbital wall.

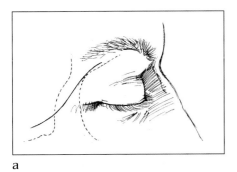

a

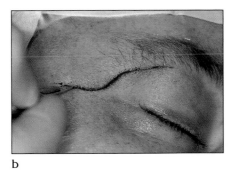

b

**Figure 17.27**
(a) A diagram demonstrating the position of a Stallard–Wright lateral orbitotomy incision in relation to the lateral orbital margin. (b) The incision being made in a patient.

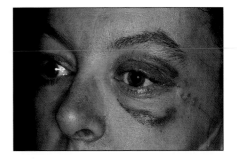

**Figure 17.28**
A patient 3 days after undergoing a lateral orbitotomy via an extended upper eyelid crease incision.

The bicoronal flap requires much more operative time and exposes the patient to risks of hair loss, greater degrees of sensory loss and the risk of a frontalis palsy. The subsequent development of male pattern baldness will expose a large scar.

## Stallard–Wright lateral orbitotomy

1. The patient is placed into a reverse Trendelenburg position.
2. The surgeon is seated at the side of the patient facing the lateral orbital margin.
3. The patient's head is turned slightly away from the surgeon.
4. The lateral orbitotomy incision is marked out. This should extend from just below the lateral aspect of the eyebrow to end in a rhytid over the anterior zygomatic arch (see Figure 17.27a)
5. A subcutaneous injection of 0.5% bupivacaine with 1:200,000 units of adrenaline is given subcutaneously along the lateral orbital margin.
6. The cornea is protected with Lacrilube ointment.
7. A skin incision is made with a No. 15 Bard Parker blade.
8. The subcutaneous tissues are dissected down to the periosteum using a cutting diathermy blade.
9. Multiple 4/0 silk traction sutures are placed (Figure 17.29).
10. Blunt dissection is used to expose the periosteum of the whole of the lateral orbital margin.
11. The periosteum is then incised with a No. 15 Bard Parker blade 2 mm lateral to the orbital rim. The incision is carried superiorly above the frontozygomatic suture and inferiorly past the superior aspect of the zygomatic arch (Figure 17.29). Posterior relieving incisions are made in the periosteum.
12. The periosteum and temporalis muscle are then reflected posteriorly using a Freer periosteal elevator exposing the lateral wall of the orbit in the temporal fossa: 2 × 2-inch gauze swabs are inserted into the temporal fossa to aid in retraction and haemostasis (Figure 17.30). These must be recorded and removed at the end of the procedure.
13. The periosteum is now very carefully reflected from the internal aspect of the lateral orbital wall (Figure 17.31). Great care should be taken to maintain the periorbita intact at this stage. The zygomaticotemporal and zygomaticofacial vessels are cauterized. The periorbita does not need to be raised beyond the frontosphenoidal suture line.
14. Incision lines are drawn on the bone approximately 5 mm above the frontozygomatic suture superiorly and just above the zygomatic arch inferiorly (Figure 17.32).

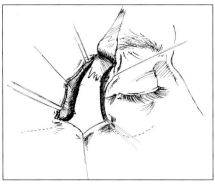

a

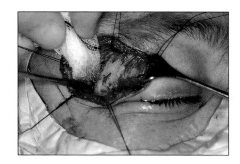

**Figure 17.30**
2 × 2-inch gauze swabs are inserted into the temporal fossa.

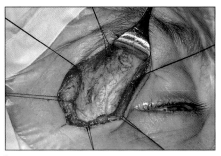

b

**Figure 17.29**
(a) The lateral orbital margin is exposed to a position approximately 2 cm above the frontozygomatic suture line superiorly and to a position level with the zygomatic arch inferiorly. (b) The periosteum is incised 2 mm lateral to the orbital rim with posterior relieving incisions at the superior and inferior aspects of the incision.

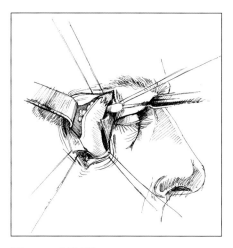

**Figure 17.31**
The periosteum is very carefully reflected from the lateral orbital margin and internal aspect of the lateral orbital wall with a fine periosteal elevator.

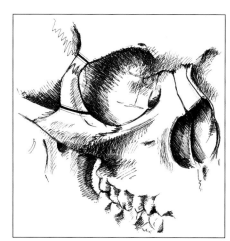

**Figure 17.32**
The position of the bone cuts is demonstrated.

15. A broad malleable retractor is inserted into the orbit to protect the orbital contents, while another is placed into the temporal fossa to protect the temporalis muscle and to prevent any swabs from being caught by the saw. An oscillating saw with an angled blade is used to cut along the incision lines (Figure 17.33a). It is important to use copious irrigation. Great care is taken to angulate the superior saw cut inferiorly to avoid any risk of entering the anterior cranial fossa. (It is preferable to place the superior incision at a slightly lower level, as the bony opening can always be enlarged if necessary with a burr and the superior drill hole repositioned.) Drill holes are now made above and below the saw cuts (Figure 17.33b).

16. The lateral orbital wall is grasped with a large bone rongeur and gently rocked in an outward direction until it fractures posteriorly (Figure 17.34). It is then removed (Figure 17.35). It is safely stored in a large saline-soaked gauze swab (Figure 17.36).

17. The irregular fracture line can be smoothed and further bone removed with a burr or a bone rongeur (Figure 17.37). The thick cancellous bone of the sphenoid is encountered, marking the posterior limit of any further bone removal.

18. Bone wax is applied to any bleeding points from the bone. The gauze swabs in the temporal fossa are removed and replaced. Haemostasis is secured before proceeding.

19. A T-shaped incision is made in the periorbita. A small initial incision is made with a No. 15 Bard Parker blade at the lower border of the lateral rectus muscle in an anteroposterior direction. This incision is enlarged posteriorly with blunt-tipped Westcott scissors. Vertical incisions are made anteriorly in a superior direction in front of the lacrimal gland and in an inferior direction to the base of the orbitotomy.

20. The periorbita is grasped and gently dissected from the orbital contents with blunt-tipped Westcott scissors.

21. The lateral rectus muscle is identified after opening the perimuscular fascial sheaths by blunt dissection with a Freer periosteal elevator. A loop of O'Donoghue's silicone tubing is gently passed around the muscle and retracted inferiorly (Figure 17.38).

22. The position of the orbital mass is confirmed by gentle digital palpation.

23. The orbital fat is gently retracted in a hand-over-hand fashion using Wright's retractors (Figure 17.20a).

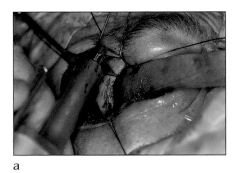
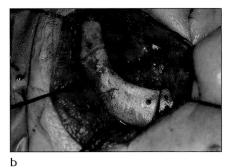
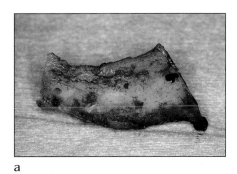

a                                          b

**Figure 17.33**
(a) Malleable retractors are used to protect the orbital contents and the temporal fossa when the saw cuts are made. The superior saw cut should be angled inferiorly. (b) Drill holes have been made above and below the saw cuts.

**Figure 17.34**
The lateral orbital bone is grasped with a large rongeur and gently rocked back and forth.

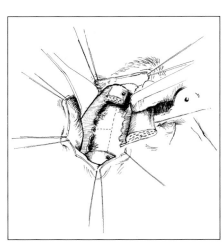
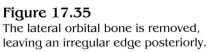
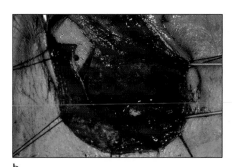

a                                          b

**Figure 17.36**
(a) The appearance of the bone removed for a lateral orbitotomy. (b) The appearance of the intact periorbita.

**Figure 17.35**
The lateral orbital bone is removed, leaving an irregular edge posteriorly.

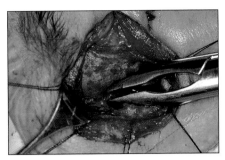

**Figure 17.37**
Bone rongeurs are used to remove further bone posteriorly, leaving a smooth edge.

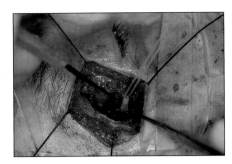

**Figure 17.38**
The lateral rectus muscle has been identified and muscle hooks used to isolate the muscle, which is then looped with silicone tubing.

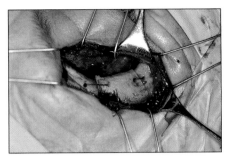

**Figure 17.39**
The bone is replaced and sutured into position with 3/0 Vicryl sutures.

24. Blunt dissection over and around the lesion is aided by placing 1/20-inch neurosurgical cottonoid patties behind the retractors, which assists in keeping the orbital fat from the surgical field (Figure 17.20b). These also absorb blood and allow gentle suction to be applied without frequent blockage of the suction tip by globules of fat. Suction of fat should be avoided to prevent the rupture of fine vessels with bleeding.
25. Fine-tipped bayonet bipolar cautery forceps are used for haemostasis.
26. Operating loupes usually provide adequate magnification but the operating microscope may occasionally be required.
27. If the lesion is encapsulated it is bluntly dissected from the surrounding orbital tissues with a Freer periosteal elevator, keeping the dissection close to the capsule to avoid inadvertent injury to orbital structures.
28. The patient's pupil should be checked at regular intervals.
29. Delivery of the lesion may be assisted by the use of a cryoprobe.
30. If the lesion is not encapsulated and cannot be removed safely, it should be biopsied or debulked as safely as possible.
31. Meticulous attention is paid to haemostasis with gentle cautery. Gelfoam and thrombin may be used but should be removed prior to closure of the orbitotomy.
32. Intravenous corticosteroid (8 mg dexamethasone) is given by the anaesthetist.
33. It may not be possible to close the periorbita at the end of the procedure. If the edges can be re-approximated, the periorbita is sutured with interrupted 5/0 Vicryl sutures.
34. The bone fragment is replaced and anchored into position with 3/0 Vicryl sutures (Figure 17.39).
35. The periosteum is reapproximated over the bone with interrupted 5/0 Vicryl sutures.
36. The swabs are removed from the temporal fossa and the bone and temporalis muscle checked for bleeding.
37. The subcutaneous tissue is closed with interrupted 5/0 Vicryl sutures.
38. The skin is closed with a continuous subcuticular 4/0 nylon suture.
39. A suction drain should be placed into the temporal fossa.
40. A pressure dressing is applied and then removed as soon as the patient is awake in the recovery room to allow a visual acuity check and inspection of the wound and globe position.

# Combined orbitotomies

The orbitotomies described may be used in combination if necessary. Access to the medial orbital apex, for example, can be improved by combining a medial orbitotomy with a lateral orbitotomy.

Small benign orbital apical lesions causing compressive optic neuropathy may be approached endoscopically via the ethmoid sinus. The posterior aspect of the lamina papyracea may be removed and the periorbita opened to allow the lesion to prolapse medially, relieving pressure on the optic nerve. This is a particularly useful approach for older patients with cardiovascular problems in whom a more formal surgical exploration carries a significant risk of visual morbidity. This approach can also be used in selected cases in order to obtain a small biopsy of a medial orbital apical lesion.

# Transfrontal orbitotomy

A lesion at the orbital apex may require an approach from above the orbit to gain adequate safe access. Such surgery is undertaken as a team approach involving a neurosurgeon. The patient must understand the risks and potential complications of such surgery: e.g. postoperative epilepsy, which may have major implications for the patient's occupation and driving. The patient should understand that a postoperative ptosis and an extraocular muscle palsy are frequently seen, but in most cases resolve spontaneously after a period of months.

A frontal craniotomy is undertaken via a bicoronal flap approach (Figures 17.40–17.42). The frontal bone flap is hinged laterally, still attached by the temporalis muscle and pericranium. The flap can include the superior orbital margin if a wider exposure is required. This provides good exposure of the medial, superior and lateral orbital apex. Lesions that involve the inferior orbital apex may require a temporal craniotomy approach, sometimes combined with a lateral orbitotomy.

For lesions confined to the orbit, an extradural approach is undertaken. For orbitocranial tumours, e.g. an optic nerve sheath meningioma, an intradural approach is required. The frontal lobe is gently retracted with self-retaining retractors (Figure 17.42). The

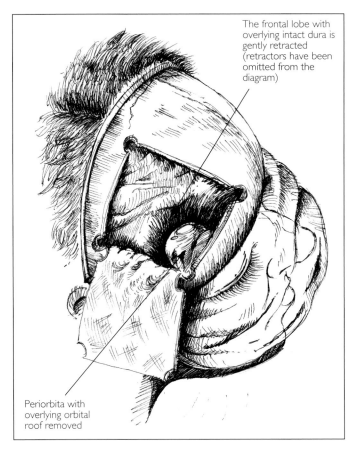

The frontal lobe with overlying intact dura is gently retracted (retractors have been omitted from the diagram)

Periorbita with overlying orbital roof removed

**Figure 17.40**
A schematic diagram of a right frontal craniotomy gaining access to the orbital apex.

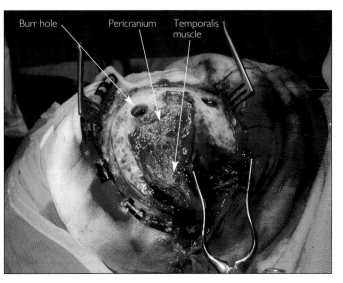

Burr hole    Pericranium    Temporalis muscle

**Figure 17.41**
A right frontal craniotomy in preparation. Burr holes are being prepared. The bone flap with attached pericranium and temporalis muscle will be hinged laterally and kept moistened in a large swab during the orbital dissection.

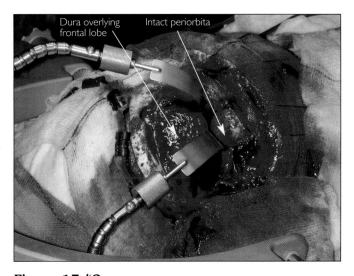

Dura overlying frontal lobe    Intact periorbita

**Figure 17.42**
The frontal lobe is very gently retracted with self-retaining retractors. The orbital roof has been removed. The periorbita is intact. This will be opened and the orbital apical lesion exposed.

orbital roof is removed to the apex of the orbit, keeping the periorbita intact. This is then opened in a similar fashion to a lateral orbitotomy. The frontal nerve is identified, running in a posteroanterior direction over the levator muscle. The orbit should be entered medial to the optic nerve to avoid damaging the cranial nerves entering the orbit via the superior orbital fissure. The orbital lesion is identified and removed in a similar fashion to that described during the course of a lateral orbitotomy. The orbital roof is then reconstructed by using either an alloplastic material or by using the inner table of the frontal bone flap.

# Postoperative management following orbital surgery

1.  Instructions are given for the patient's head to be elevated 45 degrees.
2.  The patient is instructed against any manoeuvre that could raise venous pressure with the risk of provoking haemorrhage.
3.  The dressings are removed approximately 45 min following surgery and the patient's visual acuity and pupil reactions checked hourly for 18 hours.
4.  An ice pack is applied to the periorbital area intermittently for 24 hours.
5.  *No opiates are prescribed for pain management. Any complaint of pain should be followed by the immediate examination of the patient to exclude signs of a retrobulbar haemorrhage.*
6.  The patient should be kept nil by mouth until the following day as a precaution. If a sudden retrobulbar haemorrhage were to occur causing an orbital compartment syndrome the patient would have to be returned to the operating

room immediately for the orbit to be re-explored and the source of bleeding stopped. Medical therapy to lower the intraocular pressure would be given in the interim.

7. Systemic corticosteroids are prescribed for a period of 6 days following surgery (commencing at 60 mg of prednisolone and reducing by 10 mg per day) and topical antibiotic ointment for the wound.

8. Systemic antibiotics are only used for specific indications, e.g. previous infection, foreign bodies, exposure of the paranasal sinuses.

# Further reading

1. Dutton JJ. *Atlas of clinical and surgical orbital anatomy*. Philadelphia: WB Saunders, 1994.

2. De Potter P, Shields JA, Shields CL. *MRI of the eye and orbit*. Philadelphia: JB Lippincott, 1995.

3. Housepian EM. Microsurgical anatomy of the orbital apex and principles of transcranial orbital exploration. *Clin Neurosurg* (1978) **25**:556–73.

4. Jordan DR, Anderson RL. *Surgical anatomy of the ocular adnexa: a clinical approach*. Ophthalmology Monograph 9, American Academy of Ophthalmology, 1996.

5. Kersten RC. The eyelid crease approach to superficial lateral dermoid cysts. *J Pediatr Ophthalmol Strabismus* (1988) **25**:48–51.

6. Kersten RC, Kulwin DR. Vertical lid split orbitotomy revisited. *Ophthal Plast Reconstr Surg* (1999) **15**:425–8.

7. Kersten RC, Nerad JA. Orbital surgery. In: Tasman W, Jaeger EA, eds, *Duane's clinical ophthalmology*, rev ed., Vol. 5. Baltimore: Lippincott, Williams & Wilkins, 1988, pp. 1–36.

8. Rootman J. Orbital surgery. In: Rootman J, ed., *Diseases of the orbit*, Philadelphia: JB Lippincott, 1988, pp. 579–612.

9. Rootman J, Stewart B, Goldberg RA. *Orbital Surgery, A Conceptual Approach*. Philadelphia: Lippincott-Raven, 1995.

10. Shorr N, Baylis H. Transcaruncular–transconjunctival approach to the medial orbit and orbital apex. Oral presentation at the American Society of Ophthalmic Plastic and Reconstructive Surgeons, 24th Annual Scientific Symposium, Chicago, 13 November, 1993.

# 18

# Thyroid eye disease

## Introduction

Thyroid eye disease is the most common orbital disorder and the commonest cause of unilateral or bilateral proptosis in an adult. Although it was described by Graves in 1835, the disorder remains an enigma, with many major issues remaining unresolved.

It is a very variable disorder, with a wide spectrum of clinical presentation, which can result in initial misdiagnosis. Diagnostic accuracy has been improved by advances both in laboratory investigations and orbital imaging techniques. Research continues to improve our understanding of the underlying pathogenesis of the disorder. The clinical management of patients has also been greatly improved over recent years with a better understanding of the pathophysiology of eyelid retraction, restrictive myopathy and compressive optic neuropathy. The surgical approaches to orbital decompression continue to evolve.

## Pathogenesis

Although the precise cause of thyroid eye disease continues to elude researchers, the orbitopathy and dysthyroid state appear to be associated with immunological abnormalities. It is generally believed that the orbitopathy is an organ-specific autoimmune disorder with target auto-antigens and circulating auto-antibodies, closely related to but separate from the thyroid gland disorder, which tends to affect females more commonly than males. Patients often have a history or family history of other auto-immune disorders, e.g. diabetes mellitus, pernicious anaemia, Addison's disease, myasthenia gravis. Smoking has a major adverse effect on the disease process. Patients treated with radioactive iodine may suffer a worse orbitopathy.

## Pathology

The extraocular muscles show inflammatory cell infiltration with lymphocytes, plasma cells and mast cells. Although the inferior and medial rectus muscles are more commonly affected clinically, orbital imaging demonstrates that most if not all the extraocular muscles, including the levator muscle, are involved in the disease process. The muscles undergo degenerative changes caused by the deposition of glycosaminoglycans and collagen formation, and demonstrate infiltration with fat. In the majority of patients the disease process becomes inactive after a period of 18 months to 2 years. The degenerated extraocular muscles become replaced by fat and fibrous tissue, resulting in

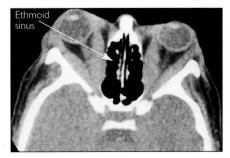

a

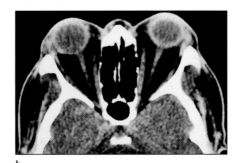

b

**Figure 18.1**
(a) Severe bilateral proptosis due to extraocular muscle enlargement with orbital apical crowding. (b) Marked bilateral proptosis in a patient with thyroid eye disease. The extraocular muscles are of normal size but the volume of orbital fat is increased. The optic nerves are stretched, with tenting of the posterior poles of the globes. The patient had a severe dysthyroid optic neuropathy.

a restrictive myopathy in severe or untreated cases. In most patients the orbital fat does not undergo significant structural changes, although in some patients the orbital fat shows marked volumetric alterations that can be responsible for marked proptosis, even in the absence of extraocular muscle enlargement, as seen on orbital imaging (Figure 18.1b).

# Pathophysiology

A single extraocular muscle or multiple extraocular muscles may be affected by the disorder, which may present symmetrically or asymmetrically. The extraocular muscle enlargement and/or orbital fat hypertrophy cause a secondary mass effect within the confines of the bony orbit. The secondary effects depend on a number of variable and interacting factors that are responsible for the wide range of clinical presentation of thyroid eye disease. These include:

1.  The volume of the orbital cavity
2.  The axial length of the globe
3.  The integrity of the orbital septum
4.  The degree and rapidity of the orbital inflammation
5.  The degree of enlargement of the extraocular muscles
6.  The degree of hypertrophy of the orbital fat
7.  The absence of lymphatics from the posterior orbital tissues.

If the orbital cavity is small, any mass effect can result in more severe degrees of proptosis and even in frank subluxation of the globe. *Patients with axial myopia tend to experience a more severe cosmetic deformity resulting from proptosis (Figure 18.2).*

The degree of proptosis, which results from the orbital mass effect, is influenced by the tightness of the orbital septum. A lax orbital septum offers little resistance to the forward movement of the globe. The degree of resultant proptosis is governed by the size of the orbital cavity, the axial length of the globe, the degree of extraocular muscle and/or orbital fat swelling, the compliance of the extraocular muscles and the length of the optic nerve. The resultant proptosis represents a spontaneous orbital decompression that may be severe enough to result in spontaneous subluxation of the globe. It may also be severe enough to cause a stretching of the optic nerve and deformation of the posterior aspect of the globe, which may cause an optic neuropathy with visual loss.

In contrast, where the orbital septum is tight, as seen in the younger patient, the globe is prevented from moving forwards and the pressure within the orbit rises. This rise in intraorbital pressure, in conjunction with swelling of the extraocular muscles in the confined bony space of the orbital apex, can result in an insidious compressive optic neuropathy. The degree of visual impairment may be out of proportion to apparent clinical extent of the disease (Figure 18.3).

The tightness of the orbital septum and the absence of deep orbital lymphatic vessels also influence the magnitude of secondary periorbital tissue oedema. If the orbital inflammation progresses rapidly, the secondary congestive changes can be severe, resulting in so-called malignant exophthalmos (see Figure 18.12).

# Epidemiology

The majority of patients (approximately 90%) present within the first 15–24 months of hyperthyroidism. A much smaller proportion (approximately 4%) of patients presenting with thyroid eye disease are hypothyroid, with the remainder being euthyroid. Men and older patients (over 50 years of age) tend to have much more aggressive disease.

**Figure 18.2**
Young Malaysian patient with marked symmetric proptosis. The patient has high axial myopia and shallow orbits.

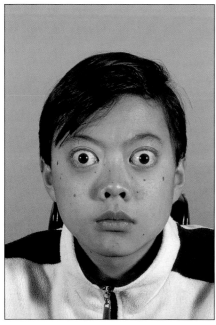

a

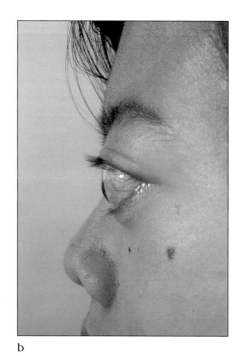

b

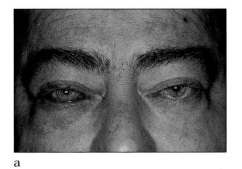
a

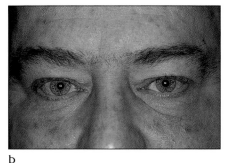
b

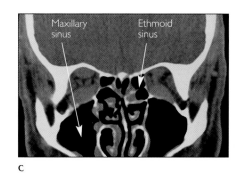
c

**Figure 18.3**
(a) Patient with bilateral severe compressive optic neuropathy unresponsive to aggressive medical therapy. (b) Patient following bilateral two-wall orbital decompression performed via subciliary skin incisions. (c) Coronal CT scan demonstrating orbital apical crowding from extraocular muscle enlargement.

# Clinical presentation

The clinical manifestations of thyroid eye disease can be very variable and may be acute or insidious in onset. Patients can be divided into two subtypes.

## Type 1

Patients with type 1 or 'noninfiltrative' orbitopathy tend to be younger and usually present with symmetric proptosis, eyelid retraction, minimal inflammatory signs and no extraocular muscle restrictions (Figure 18.4). These clinical features tend to be manifestations of hyperthyroidism and may even regress once the hyperthyroidism has been controlled. The diagnosis of thyroid eye disease in this subset of patients does not usually present a problem.

## Type 2

Patients with type 2 or 'infiltrative' orbitopathy are usually middle-aged and run a much more fulminant course. The orbitopathy is likely to be more asymmetric and the patient is likely to present with chemosis, diplopia and compressive optic neuropathy (Figure 18.5).

# Clinical symptoms and signs

The symptoms of thyroid eye disease are variable and may be nonspecific. They include ocular irritation, a foreign body sensation, tearing, photophobia, diplopia and visual impairment. Many patients with type 2 orbitopathy complain of a constant deep boring orbital pain.

The physical signs are also variable and include:

1. Proptosis
2. Eyelid retraction
3. Eyelid lag
4. Lagophthalmos
5. Periorbital oedema
6. Conjunctival and caruncular oedema
7. Injection of the vessels along the horizontal recti
8. Limitation of ocular motility
9. Exposure keratopathy
10. Superior limbic keratoconjunctivitis
11. Optic disc oedema/pallor with signs of optic nerve dysfunction
12. Choroidal folds (Figure 18.6)

> It should be noted that these physical signs, with the exception of superior limbic keratoconjunctivitis, may be observed, singly or in combination, in any orbital inflammatory disorder.

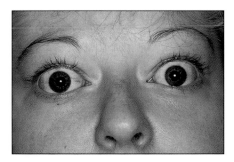

**Figure 18.4**
Young female patient with type 1 thyroid eye disease.

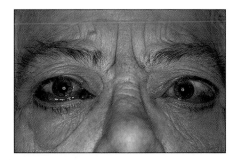

**Figure 18.5**
Older female patient with type 2 thyroid eye disease.

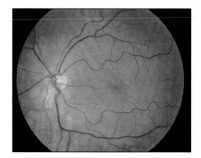

**Figure 18.6**
Choroidal folds in a patient with thyroid eye disease.

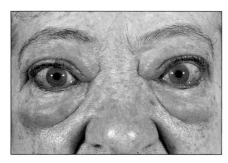

**Figure 18.7**
Patient with type 2 thyroid eye disease demonstrating typical periorbital oedema.

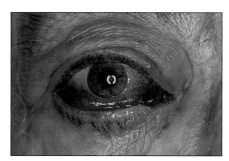

**Figure 18.8**
Patient with inferior chemosis and caruncular oedema.

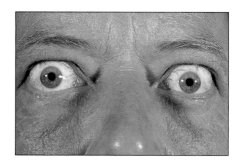

**Figure 18.9**
Marked bilateral upper eyelid retraction due to severe proptosis and infiltration of the levator muscles.

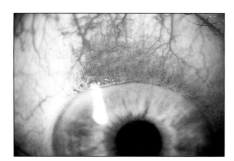

**Figure 18.10**
Superior limbic keratoconjunctivitis.

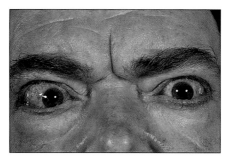

**Figure 18.11**
Male patient with severe type 2 thyroid eye disease. The severity of the myopathy should alert his clinicians to the possibility of an insidious compressive optic neuropathy. He also demonstrates a typical contraction of the procerus and corrugator supercilii muscles with marked glabellar frown lines creating a very aggressive appearance.

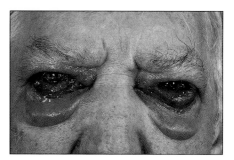

**Figure 18.12**
A male patient with severe infiltrative thyroid orbitopathy and a bilateral 'malignant exophthalmos'.

The physical signs in thyroid eye disease can alter with subtle remissions and exacerbations.

Periorbital oedema is an early sign of thyroid eye disease. The oedema is particularly prominent in the upper lids and tends to be maximal in the morning, diminishing throughout the day (Figure 18.7).

Caruncular oedema may be quite subtle. This, in conjunction with conjunctival chemosis, is a clinical measure of disease activity and response to medical therapy (Figure 18.8). Chemosis can be very marked in some patients and may interfere with the normal distribution of the tear film.

The causes of eyelid retraction in thyroid eye disease are discussed in Chapter 19 (The Management of Thyroid-Related Eyelid Retraction) (Figure 18.9). A ptosis can occasionally be seen in thyroid eye disease patients as a result of a stretching of the levator aponeurosis following marked upper eyelid oedema.

Superior limbic keratoconjunctivitis is a nonspecific ocular lesion which has no known cause but is frequently associated with thyroid eye disease when present bilaterally (Figure 18.10).

Ocular motility limitation is often variable and frequently asymmetric. Symmetrical restriction may spare the patient from diplopia but, frequently, asymmetric progression results in diplopia (Figure 18.11). The inferior recti followed by the medial recti are the most frequently affected muscles. Vertical diplopia with discomfort and pain that increases on upgaze is most frequently seen. Forced duction testing confirms restriction of motility. A rise in intraocular pressure may be noted on upgaze. *It is important not to overlook the possibility of myasthenia gravis as a cause of a changing or unusual ocular deviation in a patient with thyroid eye disease.*

Exposure keratopathy can occur due to:

- 1.   Severe proptosis
- 2.   Eyelid retraction with lagophthalmos
- 3.   Conjunctival chemosis causing dellen formation

Corneal thinning, scarring or frank ulceration can occur, resulting in severe visual morbidity (Figure 18.12).

Subluxation of the globe is a distressing situation for a patient where the eyes are so protrusive that they may prolapse out of the orbit, especially on attempting to look up. The eyelids may close behind the eye (Figure 18.13). Such patients are naturally

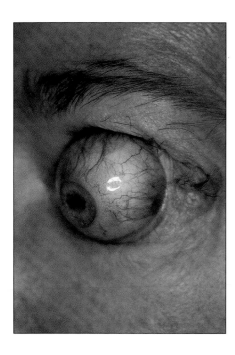

**Figure 18.13** Subluxation of the globe in a patient who has previously undergone an inappropriate lateral tarsorrhaphy.

reluctant to look up during examination of their ocular motility. Great care should be taken during the use of an exophthalmometer, which can provoke a subluxation. If subluxation should occur, the globe should be manually repositioned immediately.

*Compressive optic neuropathy can occur as an insidious complication of thyroid eye disease, often in patients without marked proptosis and often in the absence of any fundoscopic abnormalities.* Only a small percentage of patients demonstrate optic disc oedema. The incidence of optic neuropathy in patients with thyroid eye disease is approximately 4–5%. A high index of suspicion for its development should be maintained when examining patients with thyroid eye disease. In general, patients with a more severe myopathy pose the greatest risk for the development of compressive optic neuropathy.

# Patient evaluation

In the majority of patients with thyroid eye disease there is no difficulty in establishing the diagnosis, as there is a prior history of thyroid dysfunction or characteristic clinical findings. In patients with no prior history of thyroid dysfunction, thyroid function tests are performed along with antibody studies. The diagnosis can be particularly difficult to establish in the small percentage of patients who present with no prior history of a thyroid disorder or who demonstrate no abnormality of thyroid function. The assistance of an endocrinologist should be sought in the evaluation and management of all patients with suspected thyroid eye disease.

> Patients should be examined repeatedly and thoroughly with a special emphasis on tests of optic nerve function.

A number of classifications of the ophthalmic changes in thyroid eye disease have been described in an attempt to quantitate the orbitopathy. The classification by Werner was frequently used because of the easily remembered mnemonic 'NOSPECS'. Although widely used, there are many difficulties in applying this and other classifications. The preferred classification is that of Mourits (see Further Reading, Ref 2).

In the evaluation of patients with thyroid eye disease, two aspects should be considered:

- The *activity* of the disease
- The *extent* of the disease

The activity of the disease is indicated by the soft tissue symptoms and signs. It can also be determined by a 'STIR' (short tau inversion recovery) sequence magnetic resonance imaging (MRI) scan that suppresses the normal bright signal from orbital fat on T1-weighted images. The extent is determined by the effect of the disease on:

1. Optic nerve function
2. Ocular motility
3. The cornea
4. The position of the eyelids
5. The position of the globe

# Orbital imaging

A computed tomography (CT) scan of the orbit and paranasal sinuses should be performed in both axial and coronal planes. It has an important role in the evaluation of the patient with thyroid eye disease:

1. It can assist in determining the cause of decreased visual function by demonstrating orbital apical muscle enlargement and a 'crowded orbital apex syndrome'.
2. It can assist in excluding other mimicking orbital disorders or dual pathology (see Figure 18.16)
3. It provides an evaluation of the size of the orbits and the size and status of the paranasal sinuses.
4. It demonstrates the true extent of the patient's proptosis.
5. It assesses the relative contributions of extraocular muscle enlargement versus orbital fat enlargement to the patient's proptosis.
6. A coronal view demonstrates the position of the cribriform plate and its relationship to the frontoethmoidal suture line (Figure 18.14).

A crowded orbital apex is demonstrated well on coronal sections. It is important to exclude an additional pathological process as a cause of proptosis, particularly with asymmetric disease.

An axial scan can demonstrate the true extent of the proptosis and the relationship of the globe to the anterior bony opening of the orbit. Extreme stretching of the optic nerve may be seen and can represent another mechanism for optic neuropathy.

If a patient requires an orbital decompression, a preoperative CT scan is essential and should be available for examination in the

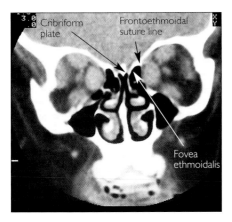

**Figure 18.14**
Coronal CT scan demonstrating
extraocular muscle enlargement. The
ethmoid sinuses are clear, with plenty
of room between the cribriform plate
and the frontoethmoidal suture line.
The lower position of the cribriform
plate should be noted.

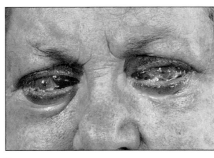

a                                    b

**Figure 18.16**
(a) Female patient with hyperthyroidism who presented with bilateral visual loss and
diplopia. A diagnosis of severe thyroid orbitopathy had been made by her general
ophthalmologist. She developed severe exposure keratopathy while undergoing
orbital radiotherapy. (b) A coronal CT scan demonstrated bilateral infiltrating orbital
masses. A biopsy confirmed the diagnosis of metastatic breast carcinoma.

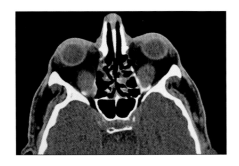

**Figure 18.15**
Bilateral orbital apical 'masses'. This
appearance on an axial CT scan is due
to the angle of the axial section
cutting across enlarged inferior rectus
muscles.

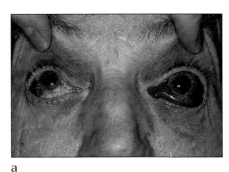

a                                    b

**Figure 18.17**
(a) A patient with a low-flow arteriovenous shunt. (b) Close-up of the left eye
demonstrating chemosis and enlargement of the episcleral vessels.

operating room during surgery. The type of orbital decompression
required by the individual patient is largely determined by the CT
scan appearances. It is important to be aware of the proximity of
the cribriform plate to the frontoethmoidal suture line (Figure
18.14). Patients with a low cribriform plate and a small fovea
ethmoidalis are at greater risk of intraoperative damage to the
cribriform plate and a subsequent cerebrospinal fluid (CSF) leak.

It is important to be aware that enlargement of the inferior
rectus muscle in thyroid eye disease can be mistaken for an
orbital apical mass on an axial CT scan, particularly in patients
with unilateral proptosis (Figure 18.15). The true cause of the
patient's proptosis is readily seen on the coronal views.

An MRI scan is useful to determine the activity of the disease
by assessing the signal from the extraocular muscles prior to
committing the patient to corticosteroids, radiotherapy and even
antimetabolites. A STIR sequence with fat suppression is particularly useful.

# Differential diagnosis

Orbital disorders that may mimic thyroid eye disease in their
clinical presentation produce inflammation and infiltration of the
orbital muscles (Figure 18.16). These disorders include:

1.  Nonspecific orbital inflammatory syndrome
2.  Arteriovenous shunts
3.  Extraocular muscle metastases
4.  Wegener's granulomatosis
5.  Sarcoidosis
6.  Amyloidosis
7.  Collagen vascular diseases

Most of these disorders should be readily differentiated on the
basis of the history, clinical appearances and imaging characteristics, e.g. an orbital myositis is usually painful, and does not spare

the tendon of insertion of the extraocular muscle(s) on orbital imaging in contrast to the myopathy of thyroid eye disease.

A low-flow arteriovenous shunt (Figure 18.17) can, however, create diagnostic confusion, as this can cause a diffuse enlargement of the extraocular muscles, as seen on orbital imaging, along with conjunctival chemosis. Distension of the episcleral vessels is not, however, confined to those over the horizontal recti and the superior ophthalmic vein, unless thrombosed, is dilated. This is best seen on axial images.

> It should be borne in mind that patients with thyroid dysfunction can develop other orbital disorders. An open mind should always be maintained and the diagnosis questioned.

## Management

The goals in the management of the patient with thyroid eye disease are to:

1. Resolve or control the orbital inflammation
2. Prevent visual loss
3. Re-establish ocular muscle balance
4. Provide cosmetic rehabilitation

In attempting to achieve these goals, the patient should be placed at minimum risk of complications.

It is important to involve an endocrinologist in the patient's management and to communicate effectively. Good control of thyroid function is important:

- There is a relationship between the severity of hyperthyroidism and the severity of the orbitopathy
- The patient's thyroid disorder must be under good control prior to any surgery

Many of the ophthalmic consequences of thyroid eye disease can be managed conservatively. The management options should be discussed carefully with the patient. Some patients require medical therapy alone, others respond to a combination of medical and surgical treatment, whereas patients with specific sequelae of the disease require surgical intervention alone.

## *Medical management*

Medical treatment consists of

- Immunosuppressive therapy – corticosteroids, antimetabolites
- Radiotherapy

Systemic corticosteroids are used for two groups of patients:

1. Patients with acute inflammatory eye disease
2. Patients with compressive optic neuropathy

Patients with acute inflammatory eye disease typically respond very quickly to steroids, but maintenance doses frequently lead to steroid complications. Patients with chronic disease do not respond to corticosteroids or alternative medical therapy.

The therapeutic threshold for compressive optic neuropathy is very high, with some patients requiring corticosteroid doses in excess of 100 mg/day. Pulsed intravenous steroids arrest the disease process more quickly. Antimetabolite agents, e.g. azathioprine, may be used in conjunction, as 'steroid sparers'. This reduces the steroid side effects but exposes the patient to the risks of further immunosuppression.

Corticosteroids are used not as the definitive form of treatment for compressive optic neuropathy by most clinicians but as a temporizing measure until radiotherapy or surgery can be employed. In a small percentage of patients, however, the orbitopathy abates and the patient can be successfully weaned off steroids without the need for further treatment. In contrast, some patients, in spite of radiotherapy and/or surgical decompression, require long-term use of corticosteroids to control continued orbital inflammation and prevent visual loss.

Radiotherapy also has favourable results in acute inflammatory disease and in compressive optic neuropathy but is ineffective in chronic disease. It is focused on the posterior orbit, sparing the globe, and has a low morbidity. A large proportion of patients respond to radiotherapy, with a resolution of soft tissue signs and symptoms. Radiotherapy itself causes some worsening of orbital inflammation before its beneficial effects are seen. It must therefore be used in conjunction with corticosteroids, which are then gradually withdrawn. It is used in some centres for the management of compressive optic neuropathy when surgical decompression is either contraindicated or has failed. It has the disadvantage that the effects are not seen for a period of 4–6 weeks. In addition, relapses may affect up to 20–30% of patients. Such patients must therefore be followed closely.

> It is extremely important to be aware of the potential serious systemic side effects of the use of corticosteroids and antimetabolites: e.g. aseptic necrosis of the femoral head; osteoporosis and pathological fractures; duodenal ulceration with gastrointestinal haemorrhage; secondary diabetes mellitus; cataracts; glaucoma; and predisposition to opportunistic infection. Patients should be carefully warned about the risks. Patients must be monitored very closely, and in conjunction with an endocrinologist, who can monitor for and treat osteoporosis.

## *Surgical management*

Surgical intervention should be approached in a specific sequence. Decompressive surgery may alter ocular muscle balance, and ocular muscle surgery may alter eyelid position. Surgery is therefore performed in sequence, recognizing that not all patients require surgery of each stage but may omit various stages. The order of surgical intervention is therefore:

1. Orbital decompression
2. Strabismus surgery
3. Eyelid repositioning surgery
4. Blepharoplasty

In some cases, however, blepharoplasties may be performed in conjunction with orbital decompression, depending on the approach.

Patients with reduced orbital compliance who demonstrate resistance to simple retropulsion of the globe will gain much less effect from any orbital decompression procedure than a patient with the same degree of proptosis who has normal orbital compliance.

Strabismus and eyelid repositioning surgery should preferably be deferred until the clinical signs are stable. Surgical intervention may, however, have to be performed urgently for severe corneal exposure or for compressive optic neuropathy unresponsive to medical therapy.

Patients must understand the possible requirement for multiple surgical procedures, which may take some considerable time to complete. Such patients need to be counselled very carefully to ensure that their expectations are realistic.

# Surgical orbital decompression

The cardinal indication for surgical decompression remains compressive optic neuropathy but, as decompressive surgery continues to evolve, the indications have become far less conservative.

## Indications

1. Compressive optic neuropathy unresponsive to medical treatment
2. Recurrent subluxation of the globe
3. Severe proptosis with exposure keratopathy
4. Cosmetic rehabilitation of unsightly proptosis
5. Constant boring orbital pain unresponsive to medical treatment
6. Reduction of proptosis prior to extraocular muscle recessions

Surgery may be urgent for the management of compressive optic neuropathy or severe exposure keratopathy or elective for the remaining indications. In general, surgery should be undertaken only after initial medical intervention.

Some patients have constant aching orbital pain due to congestion of the orbital tissues. This can be relieved by a decompression procedure in the majority of cases.

In some patients with marked proptosis, the degree of proptosis may worsen following extraocular muscle surgery undertaken to improve diplopia. In such patients, a decompression operation may be considered desirable prior to such extraocular muscle surgery.

Decompressive surgery is being requested more and more frequently to improve the aesthetic appearance of patients, as the surgical results and safety of the surgery have improved considerably over recent years (Figure 18.18). Such surgery should be regarded as 'rehabilitative' rather than 'cosmetic'. There is no doubt that the changes in appearance caused by thyroid eye disease can have a devastating psychological effect on patients and such surgery can achieve significant improvements. The goal is to restore the appearance to that which existed prior to the onset of this disease process. However, such goals are rarely achieved completely and patients must be counselled very carefully preoperatively to ensure that they have realistic expectations.

# Surgical approaches

The orbit may be decompressed by:

- Reducing the orbital contents (removal of orbital fat)
- Expanding the orbital volume (removing orbital walls/advancing the lateral orbital wall).

These decompression procedures can be used in isolation or in combination.

# Orbital fat removal

Removal of orbital fat may achieve a satisfactory reduction in proptosis in a patient without significant enlargement of the extraocular muscles who has no resistance to retropulsion of the globe clinically. This can be performed alone or it can be used to gain additional decompressive effect in patients undergoing a bony decompression. The fat may be removed in combination with an upper and/or lower eyelid blepharoplasty. The surgical approach is transcutaneous in the upper eyelid. In the lower eyelid it may be transcutaneous or transconjunctival. Better surgical exposure for removal of inferolateral orbital fat is achieved if a transconjunctival approach is combined with a lateral canthotomy and inferior cantholysis (a 'swinging eyelid' approach).

The removal of orbital fat demands extreme care and patience to avoid inadvertent damage to other intraorbital structures. Respect must be paid to meticulous haemostasis. The fat is gently teased out with gentle dissection of the delicate orbital septa. Haemostasis is facilitated by the use of a Colorado needle used on constant coagulation mode. Bipolar cautery is applied to larger vessels before these are damaged. Good retraction by an assistant is essential. The pupil should be monitored throughout the surgery and any pressure on the globe released at intervals. The patient's vision must be monitored very closely postoperatively.

## Advantages

1. This approach avoids the risk of inferior displacement of the globe
2. There is no risk of injury to structures external to the periorbita such as the dura, the lacrimal sac and the infraorbital nerve

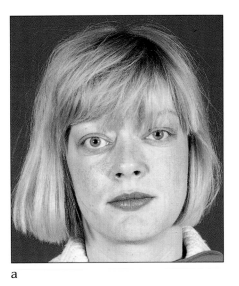
a

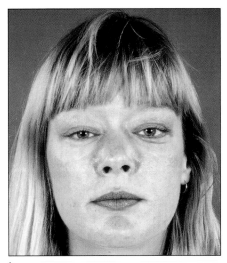
b

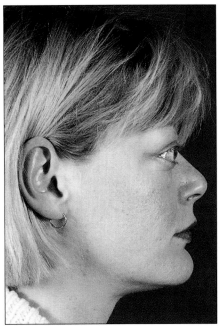
c

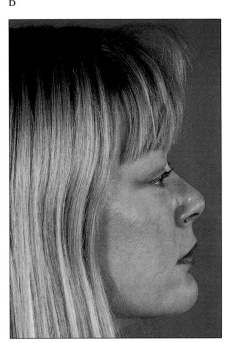
d

**Figure 18.18**
A patient before (a,c) and after (b,d) a bilateral three-wall translid orbital decompression performed for cosmetic rehabilitation.

3. The surgical incisions are minimal
4. The postoperative recovery is rapid
5. It can further improve the reduction in proptosis achieved by surgery on the orbital walls

## Disadvantages
1. The surgery is time-consuming
2. It risks damage to delicate intraorbital structures
3. Postoperative bleeding can jeopardize vision

## Increasing orbital volume

Over the years all four walls of the orbit have been resected, singly or in combination, for the purposes of orbital decompression. There is no longer any indication for surgery on the orbital roof. The choice of decompressive procedure should be tailored to the individual patient's needs based on the following:

1. The indication(s) for the surgery
2. The patient's age and general health

3. The size and status of the paranasal sinuses
4. The size of the orbits
5. The amount of proptosis
6. The relative contributions of extraocular muscle enlargement versus orbital fat swelling to proptosis
7. The orbital compliance

Patients should not be merely subjected to the surgeon's favourite operation for orbital decompression. Unless a large decompression is required for severe proptosis, a medial strut should be maintained between the medial orbital wall and the orbital floor to reduce the risk of a postoperative esotropia or frank medial globe dystopia. An orbital decompression must, wherever possible, avoid an inferior displacement of the globe, which worsens upper eyelid retraction. For this reason it is preferable not to remove the whole of the orbital floor. It is preferable to balance the medial wall decompression with a lateral wall decompression and avoid any removal of the orbital floor if possible.

*Surgery for compressive optic neuropathy should provide adequate relief of orbital apical compression.* The outcome of surgery improves with time from the decompression. In some patients this can be achieved by fat decompression alone.

The bony walls can be accessed in a variety of ways. Each of these approaches has its advantages and disadvantages.

1. Via a nasal endoscopic approach
2. Via a lower eyelid subciliary or skin crease incision
3. Via a lower eyelid transconjunctival incision ('swinging eyelid' flap)
4. Via a medial canthal ('Lynch') skin incision
5. Via a lateral canthal/lateral orbitotomy/upper eyelid incision
6. Via a bicoronal flap approach
7. Via a transantral (Caldwell–Luc) approach
8. Via a transcaruncular approach

# Applied anatomy

It is important for any surgeon who wishes to undertake a bony orbital decompression to have a sound knowledge of the anatomy of the paranasal sinuses.

# *The paranasal sinuses*

The frontal, ethmoidal, sphenoidal and maxillary paranasal sinuses vary in size and shape in different individuals. Most are rudimentary, or even absent, at birth. They enlarge considerably during the time of eruption of the permanent teeth and after puberty, and this growth is a factor in the alteration in the size and shape of the face at these times. They are lined with mucous membrane continuous with that of the nasal cavity, an important fact in connection with the spread of infections. The mucous membrane resembles that of the respiratory region of the nasal cavity, but is thinner, less vascular and more loosely adherent to the bony walls of the sinuses. The mucus secreted by the glands in the mucous membrane is swept into the nose through the apertures of the sinuses by the movement of the cilia covering the surface.

# The frontal sinuses

Two frontal *sinuses* are posterior to the superciliary arches, between the outer and inner tables of the frontal bone. They are rarely symmetrical, as the septum between them frequently deviates from the median plane. The frontal sinus is sometimes divided into a number of communicating recesses by incomplete bony partitions. Rarely, one or both sinuses may be absent, and the degree of prominence of the superciliary arches is no indication of the presence or size of the frontal sinuses. *The part of the sinus extending upwards in the frontal bone may be small and the orbital part large, or vice versa.* Sometimes one sinus may overlap in front of the other. The sinus may extend posteriorly as far as the lesser wing of the sphenoid but does not invade it. Each opens into the anterior part of the corresponding middle meatus of the nose, either through the ethmoidal infundibulum or through frontonasal duct, which traverses the anterior part of labyrinth of the ethmoid. *Rudimentary or absent at birth, the frontal sinuses are generally fairly well developed between the seventh and eighth years, but reach their full size only at puberty.*

The frontal sinuses are usually larger in males, giving the profile of the head an obliquity that contrasts with the vertical or convex outline usually seen in children and females. The arterial blood supply of the sinus is from the supraorbital and anterior ethmoidal arteries, and the venous drainage is into the anastomotic vein in the supraorbital notch, connecting the supraorbital and superior ophthalmic veins. The lymphatic drainage is to the submandibular nodes. The nerve supply is derived from the supraorbital nerve.

# The ethmoidal sinuses

The ethmoidal sinuses consist of thin-walled cavities in the ethmoidal labyrinth. They vary in number and size from 3 large to 18 small sinuses on each side, and their openings into the nasal cavity are very variable. They lie between the upper part of the nasal cavity and the orbits, and are separated from the latter by the extremely thin orbital plates of the ethmoid, the lamina papyracea. Infection can spread readily from the sinuses into the orbit and produce orbital cellulitis. On each side they are arranged in three groups – anterior, middle and posterior. The three groups are not sharply delimited from each other and one group may encroach on the territory generally occupied by another. The groups are really only distinguishable on the basis of their sites of communication with the nasal cavity. In each group the sinuses are partially separated by incomplete bony septa. The *anterior group* varies up to 11 in number and opens into the ethmoidal infundibulum or the frontonasal duct by one or more orifices; one sinus frequently lies in the agger nasi. *This is frequently encountered during external dacryocystorhinostomy (DCR) procedures and should be recognized.* The *middle group* generally comprises 3 cavities that open into the middle meatus by one or more orifices on or above the ethmoidal bulla. The *posterior group* varies from 1 to 7 in number and usually opens by one orifice into the superior meatus inferior to the superior concha, though one may open into the highest meatus (when present), and one or more sometimes opens into the sphenoidal sinus. *The posterior group is very closely related to the optic canal and optic nerve.* The sinuses usually rise above the level of the frontoethmoidal suture line forming a dome into the base of the skull referred to as the *fovea ethmoidalis* (see Figure 18.14). The size and shape of this is variable. *If this area is small there is a greater risk of damaging the cribriform plate during orbital decompression surgery.*

The ethmoidal sinuses are small at birth, growing rapidly between the sixth and eighth years and after puberty. They derive their arterial blood supply from the sphenopalatine and the anterior ethmoidal and posterior ethmoidal arteries and are drained by the corresponding veins. The lymphatics of the anterior and middle groups drain into the submandibular nodes and those of the posterior group into the retropharyngeal nodes. The ethmoidal sinuses are supplied by the anterior and posterior ethmoidal nerves, and the orbital branches of the pterygopalatine ganglion.

## The sphenoidal sinuses

The two sphenoidal sinuses lie posterior to the upper part of the nasal cavity. Contained within the body of the sphenoid bone, they are related to the optic chiasm superiorly, and the pituitary, and, on each side, to the internal carotid arteries and the cavernous sinuses. If the sinuses are small, they lie in front of the pituitary. They vary in size and shape, and, because of the lateral displacement of the intervening septum, are frequently asymmetrical. One sinus is often larger than the other and extends across the median plane behind the sinus of the opposite side. One sinus may overlap above the other, and rarely there is a communication between the two sinuses. *Occasionally, one or both sinuses may extend close to and even partially encircle the optic canal on its own side.* For this reason sphenoid sinusitis may be responsible for an optic neuropathy. When exceptionally large they may extend into the roots of the pterygoid processes or greater wings of the sphenoid, and may invade the basilar part of the occipital bone. *Occasionally there are gaps in the bony walls and the mucous membrane may lie directly against the dura mater.*

Bony ridges, produced by the internal carotid artery and the pterygoid canal, may project into the sinuses from the lateral wall and floor, respectively. *The proximity of the carotid artery must be borne in mind when attempting to decompress the optic canal through the sphenoid sinus following a fracture with a compressive optic neuropathy.* A posterior ethmoidal sinus may extend into the body of the sphenoid and largely replace a sphenoidal sinus. Each sinus communicates with the sphenoethmoidal recess by an aperture in the upper part of its anterior wall. They are present as minute cavities at birth, but their main development occurs after puberty. Their blood supply is by one of the posterior ethmoidal vessels and the lymph drain is to the retropharyngeal nodes. Their nerve supply is from the posterior ethmoidal nerves and the orbital branches of the pterygopalatine ganglion.

## The maxillary sinuses

The two maxillary sinuses, which are the largest accessory air sinuses of the nose, are pyramidal cavities in the bodies of the maxillae. The base of each is formed by the lateral wall of the nasal cavity; the apex extends into the zygomatic process of the maxilla. The roof, which forms the orbital floor, is frequently ridged by the infraorbital canal. The area medial to the infraorbital canal is particularly weak and is the usual site for the occurrence of an orbital floor blowout fracture. The size of the maxillary sinus varies in different skulls, and even on the two sides of the same skull. In some patients a large maxillary sinus may extend into the zygomatic bone (Figure 18.3c). The sinus communicates with the lower part of the hiatus semilunaris through an opening in the anterosuperior part of its base. A second orifice is frequently seen in, or immediately below, the hiatus. Both are nearer the roof than the floor of the sinus. The maxillary sinus does not reach its full size until after the eruption of all the permanent teeth. The blood supply of the sinus is by means of the facial, infraorbital and greater palatine vessels; the lymph drainage is to the submandibular nodes. The nerve supply is derived from the infraorbital and the anterior, middle and posterior superior alveolar nerves.

# Orbital decompression – surgical approaches

## *Nasal endoscopic approach*

This approach is normally utilized by an ear, nose and throat (ENT) surgeon who has expertise in endoscopic sinus surgery. The approach may also be used by the orbital surgeon in conjunction with an eyelid incision approach to assist safe orbital apical bone removal.

### Advantages

1. There is no requirement for a skin or conjunctival incision
2. The operation can be performed quickly in experienced hands
3. An excellent view of the most posterior medial orbital wall can be obtained
4. It removes the need for retraction on the globe intraoperatively

### Disadvantages

1. The middle turbinate may have to be sacrificed to proceed with the surgery losing its important physiological functions.
2. The infraorbital neurovascular bundle cannot be protected easily during removal of the medial part of the orbital floor.
3. This approach alone cannot be combined with a lateral orbital wall decompression without resorting to a skin or conjunctival incision. If a balanced decompression is required to reduce the risks of postoperative diplopia, the advantages of an endoscopic approach are removed.
4. This approach requires expensive equipment.

The endoscopic approach avoids the need for any skin incisions and is excellent for access to the orbital apex in patients with compressive optic neuropathy. It offers a major advantage in the following groups of patients:

- Those with severe proptosis and a 'tight' orbit
- Patients with high myopia
- Patients with cardiovascular disease
- Patients with peripheral corneal thinning

These patients pose problems with access to the medial orbital wall and the orbital apex. The view may be difficult. Retraction of the globe may temporarily close the central retinal artery, with the attendant risks in the patient with cardiovascular disease. Patients with peripheral corneal thinning from chronic exposure keratopathy, or scleral thinning from high myopia, pose a risk of globe rupture with aggressive retraction.

## Lower eyelid subciliary or skin crease incision

This incision permits good access, in the majority of patients, to the medial orbital wall and its apex, to the floor of the orbit and to the lateral wall of the orbit. In the older patient, access to the orbit is quicker and easier via a lower lid skin crease incision. A subciliary incision is preferable in the younger patient.

## Advantages

1. The surgical approach is familiar to the oculoplastic surgeon who performs orbital wall blowout fracture repairs
2. The eyelid affords good ocular surface protection during the surgery
3. The approach permits access to three orbital walls through the same incision
4. The approach permits the removal of orbital fat to supplement the effect of the decompression
5. The approach can be combined with a lower eyelid blepharoplasty with removal of excess skin and muscle as well as extraconal fat
6. The subcutaneous injection of adrenaline does not affect the observation of the pupil response to traction on the globe

## Disadvantages

1. The lower eyelid may retract postoperatively unless the patient complies with postoperative eyelid massage
2. The view of the orbital apex may be obscured if there is inadvertent premature opening of the periorbita
3. The view of the orbital apex can be difficult in the patient with a 'tight' orbit or high myopia

## Lower eyelid transconjunctival incision ('swinging eyelid' flap)

This approach obviates the need for a skin incision and is preferred by many oculoplastic surgeons.

## Advantages

1. A cutaneous scar is confined to the lateral canthus
2. The approach to the orbital walls can be quickly achieved
3. The surgical approach is familiar to the oculoplastic surgeon who performs orbital wall blowout fracture repairs
4. The approach permits access to three orbital walls through the same incisions
5. The approach permits the removal of orbital fat to supplement the effect of the decompression
6. The approach can be combined with a lower eyelid blepharoplasty with removal of extraconal fat

## Disadvantages

1. The approach is associated with more postoperative chemosis and discomfort, particularly at the lateral canthus
2. The pupil may become dilated following the subconjunctival injection of adrenaline, preventing monitoring of the pupil response to traction on the globe
3. The view of the orbital apex may be obscured if there is inadvertent premature opening of the periorbita
4. The view of the orbital apex can be difficult in the patient with a 'tight' orbit or high myopia

## Medial canthal (Lynch) skin incision

This approach offers no advantages over alternative approaches and has significant disadvantages, e.g. a visible obtrusive scar prone to 'bow stringing'. It necessitates the removal of the medial canthal tendon and the division of the ethmoidal arteries. Such manoeuvres are unnecessary in alternative approaches.

## Lateral canthal/lateral orbitotomy/upper eyelid incision

These incisions permit access to the lateral orbital wall in cases where a formal lateral orbitotomy and an advancement/valgus rotation of the lateral wall are required. An extended upper eyelid crease incision affords better cosmetic results than a standard lateral orbitotomy incision or an extended lateral canthotomy incision. It is uncommon to have to resort to such procedures.

## Bicoronal flap approach

A bicoronal flap is a much more invasive operation that, in an era of small incision surgery, has very few indications.

### Advantages

1. The approach affords good access to the medial wall, lateral wall and lateral portion of the floor of the orbit
2. It permits reduction of the procerus and corrugator supercilii muscles responsible for marked glabellar frown lines in patients with thyroid eye disease
3. The surgical scar is hidden behind the hairline

### Disadvantages

1. It has to be combined with other incisions to afford good access to the whole of the orbital floor
2. It requires a greater amount of operating room time
3. It requires a much longer inpatient stay
4. It commits the surgeon to performing a bilateral operation, which runs a risk, albeit small, of visual loss
5. It is associated with the risk of damage to the temporal branch of the facial nerve with a brow ptosis
6. It is commonly associated with a large area of loss of sensation in the forehead and scalp
7. In male patients, hair loss leaves a large visible scar

## Transantral (Caldwell–Luc) approach

This approach offers no advantages over alternative approaches and has significant disadvantages, e.g. a much higher risk of postoperative diplopia than alternative approaches. It is associated with significant postoperative discomfort.

## Transcaruncular approach

This approach allows ready access to the medial orbital wall, and the conjunctival incision can be extended inferiorly to gain access to the medial aspect of the orbital floor. A separate incision is required to gain access to the lateral orbital wall. This approach requires great care as the surface of the globe is exposed during the surgery.

## The eyelid approach

The eyelid approach (transcutaneous or transconjunctival) leaves a cosmetically excellent scar and permits access to the medial and lateral walls and the orbital floor. If necessary, it can be used in conjunction with an endoscope to gain an excellent view of the most posterior aspect of the medial orbital wall. Orbital fat can be safely removed via this approach. The surgery can be performed bilaterally or unilaterally depending on the patient's individual circumstances. Patients undergoing such surgery are usually in hospital for only one night. The transcutaneous eyelid approach is now described in detail.

### Preoperative preparation

The patient's thyroid function should be well controlled prior to the use of general anaesthesia. A full blood count and platelet count should be performed. A history of excessive bleeding should be excluded. All antiplatelet agents should be discontinued. Patients on anticoagulants must be admitted and transferred to intravenous heparin under the supervision of a haematologist. The preoperative CT scans must be available in the operating room.

On induction of anaesthesia the patient should be given 500 mg Diamox (acetazolamide) intravenously, which permits easier subperiosteal retraction and an improved view of the posterior aspect of the medial orbital wall. In the absence of any contraindications, the anaesthetist should be asked to induce moderate hypotension A throat pack should be placed. The patient is placed into a reverse Trendelenburg position to reduce venous pressure and the neck is extended. A nasal epistaxis tampon is placed in the nose, aiming for the medial canthus, and moistened with 5% cocaine solution. A subciliary or skin crease incision is marked using gentian violet. A volume of 3 ml of 0.5% Marcain (bupivacaine) with 1:200,000 units of adrenaline is injected into the lower eyelid, which is compressed for 5 min.

A headlight and surgical loupes must be worn throughout this surgical procedure.

### Surgical technique

1. One or two 4/0 silk traction sutures are placed through the grey line of the lower eyelid and fixated to the forehead drapes using a curved haemostat.
2. A subciliary incision is made using a Colorado needle.
3. Using a Paufique forceps the orbicularis muscle below the incision is lifted and a plane of dissection posterior to the orbicularis oculi muscle and anterior to the orbital septum is created using the Colorado needle.
4. Haemostasis is achieved using bipolar cautery when required. The orbital septum is touched at intervals to shrink away any bulging orbital fat to aid the dissection.
5. The plane of dissection is carried to the inferior orbital rim.
6. One or two Jaffe lid retractors are inserted into the wound and fixated to the drapes using a curved haemostat (Figure 18.19)

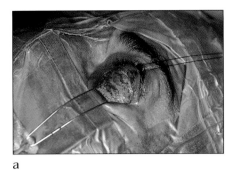 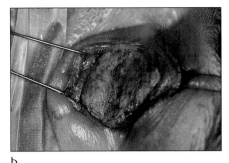

a                                                                 b

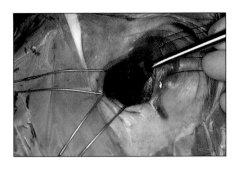

### Figure 18.19
(a) A transcutaneous lower eyelid approach to an orbital decompression. (b) The orbital septum has been maintained intact, keeping the fat out of the surgical field. The fat may be removed at this stage if it causes problems with surgical access.

### Figure 18.20
The periorbita has been reflected from the floor and medial wall of the orbit and a Sewell retractor is used to retract the orbital contents

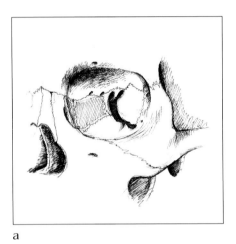 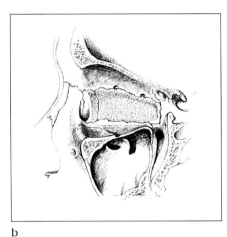

a                                                                 b

### Figure 18.21
(a) The area of bone removal from the medial wall is illustrated. The posterior extent of the bone resection is limited by the body of the sphenoid anterior to the optic foramen. (b) A side view demonstrates that the anterior and posterior ethmoidal vessels lie at the superior aspect of the medial wall resection. The posterior lacrimal crest marks the anterior limit of the medial wall resection.

7. Using the Colorado needle the periosteum is incised 2 mm below the rim, commencing medially and carrying this incision to a lower position laterally.

8. The periosteum is elevated from the underlying bone using a Freer periosteal elevator.

9. The periorbita is then elevated from the orbital floor and the orbital contents retracted using Sewell retractors (Figure 18.20).

10. A constant vessel is encountered along the centre of the orbital floor passing from the infraorbital neurovascular bundle to the orbit. This is cauterized and cut.

11. The periorbita is then elevated from the medial orbital wall until the anterior and posterior ethmoidal vessels are identified. This marks the superior limit of the medial wall dissection.

12. The dissection is continued posteriorly until the body of the sphenoid bone is encountered. This marks the posterior limit of the medial dissection (Figure 18.21).

13. The bone of the central aspect of the medial orbital wall is infractured using a curved haemostat or Freer periosteal elevator (Figure 18.22a).

14. The lamina papyracea is then removed anteriorly as far as the posterior lacrimal crest using a Kerrison rongeur, taking care not to damage the lacrimal drainage apparatus, and posteriorly as far as the body of the sphenoid using Takahashi ethmoidectomy rongeurs (Figure 18.22b). The body of the sphenoid is noted by the change of character of the bone from very thin and friable to solid. This bone lies just in front of the optic canal. (If necessary this bone can be gently burred anteriorly using a diamond burr under endoscopic control. It is now easy to pass the endoscope via the nose and direct the tip to the orbital apex under direct vision. The burr can be introduced via the eyelid wound and the tip then visualized endoscopically.)

15. The ethmoid air cells and mucosa are very carefully removed using the Takahashi rongeurs. Great care is taken to stay

Great care is taken to ensure that the periorbita is maintained intact throughout this dissection. Inadvertent damage to the periorbita will result in an immediate prolapse of orbital fat, which will obscure any further dissection, increasing the risk of complications.

It is essential to decompress the medial orbital wall to the body of the sphenoid in patients with compressive optic neuropathy. In patients undergoing a decompression for any other reason, it is safer to be conservative and not extend the dissection this far posteriorly.

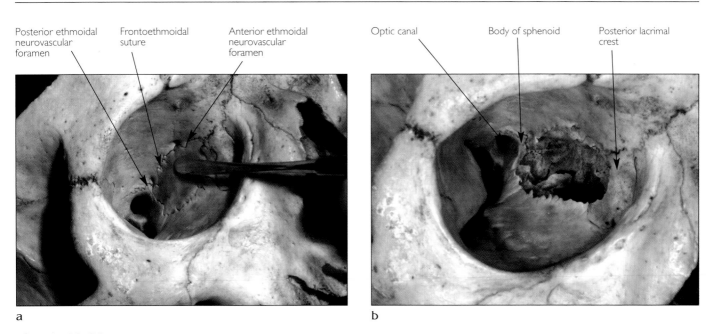

Posterior ethmoidal neurovascular foramen

Frontoethmoidal suture

Anterior ethmoidal neurovascular foramen

Optic canal

Body of sphenoid

Posterior lacrimal crest

a

b

**Figure 18.22**
(a) The medial orbital wall is removed superiorly to the level of the frontoethmoidal suture line. (b) The medial orbital wall has been removed posteriorly as far as the body of the sphenoid and anteriorly as far as the posterior lacrimal crest.

below the ethmoidal vessels. The mucosa bleeds, but once the mucosa and air cells have been exenterated the bleeding ceases. Any bleeding which obscures the view can be controlled by the gentle insertion of small patties moistened in 5% cocaine, which should be left in position for a few minutes.

16. The fovea ethmoidalis is seen to arch above the position of the frontoethmoidal suture line. More medially, lies the cribriform plate. Great care should be taken to avoid any damage to these structures, which will lead to a CSF leak. (If a CSF leak is encountered, the anaesthetist should be asked to place a lumbar drain, and the area of the leak should be patched with orbicularis muscle harvested from the lower eyelid wound.)

17. At the inferior aspect of the medial orbital wall the bony dissection is discontinued if it is intended to leave a medial strut.

18. The bone of the orbital floor is infractured using a curved haemostat medial to the infraorbital nerve. Bone is then removed from the medial half of the orbital floor using Kerrison and Takahashi rongeurs. Bone is removed to the posterior wall of the maxillary sinus (Figure 18.23). The maxillary sinus mucosa is removed from the roof of the antrum.

19. The bone is burred using a diamond burr as the dissection approaches the infraorbital neurovascular bundle. This avoids damage to the infraorbital nerve and postoperative infraorbital anaesthesia. Damage to the infraorbital vessels should be avoided as these can bleed profusely.

20. The periorbita is then elevated from the lateral aspect of the orbital floor and around the anterior aspect of the inferior orbital fissure to the lateral orbital wall.

21. The zygomaticofacial and zygomaticotemporal neurovascular bundles are cauterized and severed. The periorbita is reflected deeply into the orbit, exposing the greater wing of the sphenoid bone, and as superiorly as possible along the lateral orbital wall (Figure 18.24).

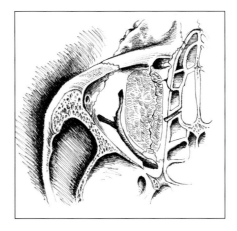

**Figure 18.23**
The area of bone removal from the medial aspect of the orbital floor is demonstrated.

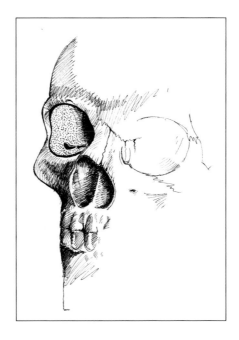

**Figure 18.24**
The area of bone which can be removed from the lateral wall and lateral part of the orbital floor is demonstrated.

22. The exposed bone of the lateral aspect of the orbital floor and the lateral orbital wall is burred away. The inferotemporal fat and temporalis fascia are exposed.
23. The periorbita is now slit from posterior to anterior along the medial orbital wall using a curved sharp blade. Great care is taken to avoid damage to the medial rectus muscle.
24. The rest of the periorbita is now opened with the curved blade. The periorbita is then widely opened using blunt-tipped Westcott scissors and the orbital fat encouraged to prolapse by applying pressure to the globe.
25. Orbital fat can be removed as required, depending on the degree of reduction in proptosis achieved.
26. The orbit is inspected for bleeding and cautery used as required.
27. The skin–muscle flap is then closed with a continuous 7/0 Vicryl suture.
28. The lower eyelid traction sutures are used as Frost sutures.
29. A compressive dressing is applied and removed the following day along with the Frost sutures.

## Postoperative management

Systemic antibiotics and a rapidly tapering course of systemic steroids are prescribed for 1 week postoperatively. Lower eyelid massage is commenced on the first postoperative day and continued for 6 weeks. The patient is instructed not to blow the nose or hold the nose if sneezing for a period of 6 weeks.

## *Potential complications*

Potential complications of orbital decompression surgery should be borne in mind when counselling patients about this surgical procedure and when taking informed consent from patients. The risks of general anaesthesia should also be considered in patients with coexistent disease, e.g. diabetes mellitus, myasthenia and cardiovascular and respiratory disease.

## 1. Diplopia

Strabismus is quoted as the most common potential complication of orbital decompression surgery but its incidence varies markedly from centre to centre. It is a common problem in patients with preoperative ocular motility restrictions. Approximately 30% of such patients have some degree of worsening of their diplopia. Approximately 10% of such patients require strabismus surgery. The results of strabismus surgery are generally very good, with a very small percentage of patients experiencing permanent and disabling diplopia. Postoperative diplopia is a very uncommon problem in patients without preoperative motility restrictions.

The risk of postoperative motility disturbances can be minimized:

- Attempt to leave a bony strut between the medial wall and the orbital floor

- Avoid excessive removal of the orbital floor
- Avoid damage to the extraocular muscles when opening the periorbita
- Avoid the origin of the inferior oblique muscle
- Pay meticulous attention to haemostasis at all stages of the procedure

## 2. Blindness

Visual loss following orbital decompression surgery is a devastating but fortunately extremely rare complication. The risks can be minimized:

- Avoid prolonged retraction on the globe
- Pay meticulous attention to haemostasis at all stages of the procedure
- Monitor the pupil at intervals
- Avoid a compressive dressing when an orbital fat decompression alone has been performed
- Monitor the patient for pain, sudden proptosis and visual disturbance every 30 min postoperatively for 12 hours when an orbital fat decompression alone has been performed
- Avoid orbital apical dissection endoscopically if the view is suboptimal
- Avoid undue traction on orbital fat during orbital fat dissection

## 3. CSF leak/meningitis

A CSF leak is a rare complication and can be readily avoided:

- Ascertain the position of the cribriform plate with respect to the frontoethmoidal suture line on a coronal CT scan.
- Ensure good visualization of the ethmoidal air cells by good haemostasis, by good traction and by avoiding damage to the periorbita with premature prolapse of orbital fat. If the view of the medial orbital wall is poor because of a 'tight' orbit, the lateral orbital wall can be decompressed first, allowing the orbital contents to shift laterally.

## 4. Haemorrhage

Blood loss from an orbital decompression should be minimal (less than 5 ml). The risk of bleeding can be minimized, as discussed in the Preoperative preparations section above. In addition:

- Ensure the medial wall dissection remains below the ethmoidal arteries
- Identify and cauterize the constant orbital floor vessels
- Avoid the use of bone rongeurs close to the infraorbital neurovascular bundle
- Identify and cauterize the zygomatic vessels

## 5. Infraorbital anaesthesia

Neurosensory defects in the distribution of the infraorbital nerve usually recover after a period of months. They are, however, disturbing to patients and can be avoided by meticulous bone removal using a diamond burr adjacent to the infraorbital neurovascular bundle. Excessive use of cautery adjacent to the nerve will cause postoperative neurosensory defects. Some degree of neurosensory deficit is inevitable if the whole of the orbital floor has to be removed in a patient with severe proptosis. In such patients the nerve should be unroofed with great care.

## 6. Orbital cellulitis

Postoperative infection is a potentially serious complication. The risk is minimized by the use of antibiotics postoperatively and by advising the patient to avoid blowing the nose for 6 weeks.

## 7. Hypoglobus

The risk of an inferior displacement of the globe and a secondary worsening of upper eyelid retraction is avoided by minimizing the degree of orbital floor decompression.

## 8. Epiphora

The lacrimal sac is prone to injury if the medial wall dissection is carried too far anteriorly.

A number of additional complications are specific to other approaches, e.g. oroantral fistula following a transantral approach.

In view of the risk, albeit small, of visual loss from an orbital decompression, the procedure should be performed on each orbit on separate occasions unless the patient poses unacceptable risks from separate general anaesthetics. Postoperative oedema and ecchymosis is minimized by a compressive dressing that is well tolerated unilaterally but is distressing for the patient when applied bilaterally. The operating time is reduced, as is any blood loss. The effects of the surgery can be seen and the surgical management of the fellow orbit modified if necessary.

It is wise to be conservative with an orbital decompression procedure. It is much easier to perform additional decompressive surgery than it is to attempt to correct the problems encountered following over-aggressive surgery, e.g. a hypoglobus.

# Ocular muscle surgery

Muscle recession is the major surgical procedure performed in cases of thyroid myopathy. The use of adjustable sutures has improved surgical results but in many cases management may be very difficult, especially after surgical orbital decompression. It is rare to obtain single vision in all fields of gaze.

# Eyelid repositioning surgery

Surgery to alleviate upper and lower lid retraction should be deferred until the eyelid position is stable and until other treatment modalities have been completed unless the patient has significant corneal exposure. The management of thyroid-related eyelid retraction is discussed in detail in Chapter 19.

It is important to emphasize to patients at the outset that the road to recovery from the disfiguring and disabling effects of thyroid eye disease may be very long (Figure 18.25).

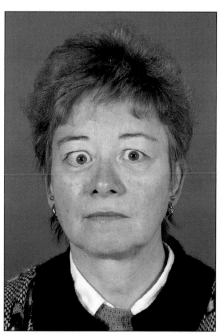 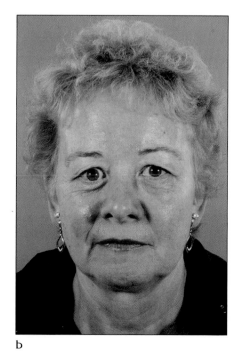

a                    b

**Figure 18.25**
(a) Patient referred with stable 'burnt out' thyroid eye disease with asymmetric proptosis, an esotropia and bilateral eyelid retraction. (b) The same patient 4 years later having undergone a bilateral decompression, strabismus surgery with adjustable sutures and a bilateral posterior approach levator recession with Müllerectomy.

# Further reading

1. Adenis JP, Robert PY, Lasudry JG, Dalloul Z. Treatment of proptosis with fat removal orbital decompression in Graves' ophthalmopathy. *Eur J Ophthalmol* (1998) **8**:246–52.

2. Bailey CC, Kabala J, Laitt R, *et al*. Magnetic resonance imaging in thyroid eye disease. *Eye* **10**:617–19.

3. Char DH. Thyroid eye disease. *Br J Ophthalmol* (1996) **80**:922–6.

4. Claridge KG, Ghabrial R, Davis G, *et al*. Combined radiotherapy and medical immunosuppression in the management of thyroid eye disease. *Eye* **11**:717–22.

5. Dutton JJ. *Atlas of clinical and surgical orbital anatomy*. Philadelphia: WB Saunders, 1994.

6. Goldberg RA. The evolving paradigm of orbital decompression surgery. *Arch Ophthalmol* (1998) **116**:95–6.

7. Goldberg RA, Kim AJ, Kerivan KM. The lacrimal keyhole, orbital doorjamb, and basin of the inferior orbital fissure. Three areas of deep bone in the lateral orbit. *Arch Ophthalmol* (1998) **116**:1618–24.

8. Goldberg RA, Peny JD, Hortaleza V, Tong JT. Strabismus after balanced medial plus lateral wall versus lateral wall only orbital decompression for dysthyroid orbitopathy. *Ophthal Plast Reconstr Surg* (2000) **16**:271–7.

9. Graham SM, Chee L, Alford MA, Carter KD. New techniques for surgical decompression of thyroid-related orbitopathy. *Ann Acad Med Singapore* (1999) **28**:494–7.

10. Lazarus JH. Relation between thyroid eye disease and type of treatment of Graves' hyperthyroidism. *Thyroid* **8**:437.

11. Mourits MP, Prummel MF, Wiersinga WM, Koornneef L. Clinical activity score as a guide in the management of patients with Graves' ophthalmopathy. *Clinical Endocrinology* (1997) **47**:9–14.

12. Paridaens DA, Verhoeff K, Bouwens D, van Den Bosch WA. Transconjunctival orbital decompression in Graves' ophthalmopathy: lateral wall approach ab interno. *Br J Ophthalmol* (2000) **84**:775–81.

13. Perros P, Kendall-Taylor P. Natural history of thyroid eye disease. *Thyroid* (1998) **8**:423–5.

14. Scott IU, Siatkowski MR. Thyroid eye disease. *Sem Ophthalmol* (1999) **14**:52–61.

15. Shorr N, Baylis HI, Goldberg RA, Perry JD. Transcaruncular approach to the medial orbit and orbital apex. *Ophthalmology* (2000) **107**:1459–63.

16. Van Ruyven RL, Van Den Bosch WA, Mulder PG, Eijkenboom WM, Paridaens AD. The effect of retrobulbar irradiation on exophthalmos, ductions and soft tissue signs in Graves' ophthalmopathy: a retrospective analysis of 90 cases. *Eye* (2000) **5**:761–4.

17. Wright ED, Davidson J, Codere F, Desrosiers M. Endoscopic orbital decompression with preservation of an inferomedial bony strut: minimization of postoperative diplopia. *J Otolaryngol* **28**:252–6.

# 19

# The management of thyroid-related eyelid retraction

## Introduction

The appropriate management of eyelid retraction in Graves' disease depends on an understanding of the pathophysiological mechanisms responsible for the eyelid malposition. Attention to the pathophysiology of the eyelid malposition permits the selection of the most appropriate intervention and improves the predictability of the outcome. In the upper and lower eyelids the pathophysiological mechanisms are:

- Adrenergic stimulation of Müller's muscle and its lower eyelid equivalent
- Pseudoproptosis due to myopia
- Proptosis
- Inflammation and fibrosis of the upper and lower eyelid retractors
- Inflammation and fibrosis of the inferior rectus muscle

These mechanisms, which may occur singly or in combination and with varying degrees of asymmetry, are now condsidered in turn.

Mild degrees of eyelid retraction caused by increased sensitivity of Müller's muscle and its lower eyelid equivalent to circulating catecholamines may resolve with treatment of the hyperthyroid state.

Axial myopia is commonly overlooked as a cause of eyelid retraction. High myopia can compound other mechanisms of eyelid retraction and make the surgical management particularly challenging (Figure 19.1).

Proptosis, similarly, acts as a wedge between the eyelids. In many patients treatment of the proptosis by orbital decompression surgery can relieve the eyelid retraction (Figure 19.2).

Inflammation and fibrosis of the upper and lower eyelid retractors can be responsible for marked degrees of eyelid retraction (Figure 19.3). Downward traction applied by the examiner to the upper eyelid margin will be met with marked resistance.

Inflammation and fibrosis of the inferior rectus muscle may cause a hypotropia with a compensatory overaction of the superior rectus/levator complex causing eyelid retraction. The degree of

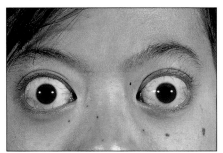

a

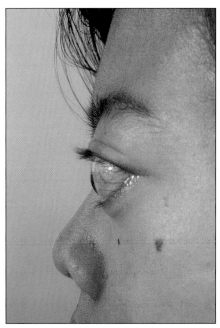

b

**Figure 19.1**
(a) Bilateral upper and lower eyelid retraction in a patient of Chinese descent. He has bilateral proptosis with shallow orbits and axial myopia (axial lengths 29 mm). (b) Lateral view demonstrating marked proptosis.

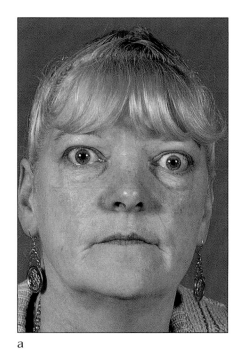

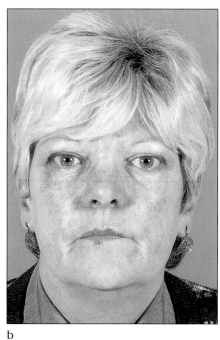

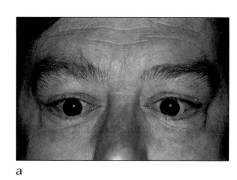

a

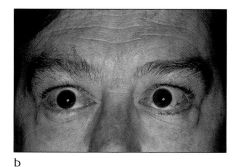

b

a                                          b

### Figure 19.2

(a) Bilateral upper eyelid retraction in a patient with moderate proptosis. (b) The postoperative appearance following a bilateral two-wall orbital decompression procedure performed via lower eyelid subciliary incisions. No eyelid repositioning surgery was required.

### Figure 19.4

This patient's upper eyelid retraction increases on upgaze due to inferior rectus contracture.

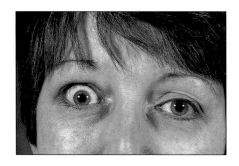

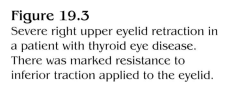

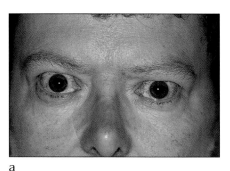

a                                          b

### Figure 19.3

Severe right upper eyelid retraction in a patient with thyroid eye disease. There was marked resistance to inferior traction applied to the eyelid.

### Figure 19.5

This patient's upper eyelid retraction is partially masked by her bilateral brow ptosis.

eyelid retraction should be assessed and compared in downgaze and upgaze. Upper eyelid retraction which worsens on upgaze is due to fibrosis of the inferior rectus muscle (Figure 19.4). Such patients also demonstrate a rise in intraocular pressure on upgaze.

## Patient evaluation

The patient should be carefully evaluated to determine the following:

- The degree of activity of the disease
- The mechanisms responsible for the eyelid retraction
- The severity of any exposure keratopathy
- The degree of eyelid retraction

In some patients the degree of upper eyelid retraction can be underestimated due to the presence of a brow ptosis and dermatochalasis or upper eyelid swelling. The brows should be gently elevated to ascertain the true position of the upper eyelids (Figure 19.5).

# Timing of surgical intervention

Eyelid surgery in thyroid eye disease should be deferred until the disease has entered a quiescent phase unless exposure keratopathy unresponsive to medical therapy requires more urgent intervention. Eyelid surgery undertaken during the active phase can compromise the outcome. In general, the thyroid status and eyelid position should be stable for a minimum period of 6 months before any eyelid surgery is undertaken.

---

As a general rule eyelid surgery should be undertaken after orbital decompression surgery and any strabismus surgery – should these be required.

---

# Orbital decompression versus eyelid surgery

It can be difficult to counsel a patient with significant proptosis about the relative merits of orbital decompression, surgery versus eyelid repositioning surgery in the absence of other clear indications for orbital decompression, e.g. compressive optic neuropathy unresponsive to medical therapy. In the presence of a significant degree of proptosis, unilateral proptosis or asymmetric proptosis, there is no question that eyelid repositioning surgery alone will not achieve a good cosmetic result for the patient (Figure 19.6). Orbital decompression surgery is, however, far more invasive than eyelid surgery alone and is associated with a number of risks. The decision should be made on an individual basis.

A patient must be carefully counselled about the aims, risks and potential complications of surgery. Unrealistic expectations will lead to an unhappy patient postoperatively. The patient should be prepared for the possibility of multiple surgical procedures to achieve the desired end result.

# Upper eyelid retraction

The upper eyelid, in contrast to the lower eyelid, does not require the use of spacers to achieve the desired position.

# Methods of upper eyelid lowering

A variety of surgical procedures have been described to manage upper eyelid retraction in Graves' disease; all these procedures aim to reduce upper eyelid retractor tone. The choice of procedure depends on the degree of eyelid retraction. The aim is to achieve a satisfactory lowering of the eyelid without a temporal flare, which can mar the cosmetic result. The procedures that are used by the author are:

- Müllerectomy (1–2 mm of retraction)
- Posterior approach levator recession (2–3 mm of retraction)
- Anterior approach levator recession (3–4 mm of retraction)
- Anterior approach Z-myotomy (> 4 mm of retraction)

# Müllerectomy

A Müllerectomy is a relatively simple surgical procedure that is useful for small degrees of eyelid retraction (1–2 mm). It can be performed under local anaesthesia.

## Surgical technique

1. A volume of 2 ml of 0.5% bupivacaine with 1:200,000 units of adrenaline is injected subcutaneously in the centre of the upper eyelid just above the eyelashes.
2. A 4/0 silk suture is passed through the grey line of the upper eyelid, which is everted over a large Desmarres retractor.
3. 2–3 ml of 0.5% bupivacaine with 1:200,000 units of adrenaline is injected subconjunctivally. The retractor is removed and pressure is applied for 5 min.
4. A conjunctival incision is made using a No. 15 Bard Parker blade across the whole of the upper eyelid just above the upper border of the tarsus (Figure 19.7).
5. The conjunctival edge is lifted with toothed forceps and the underlying Müller's muscle is opened with blunt-tipped Westcott scissors. The surgical space between the levator aponeurosis and Müller's muscle is dissected open with the Westcott scissors for a distance of approximately

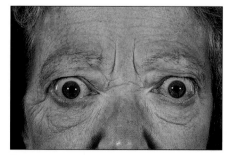
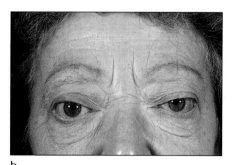

a                                    b

**Figure 19.6**
(a) Bilateral upper eyelid retraction in a patient with bilateral symmetric proptosis. (b) The patient is seen following a bilateral upper eyelid retractor recession performed without addressing the proptosis. A typically abnormal eyelid contour with lateral flare is the inevitable consequence of performing this surgery in the presence of untreated proptosis.

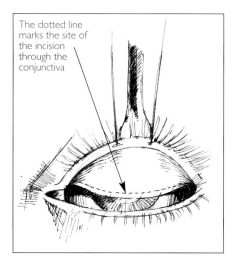

**Figure 19.7**
The conjunctival incision is made at the upper border of the tarsus with the eyelid everted over a Desmarres retractor.

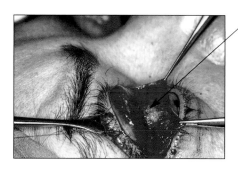

**Figure 19.8**
The surgical space between Müller's muscle and the overlying levator aponeurosis has been dissected.

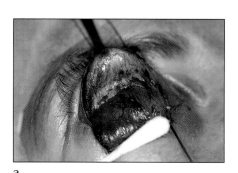

a

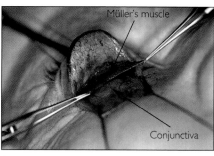

a

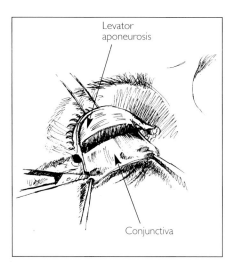

**Figure 19.9**
Müller's muscle is incised with Westcott scissors temporally and undermined.

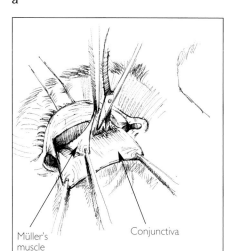

b

**Figure 19.10**
(a) Müller's muscle has been separated from the overlying levator aponeurosis. (b) Müller's muscle is dissected from the overlying levator aponeurosis.

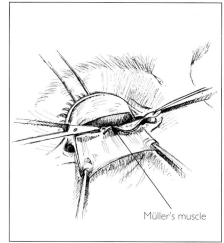

b

**Figure 19.11**
(a) Müller's muscle has been dissected from the underlying conjunctiva. (b) Müller's muscle is being resected, leaving a small residual strip undisturbed medially.

10–12 mm. Müller's muscle will contain fatty tissue and will bleed (Figure 19.8). Bipolar cautery will be required frequently.

6. An incision is then made through Müller's muscle with blunt-tipped Westcott scissors temporally (Figure 19.9).

7. A volume of 0.5–1.0 ml of 0.5% Marcain (bupivacaine) with 1:200,000 units of adrenaline is carefully injected into Müller's muscle and left for a few minutes.

8. Using 0.3 toothed forceps and blunt-tipped Westcott scissors, Müller's muscle is dissected from the underlying conjunctiva with a blunt stripping motion from the cut edge

of the conjunctiva to its superior origin from the levator (Figure 19.10).

9. Müller's muscle is excised, leaving a small residual strip nasally to avoid a medial ptosis (Figure 19.11).

Sutures are unnecessary and risk causing discomfort or a corneal abrasion.

Postoperatively the patient is prescribed topical antibiotic drops. The patient may commence eyelid traction within 2–3 days to maintain the desired height and contour of the upper eyelid. This can be continued for a period of 6–8 weeks.

# Posterior approach levator recession with Müllerectomy

This approach can be performed under local anaesthesia with intraoperative monitoring of the eyelid position, with or without intravenous sedation as required.

## Advantages

1. No sutures are required
2. The height and contour of the eyelid can be manipulated postoperatively with massage
3. The absence of a skin incision reduces the amount of postoperative eyelid oedema and permits a more rapid postoperative recovery
4. The absence of an incision through the orbicularis muscle avoids temporary denervation of the orbicularis muscle and secondary lagophthalmos

## Disadvantages

1. This approach does not permit as satisfactory a degree of exposure of the lateral horn of the levator muscle as the anterior approach
2. The skin crease cannot be adjusted or any excess upper eyelid skin removed
3. Great care must be taken to avoid iatrogenic injury to the globe

## Surgical technique

The initial aspects of this approach are identical to stages 1–9, as described for a Müllerectomy.

10. The levator aponeurosis is stripped away from the superior border of the tarsus using blunt-tipped Westcott scissors commencing temporally (Figure 19.12).
11. The patient is placed into a sitting position and the height and contour of the upper eyelid are assessed. This is repeated as required.

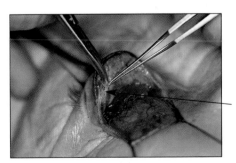

Levator aponeurosis

**Figure 19.12**
The levator aponeurosis is stripped away from the superior border of the tarsus using blunt-tipped Westcott scissors and fine-toothed forceps.

12. The stripping of the levator fibres is continued until the desired end point is reached. (This is usually a 1–2 mm overcorrection. *A greater degree of overcorrection risks a postoperative ptosis. It is much easier to undertake a further levator recession for an undercorrection than it is to have to undertake ptosis surgery for an overcorrection.*)
13. If the desired eyelid height has not been achieved the levator aponeurosis can be opened at the 'white line', exposing the preaponeurotic fat as in a posterior approach levator advancement. The lateral horn of the levator can be gently divided. Such manoeuvres, however, increase the risk of postoperative overcorrection and haemorrhage.

The traction suture is removed and ice packs are applied. Leaving the traction suture taped to the cheek risks a postoperative overcorrection.

Sutures are unnecessary and risk causing discomfort or a corneal abrasion.

Postoperatively, the patient is prescribed topical antibiotic drops. The patient may commence eyelid traction within 2–3 days to maintain the desired height and contour of the upper eyelid. This can be continued for a period of 6–8 weeks (Figure 19.13).

In determining the desired end point it is important to contrast symmetrical upper eyelid retraction with asymmetrical or unilateral upper eyelid retraction. As the upper eyelids obey Hering's law, alterations to the position of one eyelid will have an influence on the position of the fellow eyelid. This can create a challenge in achieving symmetry. In addition, the eyelid position is further influenced by the patient's own voluntary effort, by the effects of adrenaline and by the effects of oedema. *It is always preferable to aim for an undercorrection* (Figure 19.13).

# Anterior approach levator recession

This approach is required for greater degrees of eyelid retraction and can be combined with a Z-myotomy of the levator aponeurosis and muscle. It can be performed under local anaesthesia, although intravenous sedation may be required. General anaesthesia may be preferred for the more anxious patient.

## Advantages

1. This approach is familiar to surgeons performing anterior approach levator surgery for ptosis
2. It allows better access to the lateral horn of the levator and to the more proximal aspect of the levator muscle
3. It is easier to control the desired height and contour of the eyelid intraoperatively
4. It allows the skin crease to be set at the desired level
5. It allows an upper lid blepharoplasty to be performed simultaneously
6. The globe is well protected during the course of the surgery

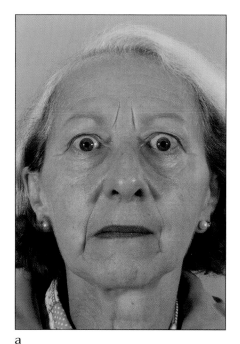

a

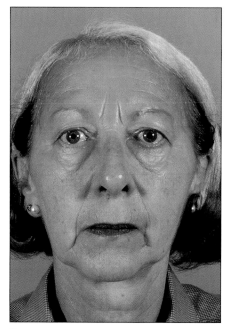

a

**Figure 19.13**
(a) Patient with bilateral symmetrical dysthyroid upper eyelid retraction.
(b) Postoperative appearance following a bilateral posterior approach levator recession with Müllerectomy.

## Disadvantages

1. This approach is associated with a longer postoperative recovery period with pretarsal eyelid oedema
2. The upper eyelid incision temporarily denervates the orbicularis oculi muscle, causing lagophthalmos
3. This approach requires more surgical time

## Surgical technique

1. A skin crease incision is marked at the desired level in the upper eyelid using gentian violet and a cocktail stick after cleansing the skin with an alcohol wipe.
2. A volume of 1–1.5 ml of 0.5% bupivacaine with 1:200,000 units of adrenaline is injected subcutaneously into the upper eyelid. It is important to avoid a deeper injection in order to prevent a haematoma and to minimize the effect on the levator function.
3. A 4/0 silk traction suture is placed through the grey line of the upper lid at the desired location of the peak of the eyelid and fixated to the face drapes using a small haemostat.
4. An upper eyelid skin crease incision is made using a Colorado needle.
5. The Colorado needle is used to dissect down through the orbicularis oculi muscle to the orbital septum. The orbicularis is dissected from the orbital septum superiorly to avoid inadvertent injury to the levator aponeurosis.
6. The orbital septum is then opened with the Colorado needle throughout the entire length of the incision and the preaponeurotic fat exposed. The preaponeurotic fat is dissected from the underlying levator aponeurosis.
7. A Jaffe lid speculum is then placed in the incision site to provide complete exposure of the levator aponeurosis.

8. The levator aponeurosis is dissected from the underlying Müller's muscle, commencing at the superior aspect of the tarsus. Great care should be taken to avoid inadvertent bleeding from the superior tarsal vascular arcade. The medial attachment of the levator to the tarsus should be left undisturbed if possible to avoid a low position of the medial aspect of the eyelid with temporal flare (Figure 19.14).
9. A volume of 0.5–1.0 ml of 0.5% bupivacaine with 1:200,000 units of adrenaline is carefully injected into Müller's muscle and left for a few minutes.
10. Using 0.3 toothed forceps and blunt-tipped Westcott scissors, Müller's muscle is dissected from the underlying conjunctiva with a blunt stripping motion from the cut edge of the conjunctiva to its superior origin from the levator.
11. Müller's muscle is excised.
12. Westcott scissors are used to strip away any subconjunctival scar tissue.
13. The levator aponeurosis is dissected to the common sheath with the superior rectus muscle recognized as a white tissue beneath the levator muscle.
14. If the procedure is being performed under local anaesthesia, the patient is placed into a sitting position and the height and contour are assessed. This is repeated as required.
15. The lateral horn of the levator is divided if necessary to overcome temporal flare, taking great care not to damage the lacrimal gland.
16. Once the desired position has been achieved, the edges of the recessed levator aponeurosis are attached to the conjunctiva using interrupted 7/0 Vicryl sutures, taking care to ensure that the sutures do not abrade the cornea (Figure 19.15).
17. Any excess upper lid skin can be removed as a standard but conservative blepharoplasty.
18. The skin crease is reformed by attaching the skin edges to the upper border of the tarsus with interrupted 7/0 Vicryl sutures.

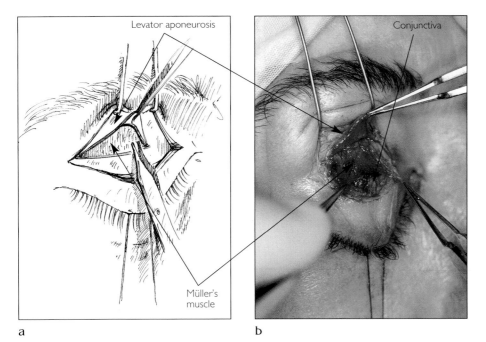
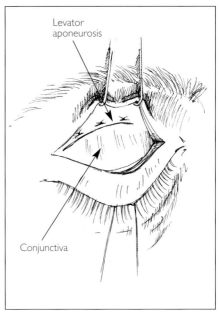

a        b

## Figure 19.14

(a) The levator aponeurosis is opened above the superior tarsal arcade to avoid bleeding. (b) Müller's muscle is exposed and excised.

## Figure 19.15

The recessed edge of the levator aponeurosis is sutured to the conjunctiva.

The end point of the surgery is the attainment of the desired eyelid height and contour, as the eyelid should remain at its intra-operative height (Figure 19.16). If the operation has been performed under general anaesthesia, adjustable sutures can be placed and the height and contour of the eyelid adjusted the following day. It is preferable, however, to perform the necessary adjustments intraoperatively under local anaesthesia.

Postoperatively, ice packs are applied and a topical antibiotic ointment. If a compressive dressing is required to prevent excess postoperative swelling, a lower lid Frost suture is placed and the dressing maintained in place for 24–48 hours. An example of a patient who has undergone this procedure following an orbital decompression is shown in Figure 19.16.

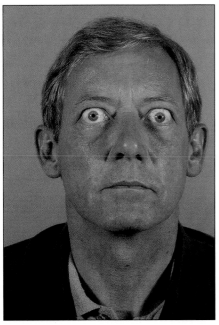
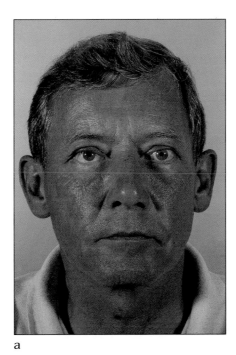

a        a

## Figure 19.16

(a) Patient with bilateral symmetric proptosis and severe upper eyelid retraction. (b) Postoperative appearance following a bilateral three-wall orbital decompression with fat excision and a bilateral anterior approach levator recession with Müllerectomy. The patient has been left with residual lateral flare in spite of extensive dissection of the lateral horns of the levator.

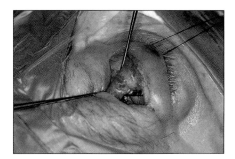

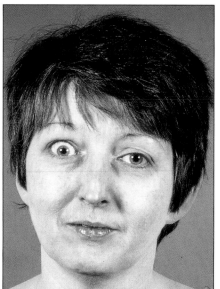

a

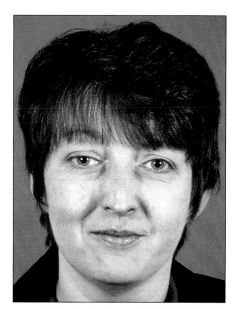

a

**Figure 19.17**
Muscle hooks have been passed beneath the enlarged belly of the levator muscle.

**Figure 19.18**
(a) A patient with severe right upper eyelid retraction (> 5 mm). (b) The postoperative result 3 months following a Z-myotomy.

## *Anterior approach Z-myotomy*

This procedure is reserved for patients with severe degrees of upper eyelid retraction. The surgery is normally performed with the patient under general anaesthesia, as the dissection can be difficult. Severe degrees of retraction are associated with widespread fibrosis, fatty infiltration and bleeding of the upper eyelid tissues. The initial aspects of this approach are identical to stages 1–13, as described for an anterior approach levator recession.

14.  The lateral horn of the levator is divided completely, taking great care not to damage the lacrimal gland.
15.  Whitnall's ligament is divided medially and laterally.
16.  A muscle hook is passed beneath the belly of the levator muscle and the levator pulled forward (Figure 19.17).
17.  The levator muscle is partially transected from one side of the muscle and from the opposite side at a higher level using the Colorado needle to prevent bleeding.

The operation is completed as for an anterior approach levator recession. A lower lid Frost suture is inserted and a compressive dressing applied for 48 hours postoperatively.

The eyelid is usually overcorrected postoperatively but should not be adjusted. The eyelid will gradually rise over the course of the next 6–12 weeks and no further adjustments should be made until all postoperative oedema has subsided and the eyelid position is static (Figure 19.18).

## Lower eyelid retraction

Surgery for the management of lower eyelid retraction is not required as frequently as that for upper eyelid retraction. Patients do not tend to be as concerned about lower eyelid retraction, as they do about upper eyelid retraction which has much more of a profound effect on a patient's ocular function and cosmesis. *Surgery for lower eyelid retraction is rarely required following successful orbital decompression surgery.*

The lower eyelid, in contrast to the upper eyelid, usually requires the use of a spacer to achieve the desired position. Although a variety of surgical procedures have been described to manage lower eyelid retraction in Graves' disease, the underlying principles are based on:

- Division of the orbital septum
- Recession of the inferior retractor complex and conjunctiva
- Placement of a spacer between the recessed inferior retractors and conjunctiva and the inferior border of the tarsus

A number of spacers are available. The ideal spacer should be sufficiently rigid to counteract the effects of gravity without adding bulk to the eyelid, and should have a mucosal surface to allow maximal recession of the conjunctiva as well as the inferior retractors.

## Spacers

- Hard palate
- Upper eyelid tarsus

Both of these spacers meet the required criteria. Synthetic materials, e.g. Gore-Tex, must be covered by the inferior palpebral conjunctiva and risk exposure and foreign body reactions. Donor sclera is no longer an acceptable material for use as a spacer because of the risk of transmissible disease.

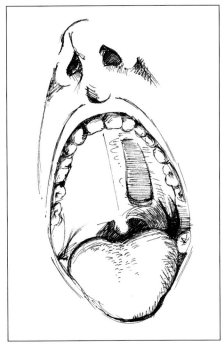

a

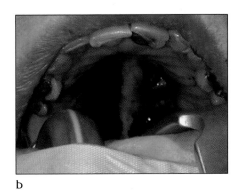

b

**Figure 19.19**
(a) An illustration demonstrating the donor site for a hard palate graft.
(b) Two hard palate grafts have been harvested, leaving the midline raphé intact.

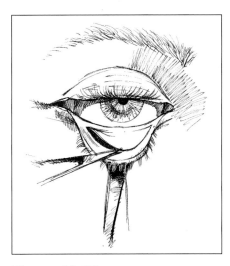

**Figure 19.20**
A conjunctival incision is made at the lower border of the tarsus.

The patient's hard palate is examined to determine its suitability for use as a spacer. Alternatively the patient's upper eyelids are everted and the height of the tarsus is assessed to determine whether or not the upper eyelid tarsus is suitable for use as a spacer. If a hard palate graft is to be used the surgery should ideally be performed under general anaesthesia whereas the surgery may be performed under local anaesthesia if upper lid tarsus is to be used.

In general, upper eyelid retraction should be addressed first and the management of lower eyelid retraction deferred until a satisfactory result has been obtained from upper eyelid surgery.

## Lower lid retractor recession with hard palate graft spacer
### Surgical technique

The hard palate graft is harvested first. A throat pack is placed and its presence recorded to ensure that this is removed prior to extubation.

1.  The hard palate is injected with 3–5 ml of 0.5% bupivacaine with 1:200,000 units of adrenaline. A Boyle Davies retractor is placed, taking care not to damage the teeth or disturb the endotracheal tube.
2.  The graft, measuring approximately 20–25 mm × 5 mm is outlined on the hard palate, avoiding the midline raphé and the soft palate (Figure 19.19). (The surgeon should be familiar with the anatomy of the greater and lesser palatine vessels. It is much easier to harvest the graft in the edentulous patient.)

3.  The hard palate is incised with a No. 15 Bard Parker blade.
4.  The graft is then dissected out in the plane of the submucosa, leaving the underlying mucoperiosteum undisturbed using a No. 66 Beaver blade.
5.  The dissection can then be completed with Westcott scissors.
6.  The submucosa of the graft is then thinned with Westcott scissors and *then wrapped in a saline-soaked gauze swab and kept in a safe location by the scrub nurse until it is required.*
7.  Neurosurgical patties moistened with 1:10,000 adrenaline are placed over the hard palate wound for 5 min.
8.  The wound is then inspected and bipolar cautery applied to any bleeding vessels.

Next, attention is directed to the lower eyelids:

1.  A volume of 3–4 mls of 0.5% Marcain with 1:200,000 units of adrenaline is injected subconjunctivally into the lower eyelid.
2.  Two 4/0 silk traction sutures are placed through the grey line of the lower eyelid and the lid is everted over a large Desmarres retractor.
3.  A conjunctival incision is made with a No. 15 Bard Parker blade at the lower border of the tarsus (Figure 19.20).
4.  The conjunctiva is dissected into the inferior fornix and onto the globe using blunt-tipped Westcott scissors. (A lateral canthotomy and inferior cantholysis can be combined with this approach to enable a lateral tarsal strip procedure to be performed if there is significant lower eyelid laxity.)
5.  The lower lid retractors are then undermined from the orbicularis muscle with Westcott scissors and dissected from the lower border of the tarsus.

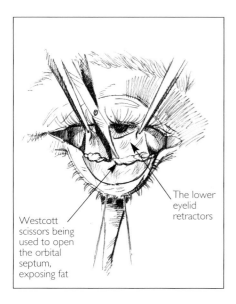

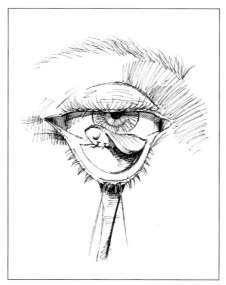

a

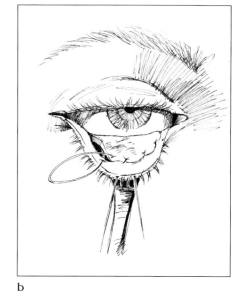

b

**Figure 19.21**
The lower eyelid retractors are
dissected free.

**Figure 19.22**
(a) The inferior aspect of the hard palate graft is first sutured to the superior
border of the recessed lower eyelid retractors. (b) The superior aspect of the
hard palate graft is then sutured to the inferior margin of the tarsus.

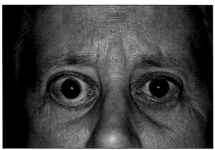

a

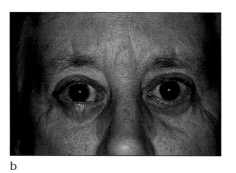

b

**Figure 19.23**
(a) A patient with right upper and
lower eyelid retraction. (b) The
postoperative appearance 6 weeks
following a right upper eyelid
posterior approach levator recession,
a lower eyelid retractor recession with
a hard palate graft and a lateral tarsal
strip procedure.

6.  The retractors are then dissected free into the inferior fornix
    and the orbital septum opened, exposing the lower eyelid
    preaponeurotic fat (Figure 19.21). The lower lid should now
    rise above the inferior limbus with gentle traction.
7.  The hard palate graft is placed into the inferior fornix with
    the mucosal surface facing the globe and sutured to the
    recessed inferior retractors and conjunctival edge with inter-
    rupted 7/0 Vicryl sutures (Figure 19.22).
8.  Three interrupted 5/0 Vicryl sutures are then passed from
    the submucosa of the mid-portion graft through the full
    thickness of the eyelid and tied over rubber bolsters.
9.  The superior margin of the graft is sutured to the inferior
    border of the tarsus using interrupted 7/0 Vicryl sutures that
    are buried to prevent any corneal irritation.

The traction sutures are taped to the forehead as Frost sutures
and a pressure dressing applied overnight. The Frost sutures are
removed the next day and topical antibiotic ointment prescribed
for 2 weeks. The bolster sutures are removed after 1 week. An

example of an early postoperative result following this surgical
procedure is shown in Figure 19.23.

The patient should be prescribed an antiseptic oral rinse for 7
days and should have a soft bland diet until the hard palate
wound has healed. This normally takes 2–3 weeks.

## Lower lid retractor recession with free tarsal graft spacer

The tarsal graft is harvested from the upper eyelid, ensuring that
a minimum of 3.5 mm of tarsus above the eyelid margin is left
undisturbed. This is described in Chapter 26 (The Use of
Autogenous Grafts in Ophthalmic Plastic Surgery). The graft is
used in a similar fashion to a hard palate graft.

This technique is better reserved for the management of
lower eyelid retraction due to causes other than thyroid eye
disease.

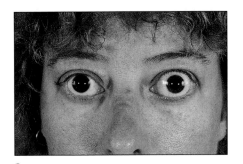

a

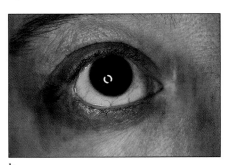

b

**Figure 19.24**
(a) A patient with proptosis and bilateral upper and lower eyelid retraction who has been inappropriately managed with lateral tarsorrhaphies. (b) A close-up of the right eye demonstrating a stretched lateral tarsorrhaphy.

# The role of a lateral tarsorrhaphy in thyroid eye disease

A lateral tarsorrhaphy can be used as an urgent procedure to protect an exposed cornea in a patient with thyroid eye disease prior to a more definitive procedure, e.g. an orbital decompression or an eyelid lengthening procedure. It is not a satisfactory procedure when performed alone as it tends to become stretched and unsightly or it may cause the lower eyelid to be drawn upwards, creating a cosmetic deformity (Figure 19.24).

A lateral tarsorrhaphy can, however, be very useful when used as an adjunct to an orbital decompression or to eyelid lengthening procedures.

The lateral tarsorrhaphy should only extend for 3–4 mm for the optimal cosmetic result. Although a variety of methods of performing the tarsorrhaphy in this situation have been described, it is preferable to undertake a very simple procedure that can be reversed if required.

## Surgical technique

1.  The upper and lower lids are injected with 2–3 ml of 0.5% Marcain and 1:200,000 units of adrenaline.
2.  The eyelid is held taut centrally and laterally with toothed forceps.
3.  A micro-sharp blade mounted in a Beaver blade handle is used to make a shallow incision for 3–4 mm along the grey line of each eyelid.
4.  Using the same blade, two incisions are made at 90 degrees to the grey line incision posteriorly. Next, using a 0.12 toothed forceps and a sharp-tipped Westcott scissors, an

0.5 mm strip of eyelid margin tissue is carefully removed posteriorly.
5.  An interrupted 5/0 Vicryl suture on a 1/4-circle needle is passed horizontally through the tarsal plates of the upper and lower lids and tied with the knot placed anteriorly away from the cornea.
6.  Interrupted 7/0 Vicryl sutures are placed through the anterior lips of the grey line incisions.

There is no requirement for any external bolsters. Topical antibiotic ointment is applied for 2 weeks. The eyelids fuse laterally. This procedure does not sacrifice normal eyelashes.

# Further reading

1.  Bartley GB. The differential diagnosis and classification of eyelid retraction. *Ophthalmology* (1996) **103**:168–76.
2.  Beatty RC, Harris G, Bauman GR, Mills MP. Intraoral palatal mucosal graft harvest. *Ophthal Plast Reconstr Surg* (1993) **9**:120–4.
3.  Cohen MS, Shorr N. Eyelid reconstruction with hard palate mucosal grafts. *Ophthal Plast Reconstr Surg* (1992) **8**:183–95.
4.  Gardner TA, Kennerdell JS, Buerger GE. Treatment of dysthyroid lower eyelid retraction with autogenous tarsus transplants. *Ophthal Plast Reconstr Surg* (1992) **8**:26–31.
5.  Goodall KL, Jackson A, Leatherbarrow B, Whitehouse RW. Enlargement of the tensor intermuscularis muscle in Graves' ophthalmopathy. *Arch Ophthalmol* (1995) **113**:1286–9.
6.  Kersten PC, Kulwin DP, Levartovksy S, *et al*. Management of lower eyelid retraction with hard palate mucosal grafting. *Arch Ophthalmol* (1990) **108**:1339–43.
7.  Lemke BN. Anatomic considerations in upper eyelid retraction. *Ophthal Plast Reconstr Surg* (1991) **7**:158–66.
8.  Putterman AM. Surgical treatment of thyroid related upper eyelid retraction: graded Müller excision and lessor recession. *Ophthalmology* (1981) **88**:507–12.

# 20

# The diagnosis and management of epiphora

## Introduction

The complaint of a watering eye is very common and may affect patients of any age. It is important to establish the true nature of the patient's complaint. The term *epiphora* refers to the overflow of tears onto the cheek. The complaint by a patient of a 'watering' or 'watery' eye or 'tearing' may not imply that tears actually overflow from the eye. There are many abnormalities that can lead the patient to seek attention for this complaint. It is important to establish the underlying cause by obtaining an accurate detailed history and by performing an appropriate clinical examination and, where indicated, supplementary investigations. It should not be assumed that this complaint automatically signifies a lacrimal drainage system obstruction.

## Applied anatomy
### The lacrimal system

The lacrimal system comprises the tear-producing glands, the lacrimal gland and accessory lacrimal glands of the conjunctiva and eyelids, the tear film, and the tear drainage system. The eyelids distribute the tears across the eye by the act of blinking and also contribute to tear drainage by means of the 'lacrimal pump' mechanism. Any abnormality of these components of the lacrimal system can give rise to the complaint of a 'watery' eye.

### The tear film

The tear film consists of three layers:

- The mucinous layer
- The aqueous layer
- The lipid layer

The mucinous layer is produced by the many goblet cells throughout the conjunctiva. The aqueous layer is produced by the lacrimal gland and by the many accessory lacrimal glands. The lipid layer serves to retard the evaporation of the aqueous layer and is produced by the sebaceous glands of the eyelids and caruncle. The tear film can be stained with a fluorescein strip and its stability observed between blinks. The tear film should remain stable for approximately 10–12 seconds under normal conditions.

There is normally a balance between tear production, tear evaporation and tear drainage. A patient who has poor tear production but a complete lacrimal drainage system obstruction will not experience epiphora. A patient who has excessive tear production, e.g. gustatory lacrimation following aberrant reinnervation of the facial nerve, but a normal lacrimal drainage system will experience epiphora. The patient with an unstable tear film may experience symptoms of ocular irritation, with reflex hypersecretion of tears by the lacrimal gland, and may suffer intermittent epiphora in spite of a normal lacrimal drainage system.

### The lacrimal gland

The lacrimal gland lies in the concavity of the lacrimal gland fossa in the superolateral aspect of the orbit. Its two lobes, the orbital and palpebral lobes, are separated by the lateral expansion (the lateral horn) of the levator aponeurosis. The orbital lobe lies within the orbit above the palpebral lobe (Figure 20.1). The palpebral lobe lies against the conjunctiva in the superolateral aspect of the superior fornix. This lobe is visible in many patients on everting the upper eyelid (Figure 20.2).

The lacrimal ductules pass through the palpebral lobe from the orbital lobe into the superolateral fornix. The ductules can be seen on slit lamp examination with the use of high magnification after applying a fluorescein strip to the conjunctiva of the superolateral fornix.

> Any surgery performed in this area, e.g. surgery to remove a congenital dermolipoma, risks damage to these ductules and a dry eye.

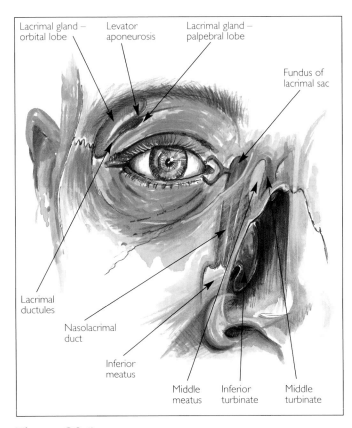

**Figure 20.1**
The anatomy of the lacrimal system.

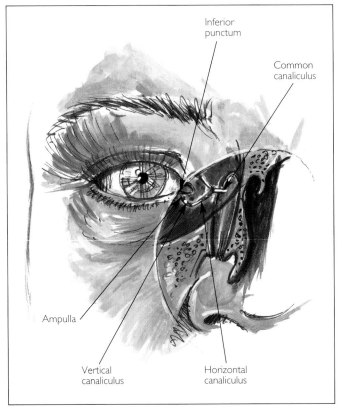

**Figure 20.3**
The anatomy of the lacrimal drainage system.

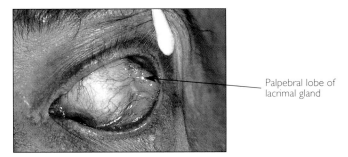

**Figure 20.2**
The palpebral lobe of the lacrimal gland visible in the patient on raising the upper eyelid.

# The lacrimal drainage system

The lacrimal drainage system comprises the superior and inferior puncta, the superior and inferior canaliculi, the common canaliculus, the lacrimal sac and the nasolacrimal duct (Figures 20.1 and 20.3).

## The puncta

The lacrimal drainage system commences with the puncta, which are situated approximately 5 mm from the medial commissure. Each punctum lies on the lacrimal papilla, a slight elevation of the eyelid margin. The inferior punctum lies in apposition to the tear meniscus and should not be visible on slit lamp examination without manual eversion of the eyelid. There are no eyelashes medial to the punctum.

A number of abnormalities of the puncta can be responsible for epiphora:

- Congenital punctual atresia (rare)
- Punctal ectropion
- Acquired punctual stenosis
- Punctal occlusion by eyelash/tumour

Acquired punctual stenosis commonly occurs with punctal ectropion and drying of the punctum.

## The canaliculi

The puncta lead to the canaliculi, which are initially vertical for approximately 2 mm and which then turn to lie horizontally for approximately 8 mm. They are approximately 1–1.5 mm in diameter. The junction of the vertical and horizontal portions of the canaliculi is referred to as the ampulla and is slightly dilated. In the majority of patients the superior and inferior canaliculi join to form a common canaliculus before entering the lacrimal sac. In a small proportion of patients the superior and inferior canaliculi enter the lacrimal sac independently. This should be borne in mind when using a pigtail probe. The canaliculi lie directly beneath the anterior limb of the medial canthal tendon before entering the lacrimal sac. This relationship is important to recall when performing a canaliculo-dacryocystorhinostomy.

# The lacrimal sac

The lacrimal sac lies within the lacrimal sac fossa (see Figure 20.30). The fossa is bounded anteriorly by the anterior lacrimal crest and posteriorly by the posterior lacrimal crest. The floor of the fossa comprises part of the maxillary bone, which usually forms the anterior two-thirds and the lacrimal bone. A vertical suture lies between these bones. This represents a weak area, which is broken at the commencement of the creation of the bony osteotomy during a dacryocystorhinostomy procedure. Occasionally, anterior ethmoid air cells may be situated very anteriorly and even extend into the anterior lacrimal crest. It is important to recognize this and differentiate friable ethmoid sinus mucosa from thin nasal mucosa.

The lacrimal sac measures approximately 12–15 mm in vertical height and is approximately 2–3 mm wide in its resting semi-collapsed state. The fundus of the sac rises above the level of the anterior limb of the medial canthal tendon. The body of the sac gives rise to a narrowed neck, which joins the nasolacrimal duct. The anterior limb of the medial canthal tendon marks the superior limit of the osteotomy in an external dacryocystorhinostomy procedure. The cribriform plate can lie within 2–3 mm of this tendon in some patients. The anterior limb of the medial canthal tendon is a firm structure and prevents distension of the fundus of the sac by fluid or mucus in the presence of a nasolacrimal duct obstruction. For this reason a mucocoele or amniocoele distends below the level of the tendon. The tendon offers no such resistance to a lacrimal sac tumour. Any enlargement of the lacrimal sac above the tendon should therefore suggest a tumour process until proven otherwise (see Figure 20.5). In infants other medial canthal lesions should be considered, e.g. an encephalocoele, a dermoid cyst, a capillary haemangioma.

# The nasolacrimal duct

The membranous portion of the nasolacrimal duct extends from the inferior aspect of the lacrimal sac and travels within the bony nasolacrimal duct to open beneath the inferior turbinate in the inferior meatus of the nose. The nasolacrimal duct is approximately 15 mm in length. A common misconception is that the duct is much longer, with the result that probes are passed too far through the system, abutting the floor of the nose or passing into the nasopharynx.

A number of valves are present within the lacrimal drainage system, which prevent the retrograde passage of tears or air. The most important are:

- The valve of Rosenmüller
- The valve of Hasner

The valve of Rosenmüller is situated at the junction of the common canaliculus and the lacrimal sac. Although not a true valve, it functions to prevent retrograde flow of tears from the lacrimal sac to the conjunctival sac. If the valve is competent in the presence of a nasolacrimal duct obstruction, a tense mucocoele or acute dacryocystitis will occur. External pressure applied to the lacrimal sac will cause pain. In contrast, if the valve is incompetent a mucocoele can be decompressed by external pressure applied to the lacrimal sac with a regurgitation of mucus through the canaliculi and puncta into the lacrimal sac.

The valve of Hasner is situated at the entrance of the nasolacrimal duct to the inferior meatus of the nose. This area represents the last portion of the lacrimal drainage system to develop embryologically. It is not uncommon for a thin membranous obstruction to occur in this region in the newborn. The vast majority of such obstructions spontaneously resolve by the age of 2 years. Failure to do so by this age warrants surgical intervention by simple probing of the nasolacrimal duct.

Other named valves are present but have no clinical significance.

# *The nose*

It is important to have a knowledge of basic intranasal anatomy to be able to examine the nose as part of the clinical evaluation of a patient presenting with epiphora and to be able to undertake endonasal lacrimal drainage procedures.

# The nasal septum

The nasal cavity is divided by the nasal septum. It is common for the nasal septum to show some minor degrees of deviation. A significant degree of deviation, e.g. following a previous nasal fracture, can prevent intranasal access. Surgery to correct such a deviation may be required to permit some lacrimal drainage surgery procedures to be performed, e.g. placement of a Lester Jones tube.

# The turbinates

The middle and inferior turbinates are important landmarks in lacrimal drainage procedures (Figure 20.4 and see Figure 20.11). The superior turbinate plays no role in lacrimal drainage surgery. The turbinates are seen as projections from the lateral wall of the nose. Their purpose is to warm and moisten air drawn through the nose. A space, the meatus, lies beneath each turbinate. *The nasolacrimal duct opens beneath the inferior turbinate into the inferior meatus.* The inferior meatus can be particularly narrow in some infants, necessitating an infracture of the inferior turbinate to gain access to the inferior meatus. The area can be directly visualized with a paediatric (2.7 mm) endoscope after decongesting the mucosa.

The middle turbinate is seen at a higher level within the nose. The anterior tip of the middle turbinate lies adjacent to the lacrimal sac. Sometimes ethmoid air cells invade the middle turbinate, a condition referred to as concha bullosa. It is very occasionally necessary to resect a small portion of the middle turbinate if it obstructs a dacryocystorhinostomy osteum. As the root of the middle turbinate joins the cribriform plate, great care should be taken if surgery is performed on the

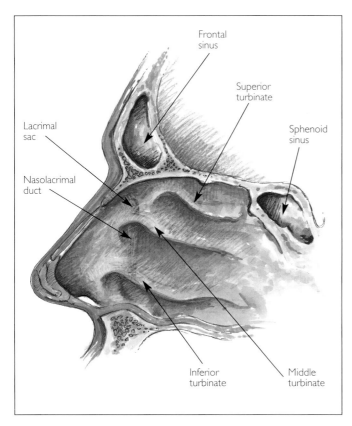

**Figure 20.4**
The relationship of the lacrimal sac and the nasolacrimal duct to the turbinates.

middle turbinate to avoid a cerebrospinal fluid (CSF) leak. The middle turbinate's function should be respected and it should never be routinely resected, e.g. during endoscopic orbital decompression surgery. The frontonasal duct from the frontal sinus drains into the middle meatus. The anterior and middle ethmoid sinuses and the maxillary sinus drain into the middle meatus.

# History

A history of irritation, foreign body sensation or allergy should alert the clinician to the possibility of reflex hypersecretion of

tears. Patients with a dry eye may paradoxically present with the complaint of epiphora due to increased reflex tear secretion. It is essential to exclude such an underlying aetiology, as such patients will not benefit from any form of lacrimal drainage surgery however well performed. The use of topical medications, e.g. glaucoma drops, should raise the suspicion of allergy with an associated lower lid dermatitis or a cicatrizing conjunctivitis with punctal or canalicular obstruction. A history of previous dacryocystitis indicates the presence of a nasolacrimal duct obstruction.

A history of previous intranasal surgery or facial trauma should alert the clinician to the possibility of a nasolacrimal duct obstruction and may require more detailed preoperative investigations, e.g. a coronal computed tomography (CT) scan to determine the presence and location of microplates or bone grafts and the position of the cribriform plate. A history of bloody tears, nasal obstruction or epistaxis should raise the suspicion of nasal, sinus or lacrimal sac malignancy or Wegener's granulomatosis (Figure 20.5). Such patients should be evaluated with the assistance of an ear, nose and throat (ENT) colleague.

A previous history of a facial palsy should alert the clinician to the possibility of 'crocodile tears', a residual incomplete blink or frank lagophthalmos.

The history taking should be tailored to the patient's age, bearing in mind the common causes of epiphora in each age group:

- Infants and children
    congenital nasolacrimal duct obstruction
    congenital anomalies of the lacrimal drainage system
- Young patients
    trauma – canalicular/lacrimal sac lacerations, nasoethmoidal fractures
    canalicular scarring – herpes simplex canaliculitis
- Middle-aged patients
    dacryoliths – *actinomyces* infection
    cicatricial disorders of the lower eyelid anterior lamella
- Older patients
    idiopathic primary acquired nasolacrimal duct obstruction
    involutional eyelid malpositions

The examination of infants and children with epiphora is considered separately under nasolacrimal duct probing and intubation below.

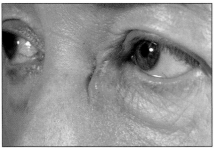

a

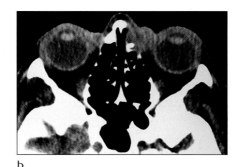

b

**Figure 20.5**
(a) Patient who presented with a history of painless epiphora who was thought to have a nasolacrimal duct obstruction and a secondary mucocoele. She was referred following a biopsy performed during an attempted DCR. The biopsy revealed a lacrimal sac carcinoma.
(b) Axial CT scan of patient demonstrating a mass in the region of the lacrimal sac.

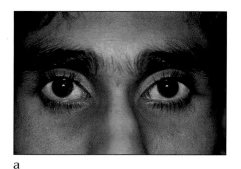
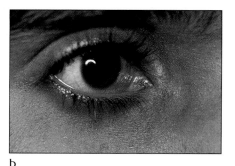

a                                                    b

**Figure 20.6**
(a) Patient referred with a long-standing history of constant epiphora. (b) A side view revealed an antero-displacement of the anterior limbs of the medial canthal tendons, drawing the puncta away from the globe. The patient has a prominent nose. The diagnosis is 'Centurion syndrome'. The treatment is a repositioning of the medial canthal tendons. Failure to recognize the true cause of the epiphora can lead to inappropriate surgical procedures.

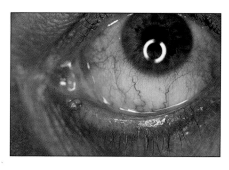

**Figure 20.7**
A papillomatous lesion obstructing the inferior punctum.

# External examination

A number of abnormalities of the eyelids may be responsible for the complaints of epiphora and can be overlooked with a cursory examination (Figure 20.6).

1. Lower lid ectropion
2. Punctal eversion/obstruction
3. Lower lid/upper lid entropion
4. Trichiasis
5. Eyelid lesions, e.g. molluscum contagiosum
6. Incomplete blink
7. Aberrant reinnervation of the facial nerve

A lower eyelid entropion may be intermittent. The patient should be asked to look down and to forcibly close the eyes to ascertain whether or not an entropion can be provoked. This also enables an assessment of orbicularis function. The medial canthus should be palpated for any intrinsic lacrimal sac lesions, e.g. a lacrimal sac mucocoele, or an extrinsic lesion compressing the lacrimal sac, e.g. an ethmoid sinus mucocoele.

## *Slit lamp examination*

Biomicroscopy should be used to exclude causes of reflex hyper-secretion of tears and tear film abnormalities or a dry eye. The puncta should be examined carefully to ensure normal position and exclude an early eversion, stenosis or obstruction by cilia or other lesions (Figure 20.7).

Stenosis of the inferior punctum is commonly associated with an early punctal ectropion. The lacrimal sac should be massaged and the puncta observed for any discharge. Reflux of mucoid material is pathognomonic for a lower lacrimal drainage system obstruction.

# Clinical evaluation of the lacrimal drainage system

The following simple clinical tests should be performed:

- Fluorescein dye disappearance test
- Syringing of the lacrimal drainage system
- Probing of the canaliculi
- Endoscopic nasal examination

## *Fluorescein dye disappearance test*

This is a very simple physiological method for assessing the lacrimal drainage system and can be used in children. A drop of 2% fluorescein is instilled into the inferior fornix of each eye. Complete disappearance of the dye after a period of 4–5 min excludes any significant lacrimal drainage system obstruction. A delayed or asymmetrical dye disappearance is an indication to progress with further clinical tests of the lacrimal drainage system. (The Jones dye tests are not used by the author, who does not find them practical to perform or useful in clinical practice.)

## *Syringing of the lacrimal drainage system*

The patient should be advised that this is not a therapeutic but a diagnostic procedure. It should be performed by the surgeon and never delegated to a nurse.

A local anaesthetic drop is instilled into the conjunctival sac and the residual fluorescein dye is washed from the conjunctival sac. Dilatation of the puncta should only be required where the puncta are stenosed. If this is necessary it should be done with great care to avoid creating a false passage. A fine lacrimal cannula on a 2 ml syringe of sterile saline is gently manipulated through the inferior punctum and along the inferior canaliculus with the eyelid pulled laterally. The cannula should be advanced following the correct anatomical line of the canaliculus and taking great care not to concertina the canaliculus, which creates a false impression of a canalicular or common canalicular obstruction (a common mistake).

Very gentle pressure should be applied to the syringe. Normal patency of the system will allow easy passage of saline to the nasopharynx with no regurgitation. Passage of saline to the nasopharynx after applying more pressure to the syringe suggests a partial obstruction of the lacrimal drainage system or the presence of a dacryolith.

Regurgitation of saline stained with fluorescein through the opposite punctum indicates patent canaliculi but suggests a distal obstruction. It excludes lacrimal pump failure as a cause of epiphora as the fluorescein reached the lacrimal sac. Regurgitation of mucoid or mucopurulent material suggests a nasolacrimal duct obstruction. Regurgitation of blood is an indication to exclude the possibility of a lacrimal sac malignancy.

## Probing of the canaliculi

If syringing of the lacrimal drainage system has suggested an obstruction, careful probing of the canaliculi using a 00 Bowman probe is undertaken. The probe should not be forced through any obstructions. If concretions are present, e.g. following chronic actinomyces infection, the surgeon may feel a gritty sensation with the probe.

If the probe enters the lacrimal sac a 'hard stop' is felt as the probe abuts bone (Figure 20.8). The presence of a 'soft stop' suggests a canalicular or common canalicular obstruction as long as the probe has not been inadvertently pushed into the side wall of the canaliculus, which creates a false impression of a 'soft stop' (Figures 20.9 and 20.10).

The site of any obstruction is determined by withdrawing the probe after grasping it by the punctum with forceps and measuring the length of the probe that is withdrawn. By using this manoeuvre a canalicular or common canalicular obstruction may be diagnosed.

> Under no circumstances should the nasolacrimal duct be probed as a diagnostic procedure in an adult.

## Endoscopic nasal examination

*It is essential to perform a nasal examination before embarking on lacrimal drainage surgery.* In an adult this is easily performed in clinic using a local anaesthetic spray and a nasal decongestant, e.g. oxymetazoline (Afrazine), xylometazoline (Otrivine), lignocaine and phenylephrine. It is essential to exclude intranasal pathology, e.g. polyps, tumours, gross deviations of the nasal septum preoperatively. This is most easily achieved with the use of a rigid nasal endoscope (Figure 20.11). The same instrument should be used to examine the rare failures following a dacryocystorhinostomy (DCR) to assist the surgeon in distinguishing between closure of the nasal ostium and common canalicular stenosis.

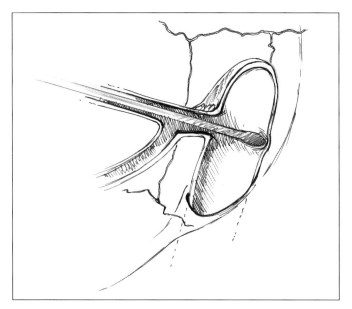

**Figure 20.8**
A 'hard stop' is felt as the lacrimal probe enters the lacrimal sac and strikes the bone on the medial aspect of the lacrimal sac.

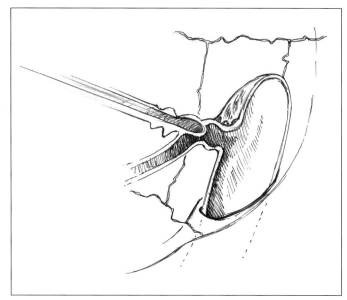

**Figure 20.9**
A 'soft stop' is felt in the presence of a canalicular or common canalicular obstruction.

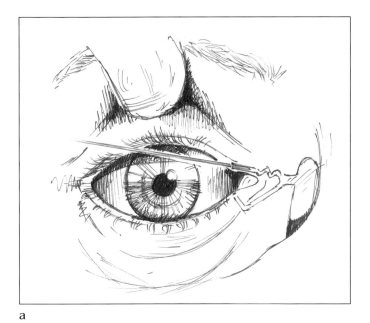

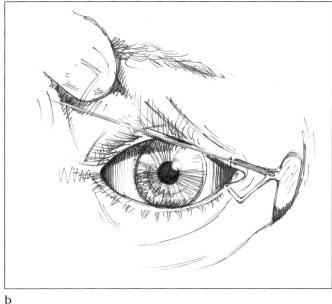

a

b

### Figure 20.10

(a) A false impression of a 'soft stop' has been caused by inadvertently pushing the end of the probe against the side wall of the canaliculus. (b) Care should be taken to ensure that the eyelid is drawn laterally and that the probe is advanced respecting the anatomical configuration of the canaliculus.

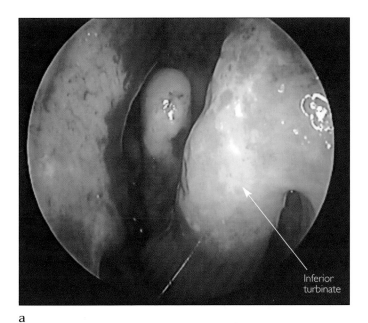

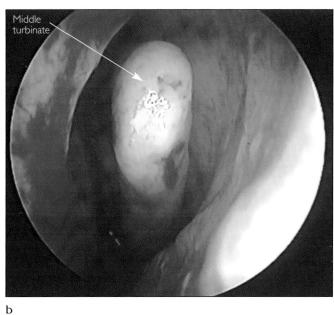

a

b

### Figure 20.11

(a) A An endoscopic view of the nose following the use of a nasal decongestant. The inferior turbinate is indicated by the arrow. The inferior meatus and the opening of the nasolacrimal duct lies under the inferior meatus. (b) The middle turbinate is indicated by the arrow. The middle meatus lies beneath this.

# Imaging

In the vast majority of patients presenting with epiphora, a good history followed by a meticulous clinical evaluation alone will suffice in enabling the surgeon to make a correct diagnosis and to determine the appropriate therapeutic option for the patient. In a minority of patients further investigations may be required:

- Dacryocystography (DCG)
- Dacryoscintigraphy
- Computed tomography (CT)

## *Dacryocystography*

This investigation provides an anatomical assessment of the lacrimal drainage system.

### Indications

1.  Suspected lacrimal sac tumour
2.  Abnormal anatomy – previous trauma, craniofacial surgery, congenital anomalies
3.  Suspected dacryoliths in a patient patent to syringing
4.  Partial or functional obstruction of the nasolacrimal duct

Superior images of the lacrimal drainage system are obtained using computerized digital subtraction dacryocystography (Figure 20.12). Additional films should be obtained 10 min after injection of dye to evaluate dye retention.

## *Dacryoscintigraphy*

This investigation provides a physiological assessment of the lacrimal drainage system. The investigation involves the instillation of a radionuclei tracer into the conjunctival sac. The lacrimal system is then imaged with a gammagram. It is a more sensitive for the diagnosis of incomplete obstructions, particularly of the more proximal system. It is very rarely required.

## *Computed tomography*

Computed tomography is required in the following situations:

1.  Following trauma
2.  To evaluate a patient with a suspected lacrimal sac malignancy (see Figure 20.5)
3.  To evaluate the infant with a medial canthal mass

## Surgical management – infants and children

## *Nasolacrimal duct probing and intubation*

Congenital lacrimal drainage system obstruction is present in approximately 3–6% of newborns. Of these, approximately 0.3% are bilateral. The most common cause is a membranous obstruction of the distal end of the nasolacrimal duct, although there is a variety of rarer anatomical variations that can also cause obstruction of the duct, e.g. a complete bony obstruction of the duct, impaction of the inferior turbinate, a duct ending within the inferior turbinate. There are a number of other congenital anomalies that must be excluded as a cause of epiphora, includ-

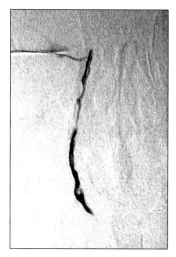 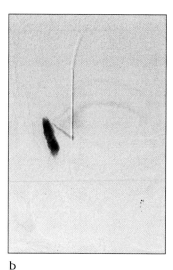

a                                          b

**Figure 20.12**
(a) Computerized digital subtraction dacryocystography (DCG) demonstrating normal right lacrimal drainage system. (b) Computerized digital subtraction DCG demonstrating a complete left nasolacrimal duct obstruction and a dilated lacrimal sac.

ing punctal atresia, congenital absence of the canaliculi, lacrimal sac fistula (see Figure 20.19) and supernumerary puncta.

Other ocular or eyelid abnormalities which can cause tearing must be excluded, e.g. buphthalmos, distichiasis.

Most infants present with epiphora and a recurrently sticky eye which has failed to respond to topical antibiotic treatment. Pressure applied over the lacrimal sac may produce a regurgitation of mucopurulent material. A frank mucocoele may be present. Dacryocystitis is unusual.

A much rarer condition of newborn infants is an amniocoele. This appears as a soft bluish mass at the medial canthus below the level of the medial canthal tendon. This may simply respond to firm pressure applied to the mass if the associated membranous obstruction of the nasolacrimal duct gives way. It is important to differentiate the lesion from a meningocoele or a capillary haemangioma as these can have very similar appearances.

### Patient assessment

In the majority of cases the diagnosis can be established from a good history and careful clinical examination. A dye disappearance test is easy to perform and causes the patient no pain or discomfort. It may demonstrate leakage through a dimple in the eyelid skin, indicating a congenital fistula. Syringing and probing can only be performed under general anaesthesia. A dacryocystogram and a CT scan may be required for patients with craniofacial anomalies.

### Management of congenital nasolacrimal duct obstruction

This should be conservative initially. The parents should be instructed to apply firm massage to the lacrimal sac in a

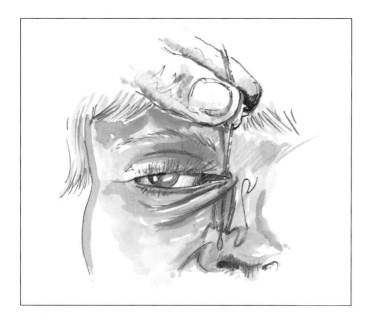

**Figure 20.13**
The technique of nasolacrimal duct probing.

downward direction after feeding. They must understand how to do this properly. Topical antibiotics can be prescribed intermittently. *Over 90% of congenital nasolacrimal duct obstructions resolve spontaneously within the first year, with the figure increasing further by the age of 24 months. Surgical intervention should therefore be deferred unless the patient is experiencing recurrent severe infections.*

## Nasolacrimal duct probing

This is performed under general anaesthesia *with the patient's airway protected.* Oxymetazoline (Afrazine) is sprayed into the patient's nostril immediately after the induction of anaesthesia. The nose is packed beneath the inferior turbinate with small neurosurgical patties moistened with oxymetazoline. The *superior canaliculus* is dilated, taking great care to avoid creating a false passage. A No. 00 or 1 Bowman probe is passed along the canaliculus while drawing the upper lid laterally, remembering the anatomical configuration of the canaliculus. Once a hard stop is felt, the probe is rotated 90 degrees into a vertical position and is then passed *inferiorly, laterally and posteriorly*, respecting the anatomical configuration of the nasolacrimal duct. It is often necessary to bend the probe slightly, particularly in the presence of a prominent brow (Figure 20.13).

Usually the membranous obstruction is felt to give way. The probe can be visualized beneath the inferior turbinate with a small endoscope (2.7 mm 0 degree). This allows confirmation that a false passage has not been created through the nasal mucosa of the lateral nasal wall or inferior turbinate, a common cause of failure.

If the inferior turbinate is found to be abnormally positioned or impacted, it can be gently infractured using the blunt end of a

Freer periosteal elevator placed under the turbinate (Figure 20.14). The turbinate is pushed towards the nasal septum. Fluorescein-stained saline can be gently irrigated through the system with a sucker lying along the floor of the nose to confirm patency of the duct. No postoperative ocular medications are required.

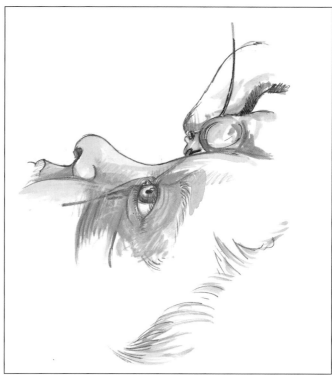

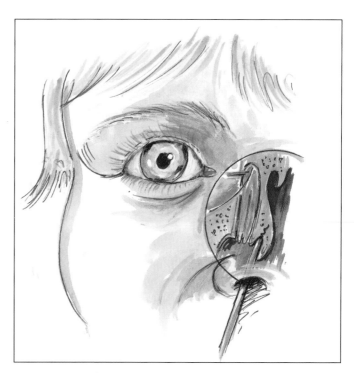

**Figure 20.14**
The technique of infracture of the inferior turbinate.

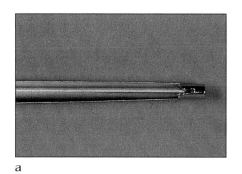

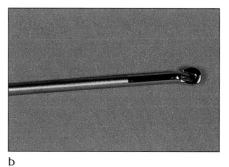

a                                    b

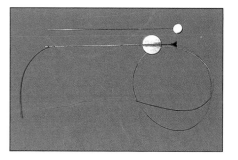

**Figure 20.15**
(a) Anderson–Hwang grooved director. (b) Crawford retrieval hook.

**Figure 20.16**
Ritleng stent with introducing probe.

## Management of a failed nasolacrimal duct probing

If a single probing has failed, the next step is to repeat the probing with placement of a silicone stent. The nose is packed beneath the inferior turbinate with small neurosurgical patties soaked in oxymetazoline. If necessary the nasal mucosa around the turbinate can be injected with 0.25% Marcain (bupivacaine) with 1:200,000 units of adrenaline. The patties are left for 5 min and removed. After probing the nasolacrimal duct, a Crawford or Ritleng silicone stent is placed, again confirming that the introducer has passed to the correct anatomical location beneath the inferior turbinate. The olive tip of the Crawford stent is easily engaged in the end of an Anderson–Hwang grooved director or a Crawford retrieval hook and withdrawn from the nose (Figure 20.15). This can be achieved in a blind fashion or with the use of a 2.7 mm endoscope.

A Ritleng stent is even simpler to remove by using a small blunt hook along the floor of the nose and hooking the nylon suture which precedes the silicone stent (Figure 20.16).

The stents are grasped with a locking Castroviejo needle holder at the tip of the inferior turbinate after spreading apart the eyelids to ensure that the stent in not under tension. A single surgeon's knot is tied tightly. The stent is released and the ends trimmed below the knot, leaving the cut ends just visible beneath the turbinate (Figure 20.17). It is unnecessary to secure the stent using any other device. The position of the stent at the medial canthus is again checked. An overly tightened stent will cause cheese-wiring of the puncta. The stent is left in place for at least 6 months and removed under a very short general anaesthetic. If the patient has only one patent canaliculus a monocanalicular Ritleng stent is used.

No postoperative ocular medications are required. The use of drops or ointments is more likely to lead to a stent prolapse.

If this procedure fails or if the patient develops a dacryocystitis, an external DCR is indicated. The operation is performed in precisely the same manner as in an adult and can be performed quite easily in infants. It is the author's preference to avoid endoscopic DCRs in infants.

If a patient presents with a completely prolapsed silicone stent, this can be removed by rotating the knot via the inferior canaliculus before cutting the stent. It is for this reason that a single surgeon's knot is used when tying the stent in the nose. The

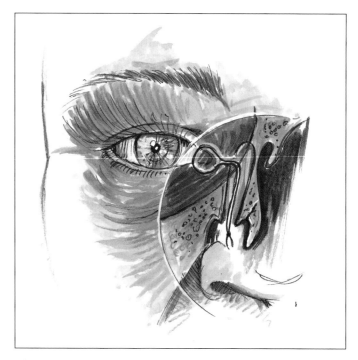

**Figure 20.17**
A stent has been placed through the lacrimal drainage system and has been tied with the knot and ends of the stent lying in the inferior meatus.

parents should be warned of this possibility and instructed to tape the stent to the side of the nose before making arrangements to be seen.

## *Dacryocystocoele*

This unusual lesion forms *in utero* when there is a combination of a congenital nasolacrimal duct obstruction and a competent valve of Rosenmüller. The lacrimal sac expands as the mucus produced within the sac is unable to escape. A medial canthal mass is visible at birth and may become infected if not treated with a degree of urgency (Figure 20.18).

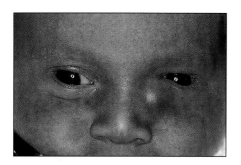

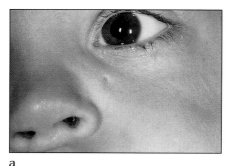

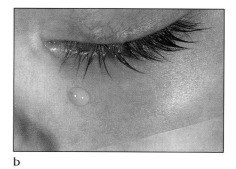

a                                                      b

**Figure 20.18**
Congenital dacryocystocoele.

**Figure 20.19**
(a) Lacrimal sac fistula seen as a small dimple below the medial canthus.
(b) Leakage of fluorescein from the fistula.

The dacryocystocoele is managed by simple probing under a short general anaesthetic. It is unwise to attempt to perform the probing without general anaesthesia as this is painful and may act as a powerful stimulant of the oculocardiac reflex.

## Lacrimal sac fistula

A lacrimal sac fistula is a rare congenital abnormality which is easily overlooked: it usually occurs in conjunction with a congenital nasolacrimal duct obstruction. Tears may be seen emanating from a tiny hole in the inferior aspect of the medial canthus. This is more easily demonstrated with a fluorescein dye disappearance test (Figure 20.19). The nasolacrimal duct obstruction is managed as described above, with placement of a silicone stent and the fistula is excised.

## Punctal atresia

This is a rare congenital abnormality in which one or more puncta are absent. An examination under general anaesthesia can be performed to ascertain whether or not the puncta are merely occluded by a surface membrane with an underlying intact canalicular system. This can be managed by a simple dilatation of the punctum using a sharp Nettleship punctal dilator. The position of the punctum can usually be identified by the position of the lacrimal papilla, which is usually visible using the operating microscope. If a single punctum is completely absent no treatment is usually required, as the patient is usually only symptomatic in cold and windy conditions. A very careful retrograde exploration of the affected canaliculus can be attempted, however, using a pigtail probe to ascertain whether or not the rest of the canalicular system distal to the absent punctum is intact. If both puncta are absent along with the canalicular system the only remaining option is to perform a conjunctivo-dacryocystorhinostomy with placement of a Lester Jones tube as soon as the patient is old enough to cooperate with aftercare of the tube (not usually prior to the age of 7 years).

# Surgical management – adults
## *Eyelid surgery*

Eyelid malpositions and trichiasis are managed according to the principles outlined in Chapters 3, 4, 5 and 6.

# *Punctoplasty*

It is rarely necessary to perform surgical procedures on the inferior punctum. Simple punctal dilatation using a Nettleship dilator usually suffices when this is combined with a procedure to correct a lower eyelid medial ectropion, e.g. a medial spindle procedure. If the effect of simple punctual dilatation is found to be temporary this can be repeated and a silicone stent placed for a few weeks. This is particularly useful if stenosis of the canaliculi is also present. This can avoid the need for a punctoplasty procedure, which can interfere with the effectiveness of the normal lacrimal pump mechanism and is irreversible. If necessary a three-snip punctoplasty can be used for severe punctal stenosis unresponsive to more simple measures. One- or two-snip punctoplasty procedures are not particularly effective.

# *Three-snip punctoplasty*

1.  The inferior punctum is approached from above, with the surgeon seated at the head of the patient
2.  Using a sharp-tipped Westcott scissors, a cut is made in the vertical portion of the canaliculus from the punctum inferiorly
3.  The scissors are turned 90 degrees and a second cut is made just posterior and parallel to the eyelid margin
4.  Holding the tissue posterior to this cut with a 0.12 Castroviejo forceps, a third cut is made, removing a triangle of canaliculus

# Dacryocystorhinostomy

Dacryocystorhinostomy (DCR) is a lacrimal drainage operation in which a fistula is created between the lacrimal sac and the nasal cavity in order to bypass an obstruction in the nasolacrimal duct. Such an obstruction may be partial or complete. The procedure can be performed via an external skin incision (external DCR) or through the nose (endoscopic DCR), either under local or general anaesthesia.

## *Indications*

1. Chronic epiphora
2. Recurrent or chronic dacryocystitis
3. Failed probings and silicone intubations in a child
4. Proposed intraocular surgery in the presence of nasolacrimal duct obstruction

## *Contraindications*

1. Acute dacryocystitis
2. Malignant lacrimal sac tumour

The procedure should not be performed on a patient with acute dacryocystitis (Figure 20.20). The infection should first be cleared with systemic antibiotics and any abscess drained via a skin incision over the lacrimal sac. Any patient in whom a lacrimal sac malignancy is suspected, e.g. a history of bloody tears, should not undergo a DCR.

The procedure is normally performed on a patient who has patent superior and inferior canaliculi although it may be successfully performed for a patient with a single patent canaliculus.

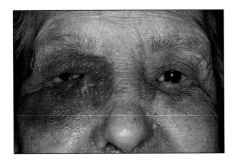

**Figure 20.20**
Acute
dacryocystitis.

## *External DCR*
### Goals and risks of the operation

Prior to scheduling a patient for an external DCR, the goals and risks of the operation are discussed with the patient. A diagram outlining the anatomical defects which need correction is presented to the patient. Pertinent features of the discussion should include:

1. The success/failure rate of the operation (the procedure should be successful in > 95% of cases)
2. The location and size of the wound (which may interfere with wearing glasses)
3. The likelihood of postoperative pain (usually minimal)
4. The need to refrain from using aspirin (and any other drugs which inhibit platelet function)
5. The possibility of postoperative epistaxis
6. The need to refrain from blowing the nose after surgery/rubbing the eye
7. The possibility of stent prolapse and its management
8. The risk of CSF leak (< 0.01%)
9. The type of anaesthesia to be recommended

Many patients, and indeed other clinicians, perceive this procedure as a relatively minor surgical intervention. It is important to dispel such misconceptions. It is not appropriate to perform such surgery on elderly patients with cardiovascular disease who are merely inconvenienced by chronic epiphora.

> It is essential to ensure that the patient does not have undiagnosed, untreated or poorly controlled hypertension

The majority of patients in the UK undergo an external DCR under general anaesthesia although the operation can easily be performed under local anaesthesia, with or without sedation, in suitably selected patients. General anaesthesia has the advantage that both the airway and the patient's blood pressure can be controlled. The anaesthetist should be asked to place a throat pack, which must be recorded and removed, at the completion of surgery. The anaesthetist must be informed prior to the use of any topical or subcutaneous agents to aid haemostasis. The majority of patients in the UK undergo this surgery on an inpatient basis because of the small risk of postoperative epistaxis within the first 12 hours following surgery.

If local anaesthesia is selected for the patient, the nostril should be sprayed with local anaesthetic solution first followed by the subcutaneous injection of local anaesthetic solution in the infratrochlear region and along the incision line. The patient may be sedated by an anaesthetist using a combination of midazolam and propofol. The patient is then prepared as under general anaesthesia as described below.

### Patient preparation

> Performing a successful DCR is greatly facilitated by a bloodless field

Appropriate identification of surgical landmarks and a respect for the integrity of the nasal mucosa are essential.

The patient should be placed in 15 degrees of reverse Trendelenburg position. The first step in performing a successful DCR is

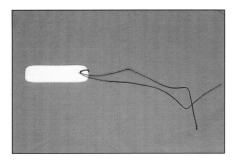

**Figure 20.21**
A nasal epistaxis tampon.

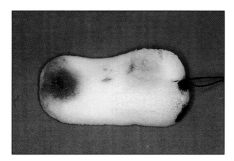

**Figure 20.22**
The appearance of the nasal epistaxis tampon after removal at the completion of the DCR.

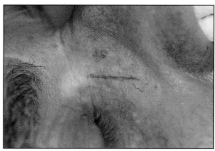

a

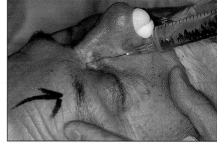

b

**Figure 20.24**
(a) The DCR incision has been marked. (b) A subcutaneous injection is given along the incision line.

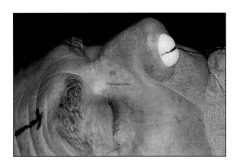

**Figure 20.23**
The correct side for surgery has been identified and marked. A diagonal incision has been marked with a cocktail stick and gentian violet. A nasal epistaxis tampon has been placed and moistened with cocaine solution. A throat pack has been placed.

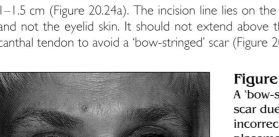

**Figure 20.25**
A 'bow-stringed' scar due to incorrect placement of the incision.

correct packing of the nose. The surgeon should wear a headlight and operating loupes. The middle turbinate must be identified and the nose packed with an epistaxis tampon lightly coated with antibiotic ointment, which is then moistened with 5% cocaine solution (or oxymetazoline in patients with cardiovascular disease) (Figure 20.21). The tampon is inserted with its superior end abutting the anterior the tip of the middle turbinate. The cocaine or oxymetazoline solution is then dripped onto the epistaxis tampon, which gradually enlarges to fill the nasal cavity. This ensures an even delivery of the cocaine to the nasal mucosa. The epistaxis tampon is soft, non-abrasive and easily removed. It soaks up any bleeding from the cut mucosal edges, facilitating posterior flap suturing (Figure 20.22).

A diagonal incision line is drawn with gentian violet applied with a cocktail stick (Figure 20.23). The line of the incision is marked halfway between the bridge of the nose and the medial canthus, starting at the level of the medial canthal tendon and directed down toward the lateral ala of the nose extending for 1–1.5 cm (Figure 20.24a). The incision line lies on the nasal skin and not the eyelid skin. It should not extend above the medial canthal tendon to avoid a 'bow-stringed' scar (Figure 20.25).

A volume of 2 ml of Marcain with 1:200,000 units of adrenaline is injected into the subcutaneous tissue and periosteum under the skin incision (Figure 20.24b).

*The surgeon should wait 10 min prior to starting the operation to allow the adrenaline to take effect.* Defatting the skin with an alcohol wipe prior to marking allows injection and prepping without losing the skin incision mark.

The operation consists of four parts:

1. Skin incision, retraction of the wound, and exposure of the lacrimal fossa
2. The osteotomy
3. The mucosal flaps and stent placement
4. The wound closure

## Incision, retraction and exposure

The surgeon sits at the patient's side. The skin incision is made using a Colorado needle. This is used to dissect bloodlessly through the orbicularis down to the underlying periosteum (Figure 20.26).

The angular vessels can be seen easily and cauterized with bipolar cautery wherever necessary to prevent bleeding. The periosteum is then incised to the bone with the Colorado needle. The periosteum is then elevated off the frontal process of the maxilla and nasal bone using blunt dissection with a Freer periosteal elevator. Next, 4/0 black silk traction sutures are used for retraction of the wound edges. The needle is passed deeply into the wound through the orbicularis and brought out just under the skin. Generally, four silk sutures are used (Figure 20.27).

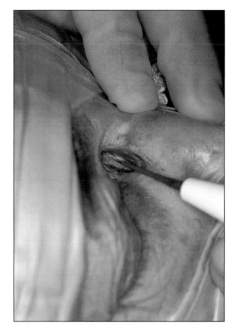

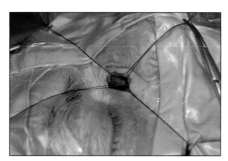

### Figure 20.27
4/0 silk traction sutures are placed to aid haemostasis and to improve exposure. These avoid the necessity for an assistant and avoid the use of rake retractors close to the globe.

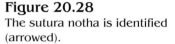

### Figure 20.28
The sutura notha is identified (arrowed).

### Figure 20.26
The skin incision and dissection to the periosteum is performed with a Colorado needle.

The sutures are clamped to the drapes. Use of the sutures greatly enhances visibility and haemostasis throughout the operation.

Next, the periosteum is elevated toward the anterior lacrimal crest. The sutura notha is located 1–2 mm anterior to the anterior lacrimal crest (Figures 20.28 and 20.29). This is an important and consistent landmark, which should be recognized. Often, bleeding from a branch of the infraorbital artery, which travels in the groove, will occur.

Bone wax should be applied for haemostasis. Once the anterior lacrimal crest has been encountered, the periorbita of the lacrimal sac is elevated from the lacrimal sac fossa floor (Figure 20.30). This should be done with great care so that the thin bone of the lacrimal sac fossa or the lacrimal sac mucosa is not violated. The dissection is facilitated using Baron's suction in the surgeon's non-dominant hand and the Freer periosteal elevator in the surgeon's dominant hand. Often, thin areas or dehiscences in the bone can be identified at this point. The periorbita of the lacrimal sac fossa is continuous with the periosteum of the nasolacrimal duct, which can be seen extending into the bony canal.

## The osteotomy

A small curved artery forceps or the blunt end of a Freer periosteal elevator is used to carefully puncture through the floor of the lacrimal fossa (Figure 20.31a). *Care must be taken not to disrupt the underlying nasal mucosa.* If a thin area cannot be identified, it is often possible to break through the suture line between the lacrimal and maxillary bones (lacrimomaxillary suture) just anterior to the posterior lacrimal crest. In some patients with

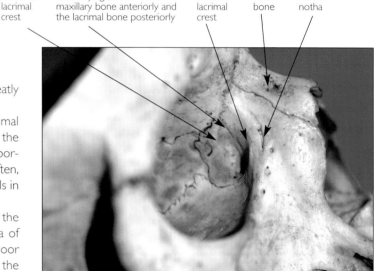

Posterior lacrimal crest — Suture lying between the maxillary bone anteriorly and the lacrimal bone posteriorly — Anterior lacrimal crest — Nasal bone — Sutura notha

### Figure 20.29
A skull viewed from the side in the position of the surgeon undertaking an external DCR.

very thick bone, a diamond burr will be required to thin down the bone before proceeding further. Once the artery forceps have broken through the bone, the jaws of the forceps are spread, enlarging the hole (Figure 20.31b). The osteum is then enlarged using a 90-degree Hardy sella punch (Figure 20.32). This punch is small and easily fits in the osteum. Occasionally, anterior ethmoidal air cells may be encountered in the posterior aspect of the osteotomy. The mucosa of the ethmoidal air cells is thin, relatively avascular and grey in contrast to the thick well-vascularized pinkish nasal mucosa. If an anterior ethmoidal air cell is encountered, the osteotomy may be placed anterior to the air cell or the air cell can be removed.

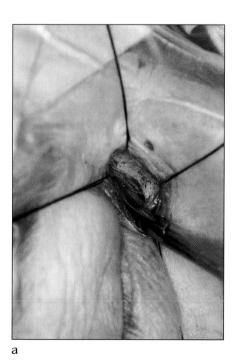

a

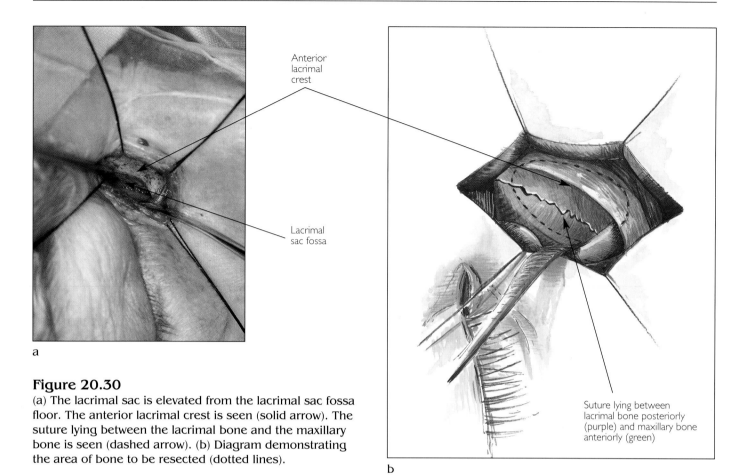

Anterior
lacrimal
crest

Lacrimal
sac fossa

Suture lying between
lacrimal bone posteriorly
(purple) and maxillary bone
anteriorly (green)

b

## Figure 20.30

(a) The lacrimal sac is elevated from the lacrimal sac fossa
floor. The anterior lacrimal crest is seen (solid arrow). The
suture lying between the lacrimal bone and the maxillary
bone is seen (dashed arrow). (b) Diagram demonstrating
the area of bone to be resected (dotted lines).

a

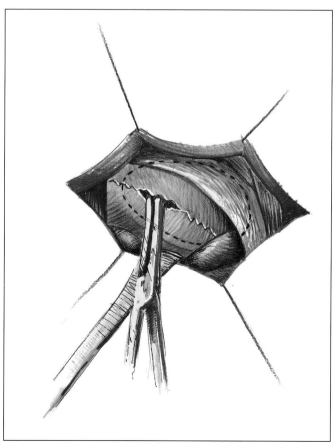

b

## Figure 20.31

(a) The floor of the lacrimal sac fossa is punctured with the
tip of a curved artery clip. (b) The tips of the artery clip are
gently opened to create sufficient room for the end of a
rongeur.

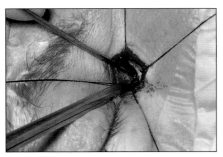

a

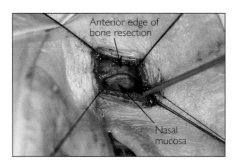

**Figure 20.33**
The osteotomy completed with nasal mucosa intact.

Anterior edge of bone resection

Nasal mucosa

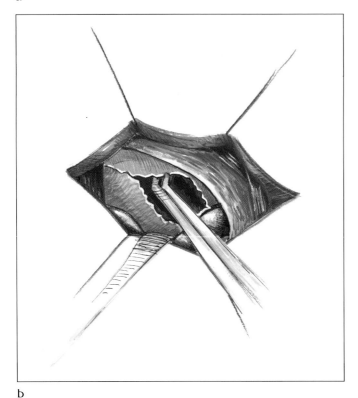

b

**Figure 20.32**
(a) A Hardy sella punch is used to begin the osteotomy. (b) The use of the punch is demonstrated diagrammatically.

The Hardy sella punch is used until the osteotomy is large enough to permit the introduction of a small Kerrison rongeur. The osteotomy into the nose is then enlarged with increasing sizes of the Kerrison rongeurs. *These bone-crunching instruments must be used delicately to avoid damage to the underlying nasal mucosa. Damage to the nasal mucosa at this point will cause a bloody surgical field for the remainder of the case and will make flap formation difficult.* The tip of the rongeur may be placed against the nasal mucosa and rotated 90 degrees. This allows the cutting edge of the rongeur to slip behind the bone without disturbing the underlying nasal mucosa.

The osteotomy is carried anteriorly removing 3–4 mm of the anterior lacrimal crest. Inferiorly, the osteotomy can be completed using a curved Belz lacrimal rongeur or a burr to remove a spine of bone between the nasal mucosa and the nasolacrimal duct. The anterior limb of the medial canthal tendon crosses over the superior one-third of the sac. Some surgeons

cut the tendon to offer better exposure of the sac. Generally, this is not necessary and the medial canthal tendon forms the superior extent of the osteotomy. Care must be taken to cut, not crack, bone in this area, thereby avoiding the risk of fractures that involve the cribriform plate. The limits of the bony osteum are slightly different in each case. The surgeon removes only the bone that is necessary to facilitate flap formation (Figure 20.33).

At this point additional Marcain and adrenaline solution is injected into the nasal mucosa. The hydrostatic effects of the local injection causing the mucosa to blanch and swell will initially stop any bleeding. Later, the effect of the adrenaline will help control bleeding. If these measures do not work, it may be necessary to pack the wound with gelfoam soaked in thrombin solution or surgicel. Bleeding from any of the bone edges is controlled by applying bone wax with the Freer periosteal elevator or cotton-tipped applicators.

## Flaps

The lacrimal sac flaps are formed by incising the lacrimal sac mucosa vertically from the fundus of the sac down into the nasolacrimal duct. The position of the incision is best defined by placing a No. 1 Bowman probe through the canalicular system into the sac. The tip of the probe can be seen tenting the sac towards the nasal mucosa. Generally, the position of the common internal punctum is in the superior aspect of the wound just below the medial canthal tendon. The incision through the lacrimal sac is made using a No. 66 Beaver blade (Figure 20.34).

An alternative is to make a horizontal incision at the junction of the sac and the nasolacrimal duct and make the vertical incision with Werb's angled scissors. The overlying periorbita of the lacrimal sac as well as the lacrimal sac mucosa must be incised to enter the sac. An incision perpendicular to the vertical incision placed at the superior and inferior extents allows the lacrimal sac mucosa to open anteriorly (the anterior lacrimal mucosal flap). The interior of the sac may now be visualized. The lacrimal probe can be seen entering the sac through the common internal punctum. The probe may be pushed medially touching the nasal mucosa. Generally, the point where the probe touches the nasal mucosa is chosen as the point of incision in the nasal mucosa. In some cases a membrane may cover the internal punctum, blocking the progress of the probe. This may be broken with a pointed Bowman probe (used carefully).

Forming the anterior and posterior flaps of the nasal mucosa is similar to forming the flaps of the lacrimal sac. The nasal mucosa is, however, much thicker than the lacrimal sac. Using a No. 66

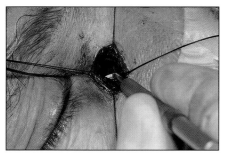

a

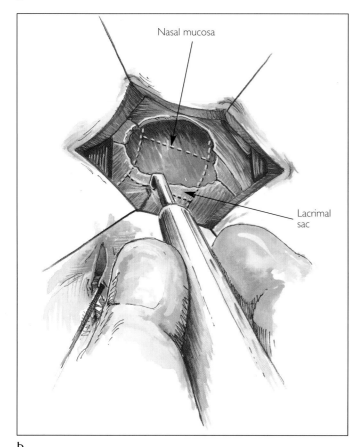

Nasal mucosa

Lacrimal sac

b

**Figure 20.34**
(a) A No. 66 Beaver blade is used to open the lacrimal sac.
(b) This is demonstrated diagrammatically.

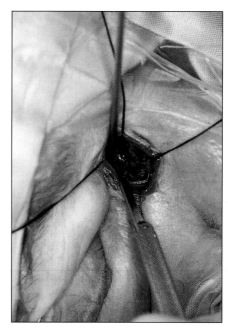

**Figure 20.35**
The nasal mucosa is opened with the No. 66 Beaver blade.

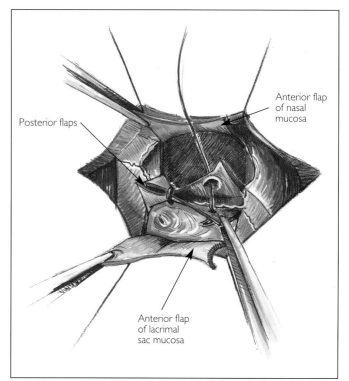

Posterior flaps

Anterior flap of nasal mucosa

Anterior flap of lacrimal sac mucosa

**Figure 20.36**
Suturing of the posterior flaps.

Beaver blade, an incision is made from the most superior aspect of the osteotomy to the most inferior aspect of the osteotomy (Figure 20.35). Again, perpendicular cuts allow the flaps to be opened anteriorly and posteriorly. Additional bone may be removed anteriorly to lengthen the anterior nasal flap if necessary. Rarely, the tip of the middle turbinate is seen to obstruct the osteum. In this case the turbinate should be injected with Marcain and adrenaline solution and the tip resected using a Kerrison rongeur. This should be done very carefully to avoid postoperative intranasal adhesions.

Next, the flaps are sutured together. A 5/0 Vicryl suture is coated with bone wax for lubrication. The 5/0 Vicryl suture on a short 1/2-circle needle is passed from the posterior nasal mucosal flap through the posterior lacrimal sac flap (Figure 20.36). This suture is carefully tied. Care is taken not to sew through the delicate flap mucosa. Single throws of these sutures are used, as these sutures will bear no tension. The surgeon should avoid pulling the suture up when tying the knot. Generally, two sutures are placed in the posterior mucosal flaps. The nasal tampon is now removed from the nose.

Crawford silicone stents are passed through the canalicular system into the nose. The stent is passed through the canalicular

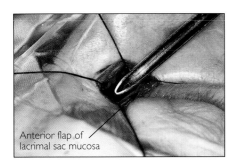

**Figure 20.37**
Quickert grooved
director.

Anterior flap of
lacrimal sac mucosa

system, through the lacrimal sac and into the osteotomy. The stent probe is retrieved using a grooved director placed into the nose via the nares (Figures 20.37 and 20.38). The stent is then pulled out through the nose. The stents is tied with a single knot.

The anterior flaps are then closed in a fashion similar to the posterior flaps (Figure 20.39).

It is important to ensure that the stent is not tight at the medial canthus by gently parting the eyelids to avoid cheese-wiring of the puncta and canaliculi (Figure 20.40).

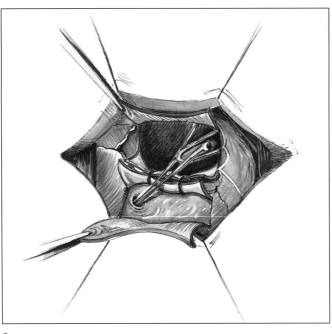

a

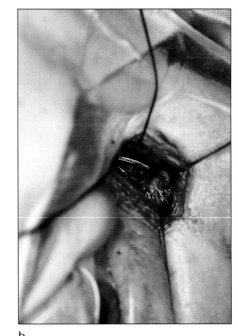

b

**Figure 20.38**
(a) Diagram
demonstrating
insertion of stent
into grooved
director.
(b) Stent being
inserted into
grooved
director.

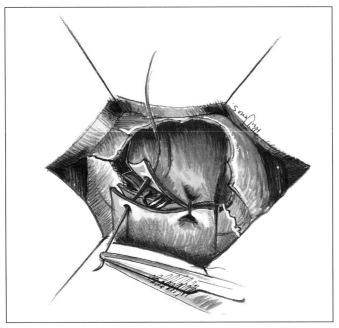

a

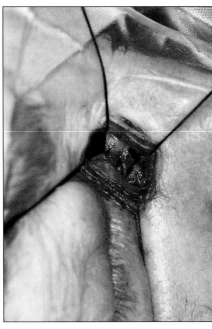

b

**Figure 20.39**
(a) Diagram
demonstrating
closure of the
anterior flaps.
(b) Anterior flaps
closed.

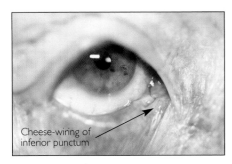

**Figure 20.40**
Cheese-wiring of inferior punctum
from over-tightened silicone stent.

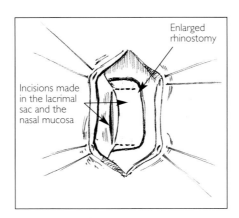

**Figure 20.41**
The nasal mucosa and scarred area of
the anastomosis are incised.

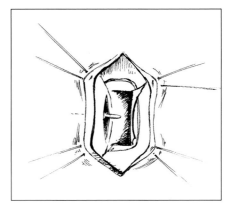

**Figure 20.42**
Scar tissue is resected with probes in
the canaliculi.

## Wound closure

It is preferable to avoid the use of subcutaneous sutures, which can predispose the patient to thickening of the wound or infection. The skin should be closed with interrupted 7/0 Vicryl sutures placed in a vertical mattress fashion.

## Postoperative care

Topical antibiotic ointment alone is used postoperatively unless the patient has had previous dacryocystitis or has a predisposition to infection, e.g. diabetes mellitus, in which case the patient should be prescribed a course of oral antibiotics. The patient should be instructed to apply wound massage postoperatively, which should be continued for 8–12 weeks.

## Redo external DCR

A repeat DCR may be required for the management of a failed DCR or a 'sump syndrome'. A 'sump syndrome' is characterized by a patent but high anastomosis with a residual dilated lacrimal sac which fills with stagnant tears and mucus. A preoperative DCG can be useful in this situation.

A skin incision is made as for a standard DCR. Skin–muscle flaps are fashioned and traction sutures are placed. A Freer periosteal elevator is used to bluntly dissect down to bone anterior to the previous osteotomy. Periosteum is then elevated off the bone and the rhinostomy enlarged. It is not uncommon to find that the original rhinostomy has not been of the correct size and in the correct position. The nasal mucosa and scarred anastomosis are incised vertically (Figure 20.41).

Bowman probes are placed into the canaliculi and scar tissue is dissected away with Westcott scissors until the ends of the probes are located. Any residual lacrimal sac is opened fully (Figure 20.42).

If any flaps can be fashioned, these should be sutured as for a standard DCR. Crawford-style lacrimal stents are placed before the anterior flaps are sutured. The wound is closed as for a DCR and the stents are left in place for a minimum period of 6 months.

If a DCR fails after being performed appropriately by the surgeon, it is usually preferable to dissect any scar tissue endoscopically. The endoscopic approach is much simpler both for the surgeon and the patient. The stents can also be placed endoscopically.

## *Endoscopic non-laser assisted DCR*

This operative approach requires skill with the use of the endoscope and good intraoperative haemostasis. It offers the patient the advantage of having no medial canthal wound and no cutaneous scar. The cosmetic deformity associated with the scar is, however, frequently overstated. With appropriate placement of the incision and postoperative wound care and massage, the cutaneous scar is barely visible in the vast majority of patients, particularly those over 50 years of age.

Young patients, particularly those at risk of hypertrophic or keloid scars, may, however, prefer to opt for an endoscopic approach. It is generally accepted that the success rate of this approach is slightly inferior to that of a standard external DCR. It is essential that the patient has undergone an endoscopic nasal examination in clinic to ensure that the procedure is technically feasible. Some patients may require other nasal procedures to enable this approach to be used, e.g. a submucosal resection of the nasal septum if this is grossly deviated.

Most patients prefer to undergo this procedure under a general anaesthetic. The operation consists of three parts:

1. Removal of a nasal mucosal flap
2. The osteotomy
3. The opening of the lacrimal sac and placement of the stent

> It is very important to gain practice inserting sharp instruments atraumatically under endoscopic control before undertaking this surgical procedure

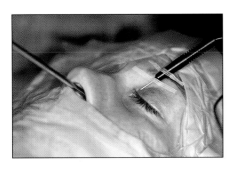

**Figure 20.43** With the endoscope turned off the retinal light pipe can be seen transilluminating the lacrimal sac fossa.

turbinate. *The surgeon should wait 10 min prior to starting the operation to allow the adrenaline to take effect.*

A 20-gauge retinal light pipe is inserted through the upper punctum and directed into the lacrimal sac (Figures 20.43 and 20.44). The nasal packing is removed. The surgeon positions himself on the right side of the operating table (or left side if left-handed) ensuring that he has an unobstructed view of the TV screen. A 0- or 30-degree endoscope is used, with the latter being preferable for a narrower nasal cavity or a deviated nasal septum.

## Patient preparation

The patient is given a nasal decongestant 2 hours and 1 hour preoperatively. Just prior to the induction of general anaesthesia the patient is given a nasal spray of 0.25% phenylephrine with 2% Xylocaine (lignocaine). After the induction of general anaesthesia 1–2 ml of 1% Xylocaine with 1:200,000 units of adrenaline are injected into the middle turbinate and lateral wall of the nose. The nose is then packed with 1/2-inch ribbon gauze soaked in 0.25% phenylephrine with 2% Xylocaine to the tip of the middle

## Removal of a nasal mucosal flap

The middle turbinate is pushed medially with the blunt end of a Freer periosteal elevator. A phacoemulsification crescent blade is used to make nasal mucosal incisions, one just posterior to the light, in the fossa behind the maxillolacrimal suture line and the other 7–8 mm anterior to the same line (Figure 20.45). This nasal mucosal flap is raised with the Freer periosteal elevator. The anterior and posterior incisions are joined horizontally superiorly and inferiorly with the crescent blade and the piece of nasal musosa is removed with forceps.

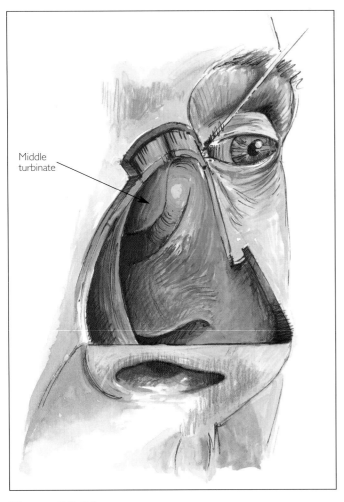

Middle turbinate

**Figure 20.44**
A diagrammatic representation of the position of the light seen from the retinal light pipe.

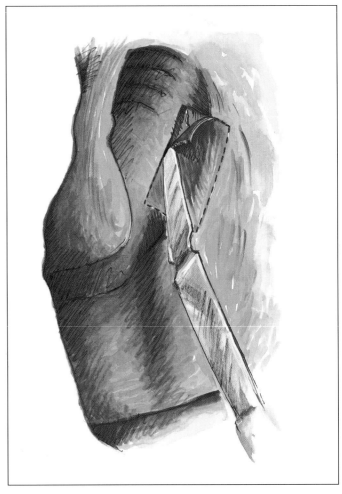

**Figure 20.45**
The nasal mucosa is carefully incised with a crescent blade.

## The osteotomy

The thinner bone posterior to the anterior lacrimal crest is raised with the Freer elevator. An up-biting Kerrison rongeur is used to take bites of bone anteriorly into the frontal process of the maxilla (Figure 20.46). The inferior two-thirds of the lacrimal sac is exposed. This procedure can also be achieved with powered instrumentation with a water-cooled burr and attached suction.

## The opening of the lacrimal sac and placement of the stent

The lacrimal sac is then opened with a sharp sickle blade. An incision is made across the superior aspect of the sac posteriorly. A vertical incision is then made from below as anterior as possible into the sac (Figure 20.47). The angle thus created is grasped with angulated forceps and torn posteriorly and inferiorly. Alternatively, the mucosa may be removed with the use of fine angulated scissors. The silicone stent is then passed in the same way as with an external DCR.

## Postoperative care

The postoperative appearance is shown in Figure 20.48. The patient is asked to irrigate the nose twice a day with a salt solution to remove dried clots. Topical steroid/antibiotic nasal drops are prescribed for 1 week. A gentle syringing of the lacrimal drainage system is undertaken the day after surgery and this is repeated after 1 week. The stent is removed after 1 month.

The endoscopic approach is advantageous for the failed DCR where the ostium has stenosed. This can be reopened with a sharp sickle blade and a stent passed relatively quickly with very little operative morbidity.

## *Endonasal laser-assisted DCR*

Advocates of endoscopic laser-assisted DCR point to a number of potential advantages of this technique.

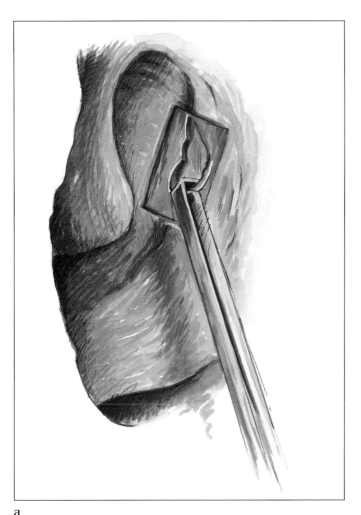

a

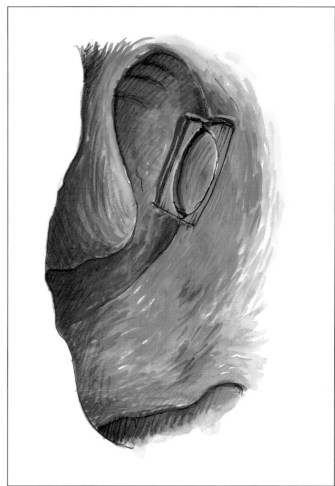

b

**Figure 20.46**
(a) Bone is carefully removed with rongeurs. (b) The inferior two-thirds of the lacrimal sac should be exposed.

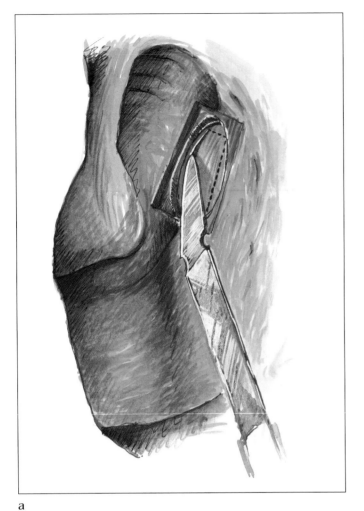

a

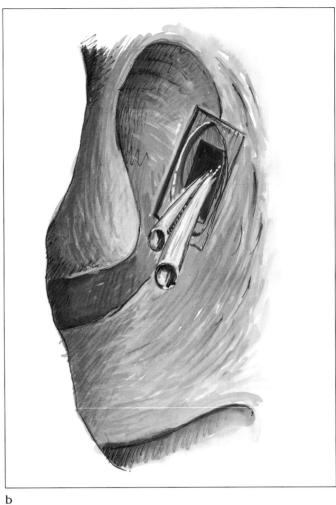

b

**Figure 20.47**
(a) The lacrimal sac is carefully incised with a crescent blade. (b) A silicone stent is placed.

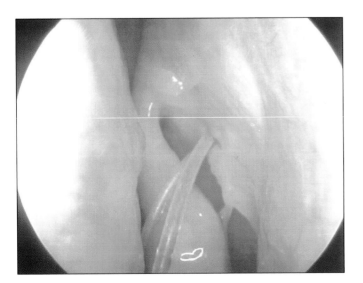

**Figure 20.48**
The postoperative appearance following an endoscopic DCR with the silicone stent in place.

# Advantages

1. Local anaesthetic day case procedure
2. Short operating time (15–30 min)
3. Minimal postoperative morbidity
4. Minimal disruption of adjacent structures
5. No cutaneous scarring
6. High patient acceptance
7. Easy revisionary surgery
8. Ideal for the patient with a bleeding diathesis

There are, however, a number of disadvantages of the procedure.

# Disadvantages

1. Low long-term success rate (less than 60%)
2. Potential risk of laser complications
3. High cost of equipment

4. Some cases require combined skills of an ophthalmologist and an ENT surgeon
5. Requires good access to the middle meatus
6. Potential morbidity in not recognizing a lacrimal sac tumour intraoperatively

## The operative procedure

The patient is prepared as described above. A 20-gauge retinal light pipe is inserted via the upper canaliculus and positioned in the lower part of the lacrimal sac, and the area is visualized endoscopically. The holmium–YAG laser probe is directed at the area of transillumination and, initially, a 7/8 mm diameter area of mucosa is ablated with the laser. The underlying bone is then lasered at a higher energy setting. The lacrimal mucosa adjacent to the area of the rhinostomy is ablated and an opening into the sac is created. The silicone stent is then placed.

## Postoperative care

This is the same as described above. Although it is hoped that the intraoperative use of topical antimetabolites may improve the success rate of this procedure, it has so far not achieved the same status as the external DCR, which has very little morbidity in the hands of the experienced oculoplastic surgeon but a very high success rate. The external DCR remains the gold standard operation by which all other procedures have to be judged.

# Canaliculo-dacryocystorhinostomy

A canaliculo-dacryocystorhinostomy is a lacrimal drainage operation in which a small section of obstructed canaliculus just lateral to the lacrimal sac is resected and the patent canaliculus anastomosed to the nasal mucosa using the lacrimal sac as a soft tissue bridge. The procedure can only be performed via an external skin incision, either under local or general anaesthesia. It cannot be performed endoscopically. For patients with a distal membranous obstruction over the common canaliculus which can be overcome with a probe, the lacrimal drainage system should be simply intubated for a period of 3–6 months.

## *Indications*

Obstruction of the common canaliculus or of the individual canaliculi just lateral to the sac with a minimum of 8 mm of patent canaliculus present.

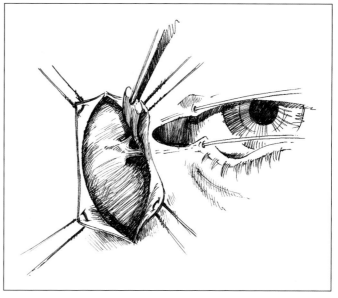

**Figure 20.49**
The anterior limb of the medial canthal tendon is disinserted from the nasal bone and reflected laterally with probes in the canaliculi helping to identify the position of the canaliculi.

## *Operative procedure*

The patient is prepared as for a standard DCR. A skin incision is made with a Colorado needle and the superficial part of the medial canthal tendon is identified and divided with a No. 15 blade just lateral to its insertion on the nasal bone.

The tendon is reflected laterally, exposing the anterior surface of the fundus of the lacrimal sac (Figure 20.49). The relationship of the canaliculi to the medial canthal tendon is demonstrated in Figure 20.50. A No. 1 Bowman's probe is placed into the superior and inferior canaliculi. The medial canthal tendon is dissected on its deep surface laterally, superiorly and inferiorly using a Freer periosteal elevator until the probes are just visible.

The periosteum is incised over the anterior lacrimal crest and reflected laterally. Next, a large rhinostomy is created. The lacrimal sac is opened anteriorly adjacent to the Bowman probes from the fundus to the commencement of the nasolacrimal duct (Figure 20.51).

The canaliculi are incised and a silicone stent passed and used to draw the canaliculi laterally. The whole of the lacrimal sac is now rotated posteriorly to form the posterior flap of the anastomosis and a large nasal mucosal flap is formed and rotated anteriorly to form the anterior flap. The lateral margins of the canaliculi are sutured to the adjacent lacrimal sac mucosa using 8/0 Vicryl sutures (Figure 20.52). The posterior flaps are then sutured and the anterior flaps sutured after the stent has been passed into the nose (Figure 20.53).

The medial canthal tendon is sutured back to its stump. The wound is closed as for a DCR but the stent is not removed for at least 6 months.

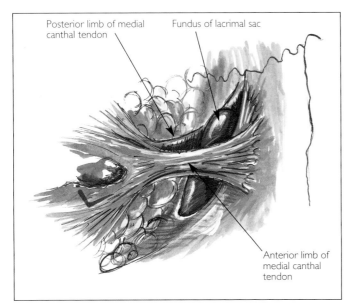

a

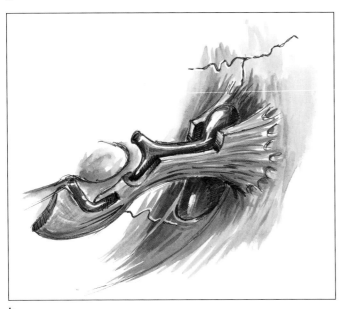

b

**Figure 20.50**
(a) The relationship of the lacrimal sac to the medial canthal tendon. (b) The relationship of the canaliculi to the medial canthal tendon, which has been partially removed.

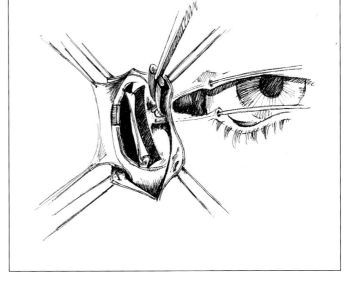

**Figure 20.51**
The lacrimal sac is opened very anteriorly creating a large posterior flap. The anterior flap is created from nasal mucosa after fashioning a large rhinostomy.

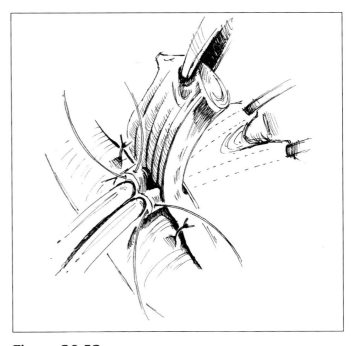

**Figure 20.52**
The lateral margins of the canaliculi are sutured to the adjacent lacrimal sac mucosa using 8/0 Vicryl sutures.

# Conjunctivo-dacryocystorhinostomy (CDCR)

This surgical procedure is an extension of a dacryocystorhinostomy (DCR) with the addition of several steps involved in the placement of a Lester Jones tube (LJ tube). Although this operation is associated with a number of potential complications, it is relatively straightforward to perform and has a success rate in experienced hands of over 95%.

## Indications

1. Symptomatic epiphora secondary to extensive scarring of both upper and lower canaliculi
2. Congenital atresia or complete absence of the canaliculi with epiphora
3. Symptomatic epiphora secondary to lacrimal pump failure, e.g. chronic facial palsy

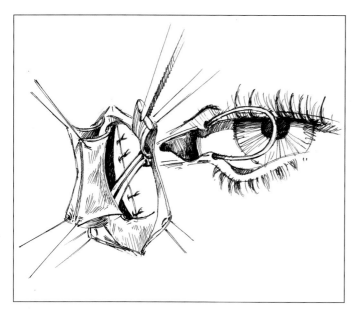

**Figure 20.53**
The posterior flaps have been sutured and the stent passed before the anterior flap is sutured.

## Patient evaluation

Each patient must be counselled about the pros, cons, risks and potential complications of this operative procedure. In particular, the patient must understand that the LJ tube is a device which is permanently implanted, committing the patient to lifelong maintenance of the tube and follow-up.

Careful patient selection is essential. Only patients whose lifestyle is adversely affected by constant epiphora and who are willing to comply with aftercare should be offered such surgery.

The patient should be carefully examined to determine whether or not additional surgical procedures will be required. Any significant eyelid malposition or medial canthal dystopia will need to be addressed. An endoscopic nasal examination must be performed to exclude intranasal abnormalities and to confirm that there is adequate space for placement of the LJ tube. Some abnormalities, e.g. elongated middle turbinate or minor degrees of nasal septal deviation, can be managed at the time of the CDCR but occasionally such abnormalities should be addressed by an ENT surgeon prior to the patient undergoing a CDCR. Occasionally a coronal CT scan will be required to evaluate the medial canthal anatomy if the patient has undergone previous craniofacial surgery, trauma or bone grafting. It is important in craniofacial anomalies to ascertain the position of the cribriform plate.

The operation itself can be performed externally or endoscopically, under general or local anaesthesia.

## External CDCR + LJ tube

The patient is prepared as for a standard external DCR. A DCR is performed to the point at which flaps of nasal and lacrimal sac mucosa are made taking care not to disrupt the medial canthal tendon. The osteotomy is made no more than 4–5 mm inferior to the lower border of the medial canthal tendon to prevent too inferior an angulation of the LJ tube. The osteotomy is made respecting an approximate 5 mm radius centred on the position of the common canaliculus. The posterior flaps are sutured.

Next, the caruncle is partially or totally resected with Westcott scissors (Figure 20.54).

An 18-gauge sharp-tipped Kirschner wire is then pushed from the bed of the caruncle to the lacrimal sac in the region of the common canaliculus to lie just anterior to the tip of the middle turbinate (Figure 20.55).

If the middle turbinate interferes with the desired placement of the wire the tip can be resected with care, avoiding twisting motions which can damage the cribriform plate and lead to a CSF leak. Next, the track is enlarged using a 2.5 mm Elliott's trephine which is slipped over the Kirschner wire (Figure 20.56). Alternatively, a Graefe knife can be used.

The length of LJ tube required is then estimated by passing a Putterman probe along the fistulous track to lie 2–3 mm from

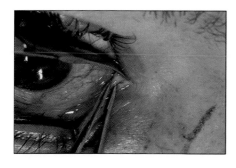

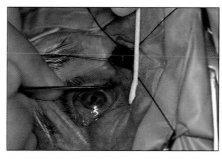

a

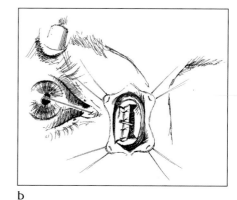

b

**Figure 20.54**
Resection of the caruncle.

**Figure 20.55**
(a) A Kirschner wire is passed through the bed of the resected caruncle. (b) The Kirschner wire is then directed through the lateral wall of the lacrimal sac in the region of the common canaliculus.

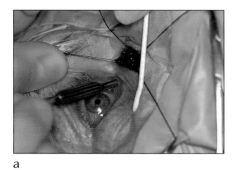

a

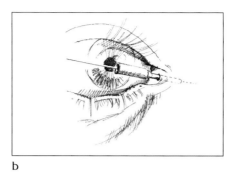

b

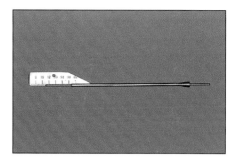

**Figure 20.56**
(a) An Elliott's trephine is slipped over the Kirschner wire. (b) The trephine is pushed through the lateral wall of the lacrimal sac.

**Figure 20.57**
A Putterman probe.

the nasal septum. The measurement of the length of tube required is provided on a scale on the probe (Figure 20.57). The tube is checked for the length and collar size (usually 3.5 or 4 mm). The track is now dilated using standard gold dilators. It is important not to over-enlarge the track, which should tightly grip the LJ tube.

An LJ tube is then slipped over a guidewire and pushed into position (Figure 20.58). The guidewire is removed and the tube pushed until the neck lies in the caruncular bed.

The position of the LJ tube in the nose should be checked using a nasal speculum and headlight or using an endoscope. If the tube is found to be too long or too short, it is removed, replaced with an alternative size and rechecked. Occasionally, an angulated tube will be required if the middle turbinate causes problems with satisfactory placement.

Next, the anterior flaps are sewn together and the tube irrigated to clear any blood clots. A 7/0 Vicryl purse-string suture is used to anchor the tube to the adjacent conjunctiva (Figure 20.59). The wound is closed as for a DCR. A firm compressive dressing is placed and not removed for 3 days.

The wound care is the same as in the case of an external DCR. Additional topical antibiotic drops are prescribed for 1 week.

# Endoscopic CDCR + LJ tube

The endoscopic CDCR has a number of advantages, which should be weighed against the disadvantages. The individual patient should be carefully assessed preoperatively to determine which approach is most suitable and to determine whether or not an ENT colleague is required to assist with any additional intranasal procedures that may be required.

## Advantages

1.  Avoids a cutaneous scar
2.  Minimally invasive, allowing more precise tissue removal
3.  Permits identification and correction of common intranasal abnormalities
4.  Allows an easier and quicker approach to reoperations

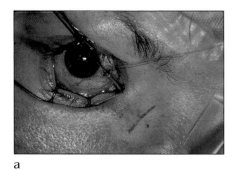

a

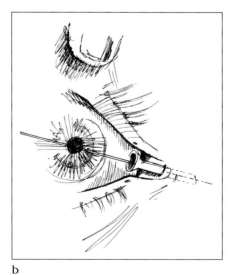

b

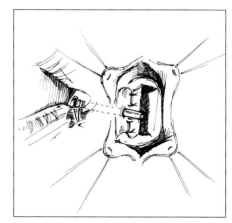

**Figure 20.58**
(a) The Lester Jones tube is passed along a blunt-tipped guidewire. (b) The Lester Jones tube is then passed over the guidewire into the nose.

**Figure 20.59**
The tube is sutured to the adjacent conjunctiva.

## Disadvantages

1. Requires meticulous intraoperative haemostasis to maintain good visualization
2. Expensive equipment
3. Unsuitable for severe bony deformities of the medial canthus

The operation is performed as for a non-laser assisted endoscopic DCR. The identification of the surgical landmarks can, however, be somewhat more challenging as a retinal light pipe cannot be placed into the lacrimal sac in cases of canalicular obstruction. In such cases the light pipe is instead placed over the caruncular bed and used to transilluminate the thin bone at the posterior aspect of the lacrimal fossa.

Once the internal rhinostomy has been completed the lacrimal sac is opened and the LJ tube is placed as described above while visualizing its position endoscopically. If a patient has previously undergone DCRs which have failed or a previous CDCR with loss of the LJ tube, the endoscopic approach is relatively simple. The rhinostomy has already been performed and placement of the LJ tube is performed as described above and the intranasal position of the tube observed endoscopically (Figures 20.60). An example of the postoperative appearance of a typical patient is shown in Figure 20.61.

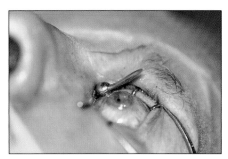

a

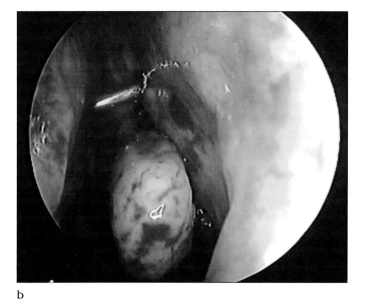

b

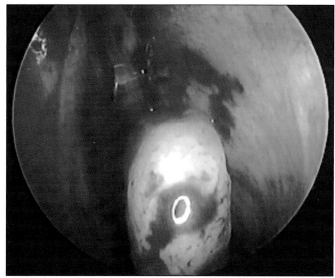

c

### Figure 20.60

(a) A gold dilator is passed via the caruncular bed. (b) The position of the dilator is observed endoscopically. In this patient the dilator is entering the nasal cavity just in front of the root of the middle turbinate. (c) This Lester Jones tube was positioned at a higher level than normal but functioned well.

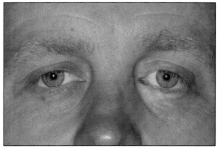

a

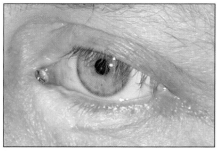

b

### Figure 20.61

(a) A patient who was referred with a lower eyelid medial cicatricial extropion and extensive canalicular scarring following trauma. A lower eyelid skin graft has been placed to reposition the eyelid and a Lester Jones (LJ) tube has been placed endoscopically. (b) A side view of the LJ tube position.

## Postoperative care

The patient is instructed to instil hypromellose drops into the eye morning and evening and, while occluding the opposite nostril with a finger, to sniff vigorously. This is done daily on a permanent basis. The patient is instructed to place two fingers over the LJ tube when sneezing and is warned about the sensation of air passing across the eye when blowing the nose. The patient is instructed to report any problems with the tube immediately as adjustments to the tube or replacement of the tube are much easier at this stage than if the patient presents some time after losing the tube, when the fistulous track has usually fibrosed. Occasionally, blocked tubes may need to be flushed through with saline via a syringe and lacrimal cannula in the clinic.

## Complications

Although there are a multitude of complications which can occur following placement of an LJ tube, the most frequently encountered problem is that of tube displacement. This needs to be managed early to avoid additional secondary ocular complications, e.g. episcleritis, corneal ulceration. Lateral migration of the tube usually indicates that the tube is too long. The tube should be removed and replaced with a more appropriately sized tube. The nose should be examined endoscopically to determine whether or not intranasal abnormalities are responsible for the migration.

Medial migration can lead to the tube becoming invisible at the medial canthus. This may be difficult to differentiate from loss of the tube, unless the medial end is visible within the nasal cavity. Rarely will a CT scan be necessary to locate the position of a displaced tube.

Granulation tissue around the tube can be controlled with topical steroids, or with surgical resection.

## Further reading

1.  Dale DL. Embryology, anatomy and physiology of the lacrimal system. In: Stephenson CM, ed. *Ophthalmic plastic, reconstructive and orbital surgery*. Boston: Butterworth–Heinemann, 1997, pp. 19–30.

2.  Linberg JV. Surgical anatomy of the lacrimal system. In: Linberg JV, ed., *Lacrimal surgery. Contemporary Issues in Ophthalmology*. New York: Churchill Livingstone, **5**:1–18, 1988.

3.  McEwen CJ, Young JDH. Epiphora during the first year of life. *Eye* (1991) **5**:596–600.

4.  Müllner K. Ritleng intubation set: a new system for lacrimal pathway intubation. *Ophthalmologica* (2000) **214**:237–9.

5.  Nowinski TS. Anatomy and physiology of lacrimal system. In: Bosniak S, ed., *Principles and practice of ophthalmic plastic and reconstructive surgery*, Vol. 2. Philadelphia: WB Saunders, 1996, pp. 731–47.

6.  Yagci A, Karci B, Ergezen F. Probing and bicanalicular silicone tube intubation under nasal endoscopy in congenital nasolacrimal duct obstruction. *Ophthal Plast Reconstr Surg (2000)* **16**:58–61.

# 21

# Blepharoplasty

## Introduction

An upper eyelid blepharoplasty may involve the removal of skin and muscle alone or this may be combined with the removal of herniated orbital fat. The procedure may be combined with an eyebrow lifting procedure or a blepharoptosis procedure. The procedure may be performed both for functional and cosmetic reasons.

A lower eyelid blepharoplasty is performed for cosmetic reasons alone and may also involve the removal of skin and muscle alone or this may be combined with the removal of herniated orbital fat.

## Applied anatomy

A thorough understanding of the surgical anatomy of the eyebrows and eyelids is essential prior to performing a blepharoplasty.

## *Upper eyelid*

The distance between the inferior aspect of the eyebrow and the upper lid skin crease on downgaze should be approximately two-thirds of the distance from the inferior aspect of the eyebrow to the eyelid margin. Likewise, the distance from the skin crease to the eyelid margin in downgaze should be one-third of the distance from the inferior aspect of the eyebrow to the eyelid margin (Figure 21.1). In general, a minimum distance of 10 mm should be left between the inferior aspect of the eyebrow and the upper eyelid skin crease.

It is important to maintain these dimensions. If an excessive amount of upper eyelid skin is removed, reducing the distance from the skin crease to the brow in the presence of a brow ptosis, an unsatisfactory result will occur, with the appearance of

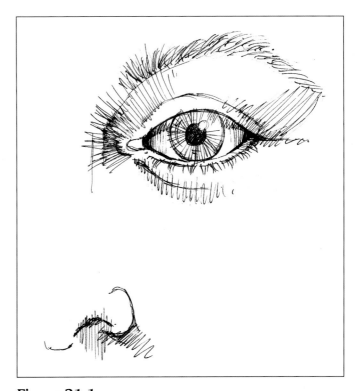

**Figure 21.1**
Topography of the eyebrow and eyelid. The palpebral aperture is almond-shaped, with the lateral canthal angle lying slightly higher than the medial canthal angle. The lateral canthal angle is generally higher in females than in males and lies approximately 5 mm from the lateral orbital margin. The upper eyelid skin crease is usually approximately 5–6 mm above the lash line in males and 7–8 mm in females.

the brow being attached to the eyelashes (Figure 21.2). This may also cause lagophthalmos (Figure 21.3).

It is important to differentiate prolapsed orbital fat from retro-orbicularis oculi fat (ROOF) that has descended, encroaching on

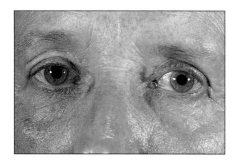

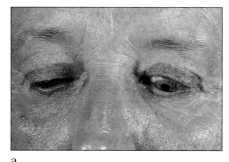

a                                              b

**Figure 21.2**
Patient following excessive left upper skin excision with worsening of brow ptosis.

**Figure 21.3**
(a) Patient demonstrating severe lag on downgaze. (b) Same patient demonstrating lagophthalmos on attempted passive eyelid closure.

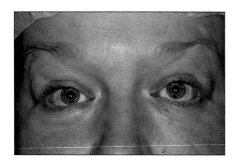

**Figure 21.4**
Patient with bilateral lateral upper eyelid 'fullness' due to spontaneous lacrimal gland prolapse.

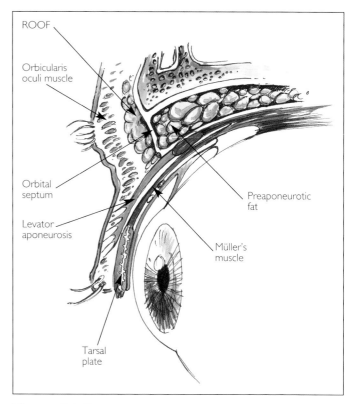

**Figure 21.5**
Diagram illustrating position of preaponeurotic fat.

the upper eyelid (see Figure 21.5). This may give rise to the appearance of upper eyelid 'fullness'. Some patients have a very prominent superolateral bony margin that can also contribute to upper eyelid 'fullness'. This can be reduced with the use of a burr at surgery for an upper eyelid blepharoplasty. Subcutaneous thickening of this area in the dysthyroid patient must be recognized. This may not be amenable to improvement by standard blepharoplasty surgery.

It is important to recognize a prolapsed lacrimal gland that may be responsible for lateral upper eyelid 'fullness' (Figure 21.4).

Some patients develop orbital fat atrophy creating an upper eyelid sulcus defect. Removal of orbital fat in such patients should be avoided to prevent a postoperative 'cadaveric' appearance.

'Fullness' in the medial aspect of the upper eyelid may be caused by a medial eyebrow ptosis. Elevation of the brow or the use of botulinum toxin is more successful at addressing this problem. Incisions in this area can leave unsatisfactory scarring. It is important to avoid the temptation to 'chase a dog ear' into this area during upper eyelid blepharoplasty surgery.

The upper eyelid skin crease represents the most superior point of attachment between the skin and the levator aponeurosis. This position is just inferior to the insertion of the orbital septum onto the levator aponeurosis. The skin crease lies at a higher level in females, approximately 7–8 mm from the lash line, compared with 5–6 mm in males. It is important not to raise the skin crease in males to avoid a feminization of the eyelid appearance.

The skin crease shows racial differences. In the Oriental eyelid the orbital septum attaches to the levator aponeurosis at a lower

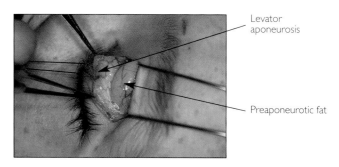

**Figure 21.6**
Intraoperative photograph demonstrating levator aponeurosis lying immediately beneath the preaponeurotic fat.

level, allowing the preaponeurotic fat to descend into the lower reaches of the eyelid, preventing the levator aponeurosis from forming a high skin crease.

Beneath the skin lies the very vascular orbicularis muscle. Local anaesthetic injections should be placed immediately beneath the skin, avoiding the orbicularis muscle, which prevents the occurrence of a haematoma. Deep to the orbicularis muscle above the skin crease lies the orbital septum. This originates from the arcus marginalis along the superior orbital margin. This firm attachment can be utilized to differentiate it from the levator aponeurosis. The orbital septum is a multi-layered structure with a variable thickness. Its multi-layered structure is readily apparent when it is dissected with a Colorado needle.

Posterior to the septum lies the preaponeurotic orbital fat. Pressure applied to the lower eyelid can force the fat to prolapse, which helps to differentiate this from descended retro-orbicularis fat and from fatty infiltration of the levator and/or Müller's muscle. The preaponeurotic fat is a key landmark in upper eyelid surgery. The levator aponeurosis lie immediately beneath it (Figures 21.5 and 21.6).

There are two main fat pads in the upper eyelid: a central pad and a nasal pad. The nasal fat pad generally paler. It is extremely important to be able to distinguish the lacrimal gland from the orbital fat.

The levator muscle gives rise to the levator aponeurosis at the level of Whitnall's ligament. The aponeurosis inserts onto the anterior surface of the superior two-thirds of the tarsus. The medial and lateral horns of the aponeurosis insert in the region of the medial and lateral canthal tendons. The lateral horn divides the lacrimal gland into orbital and palpebral lobes. Intraoperative damage to the medial horn can give rise to a lateral shift of the tarsus with an eyelid peak lying lateral to the pupil.

Whitnall's ligament supports the levator muscle complex and should not be disturbed during surgery. It is a variably developed structure that runs from the lacrimal gland to the region of the trochlea (Figure 21.7).

## *Lower eyelid*

The lower eyelid can be considered to consist of three lamellae:

- Anterior – skin and orbicularis oculi muscle
- Middle – orbital septum and inferior eyelid retractors
- Posterior – tarsus and conjunctiva

The orbital septum extends from the arcus marginalis of the inferior orbital margin to the inferior border of the tarsus (Figure 21.8). The tarsus in the lower eyelid is approximately 4–5 mm in height.

The lower eyelid retractors are analogous to the levator aponeurosis in the upper eyelid. The inferior tarsal muscle is analogous to Müller's muscle in the upper eyelid. The lower eyelid retractors, collectively referred to as the capsulopalpebral fascia, run from the inferior rectus muscle and split to envelop the inferior oblique muscle. This then inserts into the inferior border of the tarsus (Figures 21.8 and 21.9).

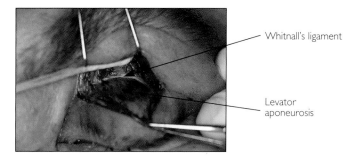

**Figure 21.7**
Whitnall's ligament.

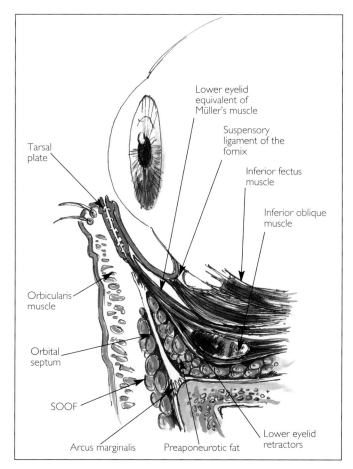

**Figure 21.8**
Diagram illustrating the anatomy of the lower eyelid region.

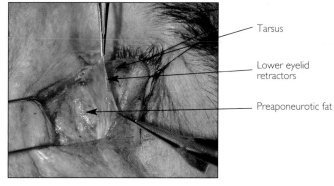

**Figure 21.9**
The lower eyelid retractors,

Isolated shortening of the anterior lamella of the lower eyelid results in ectropion, of the middle lamella results in eyelid retraction with scleral show (Figure 21.10), and of the posterior lamella results in entropion.

The lower eyelid skin crease is variable but usually situated approximately 4–5 mm below the eyelid margin. The lateral canthal angle normally sits approximately 1.5 mm higher than the medial canthal angle.

There are three fat pads in the lower eyelid: medial, central and lateral. These lie between the capsulopalpebral fascia and the orbital septum. The inferior oblique muscle lies between the medial and central fat pads (Figure 21.11).

Fat extends below the inferior orbital margin posterior to the orbicularis oculi muscle and just anterior to the periosteum as the suborbicularis oculi fat (SOOF). With increasing age, the orbicularis oculi muscle and the SOOF move inferiorly, leading to a double convexity of the lower eyelid. The superior convexity is caused by a herniation of orbital fat through a weakened orbital septum above the inferior orbital margin. The orbital margin itself is responsible for the horizontal concavity and the SOOF, which has moved inferiorly, is responsible for the second convexity.

The orbitomalar ligament connects the skin over the inferior orbital margin to the periosteum of the inferior orbital margin, creating the malar fold.

# Upper eyelid blepharoplasty

The goals of an upper eyelid blepharoplasty are:

1. To remove an appropriate amount of excess upper eyelid skin and muscle
2. To remove herniated orbital fat where appropriate
3. To create a symmetrical upper lid skin crease at an appropriate height
4. To avoid visible scarring
5. To avoid a secondary lagophthalmos

An additional goal in the Oriental patient is to create a visible upper eyelid crease, a so-called Westernization procedure.

## *Preoperative patient evaluation*

### History

A careful history should be obtained, as outlined in Chapter 22 on eyebrow ptosis. The patient's complaints, goals and expectations should be determined. The patient may be concerned about:

- An overhang of excess upper eyelid skin causing functional problems
- Excess upper lid skin causing cosmetic problems
- Upper lid fat herniation
- Upper lid 'fullness'

### Examination

The patient should undergo a complete ophthalmic examination. The patient's best corrected visual acuity should be recorded. The palpebral fissures should be measured and the position of the skin crease noted. Any asymmetries should be noted. Any frontalis overaction should be noted and the position and shape of the brows noted after preventing frontalis overaction. *The secondary effects of brow ptosis on the upper eyelids must be recognized* (Figure 21.12).

An assessment of tear production and the tear film should be documented. The degree of eyelid laxity is assessed. Any herniation of orbital fat is noted. The degree of excess upper eyelid skin is assessed. The skin quality and degree of actinic damage is assessed.

Any proptosis or pseudoproptosis due to a large globe is noted. It may be more difficult to achieve the surgical goals in

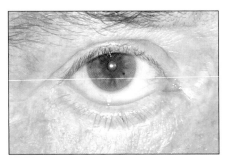

**Figure 21.10**
Middle lamellar scarring following lower eyelid blepharoplasty, resulting in lower eyelid retraction.

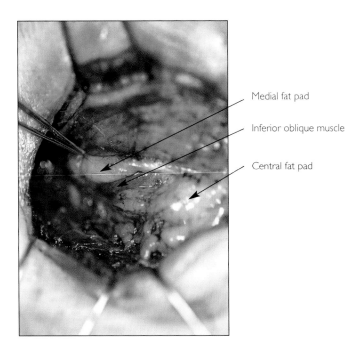

Medial fat pad

Inferior oblique muscle

Central fat pad

**Figure 21.11**
The inferior oblique muscle lying between the medial and central fat pads.

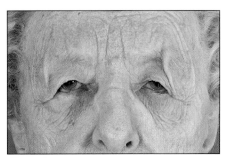

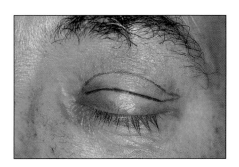

**Figure 21.12**
Marked bilateral brow ptosis,
dermatochalasis and
pseudoblepharoptosis.

**Figure 21.13**
The desired position of the upper
eyelid skin crease has been marked
with a cocktail stick dipped into a
gentian marker block. The skin above
the crease has been gently pinched
while asking the patient to passively
close the eye. The markings are not
taken medially beyond the limit of the
skin crease. Laterally, a small 'wing'
has been added to prevent a 'dog
ear'. A distance of at least 10 mm has
been left between the inferior aspect
of the brow and the superior aspect
of the blepharoplasty.

such a patient. *The patient should be examined specifically to exclude the possibility of thyroid eye disease.*

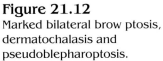

Preoperative photographs must be taken

# Surgical technique

Marking the upper eyelid skin crease

This is the first very important step in a successful upper eyelid blepharoplasty. The upper eyelid skin is defatted with an alcohol wipe and the skin crease marked with a cocktail stick impregnated with gentian violet solution. A calliper should be used to measure the height of the crease. The fellow eyelid should be marked simultaneously, ensuring precise symmetry. The skin crease should be marked at a lower level in a male patient.

The skin above the crease centrally is gently pinched with a pair of fine-toothed forceps. Great care should be taken to ensure that the eyelids can close passively. Any temptation to remove more than 10 mm of skin should be resisted, particularly in the presence of uncorrected brow ptosis. The superior aspect of the pinched skin is marked and an ellipse is marked. The relative dimensions of this area divided into thirds should be remembered to maintain a good aesthetic appearance. In general, at least 10–12 mm of skin should be left between the inferior aspect of the eyebrow and the skin crease. (Figure 21.13). *It is important not to carry the incision markings into the medial canthal area to avoid webbed scars.*

If there is no temporal hooding of skin, the lateral aspect of the incision should be kept within the orbital margin. If there is temporal hooding, a lateral wing can be added to the crescent, leaving the resulting scar running in a superolateral direction Figure 21.13.

# Anaesthesia

The procedure may be undertaken under either general or local anaesthesia. Local anaesthesia is advantageous as it allows voluntary levator muscle function to be used to assist in the identification of eyelid structures. This is particularly important when an upper eyelid blepharoplasty is being performed in conjunction with a levator aponeurosis advancement procedure.

Approximately 3 ml of 0.5% Marcain (bupivacaine) with 1:200,000 units of adrenaline is injected with a single injection just beneath the skin. The needle is inserted temporally and advanced nasally while slowly injecting the solution: 10 min is allowed for the adrenaline to take effect.

# Surgical procedure

A 4/0 silk traction suture is inserted along the grey line and placed on traction. The skin incisions are made along the markings with a Colorado needle. The incision is deepened through the orbicularis muscle to the plane of the orbital septum. A myocutaneous flap is developed and dissected off the orbital septum. If the patient merely requires the removal of excess skin and orbicularis muscle for functional reasons, the skin can be closed with a simple continuous 7/0 Vicryl suture. A lateral wing is closed with simple interrupted 7/0 Vicryl sutures. This surgical procedure is very quick and simple to perform and does not expose the patient to the small risks of postoperative intraorbital haemorrhage.

If the patient requires the removal or redraping of orbital fat, the orbital septum is opened along its entire length. The fat is allowed to prolapse. This can be sculpted with the Colorado needle and any larger vessels cauterized with bipolar cautery. Great care should be taken if the fat is clamped with a curved artery clip to avoid anterior traction that can lead to the rupture of posterior orbital vessels.

The type of skin closure is determined by the type of skin crease that is required. If this is to be a soft less well-defined crease the skin can be closed as above. If a higher well-defined crease is required, usually in a female, the skin is closed with interrupted 7/0 Vicryl sutures that incorporate a bite of the underlying levator aponeurosis. It is sometimes advantageous to remove a strip of orbicularis muscle from the inferior skin wound edge but this can lead to bleeding, particularly if the effects of the adrenaline have begun to wear off.

# Lower eyelid blepharoplasty

The goals of a lower eyelid blepharoplasty are:

1. To remove an appropriate amount of excess lower eyelid skin and muscle
2. To remove herniated orbital fat where appropriate
3. To avoid middle lamellar scarring and eyelid retraction
4. To address any associated lower eyelid laxity
5. To avoid any postoperative ectropion and secondary epiphora

# Preoperative patient evaluation

## History

A careful history should be obtained, as outlined in Chapter 22 on eyebrow ptosis. The patient's complaints, goals and expectations should be determined. The patient may be concerned about:

- Skin redundancy
- Lower lid fat herniation
- Wrinkles

## Examination

As for an upper eyelid blepharoplasty, the patient should undergo a complete ophthalmic examination. The patient's best-corrected visual acuity should be recorded. The palpebral fissures should be measured and the position of the lower eyelid with respect to the inferior limbus noted. Any asymmetries should be noted. The patient's lower lid appearance at rest and smiling should be compared.

An assessment of tear production and the tear film should be documented. The degree of lower eyelid laxity is assessed. Any herniation of orbital fat is noted. The skin quality and degree of actinic damage is assessed.

The degree of lower eyelid laxity is assessed. This can be quite subjective but, as a general rule, if the lower eyelid can be distracted from the globe by more that 6–8 mm or if the eyelid does not return to its position after release without a blink, the eyelid can be considered to have sufficient laxity to warrant a lower eyelid tightening procedure.

Any proptosis or pseudoproptosis due to a large globe is noted. It may be more difficult to achieve the surgical goals in such patient. *The patient should be examined specifically to exclude the possibility of thyroid eye disease.*

Preoperative photographs must be taken

# Surgical approaches

A blepharoplasty procedure should ideally be tailored to the individual requirements of a patient. The surgical approach selected depends on a preoperative assessment of fat herniation, the presence of a lower lid double convexity, the amount of excess lower eyelid skin, the degree of static wrinkling and actinic damage and the degree of lower eyelid laxity. The procedure may be performed in conjunction with another surgical procedure, e.g. an orbital decompression procedure in thyroid eye disease.

There are two main surgical approaches:

- Transcutaneous lower lid blepharoplasty
- Transconjunctival lower lid blepharoplasty

These procedures can be supplemented by other techniques to enhance the result:

1. Horizontal eyelid tightening procedure
2. Pinch technique skin resection
3. $CO_2$ laser resurfacing
4. Botulinum toxin injections
5. SOOF lifting

Patients with fat herniation and significant excess skin are candidates for a traditional transconjunctival blepharoplasty. A transconjunctival approach is preferred for patients with fat herniation but no significant skin excess. This approach avoids an external scar and is also ideal for patients who have previously undergone a transconjunctival blepharoplasty but who require revision surgery for residual fat herniation. It can be combined with $CO_2$ laser resurfacing to deal with skin wrinkling in those patients who are prepared to cooperate with the more onerous postoperative care. Patients with a lower eyelid double convexity should be managed by the technique of fat redraping over the inferior orbital margin after opening of the orbital septum at its junction with the arcus marginalis.

# Surgical technique

Lower eyelid blepharoplasty can be performed under local or general anaesthesia. Local anaesthesia affords the surgeon the opportunity of asking the patient to look up and to open the mouth to avoid excessive skin resection during a transcutaneous blepharoplasty. The patient should be draped using non-adhesive drapes to allow free movement of the lower eyelid and cheek.

## Transcutaneous blepharoplasty

Approximately 3 ml of 0.5% Marcain with 1:200,000 units of adrenaline is injected with a single injection just beneath the skin. The needle is inserted temporally and advanced nasally while slowly injecting the solution: 10 min is allowed for the adrenaline to take effect.

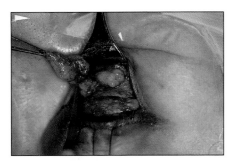

**Figure 21.14**
Lower lid fat being removed with a
Colorado needle during a
transcutaneous lower eyelid
blepharoplasty. The photograph
demonstrates the surgeon's view
while seated at the head of the
operating table.

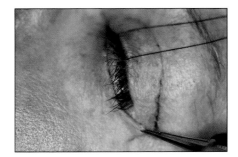

**Figure 21.15**
An upper eyelid blepharoplasty has
been completed and the wound
closed with interrupted 7/0 Vicryl
sutures. A lower eyelid skin–muscle
resection has been performed after
asking the patient to look up and to
open the mouth. The skin–muscle flap
is being drawn laterally to determine
the degree of lateral 'dog-ear'
resection required. It is important to
avoid drawing the skin–muscle flap up
to vigorously or a rounded defect will
occur as well as an over-resection.

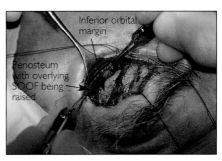

**Figure 21.16**
A subperiosteal dissection for a SOOF
lift.

A 4/0 silk traction suture is placed through the grey line of the lower eyelid and fixated to the head drape with a curved artery clip. A strictly subciliary incision is made with a Colorado needle commencing just beneath the punctum and extending to the lateral canthus where it is continued within a 'laughter line' for a few millimetres.

A skin–muscle flap is dissected from the underlying orbital septum. The orbital septum is then opened horizontally along its whole length. Gentle pressure on the globe allows the orbital fat to prolapse. The fat is then very carefully excised with strict attention to meticulous haemostasis (Figure 21.14). Excessive use of cautery, however, should be avoided to prevent postoperative middle lamellar scarring and eyelid retraction.

No undue traction should be exerted on the fat. The fat removal is commenced on the lateral fat pad, moving to the central and then to the nasal fat pads. The residual fat should be left flush with the orbital margin to prevent over-resection which can lead to hollowing and a 'cadaveric' look.

The skin–muscle flap is then draped over the lower eyelid margin while at the same time asking the patient to look up and to open the mouth. The amount of excess skin is carefully determined. Great care should be taken to avoid over-resection of skin and orbicularis. This is crucial to avoid lower eyelid retraction and rounding of the lateral canthus with scleral show (Figure 21.15). The skin is closed with a continuous 7/0 Vicryl suture. If the patient has a prominent orbicularis muscle, a small strip can be removed prior to skin closure.

In the presence of mild malar festoons the skin–muscle flap dissection is extended beyond the inferior orbital margin. To support the flap after resection of the skin and orbicularis excess, a nonabsorbable suture is used to suspend the lateral orbicularis to the periosteum of the lateral orbital rim. In the presence of a more marked malar festoon, a SOOF lift is performed. The SOOF is mobilized, taking care to avoid damage to the infraorbital nerve. A small lift can be performed via a preperiosteal dissection whereas a more extensive lift requires a subperiosteal dissection (Figure 21.16). The SOOF is then sutured to the arcus marginalis with nonabsorbable sutures or fixated to the orbital margin using Prolene sutures passed though drill holes.

If there is a significant degree of eyelid laxity present preoperatively, a lower eyelid tightening procedure is required to address this. Mild laxity can be managed with a 5/0 Vicryl suture placed through the inferior limb of the lateral canthal tendon and passed through the periosteum of the lateral orbital rim (Figure 21.17). Greater degrees of laxity require a formal lateral tarsal strip procedure.

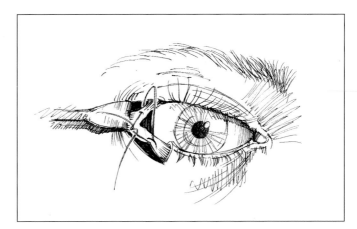

**Figure 21.17**
Lateral canthal tightening suture.

# Transconjunctival blepharoplasty

Approximately 3 ml of 0.5% Marcain with 1:200,000 units of adrenaline is injected into each fat pad via the conjunctiva medially, laterally and centrally: 10 min is allowed for the adrenaline to take effect.

A corneal protector is placed. A 4/0 silk traction suture is placed through the grey line of the lower eyelid that is then everted over a Desmarres retractor. A conjunctival incision is made with a Colorado needle 3 mm below the inferior border of the tarsus from the level of the punctum to the lateral canthus. The incision is deepened through the lower eyelid retractors. The Desmarres retractor is then placed into the inferior fornix and 4/0 silk traction sutures are placed through the conjunctiva and lower eyelid retractors. These sutures are fixated to the head drape with a curved artery clip to protect the cornea.

Pressure applied to the globe allows the orbital fat pads to herniate into the wound. The fat is removed as described above (Figure 21.18). The Desmarres retractor is removed and the eyelids inspected to ensure adequacy of fat removal and symmetry. The conjunctival edges along with the eyelid retractors are sutured together with interrupted 8/0 Vicryl sutures.

# Postoperative care

Postoperative care is similar for both upper and lower eyelid blepharoplasties. If the surgery has been performed under general anaesthesia it is wise to apply a compressive dressing for 30 min until the patient has recovered. This prevents oozing into the eyelids when the patient performs a Valsalva manoeuvre following extubation. The dressings are then removed and ice packs applied intermittently.

It is preferable to keep the patient in hospital overnight, which restricts the patient's activity and allows monitoring for pain, proptosis, bleeding and visual deterioration. A postoperative orbital haemorrhage is a potentially blinding complication. There is insufficient time available to perform the emergency surgery required to manage this complication if the patient has been discharged home.

The patient should be given careful instructions about wound care. Following a lower eyelid transcutaneous blepharoplasty, lower eyelid massage may be commenced within 48 hours to prevent wound contracture and to reduce postoperative oedema. Following an upper eyelid blepharoplasty, the patient should be instructed to use topical lubricant drops for 4–6 weeks postoperatively, as the reflex blink will be temporarily impaired. Skin sutures may be removed after 2 weeks.

# Complications of blepharoplasty surgery

A number of complications can occur following blepharoplasty surgery. Fortunately, serious complications are rare:

1. Blindness
2. Lower eyelid retraction
3. Rounding of the lateral canthus
4. Lower eyelid ectropion
5. Hollowing of the eyelids
6. Epiphora
7. Lagophthalmos
8. Asymmetrical upper lid creases
9. Diplopia
10. Ptosis
11. Chemosis

Many of these complications can be avoided by careful preoperative patient evaluation and selection of the most appropriate surgical procedure for the patient as outlined above (Figure 21.19).

Rounding of the lateral canthus occurs following the resection of skin and orbicularis muscle as a triangle laterally. This should be avoided. Mild lower eyelid retraction may be managed conservatively with postoperative eyelid massage. A SOOF lift combined with a lateral canthal resuspension may prevent the need for a

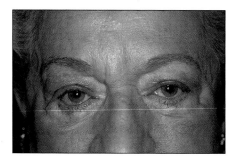

**Figure 21.19**
A dissatisfied patient referred following a bilateral lower eyelid blepharoplasty. She has bilateral epiphora due to a bilateral cicatricial ectropion following an over-resection of skin and orbicularis muscle. The lower eyelid laxity has not been addressed. The lower eyelids are retracted with inferior scleral 'show'. The lower eyelid herniated fat has been asymmetrically and incompletely removed. There is a hollowing over the inferior orbital rims and marked hollowing over the lateral orbital rims. She has a right lower eyelid 'festoon'.

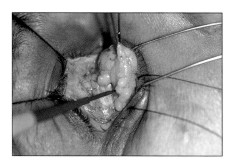

**Figure 21.18**
Transconjunctival fat excision.

By far the most serious complication of blepharoplasty surgery is blindness. This is usually due to the sudden occurrence of a postoperative orbital haemorrhage. Although rare, this is a devastating complication of an operation performed most commonly to improve a patient's cosmetic appearance. The patient should be counselled about such a risk preoperatively. It is important to ensure that all risk factors for bleeding are addressed preoperatively. No patient should undergo blepharoplasty surgery if hypertension is uncontrolled, if there is a history of a bleeding disorder or if the patient is taking antiplatelet drugs. The patient must be given postoperative instructions about restrictions on activity following surgery. The patient must be able to return to hospital immediately in the event of any sudden orbital pain, proptosis or decrease in vision.

If a patient develops a sudden orbital haemorrhage with proptosis, subconjunctival haemorrhage and decreased visual acuity, the wound must be opened immediately to drain the haematoma and a lateral canthotomy and cantholysis should be performed. Intravenous acetazolamide should also be given and, if necessary, intravenous mannitol.

skin graft following an over-resection of skin. Middle lamellar contracture may, however, require division of the scar tissue and placement of a hard palate graft. A frank ectropion occurs when significant lower eyelid laxity has not been addressed. This will usually require a lateral canthal tightening procedure, combined with a skin graft.

Hollowing of the eyelids occurs if too much orbital fat is removed, particularly in older patients with very thin eyelid skin. In the lower eyelids, care should be taken to resect the fat flush with the inferior orbital margin and to avoid pulling the fat anteriorly.

Epiphora following blepharoplasty surgery may occur as a consequence of lagophthalmos and/or a malposition of the inferior puncta. A subtle vertical positioning of the inferior punctum may result in epiphora. This may occur some years after surgery, as the lower eyelid tarsoligamentous support becomes more lax.

Lagophthalmos following an upper eyelid blepharoplasty is avoided by ensuring a conservative skin resection in the upper eyelids. Overzealous resection may require a skin graft if exposure symptoms do not respond to conservative treatment.

The appearance of the upper eyelid skin creases has a profound effect on the cosmetic outcome of an upper eyelid blepharoplasty. The skin crease should be higher in a female and well defined, in contrast to a male in which this should be lower and more subtle. Complications are avoided by meticulous preoperative planning and marking. Postoperatively, it is easier to raise a skin crease that is unsatisfactory than it is to lower it.

Diplopia is a rare complication following lower eyelid blepharoplasty, and is usually due to surgical trauma to the inferior oblique muscle. A good knowledge of anatomy, a meticulous surgical resection of orbital fat and the avoidance of excessive use of cautery should prevent such a complication.

Ptosis may occur if the levator muscle, the horns of the levator muscle complex or Whitnall's ligament are damaged during surgery: these tissues should be carefully identified and avoided. Any pre-existing ptosis should be addressed at the time of an upper eyelid blepharoplasty.

Chemosis, which is more commonly seen following a transconjunctival blepharoplasty, usually resolves after 10–14 days following the liberal use of topical antibiotics. On rare occasions, it lasts for some months postoperatively.

# Further reading

1.  Aiache AE, Ramirez OH. The suborbicularis oculi fat pads: an anatomic and clinical study. *Plast Reconstr Surg* (1995) **95**:37–42.

2.  American Academy of Ophthalmology. *Basic and clinical science course: orbit, eyelids and lacrimal system*, section 7. San Francisco: American Academy of Ophthalmology, 1998–99, pp. 13–28, 119–28, 199–206.

3.  Dutton JJ. *Atlas of clinical and surgical orbital anatomy*. Philadelphia: WB Saunders, 1994.

4.  Aiache AE, Ramirez OH. The suborbicularis oculi fat pads: an anatomic and clinical study. *Plast Reconstr Surg* (1955) **95**:37–42.

5.  May JW, Fearon J, Zingarelli P. Retro-orbicularis oculi fat (ROOF) resection in aesthetic blepharoplasty: 6 year study in 63 patients. *Plast Reconstr Surg* (1990) **86**:682–9.

6.  Kikkawa DO, Lemke BN, Dortzbach RK. Relations of the superficial musculoaponeurotic system to the orbit and characterization of the orbitomalar ligament. *Ophthal Plast Reconstr Surg* (1996) **12**:77–88.

7.  Hoenig JA, Shorr N, Shorr J. The suborbicularis oculi fat in aesthetic and reconstructive surgery. *Int Ophthal Clin* (1997) **37**:179–91.

8.  Hanira ST. Arcus marginalis release and orbital fat preservation in midface rejuvenation. *Plast Reconstr Surg* (1995) **96**:354–62.

9.  Baylis HI, Long JA, Groth MJ. Transconjunctival lower eyelid blepharoplasty: technique and complications. *Ophthalmology* (1989) **96**:1027–32.

# 22

# Eyebrow ptosis

## Introduction

The position of the eyebrows affects facial expression and influences the way in which a patient's mood and personality are judged by others. There are a variety of eyebrow shapes. In general the female brow has a higher arch than a male's, which tends to be flatter (Figure 22.1). The brow position becomes lower with age from the effects of both gravity and the depressors of the brow (the corrugator supercilii, depressor supercilii, procerus and orbicularis oculi muscles) (Figure 22.2).

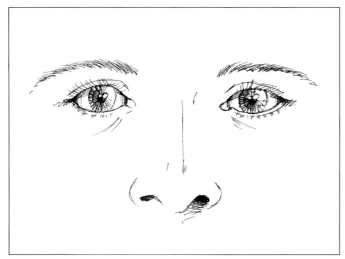

a

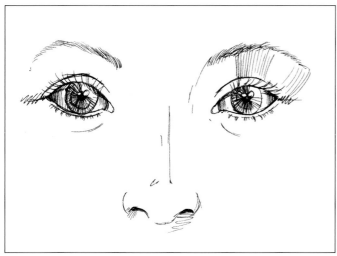

b

**Figure 22.1**
(a) Typical male brow. (b) Typical female brow.

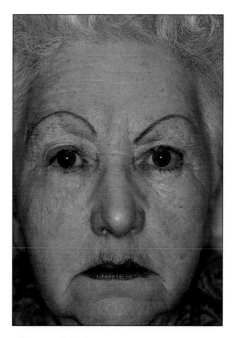

**Figure 22.2**
Female patient with bilateral brow ptosis who has undergone a reconstruction of a right lateral lower eyelid Mohs' surgery defect. She has a bilateral brow ptosis that she has camouflaged by shaving the eyebrows and drawing in herself the desired position of her brows.

Patients often attempt to raise the brows by using the frontalis muscle that leads to deep forehead furrows. This action eventually becomes involuntary. Brow ptosis creates a redundancy in the upper eyelids and medial and lateral canthi. This can lead to the appearance of upper eyelid dermatochalasis, hooding of the eyelids temporally and skin redundancy medially. It is important to recognize brow ptosis and to determine the most appropriate management. This may also include accepting the brow ptosis but modifying an upper eyelid blepharoplasty to prevent the brow from being drawn down more to meet the upper eyelid incision. This can lead to a very unsatisfactory postoperative appearance.

# Applied anatomy

## Eyebrow

The position of the eyebrows is influenced by five muscle groups (Figure 22.3):

- Elevator: the occipitofrontalis muscle
- Depressors: the corrugator supercilii, procerus, depressor supercilii and the orbicularis oculi muscles.

The occipital and frontal muscle bellies are connected via the galea aponeurotica. The occipital muscle arises from the nuchal line of the occipital bone. The frontalis muscle originates from the galea aponeurotica in the region of the coronal suture and inserts into the subcutaneous tissue of the brow, where it interdigitates

with the orbicularis oculi and corrugator supercilii muscles. *The frontalis muscle is innervated by the frontal branch of the facial nerve.* Contraction of the muscle raises the brow and causes horizontal furrows in the forehead.

The corrugator supercilii muscle arises from the nasal process of the frontal bone. The muscle passes superolaterally to insert into the medial one-third of the eyebrow. The muscle is innervated by the frontal branch of the facial nerve. Contraction of the muscle draws the brows medially and inferiorly, creating vertical folds in the glabellar region. The depressor supercilii muscle is less well defined, lying just lateral to the corrugator supercilii.

The procerus muscle originates from the lateral aspect of the nasal bone and inserts into the medial aspect of the brow. It is innervated by the zygomatic branch of the facial nerve. Contraction of the muscle draws the brows inferiorly, creating horizontal folds in the glabellar region.

The orbicularis oculi muscle is arbitrarily divided into three parts:

- Pretarsal
- Preseptal
- Orbital

The orbital part is primarily responsible for voluntary forced closure of the eyelids and depression of the brow. This part of the muscle arises from the frontal process of the maxilla and orbital process of the frontal bone. Its concentric fibres are closed linked with the insertion of the frontalis muscle. The superior part of the muscle is innervated by the frontal branch of the facial nerve, whereas the inferior part is innervated by the zygomatic branch.

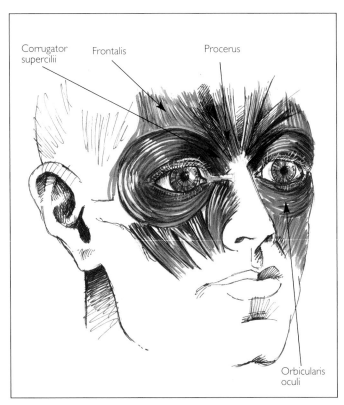

**Figure 22.3**
The muscle groups influencing the position of the eyebrows.

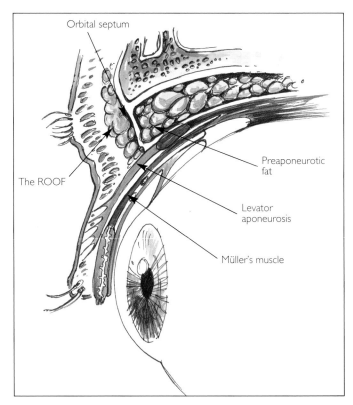

**Figure 22.4**
Diagram demonstrating position of the retro-orbicularis oculi fat (ROOF) pad.

A fat pad lies posterior to the orbicularis muscle and the inferior aspect of the frontalis muscle. This is referred to as the retro-orbicularis oculi fat (ROOF) pad (Figure 22.4). With age, this fat pad can descend into the preseptal plane of the upper eyelid. The posterior boundary of the fat pad continues into the eyelid as the orbital septum.

The muscles of the eyebrow are maintained in contact with the underlying periosteum by a firm attachment on the posterior aspect of the fat pad. The fat lying anterior to these periosteal attachments allows vertical movement of the overlying skin and muscle. These attachments are weaker laterally, giving rise to a greater degree of temporal brow ptosis with age.

> To avoid injury to the facial nerve in the temple region, dissection should be made along the deep temporal fascia

## Scalp

The central scalp consists of five layers:

- Skin
- Subcutaneous fibrofatty tissue
- Galea aponeurotica
- Loose areolar tissue
- Pericranium

## Temple

The temple consists of the following layers:

- Skin
- Subcutaneous tissue
- Temporalis muscle

The temporalis muscle is covered by a number of layers of fascia:

- The superficial temporal fascia
- The subgaleal fascia
- The deep temporal fascia

The superficial temporal fascia is continuous with the galea aponeurotica. It contains the frontal branch of the facial nerve and the superficial temporal artery (Figure 22.5). A loose areolar layer, the subgaleal fascia, separates the superficial temporal fascia from the deep temporal fascia. The deep temporal fascia is easily recognized by its thick white glistening surface.

A few centimetres above the zygomatic arch the deep temporal fascia splits into two layers: the intermediate temporal fascia and the deep layer of the deep temporal fascia. These insert onto the anterosuperior and posterosuperior aspects of the zygomatic arch, respectively. Between these two layers lies a fat pad (Yasargil's fat pad) (Figures 22.5 and 22.6).

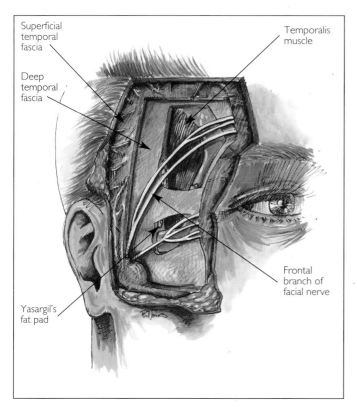

**Figure 22.5**
Diagram demonstrating the relationships of the various layers of fascia in the temple in relation to the course of the frontal and zygomatic branches of the facial nerve.

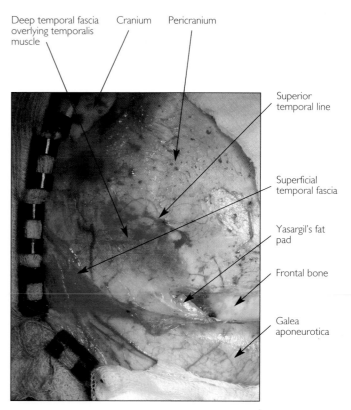

**Figure 22.6**
Intraoperative photograph during bicoronal flap dissection demonstrating layers of fascia in the right temple.

## *Facial nerve*

> A detailed knowledge of the anatomy of the facial nerve is essential for the surgeon operating in this region

The facial nerve exits the stylomastoid foramen and enters the parotid gland. It divides in a variable pattern into distal branches. Three to five branches cross the zygomatic arch. The most posterior branch is always anterior to the superficial temporal vessels. The anterior hairline at the level of the lateral canthus represents the junction of the posterior and middle branches of the nerve. The most anterior branch crosses the zygomatic arch approximately 2 cm posterior to the posterior aspect of the lateral orbital margin. In the temple the nerve runs in the superficial temporal fascia. In the brow region the frontal branch runs approximately 2 cm above the brow. The nerve is most vulnerable to injury over the zygomatic arch (Figure 22.7).

# Preoperative patient evaluation

## *History*

The patient's complaints should be carefully noted. The patient may complain of drooping eyelids, a loss of the superior visual field, headaches, ocular discomfort, or a tired appearance commented on by friends or relatives.

The complaint of droopy upper eyelids may simply be due to severe dermatochalasis causing a pseudoptosis with the underlying eyelid height being normal. The lid position should be carefully evaluated, however, as a true ptosis may also be present. Similarly, a severe dermatochalasis, often combined with a brow ptosis, may obstruct the patient's superior visual field.

Patients who have a moderate to severe brow ptosis and dermatochalasis are obliged to use their frontalis muscle to overcome the superior visual field defect. Such patients commonly develop deep forehead furrows (Figure 22.8). This leads to fatigue of the frontalis muscle, which in turn can cause a headache.

Occasionally, upper eyelid dermatochalasis and lateral brow ptosis can lead to a secondary mechanical misdirection of eyelashes, causing chronic discomfort.

The cosmetic effects of upper eyelid dermatochalasis and brow ptosis can lead to complaints of a tired appearance. Lower eyelid fat herniation can also lead to complaints of a tired appearance.

Patients should be specifically questioned about previous eyelid surgery. Patients who have previously undergone a cosmetic blepharoplasty or a facelift may omit such information, particularly if accompanied by a new partner. A history of contact lens wear, dry eye, facial palsy or thyroid dysfunction identifies a patient at risk of exposure keratopathy symptoms following an upper lid blepharoplasty. It is important to exclude a bleeding disorder, as a postoperative haemorrhage following a blepharoplasty is potentially sight-threatening. Allergies should be excluded. The use of aspirin or nonsteroidal anti-inflammatory agents (NSAIAs) should be discontinued.

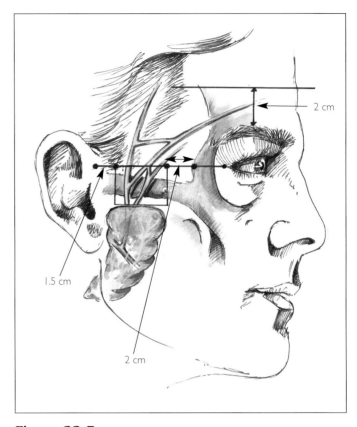

**Figure 22.7**
Diagram demonstrating course of the frontal branch of the facial nerve. The nerve is most vulnerable to injury as it crosses the zygomatic arch, where it lies just beneath the subcutaneous fat.

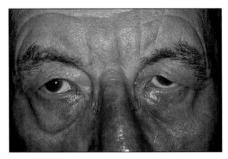

**Figure 22.8**
Bilateral brow ptosis, upper eyelid dermatochalasis and lower eyelid fat herniation. This patient complained of visual field limitation and headache towards the evening.

## *Examination*

The patient should undergo a complete ophthalmic examination. The patient's best-corrected visual acuity should be recorded. The palpebral fissures should be measured and the position of the skin crease noted. Any asymmetries should be noted. Any frontalis overaction should be noted and the position and shape of the brows noted after preventing frontalis overaction. The secondary effects of brow ptosis on the upper eyelids must be recognized.

An assessment of tear production and the tear film should be documented. The degree of eyelid laxity is assessed. Any herniation of orbital fat is noted. The degree of excess upper eyelid skin is assessed. The skin quality and degree of actinic damage is assessed.

## Surgical planning

The options for surgical and non-surgical management should be outlined. Some patients, in particular dysthyroid patients with medial brow ptosis and deep glabellar frown lines, may prefer the use of botulinum toxin instead of surgery. This is highly effective for such patients, whose glabellar furrows can create an aggressive appearance. It has the disadvantage, however, of being expensive and temporary in its effects. It has to be repeated every 3–4 months. The goals, limitations, risks and potential complications of surgery should be fully discussed with the patient. The limitations of upper eyelid blepharoplasty performed alone in the presence of significant brow ptosis should be explained. Under these circumstances an upper eyelid blepharoplasty should be very conservative to prevent further lowering of the brow and an unsatisfactory appearance. Patients should be carefully questioned to ascertain their expectations of surgery.

## Surgical procedures for the management of brow ptosis

The surgical approaches to the management of eyebrow ptosis are:

1. The direct brow lift
2. The 'gull-wing' direct brow lift
3. The mid-forehead brow lift
4. The temporal eyebrow lift
5. The transblepharoplasty browpexy
6. The eyebrow suspension procedure
7. The coronal forehead and brow lift
8. The endoscopic brow lift

## The direct brow lift

The direct brow lift is a simple surgical technique that is suitable for older patients in whom the surgical scar can be hidden within natural creases (Figures 22.9 and 22.10). It can be performed quickly under local anaesthesia and can be combined with an upper lid blepharoplasty.

With the patient in a sitting position, the proposed incision is marked just above the eyebrow. The brow is then mechanically elevated to the desired level and then released. A mark is then made on the forehead at a point that represented the leading edge of the raised brow (Figure 22.11). A slight overcorrection is desirable. An elliptical incision is then drawn out (Figure 22.12).

The shape of the proposed area for excision can be adjusted according to the desired shape of the brow. For a marked temporal brow ptosis, the incision can be modified and kept over the lateral brow only (Figure 22.13).

The marked out area is infiltrated with 0.5% Marcain (bupivacaine) with 1:200,000 units of adrenaline. A perpendicular incision is made with a No. 15 Bard Parker blade down to the level of the frontalis muscle. Great care should be taken medially to avoid any damage to the supraorbital neurovascu-

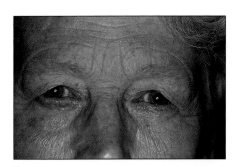
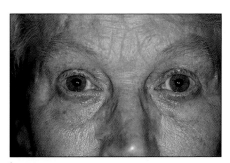

a                    b

**Figure 22.9**
(a) Female patient with bilateral brow ptosis and upper eyelid dermatochalasis. (b) The patient 12 months following bilateral direct brow lift and upper lid blepharoplasty.

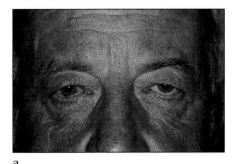
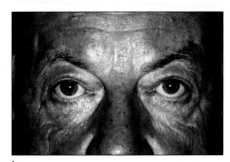

a                    b

**Figure 22.10**
(a) Male patient with bilateral brow ptosis and dermatochalasis. (b) The patient 12 months following a bilateral temporal direct brow lift and conservative upper eyelid blepharoplasties. The skin creases have been set in a low position to avoid 'feminizing' the upper lid appearance. The patient should be warned about the alteration in the shape of the eyelid following this procedure.

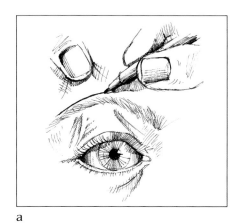
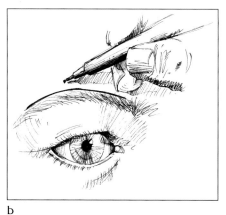

**Figure 22.11**
(a) The brow is lifted to the desired level and released. (b) A mark is made on the forehead at the leading edge of the raised brow position.

a                                      b

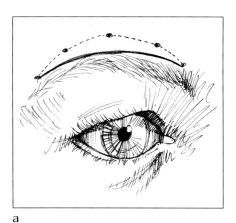
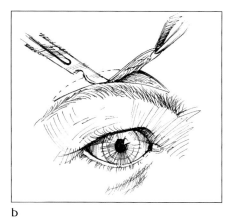

**Figure 22.12**
(a) This is repeated at three points and the marks joined into a continuous ellipse. (b) The skin and subcutaneous tissue are excised with a No. 15 Bard Parker blade A continuous intracuticular suture is used to approximate the skin edges.

a                                      b

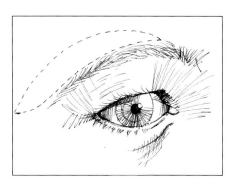
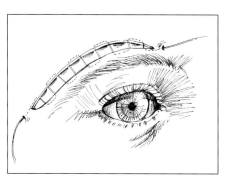

**Figure 22.13**
Temporal direct brow lift.

lar bundle. The ellipse of tissue is excised and the wound is closed with deep buried interrupted subcutaneous 4/0 Vicryl sutures. A running intracuticular 6/0 Novafil suture is used to close the skin. The skin closure is reinforced with sterile adhesive tape.

## The 'gull-wing' direct brow lift

This surgical procedure extends the direct brow lift into the glabellar region in a 'gull-wing' fashion (Figure 22.14). It is suitable for older patients who have a marked brow ptosis that affects the medial aspect of the brows in addition to the lateral aspect.

## The mid-forehead lift

This procedure is infrequently used and reserved for patients with isolated medial brow ptosis with prominent glabellar frown lines who have thin, non-sebaceous type of skin with marked forehead furrows. It allows access to the depressors of the brows, which can be dissected and weakened.

## The temporal eyebrow lift

The temporal lift is used for moderate degrees of temporal brow ptosis. It does not address any medial brow ptosis and is now

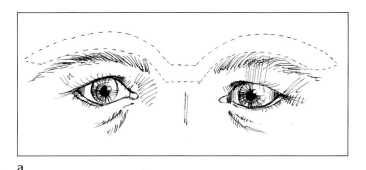

a

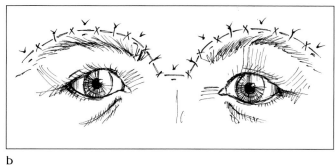

b

**Figure 22.14**
(a) A 'gull-wing' direct brow lift marked out. (b) A 'gull-wing' direct brow lift sutured.

rarely performed alone. It can, however, be used in combination with an endoscopic brow lift. This involves an incision along the standard coronal line down to the level of the deep temporal fascia. Blunt dissection is performed to the level of the lateral orbital margin. It is important to avoid damage to the frontal branch of the facial nerve that lies within the flap. The flap is mobilized and advanced. A full-thickness resection of redundant scalp is performed. The wound is closed with buried interrupted subcutaneous 4/0 Vicryl sutures and the skin is closed with staples.

## The transblepharoplasty browpexy

This procedure does not raise the brows but stabilizes the brows centrally and laterally to prevent descent of the brow following an upper lid blepharoplasty. Once redundant skin and orbicularis muscle have been removed in an upper lid blepharoplasty, the dissection is continued superiorly posterior to the orbicularis muscle to a level 1–2 cm above the superior orbital margin. This dissection is limited to the central and lateral brow to avoid any damage to the supraorbital neurovascular bundle. The brow is then fixated to the frontal periosteum with a nonabsorbable suture passed through the muscular layer of the flap, taking care to avoid any dimpling of the overlying skin.

## The eyebrow suspension procedure

This procedure is suitable for the older patient in whom the visible scarring of a direct or mid-forehead lift is unacceptable. It is relatively quick to perform. The surgical technique is similar to a frontalis suspension procedure for blepharoptosis using a double triangle. Small stab incisions are made just above the brow medially and laterally. Further stab incisions are made just

in front of the hairline medially and just behind the hairline temporally. A 2.0 Gore-Tex suture is used and passed through the subcutaneous tissue above the brow using a Wright's ptosis needle. The ptosis needle is then passed inferiorly from the superior wounds in a plane just above the galea medially and just above the deep temporal fascia laterally. The suture is withdrawn and tied. It is fixated to the adjacent galea and deep temporal fascia with a 5/0 Ethibond suture to prevent migration.

## The coronal forehead and brow lift

The coronal lift is effective in raising the brow medially and laterally. It reduces glabellar furrows and smoothes the forehead. It involves an extensive incision, however, and leaves an area of sensory loss posterior to the incision. Its use is reserved for women in whom the extensive scar is hidden behind the hairline. The incision can, however, be modified into a pretrichial incision for the patient with a high forehead. The coronal lift is now less frequently used with the advent of the minimally invasive endoscopic brow lift.

## The endoscopic brow lift

This procedure accomplishes the same goals as the coronal lift but with small incisions. It is time-consuming and requires special surgical instrumentation.

## 1. Incisions

The incision sites are selected according to the contour of the patient's forehead. If the forehead is particularly curved, the incision sites are moved forward or an additional small mid-forehead incision is added (Figure 22.15). A curved forehead can otherwise lead to difficulty in accessing and visualizing the area of the eyebrow depressors.

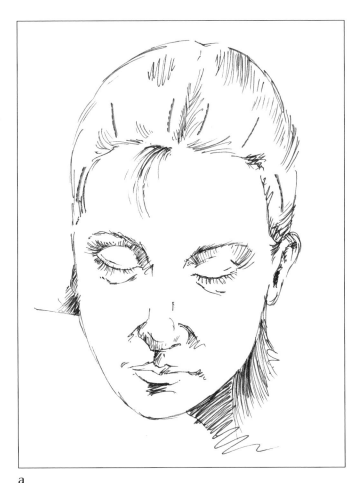

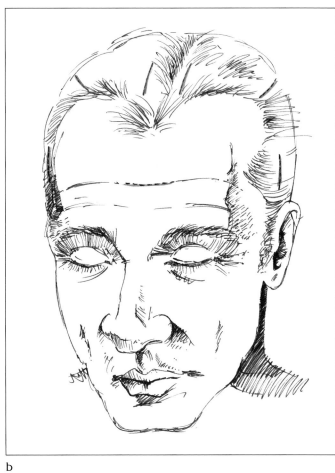

a

b

**Figure 22.15**
(a) Typical incision sites for endoscopic brow lift. (b) Additional mid-forehead incision in a male with a receding hairline.

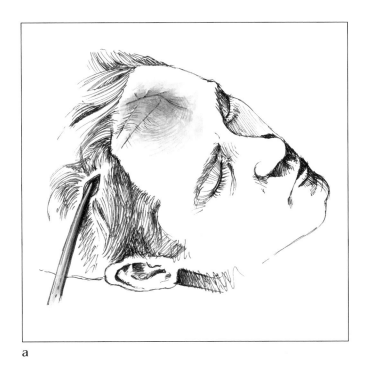

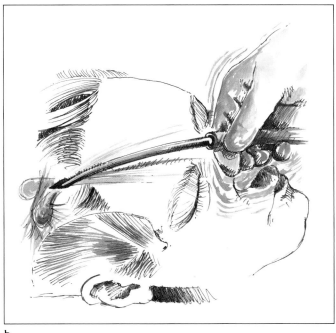

a

b

**Figure 22.16**
(a) 'Blind' subperiosteal dissection over the forehead. (b) 'Blind' subperiosteal dissection to the superior temporal line temporally.

## 2. Anaesthesia

The procedure is performed under general anaesthesia. The proposed incision sites are infiltrated with 0.5% Marcain with 1:200,000 units of adrenaline. A litre solution of lactated Ringer's solution is injected with 50 ml of 1% lignocaine, 1 ml of 1:1000 units of adrenaline and 1000 units of Hyalase (hyaluronidase); 200 ml of this solution is injected throughout the forehead and temple above the zygomatic arch and left for 10 min.

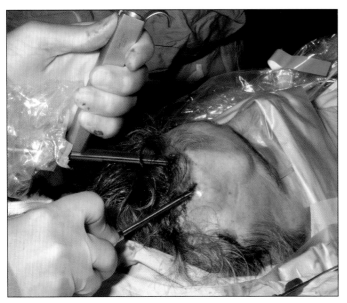

**Figure 22.17**
(a) Endoscopic brow lift. The endoscope has been inserted into a visualization pocket maintainer. The periosteal elevator is being held in the right hand.

## 3. Visualization pocket

The scalp incisions are made with a Colorado needle, which prevents bleeding from the incision sites. The central incisions are carried down to the periosteum. Through these incisions a large periosteal elevator is inserted and used to elevate the periosteum in a blind fashion both anteriorly to 2 cm above the brows, posteriorly to the superior nuchal line and temporally to the superior temporal line (Figure 22.16).

The temporal incisions are carried down to the deep temporal fascia. A pocket is developed anteriorly over the deep temporal fascia by blunt dissection with a Freer elevator. This dissection plane is very important, as the frontal branch of the facial nerve lies above this. Inadvertent damage to this nerve will result in a brow palsy and weakness of the superior orbicularis muscle. The 4 mm 0 degree endoscope, protected by a rigid irrigation sleeve with an attached handle enabling the surgeon to lift the forehead and maintain an optical space, is inserted into the pocket and the dissection plane progressed with a larger dissector (Figure 22.17).

## 4. Dissection of the conjoint fascia

The conjoint fascia is approached from the temporal incision and dissected off the superior temporal line (Figure 22.18). An optical cavity continuous with the subperiosteal dissection in the forehead is now present. The endoscope is now transferred to the central incisions and the subperiosteal dissection continued to the arcus marginalis and root of the nose.

## 5. Release of the periosteum

The periosteum is now carefully incised just above the superior orbital margin with a sharp curved periosteal elevator (Figure 22.19). Great care should be taken to avoid injury to

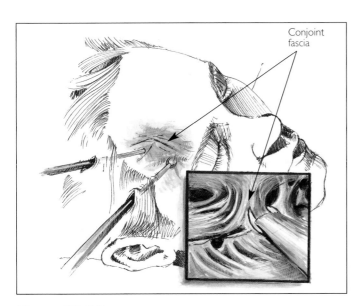

**Figure 22.18**
The conjoint fascia is dissected from the temporal approach. Inset: endoscopic view.

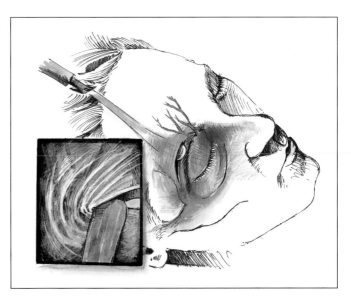

**Figure 22.19**
Opening of the periosteum 1–2 cm above the arcus marginalis. Inset: endoscopic view.

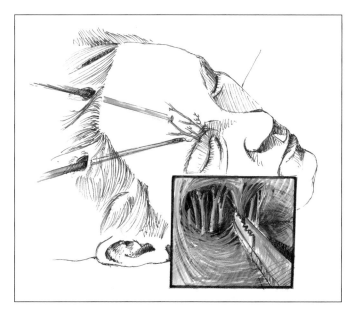

**Figure 22.20**
Endoscopic dissection of the brow depressors, taking care to avoid damage to adjacent nerves and vessels.

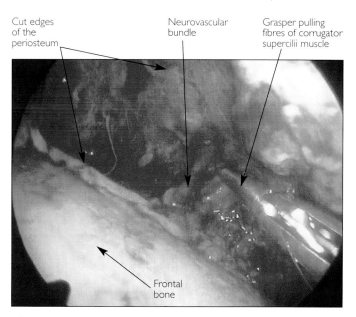

Cut edges of the periosteum

Neurovascular bundle

Grasper pulling fibres of corrugator supercilii muscle

Frontal bone

**Figure 22.21**
Intraoperative endoscopic dissection of corrugator supercilii muscle.

the supraorbital and supratrochlear neurovascular bundles. The periosteum is bluntly dissected, exposing the depressors of the brow.

## 6. Muscle modification

The corrugator supercilii muscles are gently dissected with endoscopic scissors and graspers (Figures 22.20 and 22.21). Sensory nerve branches within the corrugator supercilii should be preserved. Next, the procerus muscle over the root of the nose is incised and weakened. Overly aggressive removal of these muscles will leave a depression in the brow. An injection of botulinum toxin temporarily prevents the action of the depressors and allows the forehead to settle into its new position with the unopposed action of the occipitofrontalis muscle.

## 7. Suspension and fixation of the forehead

A variety of fixation methods have been described. The author's preference is to use small microplates centrally and paracentrally to which the scalp is attached subcutaneously with 2.0 Gortex sutures. Small bone tunnels may be drilled instead, through which the sutures are passed and tied. Alternatively, 14 mm screws may be inserted into the scalp to a depth of 4 mm, leaving the screws protruding through the wounds, which are stapled posteriorly, holding the forehead advanced. Temporally, the superficial temporal fascia is sutured to the deep temporal fascia with nonabsorbable sutures. A firm compressive dressing should be applied. A drain is normally omitted unless any bleeding has been encountered.

# Complications of brow lift surgery

A number of complications can occur from this surgery.

## 1. Facial nerve trauma

A meticulous surgical technique and a very good knowledge of anatomy of the temporal region will avoid iatrogenic damage to the frontal branch of the facial nerve.

## 2. Sensory nerve trauma

Care must be taken to recognize and avoid damage to the supraorbital and supratrochlear nerves.

## 3. Haematoma

Great care should be taken to avoid damage to the sentinel vessel just above the zygomatic arch and to the supraorbital and supratrochlear vessels to prevent the occurrence of a postoperative haematoma. If a haematoma occurs this should be drained and the bleeding vessel identified and cauterized.

## 4. Scarring

The incisions should be camouflaged appropriately and closed very carefully to avoid unsightly scars. The type of brow lift selected will influence the position and degree of resultant scarring. It is important to select the type of procedure that is most appropriate for the individual patient.

## 5. Alopecia

Care must be taken to avoid superficial dissection and overuse of cautery in the region of scalp hair follicles to prevent undue hair loss.

# Further reading

1.   Dutton JJ. *Atlas of clinical and surgical orbital anatomy*. Philadelphia: WB Saunders, 1994.

2.   Jordan DR, Anderson RL. The facial nerve in eyelid surgery. *Arch Ophthalmol* (1989) **107**:1114–15.

3.   Lemke BN, Stasior OG. The anatomy of eyebrow ptosis. *Arch Ophthalmol* (1982) **100**:981–6.

4.   Shorr N, Hoenig JA. Brow lift. In: Levine M, ed., *Manual of oculoplastic surgery*. Newton, MA: Butterworth-Heinmann, 1996, pp. 47–62.

5.   Tardy ME, Willianis EF, Boyee PG. Rejuvenation of the aging eyebrow and forehead. In: Putterman AE, ed., *Cosmetic oculoplastic surgery*. Philadelphia: WB Saunders, 1994.

# 23

# Enucleation and evisceration

## Introduction

The removal of an eye and the subsequent management of the anophthalmic socket still pose a considerable challenge for the ophthalmic surgeon in spite of many recent advances in orbital implant materials. Good results from such surgery are not easy to achieve consistently and a poor result can have profound psychological implications for the patient for the rest of his/her life. The preoperative counselling of a patient who requires an enucleation demands time and considerable compassion on the part of the ophthalmic surgeon. Close collaboration between the ophthalmic surgeon and the ocularist is essential and should commence preoperatively whenever possible.

The goals of an enucleation or an evisceration are to achieve the following:

- A healthy quiet comfortable socket free of discharge which can be fitted with a stable ocular prosthesis that mimics the fellow eye in appearance and movement
- A symmetric appearance without enophthalmos or an upper eyelid sulcus deformity
- An absence of upper or lower eyelid malposition
- Normal eyelid closure over the ocular prosthesis

To achieve these goals, the enucleation must be approached in the same manner as any intraocular procedure and must be performed meticulously.

## Indications for enucleation

There are a number of indications for enucleation:

1. A blind painful eye, e.g. following rubeosis iridis, failed retinal reattachment surgery
2. A blind unsightly eye, e.g. buphthalmos, phthisis bulbi
3. An intraocular tumour, e.g. a large choroidal melanoma

4. Severe ocular trauma and a high risk of sympathetic ophthalmia

It is important to consider alternatives to enucleation. The movement of a blind (or partially sighted) eye, a microphthalmic or phthisical eye can be more natural than that of an orbital implant and may tolerate a cosmetic shell or cosmetic contact lens. A painful eye may respond to simple surgery to relieve the pain, e.g. cyclo-destructive procedures or a conjunctival flap, and may also then tolerate a cosmetic shell or contact lens.

## Preoperative preparation

The majority of patients undergo an enucleation as an elective procedure. The operation is rarely performed as an emergency. The patient should be advised about:

1. The advantages, disadvantages, risks and potential complications of an enucleation procedure
2. The advantages, disadvantages, risks and potential complications of the use of any orbital implant
3. The implant options
4. The options regarding implant wrapping materials
5. The choice of anaesthesia
6. Postoperative pain and its management
7. The postoperative compressive dressing
8. The use of a temporary suture tarsorrhaphy
9. The use of a postoperative conformer
10. The likelihood of a temporary postoperative ptosis
11. The role of the ocularist and the timing of the fitting of the ocular prosthesis

Informed consent should be obtained after the patient has had time to consider the options.

The patient should discontinue aspirin and any other antiplatelet drugs if medically permissible at least 2 weeks preoperatively. Likewise, anticoagulants should only be altered or discontinued after discussion with the patient's haematologist. Any bacterial conjunctivitis should be treated preoperatively and topical steroids used to reduce any conjunctival inflammation.

> A computed tomography (CT) scan of the orbits and paranasal sinuses should be performed if a patient has previously suffered orbital trauma to exclude the possibility of a missed orbital wall blowout fracture

# Orbital implant materials

Enucleation (or evisceration) of an eye creates an orbital volume deficit. This necessitates the replacement of the equivalent spherical volume of approximately 6 ml (depending on the size of the globe). This can be partially compensated for by the placement of an orbital implant. An 18 mm spherical implant has a volume of only 3.1 ml. The average ocular prosthesis must then be over 2 ml to make up the difference. The advantage of using a larger orbital implant is to keep the prosthesis as light as possible. This will reduce the incidence of inferior displacement of the lower eyelid by gravitational force on the prosthetic eye. This advantage, however, must be balanced against the disadvantages of the use of a larger implant:

- Increased pressure on the conjunctival wound with a risk of dehiscence and implant exposure or extrusion
- A longer period of time required for vascularization of a porous implant
- Insufficient room for placement of a motility peg in the case of a porous implant
- Insufficient room for the ocularist to fit an ocular prosthesis with sufficient thickness to adequately mimic the presence of an anterior chamber

If no orbital implant is placed, or if the implant is of insufficient size, the ocular prosthesis will have to be made larger than is desirable in an attempt to reduce the volume deficit, which manifests itself by an enophthalmic appearance and an upper eyelid sulcus deformity. The lower lid eventually becomes stretched, the ocular prosthesis becomes inferiorly and posteriorly displaced, the levator palpebrae superioris loses its fulcrum of action, and the upper eyelid sulcus deformity becomes more exaggerated. The patient then exhibits features referred to as *the post-enucleation socket syndrome (PESS)* (Figure 23.1).

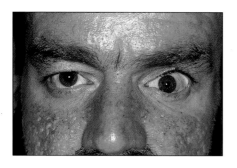

**Figure 23.1** A patient exhibiting features of a postenucleation socket syndrome.

# Primary orbital implant

The ideal time for orbital implantation is at the time of enucleation/evisceration unless primary implantation is contraindicated, e.g. in the case of severe ocular and orbital trauma or of infection. The overall results are superior and there is a much-reduced need for subsequent surgical procedures.

Controversy has raged about the use of evisceration versus enucleation. Some ophthalmologists prefer evisceration to enucleation because, in the hands of the general ophthalmologist, it may offer a more functional and cosmetically acceptable orbit compared with enucleation. Evisceration tends to produce less disruption of the orbital tissues and the physiological dynamics of muscle function, and the orbital volume can be maintained very close to its original state. It has the advantage that it can be performed very quickly under local anaesthesia and it is therefore ideal for elderly patients with blind painful eyes. It should be noted, however, that evisceration, although a faster and simpler surgical procedure, has the following potential disadvantages:

- The possible dissemination of an unsuspected intraocular tumour *(all globes with opaque media should be subjected to an ultrasound examination prior to surgery)*
- An inadequate pathological specimen is provided
- A phthisical globe will not accept an adequately sized implant
- There is concern about the possible risk, albeit small, of sympathetic ophthalmia

# Secondary orbital implant

An implant can be inserted secondarily into the anophthalmic socket but the surgical procedure is more difficult and the results are less predictable. Patients undergoing secondary orbital implantation are more likely to require additional surgical procedures to address a residual volume deficit, conjunctival adhesions/cysts and eyelid malpositions. Similarly, removal of an extruding, exposed or migrated implant with an implant exchange can be difficult.

# Choices of implant

Over the years, many different implant materials have been used, the first being glass. Many materials have followed, including cartilage, fat, bone, cork, aluminium, wood, silk, ivory and paraffin! Many of these orbital implants were associated with numerous problems and have been abandoned. Until the arrival of hydroxyapatite and porous polyethylene, acrylic and silicone materials were the most commonly used, with the most common configuration being spherical. Orbital implants can be classified as non-integrated or integrated.

# Non-integrated implants

Non-integrated implants have no direct attachments to the extraocular muscles and are usually single spheres of inert material (silicone or methylmethacrylate) buried beneath the conjunctiva and Tenon's capsule in the muscle cone. The rectus muscles may or may not be incorporated into the soft tissue closure anterior to the implant. Such implants may be inserted behind the posterior layer of Tenon's capsule within the intraconal fat space. Such implants commonly migrate within the orbit, causing secondary problems with fitting and stability of the ocular prosthesis. They have largely been abandoned for use after enucleation but are still useful for elderly patients undergoing an evisceration (Figure 23.2).

# Integrated implants

Integrated orbital implants may be further classified as buried or exposed.

**Buried integrated implants.** These may have either a spherical or an irregular shape. The spherical implants may be wrapped in donor sclera, fascia lata, temporalis fascia or Vicryl or Mersilene mesh to which the extraocular muscles can be sutured. Some spherical implants may be left unwrapped, and the muscles sutured directly to the implant material, such as the porous polyethylene (Medpor) implant. In buried integrated orbital implants with an irregular surface, muscle attachment is achieved by passing the muscles through tunnels in the implant (Allen, Castroviejo implants – Figure 23.3) or through grooves in the implant created by mounds on the anterior aspect (Iowa and Universal implants). The Roper Hall implant has a magnetic strip incorporated into the centre of the implant to enable a magnetic coupling to occur with a metallic strip inserted into the prosthesis (Figure 23.4).

**Exposed integrated implants.** These have the muscles directly attached to the implant and a portion of the implant is exposed to the outside environment (an Arruga implant). The exposed portion is in the form of a projection or an indentation,

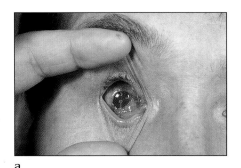

a

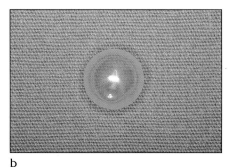

b

**Figure 23.2**
(a) A simple acrylic spherical orbital implant extruding. (b) The implant following removal.

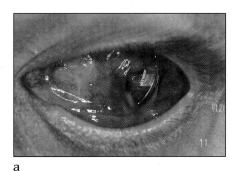

a

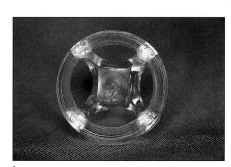

b

**Figure 23.3**
(a) An extruding Castroviejo orbital implant. (b) The implant following removal.

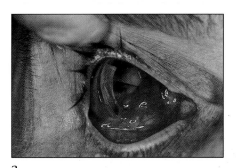

a

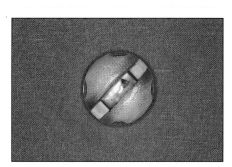

b

**Figure 23.4**
(a) An extruding magnetic orbital implant. (b) The implant following removal.

which permits the implant to be directly coupled to a prosthetic eye with its posterior projection (Figure 23.5).

Although these implants provided excellent motility, this benefit was outweighed by their disadvantage of chronic infections and extrusion. The exposed integrated implant violates two basic surgical principles:

- A wound must be completely epithelialized to avoid breakdown
- A foreign body left partly exposed will eventually extrude or become infected.

Such implants have been abandoned.

The orbital implants currently used today are mainly:

1. 'Baseball' implant
2. Hydroxyapatite implant
3. Porous polyethylene implant
4. Bioceramic implant
5. Simple acrylic sphere implant
6. Simple silicone sphere implant
7. Universal implant
8. Castroviejo implant
9. Dermis fat graft implant

*The most promising implants available today are the hydroxyapatite implant, the porous polyethylene (Medpor) implant and the aluminium oxide (Bioceramic) implant.* The hydroxyapatite implant has gained enormous popularity since its introduction several years ago and is rapidly becoming the implant of choice among many leading oculoplastic surgeons in many countries (Figure 23.6).

A synthetic form of hydroxyapatite is also available. Medpor has been introduced more recently and is likewise gaining in popularity. The Bioceramic implant has recently been marketed and is also purported to offer yet further advantages over other porous implants. These implants are all available in 14 mm to 22 mm sizes.

Hydroxyapatite is an inorganic salt of calcium phosphate similar to the inorganic portion of normal human bone. There are several advantages to these orbital implants. The materials have the capacity to develop complete fibrovascular ingrowth. The time taken for this to occur depends on a number of factors:

- The size of the implant
- The use of the implant – as a primary, secondary or exchange implant
- The wrapping material used

The porous hydroxyapatite implant can be directly coupled with the ocular prosthesis to improve movement by means of a small methylmethacrylate peg, which fits into a hole drilled into the buried implant. The conjunctiva will grow down the sides of this drilled hole only if the implant is fully vascularized. Alternatively, a titanium-sleeved peg can now be screwed into the implant after creating a central guide hole with a series of free needles of increasing size. Likewise, a titanium motility peg system is now available for the Medpor implant.

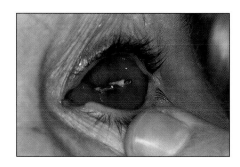

**Figure 23.5**
An Arruga orbital implant.

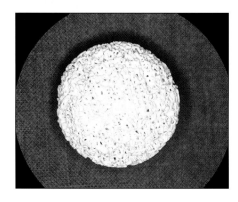

**Figure 23.6**
The hydroxyapatite orbital implant.

The time to complete vascularization varies from 4 to 12 months. The vascularization of the implant may be determined by a computed tomography (CT) scan with contrast, a magnetic resonance imaging (MRI) scan with gadolinium or a technetium-99m bone scan. Alternatively, a minimum safe waiting period may be allowed before proceeding with the second stage: e.g. 6 months for primary implants and 12 months for secondary implants.

These implants have been heavily marketed on the basis of a number of purported advantages over other implants.

## *Advantages*

1. Once the implant has become vascularized it 'cannot' extrude
2. The risk of migration of the implant within the orbit is reduced
3. The implant permits better movement of the ocular prosthesis
4. The motility peg allows the weight of the ocular prosthesis to be borne by the implant rather than by the lower eyelid, reducing the chances of instability of the artificial eye and the need for lower eyelid tightening procedures later
5. The implant is quickly and easily inserted and has a low complication rate in the hands of an experienced surgeon

## *Disadvantages*

The implant has a number of disadvantages. These include the additional costs involved: the cost of the implant, the requirement and expense of the second stage procedure to place a motility peg, and the required modifications to the ocular prosthesis. Additional expense may also be incurred if scans are used to determine whether or not the implant is vascularized and safe to drill. A small proportion of patients will require management of minor complications, e.g. removal of foreign body granulomas associated with the motility peg.

## Results

The results of primary implantation tend to be very good. The results of secondary implantation are less predictable as the socket anatomy has been disrupted and the eye muscles are retracted, scarred and difficult to locate at the time of surgery. In experienced hands, however, the results are usually good but the degree of movement is very variable from patient to patient.

## Rationale for implant use

Hydroxyapatite is a relatively expensive implant material. The successful use of this material in most surgeons' hands appears to require the use of a wrapping material (unless used in conjunction with evisceration) that:

- Adds expense (Vicryl mesh)
- Carries a risk for viral disease transmission (donor sclera)
- Incurs further surgical morbidity (autologous fascia)

The early complication rate of hydroxyapatite implants appears to be higher than that of other materials. Particular problems with implant exposure have been the subject of a number of publications and the potential advantages with regard to late complications, such as migration and extrusion, await the test of time. Its main advantage lies in its ability to accept a motility peg to enhance movement of the ocular prosthesis. In some series, however, as few as 12% of hydroxyapatite implant patients are fitted with a motility peg. The assumption is, therefore, that the majority of patients are satisfied with the initial motility achieved. Nonetheless, there is no evidence that when similar techniques are used unpegged hydroxyapatite implants have superior motility to solid sphere implants. Further, there is no anatomical basis for this to be so. Although the superior motility of the pegged hydroxyapatite implant is continually alluded to, there has yet to be a double-blind study to confirm this. There is little evidence to support the use of this more expensive implant in patients who do not wish to undergo the extra time and expense required to fit a motility peg. It seems reasonable to reserve the use of hydroxyapatite implant for patients who desire the enhanced motility the peg offers (in full knowledge of what is involved — including the increased incidence of severe postoperative pain).

Concern has also been raised as to whether the hydroxyapatite system of motility enhancement will stand the test of time, and we can only wait and see whether such a system is sustainable over a lifetime.

Similar criticism can be levelled at the Medpor implant, although this implant does offers the advantage that it can readily accept direct suturing, which obviates the need for a wrapping material. The implant is smooth, in contrast to the rough brittle surface of the hydroxyapatite implant. The ability of the implant to accept direct suturing without the necessity for a wrapping material is certainly an attractive quality. Long-term results of the placement of motility pegs in Medpor implants are not yet available, however, and concerns have been raised about the implant's pore size and completely porous nature and its hydrophobic surface characteristics. There are reports of implant exposure requiring further surgery, which therefore raises concerns about the wisdom of utilizing the implant without a wrapping material as a preventative measure. Modifications of the implant shape have been described to reduce the problems of residual upper lid sulcus deformity. Some surgeons have placed this implant with a motility peg already inserted. This is then 'externalized' later; this fails to recognize, however, that the implant can alter position and that the peg placement should be determined by the ocularist and not by the surgeon.

## Alternative implants

1. 'Baseball' implant – this remains a simple cheap but effective primary implant. The acrylic sphere is wrapped in donor sclera (or autogenous fascia, or Mersilene mesh) and buried behind posterior Tenon's fascia (Figure 23.7 and 23.8). It is of use in older patients who do not wish to take advantage of the second stage peg placement of the hydroxyapatite or Medpor implants.

2. Simple acrylic sphere implant – this is easily placed at the time of an evisceration, although the use of a subconjunctival patch of sclera or autogenous fascia will reduce the risk of implant exposure and/or extrusion.

3. Simple silicone sphere implant – silicone has achieved a certain notoriety with patients and is used infrequently. It is used in the same way as a simple acrylic sphere implant.

4. Universal implant – this remains a primary implant of choice in many centres in the United States for both enucleation and evisceration. It has a good track record, with few complications, although its placement is not as simple.

5. Castroviejo implant – this implant is still used in a number of centres in the United Kingdom but is associated with long-term problems with tilting and extrusion of the implant; its use is not to be recommended.

6. Dermis fat graft – this autogenous implant is still useful for the surgical rehabilitation of sockets which have conjunctival

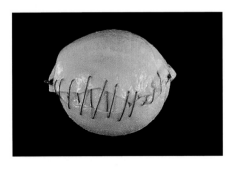

**Figure 23.7**
A 'baseball'
orbital implant.

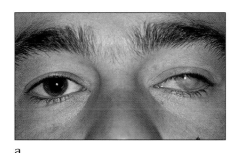
a

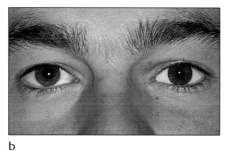
b

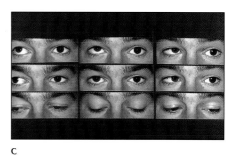
c

**Figure 23.8**
(a) A patient with a blind painful unsightly eye. (b) The patient following an enucleation with placement of a primary 'baseball' orbital implant. (c) The patient demonstrating a fair range of motility of the artificial eye.

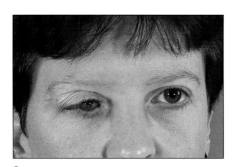
a

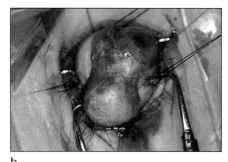
b

**Figure 23.9**
(a) Patient presenting with a right blind painful eye. She gave a history of multiple previous glaucoma surgeries and a lateral tarsorrhaphy. (b) The enucleation of the globe was difficult due to the presence of a large glaucoma drainage valve and due to conjunctival adherence to the sclera. The patient required a mucous membrane graft.

lining problems in addition to volume deficits, although some surgeons use such implants for primary cases where other implants would have a higher risk of exposure or extrusion, e.g. in acute trauma, following extrusion of other implants.

The search for the ideal implant material and design will continue. The surgeon faced with the patient requiring an enucleation or evisceration currently has a number of implants to choose from and should select the implant most appropriate to the individual patient. The choice will be influenced by a number of factors:

- The age and general health of the patient
- Consideration of cost
- The willingness of the patient to undergo a second-stage procedure
- The relative expertise of the surgeon
- The risk factors for implant extrusion

It should be recognized that the following situations represent a higher risk of implant exposure or extrusion:

1. Previous failed retinal reattachment surgery
2. Previous failed glaucoma surgery, with or without the use of antimetabolites (Figure 23.9)
3. Acute trauma
4. Cicatrization of the eyelids and conjunctiva

It should be recognized that the success of orbital implant surgery is highly dependent not only on the appropriate choice of implant but also on meticulous surgical technique and postoperative care and follow-up. This includes the use of an appropriate surgical conformer and the skilled fitting of an ocular prosthesis at the correct time. Long-term follow-up is a commitment which must be made for the patient. Most subsequent socket problems can be prevented or managed easily only with appropriate follow-up. Although orbital implant surgery can be performed by general ophthalmic surgeons, such surgeons must recognize the need to be able to manage and prevent secondary socket and adnexal problems. It is for this reason that socket surgery is fast becoming the realm of the oculoplastic surgeon alone. No surgeon undertaking such surgery can fail to acknowledge the major role the ocularist plays in the management of the patient. Ideally, the surgeon and ocularist should work in very close cooperation in the same clinic environment.

# Anaesthesia

The majority of enucleations are performed under general anaesthesia, but the operation can be performed under local anaesthesia, depending on the patient's preference and the patient's general medical status. The anaesthetist should be warned about the possible need to harvest a mucous membrane graft. The patient's airway can then be protected with a throat pack, the presence of which should be clearly marked, and the intubation tubing moved to the side of the mouth, allowing easy access to the upper and lower lips.

It is essential to have an anaesthetist in attendance during enucleation under local anaesthesia because of the risk of severe bradycardia from the oculocardiac reflex. A para-bulbar injection of 7 ml of 0.5% Marcain (bupivacaine) with 1:200,000 units of adrenaline mixed with Hyalase (hyaluronidase) is given. Great care should be taken in the case of myopic eyes with an axial length exceeding 26 mm and with eyes which have retinal explants or glaucoma valves.

An evisceration can be performed very quickly and is more commonly performed under local anaesthesia.

# Enucleation: surgical technique

> The surgeon must identify the correct eye to be removed prior to the induction of general anaesthesia. In the case of an intraocular malignancy, the pupil of the affected eye must be dilated an hour prior to surgery and the affected eye confirmed by indirect ophthalmoscopy. The surgeon must mark the affected eye and be personally responsible for the prepping and draping of the patient. The surgeon must also ensure that the fellow eye is taped closed and fully protected from inadvertent injury during the course of the surgery.

The face, eyelids and conjunctival sac should be thoroughly prepared with an antiseptic agent and a cataract drape applied. A Clarke's eyelid speculum is placed to exclude the eyelashes from the surgical field (Figure 23.10).

Using a Moorfield's forceps and blunt-tipped Westcott scissors, a 360-degree peritomy is performed taking care to preserve as much conjunctiva as possible (Figure 23.11). This may be difficult following previous failed retinal reattachment surgery.

Steven's scissors are used to bluntly dissect the four quadrants between the recti muscles (Figure 23.12).

The rectus muscles are hooked using a muscle hook. Westcott scissors are used to dissect off adjacent Tenon's tissue and the intermuscular septa. Each rectus muscle is then tagged at its insertion using 5/0 double-armed Vicryl sutures in a locking fashion (Figure 23.13).

The muscles are then disinserted from the globe, leaving a short muscle stump at the medial and lateral rectus insertions. Each of the sutures is tagged with a bulldog clip. The inferior oblique muscle is then hooked using a tenotomy hook and the entire muscle belly exposed. The muscle is stretched out using two von Graefe muscle hooks and the muscle tagged with a 5/0 double-armed Vicryl suture in a locking fashion and divided close to its insertion on the globe using Westcott scissors. Next, the superior oblique tendon is identified and hooked using a von Graefe muscle hook. The tendon is cut using Westcott scissors.

A 4/0 silk suture is then placed through the stumps of the medial and lateral recti muscles. Forward traction is placed on the globe using the silk sutures, and enucleation scissors are used to cut the optic nerve. Alternatively, a snare may be used but its use may be contraindicated in the presence of a soft globe (the snare may transect the globe), if a large corneal section or penetrating keratoplasty has been performed (the globe may rupture), or if a long length of optic nerve is required (enucleation for retinoblastoma).

The globe is removed carefully cutting any residual Tenon's fibres still adherent to the globe. The site is then packed tightly with two moistened 2 × 2 swabs: 5 min are allowed for haemostasis. *The enucleated globe is inspected thoroughly before being sent for histopathological examination.* The swabs are then

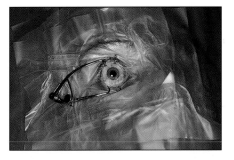

**Figure 23.10**
The preparation of a globe for an enucleation.

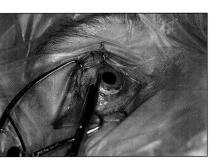

**Figure 23.11**
A 360-degree peritomy is performed at the limbus with great care to avoid any loss of conjunctiva.

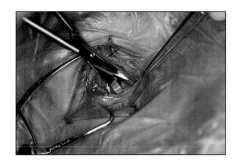

**Figure 23.12**
Steven's scissors are used for blunt dissection between the recti.

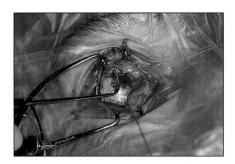

**Figure 23.13**
A double armed 5/0 Vicryl suture has been placed through the lateral rectus muscle 5 mm posterior to its insertion.

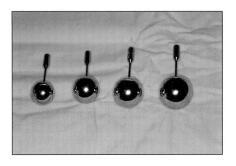

**Figure 23.14**
Orbital implant sizing spheres.

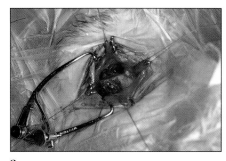

a

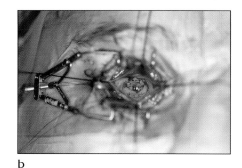

b

**Figure 23.15**
(a) The appearance of the socket following enucleation. The extraocular muscles can be seen to exit between anterior and posterior Tenon's fascia. (b) The posterior Tenon's fascia has been opened, exposing the intraconal fat space.

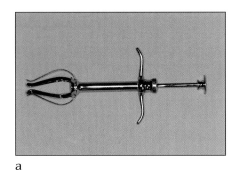

a

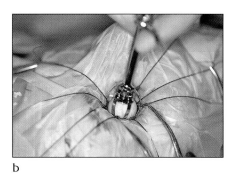

b

**Figure 23.16**
(a) A Carter sphere injector. (b) The implant is injected into the intraconal fat space.

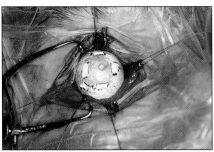

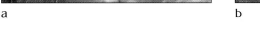

a

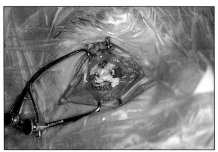

b

**Figure 23.17**
(a) In this example a hydroxyapatite implant has been wrapped in donor sclera and windows cut for the attachment of the extraocular muscles. (b) The recti and inferior oblique muscles have been sutured to the sclera.

removed and the site inspected for any bleeding. Any residual bleeding vessels are cauterized using bipolar cautery.

If the patient is deemed unsuitable for an orbital implant, the horizontal and vertical recti are simply tied to each other in a cruciate fashion. The conjunctiva is closed with interrupted 7/0 Vicryl sutures. A sterile surgical conformer of appropriate size and shape is inserted into the conjunctival sac. Topical antibiotic ointment is instilled into the conjunctival sac and a pressure dressing applied. This is not removed for a minimum of 72 hours.

If an orbital implant is to be inserted, the appropriate size is determined with the use of sizing spheres (Figure 23.14).

First, posterior Tenon's fascia is identified and then opened by blunt dissection, exposing the intraconal fat space: 4/0 silk traction sutures are placed through the posterior Tenon's fascia (Figure 23.15). If posterior Tenon's fascia cannot be closed over the surface of the sizing sphere without undue tension, a smaller sphere should be substituted.

The implant of appropriate size is then wrapped in the material which has been selected by the patient during the preoperative consultation, e.g. donor sclera, Vicryl mesh, autogenous fascia lata, temporalis fascia. It is then inserted into the intraconal fat space behind posterior Tenon's fascia using a Carter sphere injector (Figure 23.16).

The recti and the inferior oblique muscle are attached to the implant as shown in Figure 23.17.

The posterior Tenon's fascia is then closed with interrupted 5/0 Vicryl sutures. In those patients at increased risk of implant exposure, such as following trauma, patch graft of donor sclera or autogenous fascia is then placed over the suture line to reduce any risk of implant exposure. Next, the anterior Tenon's fascia is closed with interrupted 7/0 Vicryl sutures and, finally, the conjunctiva is closed likewise (Figure 23.18).

A sterile surgical conformer of appropriate size and shape is inserted into the conjunctival sac, ensuring that the eyelids will close passively over the conformer without creating tension on the

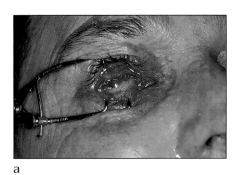

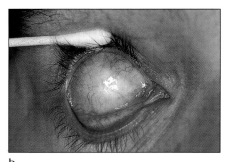

a                                                        b

**Figure 23.18**
(a) The appearance of the socket at the completion of surgery. (b) A patient in whom a subconjunctival patch graft has been placed seen 3 years following surgery. The socket is quiet and the patch graft clearly visible.

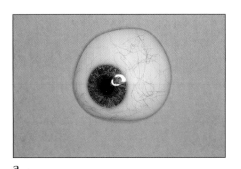

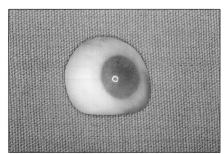

a                                                        b

**Figure 23.19**
(a) A recently polished artificial eye. (b) A neglected artificial eye with a poor appearance and a rough surface. The patient had a chronically discharging socket.

conjunctival suture line. If there is any concern about the possibility of excessive postoperative swelling, a temporary suture tarsorrhaphy should be undertaken using a central 4/0 nylon suture passed through tarsorrhaphy tubing. A retrobulbar injection of 5 ml of 0.5% Marcain and 1:200,000 units of adrenaline is given to aid postoperative analgesia. An intravenous injection of a broad-spectrum antibiotic is given along with an anti-inflammatory agent and an opiate analgesic. Topical antibiotic ointment is instilled into the conjunctival sac and a pressure dressing and bandage are applied. These are not removed for a minimum of 5 days.

## Postoperative management

The patient is discharged on a 1-week course of systemic antibiotic, a 2-week course of a systemic anti-inflammatory agent and an analgesic. Topical antibiotics are instilled for 4 weeks after removal of the dressing 5–7 days postoperatively. The patient should not be fitted with an artificial eye until a minimum of 8 weeks have passed to allow sufficient wound healing and complete resolution of postoperative oedema. If the artificial eye is fitted too soon after surgery the risk of implant exposure is increased. In addition, the artificial eye will not fit the socket properly once complete resolution of postoperative orbital oedema has occurred.

The patient should remain under the care of the ocularist, who will ensure that the artificial eye is polished on an annual basis and that topical lubricants are prescribed whenever a patient has an incomplete blink (Figure 23.19). The socket is examined to exclude implantation cysts, papillary conjunctivitis and implant exposure. Failure to maintain the artificial eye will risk conjunctival inflammation, discharge, conjunctival breakdown and implant exposure.

## *Complications*
### Implant exposure

Exposure of any orbital implant can usually be managed successfully in the absence of infection. The conjunctiva and anterior Tenon's tissue should be undermined and a patch graft placed, e.g. donor sclera, autogenous fascia or hard palate. If a large area is exposed or if there is evidence of infection the implant should be removed and replaced with a dermis fat graft (Figures 23.20 23.21).

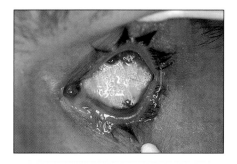

**Figure 23.20**
Large area of exposure of an hydroxyapatite orbital implant in a diabetic patient.

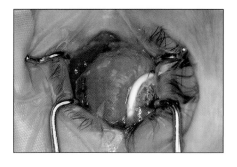

**Figure 23.21**
An infected extruding custom-wrapped synthetic hydroxyapatite orbital implant.

## Over-sized implant

If the implant size was correctly selected at surgery, the situation may improve spontaneously with time. If, however, there is insufficient room for a satisfactory artificial eye, the implant can be explored and debulked with a burr, or the lateral wall of the orbit may be decompressed by internal burring.

## Orbital haematoma

A postoperative orbital haematoma can seriously compromise a patient's outcome following an enucleation (Figure 23.22). This can predispose to socket contracture. Precautions should be taken to ensure that such an occurrence is prevented by attention to detail: the discontinuation of preoperative medications which predispose to bleeding, the preoperative management of hypertension, a meticulous surgical technique with strict attention to intraoperative haemostasis and the use of a compressive dressing postoperatively.

## Motility peg placement

If the movement of the patient's artificial eye is unsatisfactory in spite of good movement of the orbital implant, a motility peg can be placed. This should be done in consultation with an ocularist who is best placed to determine the appropriate location for the peg. *It is unwise to place a motility peg in any patient who has socket inflammation and excessive discharge, papillary conjunctivitis, lagophthalmos, or an implant which is lying in an eccentric position in the socket.*

Preoperatively, a wax drilling template is made by the ocularist. This is placed in the socket, with the patient in a sitting position. A mark is made with gentian violet through the hole in the template, which is then removed (Figure 23.23).

The patient's artificial eye is soaked in iodine. A retrobulbar local anaesthetic injection is given and the patient prepped and draped using a cataract drape. It is important to avoid conjunctival oedema from an excessive volume of local anaesthetic.

A Clarke's speculum is placed and the conjunctiva cauterized at the position indicated by the gentian violet using a disposable cautery. Next, a hole is made in the implant using a series of needles of gradually increasing size. These are mounted on a holder and are screwed into the implant in a vertical orientation, aiming towards the apex of the orbit (Figure 23.24).

Finally, once the hole is of sufficient size and depth, the titanium-sleeved peg is screwed into the implant with a small screwdriver to lie flush with the conjunctiva. A temporary flat-headed peg is inserted into the sleeved peg. All deposits of hydroxyapatite dust are then removed from the conjunctival sac with careful irrigation. The patient's artificial eye is replaced. The patient is warned preoperatively that the eye will not fit correctly until it has been modified at the next appointment with the ocularist 2 weeks later, when the permanent round-

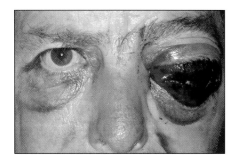

**Figure 23.22**
A massive orbital haematoma following an enucleation in a patient taking anticoagulants which were not discontinued preoperatively.

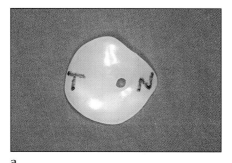

a

b

**Figure 23.23**
(a) A wax drilling template marked N for nasal and T for temporal orientation.
(b) The wax template has been placed in the socket and a mark on the conjunctiva made with gentian violet.

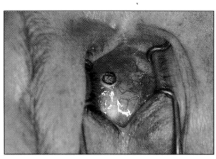

a

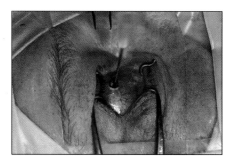

b

**Figure 23.24**
(a) The conjunctiva has been cauterized over the marked area using a disposable thermal cautery.
(b) A green needle is being used to create a hole in the hydroxyapatite orbital implant.

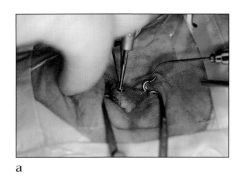
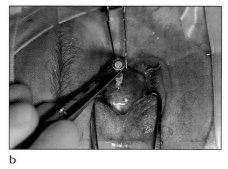
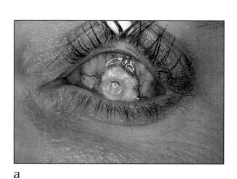

a                                    b

**Figure 23.25**
(a) A burr is being used to drill a hole into a hydroxyapatite orbital implant. Correct orientation of the burr is essential. (b) A flat-headed temporary peg is placed into the hole in the implant.

**Figure 23.27**
A modified posterior surface of an artificial eye.

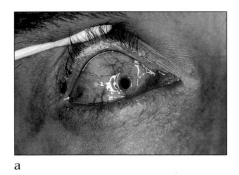
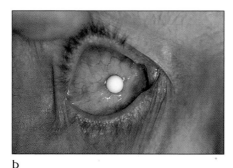

a                                    b                                    a

**Figure 23.26**
(a) The appearance of the hole 2 weeks after drilling. (b) A permanent round-headed motility peg.

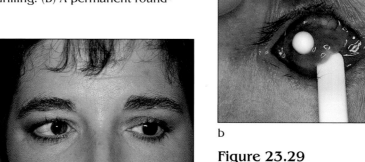

a                                    b

b

**Figure 23.28**
A patient with a secondary pegged hydroxyapatite orbital implant placed following removal of an extruding Castroviejo orbital implant.

**Figure 23.29**
(a) Exposure of a hydroxyapatite implant which was drilled before the implant was adequately vascularized. (b) A foreign body granuloma lying beneath the head of a motility peg.

headed peg is placed and the posterior surface of the artificial eye is hollowed out to accept it. A pressure dressing is applied for 24 hours.

If the titanium pegging system is deemed too expensive, the alternative is to use an acrylic peg, which is placed after drilling the implant. A 2.5 mm diamond burr is used to create a hole (Figure 23.25). It is extremely important to ensure that the burr is orientated correctly before the drilling procedure is commenced. A 3 mm burr is then used to enlarge the hole, which is drilled to a depth of 10 mm. A temporary flat-headed peg is placed, which is replaced with a permanent round-headed peg 2 weeks later when the drilling hole has become lined with conjunctiva (Figures 23.25 and 23.26).

The posterior aspect of the artificial eye is modified by the ocularist to accept the head of the permanent motility peg (Figures 23.27 and 23.28).

## Complications

Most complications are usually minor and are avoided by attention to detail both in selecting the appropriate patients for the procedure and in the surgery itself (Figure 23.29). A peg should not be placed until the implant is fully vascularized. Imaging techniques are not entirely reliable. It is preferable to delay the procedure for a sufficient length of time.

# Dermis fat graft: surgical technique

A standard enucleation is performed as described above. The dermis fat graft is harvested and trimmed to size (Figure 23.30). It is inserted into the intraconal fat space and the extraocular muscles are inserted onto the anterior surface of the dermis. The dermis may be left partially exposed if the patient has a conjunctival deficiency with the conjunctiva being tacked down to the dermis with interrupted 7/0 Vicryl sutures (Figure 23.31).

A surgical conformer is placed and the postoperative care is as described above.

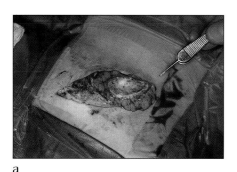

a

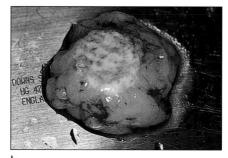

b

**Figure 23.30**
(a) A dermis fat graft is harvested from the abdominal wall or from the buttock. (b) The fat graft is trimmed and then compressed in a dry swab to dehydrate it before insertion into the socket.

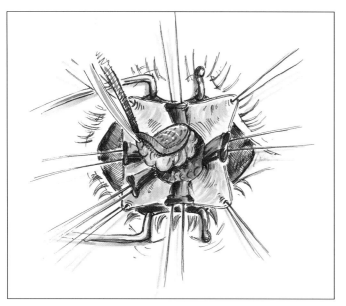

a

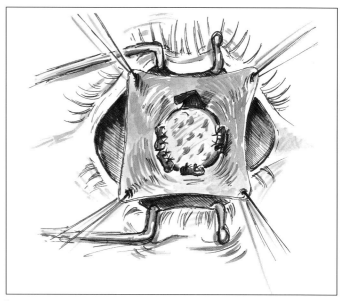

b

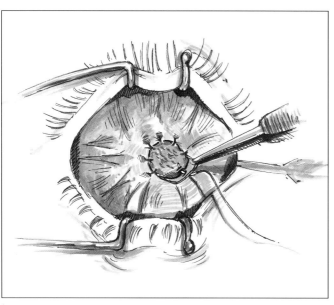

b

**Figure 23.31**
(a) The dermis fat graft is inserted into the socket. (b) The extraocular muscles attached to the dermis. (c) The conjunctival edges are sutured to the anterior surface of the dermis.

# Evisceration: surgical technique

As for an enucleation, the surgeon must identify the correct eye to be eviscerated prior to the induction of general anaesthesia or the injection of a local anaesthetic. The surgeon must mark the affected eye and be personally responsible for the prepping and draping of the patient.

The face, eyelids and conjunctival sac should be thoroughly prepared with an antiseptic agent and a cataract drape applied. A Clarke's eyelid speculum is placed to exclude the eyelashes from the surgical field. Using a Moorfield's forceps and Westcott scissors, a 360-degree peritomy is performed. A small full-thickness peripheral corneal incision is made with a No. 15 Bard Parker blade. The cornea is then removed using Westcott scissors with one blade inserted into the anterior chamber (Figure 23.32).

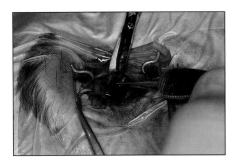

**Figure 23.32** The cornea being removed for an evisceration.

The intraocular contents are removed with an evisceration spoon. These contents and the cornea are sent for histopathological examination. The scleral shell is thoroughly cleaned out with cotton-tipped applicators soaked in absolute alcohol followed by thorough saline rinses. The interior of the scleral shell is inspected to ensure all uveal remnants have been removed. Bipolar cautery is used to seal any bleeding vessels.

Horizontal relieving incisions are made in the scleral rim. If the patient is deemed unsuitable for the use of an orbital implant a surgical conformer of appropriate size is inserted and a compressive dressing applied. This is maintained in place for 3 days. If an orbital implant is to be inserted the appropriate size is determined with the use of sizing spheres. A spherical implant appropriate to the patient is inserted into the scleral shell. (If this is a modern porous implant, four longitudinal scleral incisions are made between the recti with a No. 15 Bard Parker blade.) The sclera is closed with interrupted 5/0 Vicryl sutures, creating an overlap of the sclera.

A patch graft of donor sclera or autogenous fascia is then placed over the suture line to reduce any risk of implant exposure. Next, the anterior Tenon's fascia is closed with interrupted 7/0 Vicryl sutures and, finally, the conjunctiva is closed likewise. A sterile surgical conformer of appropriate size and shape is inserted into the conjunctival sac, ensuring that the eyelids will close passively over the conformer without creating tension on the conjunctival suture line. If there is any concern about the possibility of excessive postoperative swelling, a temporary suture tarsorrhaphy should be undertaken using a central 4/0 nylon suture passed through tarsorrhaphy tubing. If the patient is under general anaesthesia, a retrobulbar injection of 5 ml of 0.5% Marcain and 1:200,000 units of adrenaline is given to aid postoperative analgesia. An intravenous injection of a broad-spectrum antibiotic is given along with an anti-inflammatory agent and an opiate analgesic. Topical antibiotic ointment is instilled into the conjunctival sac and a pressure dressing and bandage are applied. These are not removed for a minimum of 5 days.

## *Postoperative management*

This is the same as following an enucleation.

## Further reading

1. Mark Cepela, MD, Scott Teske, FRACO, FRACS: Orbital implants (Review article). *Curr Opin Ophthalmol* (1996) **7**:38–42.

2. Dutton JJ. Coralline hydroxyapatite as an ocular implant. *Ophthalmology* (1991) **98**:370–7.

3. Kim YD, Goldberg RA, Shorr N, Steinsapir KD. Management of exposed hydroxyapatite orbital implants. *Ophthalmology* (1994) **101**:1709–15.

4. Shields JA, Shields CL, De Potter P. Hydroxyapatite orbital implant after enucleation – experience with 200 cases. *Mayo Clin Proc* (1993) **68**:1191–5.

5. Kaltreider SA, Newman SA. Prevention and management of complications associated with tbe hydroxyapatite implant. *Ophthal Plast Reconstr Surg* (1996) **12**:18–31.

6. Goldberg RA. Who should have hydroxyapatite orbital implants? (editorial) *Arch Ophthalmol* (1995) **113**:566–7.

7. Ashworth JL, Rhatigan M, Sampath R, Brammar R, Sunderland S, Leatherbarrow B. The hydroxyapatite orbital implant: a prospective study. *Eye* (1996) **10**:29–37.

8. De Potter P, Shields CL, Shields JA, Flanders AE, Rao VM. Role of magnetic resonance imaging in the evaluation of the hydroxyapatite orbital implant. *Ophthalmology* (1992) **99**:824–30.

9. Jordan DR, Allen LH, Ells A, et al. The use of Vicryl mesh (polyglactin 910) for implantation of hydroxyapatite orbital implants. *Ophthal Plast Reconstr Surg* (1995) **11**: 95–9.

10. Edelstein C, Shields CL, De Potter P, Shields JA. Complications of motility peg placement for the hydroxyapatite orbital implant. *Ophthalmology* (1997) **104**:1616–21.

11. Codere F. Hydroxyapatite implants: a rational approach (editorial). *Can J Ophthalmol* (1995) **30**:235–7.

12. Rubin PA, Popham JK, Bilyk JR, Shore JW. Comparison of fibrovascular ingrowth into hydroxyapatite and porous polyethylene orbital implants. *Ophthal Plast Reconstr Surg* (1994) **10**:96–103.

13. McNab A. Hydroxyapatite orbital implants. Experience with 100 cases. *Aust N Z J Ophthalmol* (1995) **23**:117–23.

14. Shields CL, Shields JA, De Potter P, Singh AD. Lack of complications of the hydroxyapatite orbital implant in 250 consecutive cases. *Trans Am Ophthalmol Soc* (1993) **91**:177–89.

15. Karesh JW, Dresner SC. High-density porous polyethylene (Medpor) as a successful anophthalmic socket implant. *Ophthalmology* (1994) **10**:1688–95.

16. Edelstein C, Shields CL, De Potter P, Shields JA. Complications of motility peg placement for the hydroxyapatite orbital implant. *Ophthalmology* (1997) **104**:1616–21.

17. Migliori ME, Putterman AM. The domed dermis-fat graft orbital implant. *Ophthal Plast Reconstr Surg* (1991) **7**:23–30.

18. Jordan DR, Anderson RL. The universal implant for evisceration surgery. *Ophthal Plast Reconstr Surg* (1997) **13**:1–7.

19. Levine MR, Pou CR, Lash RH: Evisceration: Is sympathetic ophthalmia a concern in the new millenium? *Ophthal Plast Reconstr Surg* (1999) **15**:4–8.

20. Flanders AE, De Potter P, Rao VM, Tom BM, Shields CL, Shields JA. MRI of orbital implants. *Neuroradiology* (1996) **38**:273–7.

21. Goldberg RA, Holds JB, Ebrahimpour J. Exposed hydroxyapatite orbital implants. Report of six cases. *Ophthalmology* (1992) **99**:831–6.

22. Nunery WR, Heinz GW, Bonnin JM, Martin RT, Cepela MA. Exposure rate of hydroxyapatite spheres in the anophthalmic socket: histopathologic correlation and comparison with silicone sphere implants. *Ophthal Plast Reconstr Surg* (1993) **9**:96–104.

23. Buettner H, Bartley GB. Tissue breakdown and exposure associated with hydroxyapatite orbital implants. *Am J Ophthalmol* (1992) **113**:669–73.

24. Dortzbach RK Holds JB. Theoretical considerations in the placement of hydroxyapatite orbital implants (letter). *Ophthal Plast Reconstr Surg* (1997) **13**:147–51.

25. Ashworth JL, Brammar R, Leatherbarrow B. A clinical study of the hydroxyapatite orbital implant. *Eur J Ophthalmol* (1997) **7**:1–8.

26. Ashworth JL, Brammar R, Inkster C, Leatherbarrow B. A study of the hydroxyapatite orbital implant drilling procedure. *Eye* (1998) **12**:37–42.

27. Smit TJ, Koornneef L, Zonneveld FW, Groet E, Otto AJ. Computed tomography in the assessment of the post enucleation socket syndrome. *Ophthalmology* (1990) **97**:1347–51.

# 24

# Exenteration

## Introduction

Exenteration is a surgical procedure that involves the removal of all the soft tissue contents of the orbit. Exenteration is classified as:

- Total
- Subtotal
- Extended

In a total exenteration all of the soft tissues of the orbit and periocular adnexa are removed. In a subtotal exenteration the eyelid skin is preserved. An extended exenteration involves resection of adjacent structures, e.g. paranasal sinuses. The extent of the surgical resection is dictated by the extent of the disease process.

This mutilating procedure is used for the management of a number of benign as well as malignant conditions which are not amenable to other treatment modalities.

## *Malignant disorders*

1. Malignant eyelid tumours with orbital involvement, e.g. basal cell or squamous cell carcinoma
2. Malignant eyelid tumours beyond simple surgical excision, e.g. extensive sebaceous carcinoma
3. Malignant conjunctival lesions, e.g. extensive melanoma
4. Orbital invasion by malignant paranasal sinus tumours
5. Primary malignant orbital tumours, e.g. lacrimal gland carcinomas

## *Nonmalignant disorders*

1. Benign orbital tumours, e.g. aggressive orbital meningioma
2. Life-threatening infection, e.g. sino-orbital mucormycosis

3. Severe nonspecific orbital inflammatory disease with intractable pain and blindness
4. Severe orbital deformity, e.g. neurofibromatosis
5. End-stage socket contracture

Patients who are to undergo an orbital exenteration should be managed by a multidisciplinary team which may include:

1. Orbital surgeon
2. Ear, nose and throat (ENT) surgeon
3. Plastic surgeon
4. Neurosurgeon
5. Radiologist
6. Radiotherapist
7. Oncologist
8. Mohs' micrographic surgeon
9. Pathologist
10. Ocularist
11. Psychologist
12. Oculoplastic nurse practitioner

## Preoperative evaluation

This comprises:

- Permanent histological sections
- Physical exam
- Radiology
- Mohs' micrographic surgery may be warranted to gain clearance of the epithelial margins in basal cell carcinomas (BCCs)
- Squamous cell carcinomas (SCCs)

As the operation may be associated with significant blood loss, typed and cross-matched blood should be made available. The patient should have a full blood count, platelet count and coagulation profile performed preoperatively. All antiplatelet agents should be discontinued 3 weeks prior to surgery. The assistance of a haematologist should be sought for the management of any patient who takes anticoagulants.

# Preoperative patient preparation

Most exenterations are performed as elective procedures. The patient should be very carefully counselled by senior experienced members of the team about the diagnosis, prognosis, nature of the surgery, its goals, risks and potential complications. The patient should be warned about inevitable anaesthesia of the forehead postoperatively. The options for surgical reconstruction of the exenterated socket should be discussed and determined according to the patient's wishes as well as the patient's age and general health. In determining the method of orbital reconstruction in the case of patients with a malignancy, the likelihood of recurrent disease must be taken into consideration.

The patient must be carefully prepared for the ensuing cosmetic deformity. Photographs of other patients who have undergone a similar exenteration may be helpful to use along with samples of typical orbital prostheses or methods of cosmetic camouflage.

The oculoplastic nurse practitioner should be on hand to explain her role in postoperative wound care and in co-ordinating aftercare in the community following discharge from hospital.

The pathologist should be consulted preoperatively and the possible need for frozen-section control of the resection margins discussed.

# Anaesthesia

General anaesthesia is preferable for this procedure although local anaesthesia with sedation can be used for the patient who is medically unfit. For local anaesthesia, 5 ml of 0.5% Marcain (bupivacaine) and 1:200,000 units of adrenaline is given with Hyalase (hyalurinodase) as a retrobulbar injection. In addition, a further 10–12 ml of 0.5% Marcain and 1:200,000 units of adrenaline are given as a series of subcutaneous injections around the orbital margin and as specific nerve blocks around the supratrochlear, supraorbital, infratrochlear, anterior ethmoidal, infraorbital, zygomaticofacial and zygomaticotemporal nerves. If the patient is under general anaesthesia 10–12 ml of 0.5% Marcain and 1:200,000 units of adrenaline is given as a series of subcutaneous injections around the orbital margin.

The anaesthetist should be warned that the dissection of the socket can provoke the oculocardiac reflex, inducing a severe bradycardia and occasionally asystole. The anaesthetist may wish to use glycopyrrolate or atropine prior to the dissection.

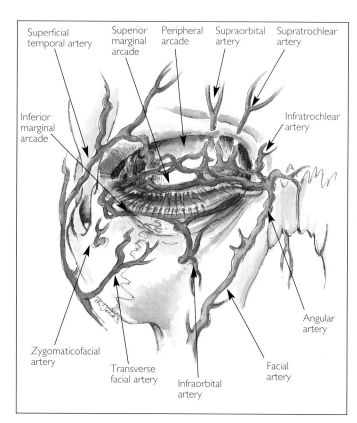

**Figure 24.1**
Vascular anatomy of the eyelids and periorbital region.

# Applied surgical anatomy

The surgeon must have a thorough knowledge of orbital anatomy in order to facilitate an expeditious exenteration that avoids excessive haemorrhage and other potentially serious complications. In particular, the surgeon should be aware of the following:

1.  The anatomical position of all the major orbital blood vessels (Figures 24.1 and 24.2)
2.  The points of increased periosteal attachment within the orbit
3.  The potential weak areas in the bony orbital walls, e.g. the orbital roof in the elderly (Figure 24.3)
4.  The position of the superior and inferior orbital fissures

# Surgical technique

The surgeon must identify the correct side to be exenterated prior to the induction of general anaesthesia. The surgeon must mark the correct side and be personally responsible for the prepping and draping of the patient. The surgeon must also ensure that the fellow eye is taped closed and fully protected from inadvertent injury during the course of the surgery.

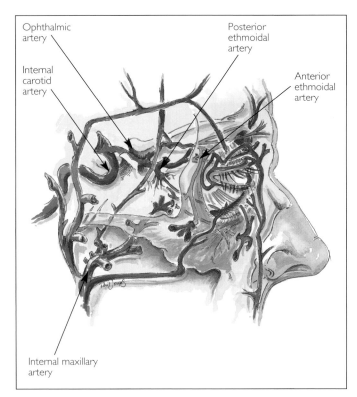

**Figure 24.2**
Vascular anatomy of the orbit and periorbital region.

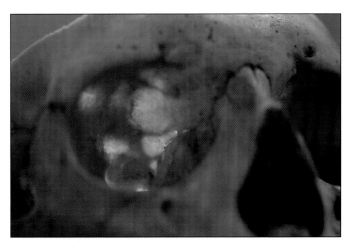

**Figure 24.3**
Transillumination of a skull demonstrating how thin the roof of the orbit (floor of the anterior cranial fossa) can be in some patients.

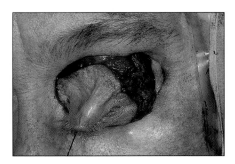

**Figure 24.4**
A total exenteration in progress.

The patient's computed tomography (CT) and/or magnetic resonance imaging (MRI) scans should be placed on the viewing screen in the operating room to be referred to if necessary during the course of the surgery.

## Total exenteration

The proposed skin incision is marked with gentian violet around the orbital margin. The eyelids are sutured together with two 2/0 silk sutures and the sutures held with an artery clip (Figure 24.4). Next, the skin and superficial subcutaneous tissues are incised with a No. 15 Bard Parker blade. The skin edges are firmly retracted and the blade is exchanged for a cutting diathermy blade, which is used to carry the dissection down to the periosteum of the orbital rim. Careful attention is paid to haemostasis with the monopolar diathermy blade. The larger vessels that are encountered are cauterized with bipolar cautery forceps.

The periosteum at the orbital margin is then incised and elevated, with a Freer periosteal elevator, taking care not to disrupt it and provoke a prolapse of orbital fat. Jaffe retractors are placed around the orbit to retract the soft tissues. The periosteum is elevated from the orbital walls, beginning superotemporally. The Freer elevator should be used with great care along the orbital roof as dehiscences in the bone are frequent in the elderly. *This dissection must not be performed blind as this risks damage to the dura mater with a subsequent cerebrospinal fluid (CSF) leak. It is important to avoid the use of monopolar cautery along the orbital roof as this also risks causing a CSF leak in the presence of any bony defects.*

The dissection is continued inferotemporally. The lateral canthal tendon is incised with the diathermy blade. The zygomaticotemporal and zygomaticfacial vessels are cauterized as they are encountered. Any bleeding from the bone is managed with bone wax.

The dissection is then continued across the floor of the orbit. A constant vessel is encountered approximately 8 mm posterior to the inferior orbital margin. This is cauterized. Great care is taken to avoid inadvertent injury to the infraorbital neurovascular bundle. The infraorbital nerve may lie exposed along the floor of the orbit. The cutting diathermy is used to dissect tissue across the anterior portion of the inferior orbital fissure.

As the dissection approaches the medial canthus, the angular vessels are cauterized. The anterior limb of the medial canthal tendon is incised with the diathermy blade, the lacrimal sac is rotated posteriorly and laterally and the posterior limb of the medial canthal tendon is incised. The nasolacrimal duct is severed. The periosteum is raised from the medial orbital wall with a Freer elevator taking great care not to fracture the lamina papyracea. The anterior and posterior ethmoidal vessels are identified as they pass through the periosteum to their respective foramina and cauterized. Superomedially, the trochlea is elevated along with the periosteum.

Once the dissection has approached the apex of the orbit, the periosteum is incised with the diathermy blade medially and laterally. Two large curved artery clips are applied across the apical orbital tissues, one medially and one laterally (Figure 24.5).

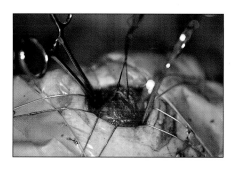

**Figure 24.5**
Two large curved artery clips are placed across the posterior orbital tissues prior to completion of the exenteration. (In this case a subtotal exenteration.)

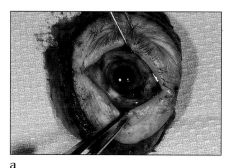

a                    b

**Figure 24.6**
(a) An exenteration specimen. (b) The exenterated orbit at the completion of surgery.

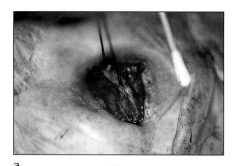

a

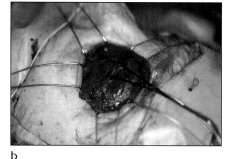

b

**Figure 24.7**
(a) A skin incision has been made 2 mm above and below the lash line. (b) The skin and orbicularis muscle has been dissected from the underlying orbital septum. Multiple Jaffe eyelid retractors have been placed to aid exposure of the orbital rim.

Curved enucleation scissors are used to excise the tissues anterior to the clips while pulling anteriorly on the traction sutures. Alternatively, a snare may be used.

The extent of the exenteration performed is dictated by the clinical requirements. The exenteration can be modified to a less extensive procedure or to a more radical resection that involves the removal of orbital walls and paranasal sinuses.

Bipolar cautery is applied to the stump of tissue at the orbital apex (Figure 24.6). Bone wax may be required for any bleeding vessels that perforate the orbital walls. Gelfoam soaked with thrombin is applied to the socket and swabs moistened with 1:10,000 adrenaline are placed over this with pressure for 5 min.

In cases where the indication for exenteration is a malignancy, the socket is carefully inspected for any residual tumour tissue. The adequacy of resection may be judged with the aid of frozen-section control. The resection of additional orbital apical tissue may be required.

The stump of the nasolacrimal duct is oversewn with inter-rupted 5/0 Vicryl sutures. If the socket is to be left to heal by granulation, a Lyofoam pack is placed into the socket and a firm pressure dressing applied for 1 week.

Postoperatively, the socket is cleaned daily for 2 weeks and Lyofoam gently reapplied. The frequency of the wound care is gradually reduced over the course of the next month. The wound can be left exposed and camouflaged with a Cartella shield once the discharge has ceased. The patient is discouraged from inspecting the exenterated socket until this has completely healed. This may take 2–4 months. An orbital prosthesis should not be fitted until the socket has completely healed.

## Subtotal exenteration

In a subtotal exenteration the eyelid skin is preserved. The skin incision is placed 2 mm behind the lash line and undermined to the arcus marginalis of the orbit (Figure 24.7). The exenteration is completed as for a total exenteration and the skin is then draped into the exenterated socket. The socket usually heals within 3 to 4 weeks.

## Extended exenteration

In an extended exenteration, adjacent structures, such as paranasal sinuses, orbital bones and intracranial structures, may be resected, depending on the extent of the patient's disease process. Such a procedure is performed by a multidisciplinary team and is beyond the scope of this text.

## Orbital reconstruction

There are a number of reconstructive options for the manage-ment of the exenterated socket. The suitability of these options must be determined for each individual patient.

## Spontaneous granulation

This approach can yield good results, particularly in the case of elderly patients for whom more lengthy operative procedures are unsuitable (Figures 24.8 and 24.9).

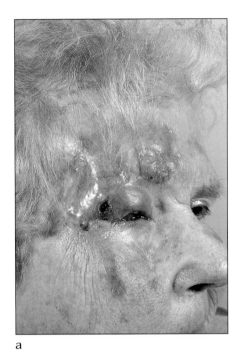

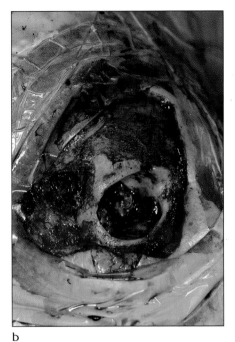

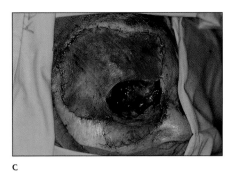

c

**Figure 24.8**
(a) Elderly female patient with neglected squamous cell carcinoma of the periorbital region with orbital invasion. (b) An extensive resection of the tumour and a total exenteration. (c) A split-thickness skin graft has been placed over the forehead, temple and cheek wounds. The socket has been left to granulate.

a                                    b

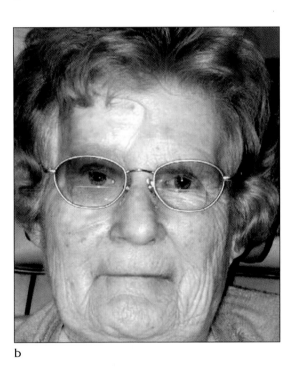

**Figure 24.9**
(a) The appearance of the socket 2 months postoperatively. (b) The appearance of the patient fitted with an orbital prosthesis.

a                                    b

## Advantages

This approach is simple and facilitates easy examination of the socket where the possibility of tumour recurrence exists. It reduces the operating time. Once healed, the socket cavity can be covered with a patch or fitted with a silicone prosthesis, which is held in position either by a spectacle mount or by a tissue adhesive.

## Disadvantages

The healing period is prolonged and requires frequent dressing changes. Spontaneous fistulae communicating with the ethmoid sinus can occur. The eyebrow can be drawn inferiorly by wound contracture.

## *Split-thickness skin graft*

The graft is harvested from the thigh with a dermatome set to 1/16 inch. The width of the required graft is determined and the appropriate blade chosen for the dermatome. The thigh is prepped and draped. Glycerine is used to lubricate the skin. The skin is then flattened with the edge of a small skin graft board in front of the dermatome. The skin graft is then harvested and the

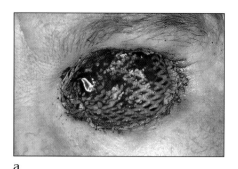
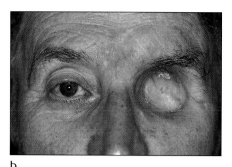
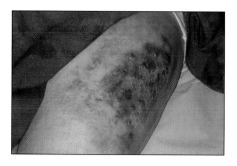

a                                    b

**Figure 24.10**
(a) A meshed split-thickness skin graft placed into the socket and sutured to the skin at the orbital margin. (b) The appearance of the healed socket 1 month postoperatively.

**Figure 24.11**
A poorly healing skin graft donor site in an elderly patient. The wound took 3 months to heal.

thigh wound covered with a Granuflex dressing. A piece of Gamgee and a bandage are also applied to aid haemostasis and to reduce the amount of exudate. This dressing should be changed if any exudate leaks from it. Once the wound is dry, a nonadherent dry dressing can be used to protect the area from clothing. The area should be massaged with Vaseline.

The skin graft is passed through a meshing device, which expands the graft and assists the egress of serosanguinous fluid. The graft is inserted into the socket and the edges of the graft are sutured to the skin edges around the socket (Figure 24.10a). The socket cavity is packed with Lyofoam and a compressive dressing applied. This is left undisturbed for 7 days.

Once the dressing has been removed, the socket is cleaned and Lyofoam again used if the socket is wet or if there is a fistula to a paranasal sinus. This is changed twice a week. In the absence of a sinus fistula, alginate sheet dressings can be used and changed twice a week until the socket has healed. Any adherent debris can be removed with hydrogen peroxide.

A piece of Lyofoam is rolled into a ball and inserted into the socket cavity, holding the graft against the orbital walls. A pressure dressing is then applied for 1 week. Postoperatively, the graft should be cleaned on a daily basis until healed and any debris gently removed using hydrogen peroxide on cotton-tipped applicators.

## Advantages

The use of a skin graft shortens the healing period. It prevents undue wound contracture and helps to maintain the depth of the socket, enabling suitable fitting of an orbital prosthesis. It also facilitates easy examination of the socket where the possibility of tumour recurrence exists.

## Disadvantages

This approach requires a separate donor site and is associated with pain and potential morbidity (Figure 24.11).

The skin graft may fail in patients who are at risk of poor healing, e.g. diabetic patients, following previous radiotherapy.

# Local flaps

A local flap, e.g. a temporalis muscle transposition flap, may be used in patients who do not pose a risk of tumour recurrence.

## Advantages

The flap can be used to make the socket deformity shallower in a patient who does not want to wear a prosthesis. It can be combined with a split-thickness skin graft.

## Disadvantages

The procedure leaves a secondary depression in the temple. The temporal branch of the facial nerve may be damaged, resulting in a brow ptosis.

Other local flaps, e.g. a median forehead flap, may be used to cover a sino-orbital fistula.

# Free flaps

A free flap, e.g. a rectus abdominis free flap, is particularly useful for the reconstruction of the defects from an extended exenteration.

## Advantages

The free flap can prevent the severe cosmetic disfigurement of an extended exenteration with exposed sinus cavities.

## Disadvantages

These procedures are difficult to perform and extremely time-consuming. There is a risk of flap failure and donor site

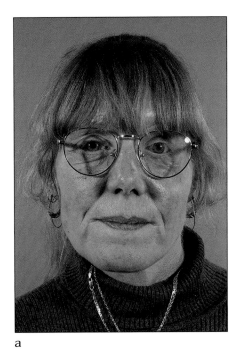 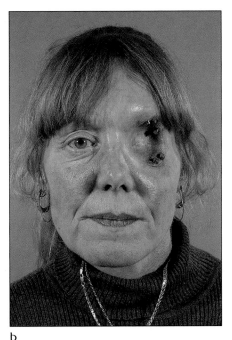

a                          b

**Figure 24.12**
(a) A patient who has undergone an exenteration followed by a 2-stage osseointegration procedure wearing a light-weight orbital prosthesis. (b) The patient demonstrating her osseointegrated implants.

morbidity. If the flap is too bulky, it may prevent the successful wearing of an orbital prosthesis.

## Osseointegration technique

Osseointegrated titanium implants permit direct coupling of an orbitofacial prosthesis to the bony orbital margins. This is a two-stage procedure. In the first stage titanium screws are implanted into the superior, lateral and inferior orbital bony margins. These are covered by soft tissue and left to integrate with the bone. At the second stage, performed approximately 6 months later, the implants are exposed and titanium cylinders (abutments) are attached to the implants. A series of bars or magnetic devices are attached to the abutments. These allow firm fixation of the prosthesis (Figure 24.12).

### Advantages

This technique allows reliable alignment of the prosthesis and good retention. Removal and reattachment of the prosthesis by the patient are relatively easy. The prosthesis can be made light and much easier to blend with the surrounding skin. The cosmetic results can be excellent for the carefully selected patient. The patient will usually require the additional use of tinted spectacles as additional camouflage.

### Disadvantages

The technique is time-consuming and expensive. The implants must be kept meticulously clean to avoid inflammation or infec-

tion and ultimately loss of the implants. Extra implants may be used as 'sleepers' to be used in the event of loss of any implants.

## Prosthetic options

Many patients abandon orbital and orbitofacial prostheses for a number of reasons:

1.  An unnatural appearance with an absence of blinking and ocular movements
2.  Intolerance to local tissue adhesives
3.  Difficulty camouflaging the edges of the prosthesis
4.  Rapid degradation of the prosthesis
5.  Expense

A simple alternative is the use of a standard black 'pirate' patch. For female patients individual customized patches can be obtained. Spectacles with an opaque lens and a side shield may also be preferred by some patients.

## Further reading

1.  Dutton JJ. *Atlas of clinical and surgical orbital anatomy.* Philadelphia: WB Saunders, 1994.
2.  Nerad JA. Osseointegration for the exenterated orbit. In: Bosniak S, ed., *Principles and practice of ophthalmic plastic and reconstructive surgery.* Philadelphia: WB Saunders, 1996, pp. 1150–60.
3.  Nerad JA, Carter KD, LaVelle WE, Fyler A, Branemark PI. The osseointegration technique for the rehabilitation of the exenterated orbit. *Arch Ophthalmol* (1991) **109**:1032–8.

# 25

# Socket reconstruction

## Introduction

The optimal time to achieve the best functional and cosmetic result for the anophthalmic patient is at the time of enucleation. Preoperative planning and a meticulous surgical approach will minimize the risks of complications and reduce the need for secondary surgical reconstruction. Nevertheless, secondary socket surgery represents a significant workload for the oculoplastic surgeon and can be extremely challenging.

Most socket reconstructive surgery is required to address the following problems:

- A volume deficit following loss of the globe
- Contracture of the socket
- Orbital implant exposure, extrusion, malposition

Many patients have additional eyelid malpositions which also require surgery. The patient must be carefully assessed and counselled about the nature of any proposed surgery, its risks and potential complications. The surgery may have to be carried out in stages. The patient may have to accept a lengthy period of time without an ocular prosthesis. Such surgery can have profound effects on a patient professionally, socially and emotionally. It is important to ensure that the patient has realistic expectations of the surgery.

## Patient evaluation

### History

The patient's current complaints must be documented, e.g. pain, discomfort, discharge, instability of the ocular prosthesis, poor movement of the ocular prosthesis, poor cosmetic appearance. The following details should be obtained:

1. The date of the enucleation/evisceration
2. The indication for the enucleation/evisceration
3. The type and size of any orbital implant
4. The nature of any previous socket or eyelid surgery
5. A history of prior radiotherapy treatment
6. A history of previous trauma

### Examination

The patient should be examined initially with the ocular prosthesis in place. Any features of the post-enucleation socket syndrome (PESS) are noted (enophthalmos, an upper eyelid sulcus deformity, ptosis or eyelid retraction, laxity of the lower eyelid, a backward tilt of the ocular prosthesis) (Figure 25.1).

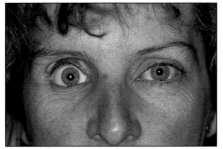
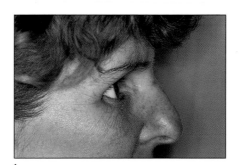

a
b

**Figure 25.1**
(a) A young patient who has the typical features of a post-enucleation socket syndrome. (b) A lateral view of the patient demonstrating a typical backward tilt to the prosthesis.

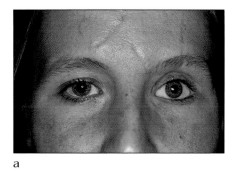 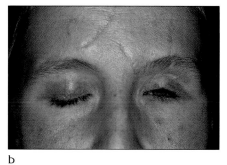 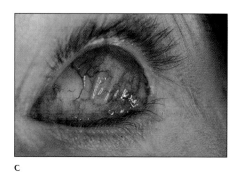

a        b        c

### Figure 25.2
(a) An anophthalmic patient with left upper eyelid retraction and an upper eyelid sulcus defect. (b) The same patient demonstrating lagophthalmos. (c) Examination of the socket reveals that superior fornix adhesions are the cause of her lagophthalmos.

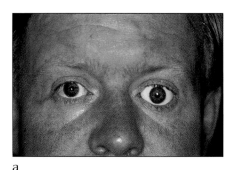 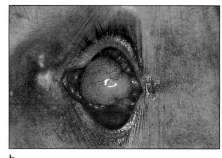

a        b

### Figure 25.3
(a) This patient complained of poor cosmesis and instability of his artificial eye. (b) Examination of his socket revealed a large conjunctival inclusion cyst.

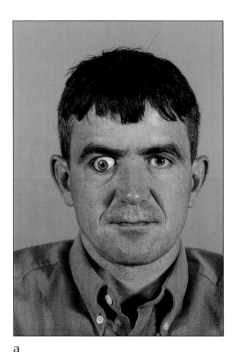 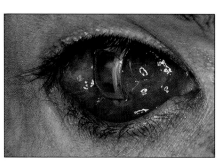 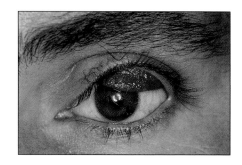

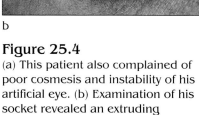

b

### Figure 25.4
(a) This patient also complained of poor cosmesis and instability of his artificial eye. (b) Examination of his socket revealed an extruding Castroviejo orbital implant.

### Figure 25.5
This patient complained of discomfort and a mucus discharge. His artificial eye had not been polished for a number of years. Eversion of the upper eyelid revealed a papillary conjunctivitis.

a

Any eyelid malpositions or lagophthalmos are noted (Figure 25.2). The degree of movement of the ocular prosthesis is ascertained. The prosthesis is then removed, noting any instability. The artificial eye is examined for scratches, surface deposits or other blemishes. Its size and shape are noted.

The socket is examined carefully. Any discharge, bleeding, conjunctival inflammation, implant exposure, granulomas, cysts, or adhesions are noted (Figures 25.2–25.4).

The fornices are examined and the upper eyelid everted to exclude the presence of papillae (Figure 25.5). The socket is gently palpated with a gloved finger to confirm the presence of an implant. The patient is asked to look in all directions as the socket is observed to ascertain the positions of the ocular muscles and the degree of movement. In particular, the position of the inferior rectus muscle is determined. These positions are documented. If the patient has a ptosis, the patient should be examined thoroughly to determine the underlying cause. A patient who complains of tearing and discharge should be examined to exclude the possibility of an associated obstruction of the lacrimal drainage system.

# Correction of an orbital volume deficiency

Patients who present with a typical PESS may benefit from secondary orbital implant surgery, but the surgical procedure is more difficult and the results are less predictable than primary orbital implantation. Patients undergoing secondary orbital implantation are more likely to require additional surgical procedures. Although the volume deficiency improves following surgery, there is commonly a variable recurrence of the upper lid sulcus defect some months following surgery once postoperative orbital oedema has completely resolved.

The type of orbital implant to be used needs to be determined by taking a number of factors into consideration:

- The age and general health of the patient
- The state of the socket
- The size, nature and complications of any orbital implant already present
- The degree of movement of the extraocular muscles
- The state of the ocular adnexa
- The cost

The orbital implants of choice for secondary orbital implantation are:

1. 'Baseball' implant
2. Hydroxyapatite implant
3. Porous polyethylene implant
4. Bioceramic implant
5. Dermis fat graft implant

The 'baseball implant' is of use in older patients who do not wish to take advantage of the second-stage placement of a motility peg. The implant can improve a volume deficiency but the motility results are unpredictable. If the degree of movement of the implant is good but that of the overlying ocular prosthesis poor, this has to be accepted.

One of the modern porous implants is ideally reserved for a patient who would wish to undergo a second-stage placement of a motility peg if the movement of the artificial eye were poor in spite of acceptable movement of the implant itself. This type of implant is ideal for the patient who has an old extruding/tilted implant. An implant exchange is performed in the absence of any socket infection. The use of this type of implant is ill-advised, however, following prior radiotherapy, in the presence of severe conjunctival inflammation or socket contracture, or for the reconstruction of badly disorganized sockets.

The dermis fat graft is preferred for the reconstruction of the socket which has mild to moderate contracture in addition to a volume deficiency. It is the implant of choice for the reconstruction of badly disorganized sockets, and when complications have necessitated the removal of a porous implant or infected synthetic implant.

# *Preoperative preparation*

The patient should be advised about:

1. The advantages, disadvantages, risks and potential complications of a secondary implant procedure
2. The implant options
3. The options regarding implant wrapping materials
4. Postoperative pain and its management
5. The postoperative compressive dressing
6. The use of a temporary suture tarsorrhaphy
7. The use of a postoperative conformer
8. The likelihood of a temporary postoperative ptosis
9. The role of the ocularist and the timing of the fitting of the ocular prosthesis

Informed consent should be obtained after the patient has had time to consider the options.

The patient should discontinue aspirin and any other antiplatelet drugs if medically permissible at least 2 weeks preoperatively. Likewise, anticoagulants should only be altered or discontinued after discussion with the patient's haematologist. Any bacterial conjunctivitis should be treated preoperatively and topical steroids used to reduce any conjunctival inflammation. It is preferable for the patient to refrain from wearing an old ocular prosthesis and to wear a surgical conformer for at least 2 weeks prior to surgery.

---

A computed tomography (CT) scan of the orbits and paranasal sinuses should be performed if a patient has previously suffered orbital trauma to exclude the possibility of a missed orbital wall blowout fracture (Figures 25.6–25.8). If a significant fracture is discovered, this should be repaired before undertaking a secondary orbital implant procedure.

---

# Secondary orbital implant procedure: surgical technique
## *Spherical implant*

The anaesthetist should be warned that the dissection of the socket can provoke the oculocardiac reflex, inducing a severe bradycardia and, occasionally, asystole. The anaesthetist may wish to use glycopyrrolate or atropine prior to the dissection. Prior to the induction of general anaesthesia it is very important that the surgeon examine the patient's socket while asking the patient to

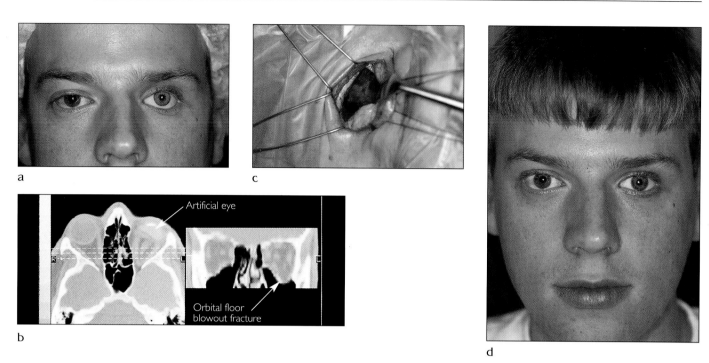

## Figure 25.6

(a) A patient with a post-enucleation socket syndrome referred for a secondary orbital implant procedure. He had undergone an enucleation of a badly ruptured globe following blunt trauma without the placement of an orbital implant. (b) A preoperative CT scan revealed a previously overlooked orbital floor and a minor anterior medial wall blowout fracture. (c) The appearance of the orbital floor fracture seen intraoperatively. (d) The postoperative appearance of the patient following repair of the orbital floor blowout fracture with placement of an orbital floor Medpor implant, the secondary implantation of an hydroxyapatite orbital implant and the fitting of a custom-made artificial eye.

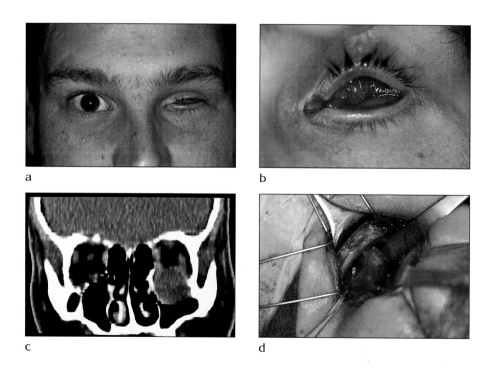

## Figure 25.7

(a) A patient referred for the management of a post-enucleation socket syndrome following a history of blunt trauma. (b) The appearance of his contracted anophthalmic socket. (c) His preoperative CT scan revealed the presence of an extensive orbital floor blowout fracture with the left globe subluxated into the maxillary sinus. (d) The intraoperative appearance of the globe seen below the inferior orbital margin.

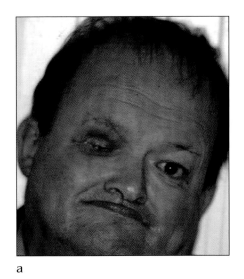

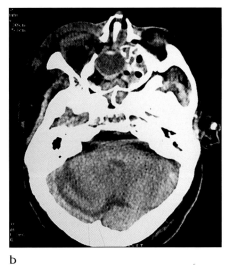

a                              b

**Figure 25.8**
(a) A patient referred following severe blunt trauma to the orbit with an apparent anophthalmos. (b) A CT scan revealed that the right globe was completely subluxated into the ethmoid sinus.

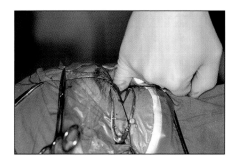

**Figure 25.9**
Blunt dissection of socket adhesions with a finger.

look up and down. The position of the inferior rectus muscle is marked on the conjunctiva using gentian violet. This is to avoid the possibility of placing the orbital implant beneath the inferior rectus muscle.

> The surgeon must also ensure that the fellow eye is taped closed and fully protected from inadvertent injury during the course of the surgery.

The face, eyelids and conjunctival sac should be thoroughly prepared with an antiseptic agent and a cataract drape applied. A Clarke's eyelid speculum is placed to exclude the eyelashes from the surgical field. A volume of 3 ml of 0.5% Marcain (bupivacaine) with 1:200,000 units of adrenaline is injected subconjunctivally. A horizontal incision is made through the conjunctiva above the inferior rectus muscle using a No. 15 Bard Parker blade. The conjunctiva is dissected into the inferior fornix and then 8–10 mm into the superior fornix, taking great care not to damage the underlying levator aponeurosis; 4/0 silk traction sutures are then placed through the superior and inferior edges of the conjunctiva and fixated to the drapes with artery clips.

The central Tenon's fascia is then incised centrally with sharp straight scissors and then blunt-tipped straight scissors are opened to expose the intraconal fat. A finger is inserted into the socket to ascertain whether any adhesions are present (Figure 25.9). Any adhesions found are dissected bluntly to avoid damage to the nerve supply to the extraocular muscles.

Four 4/0 silk traction sutures are placed through the Tenon's fascia and fixated to the drapes with artery clips. A double-armed 5/0 Vicryl suture is placed through the approximate anterior positions of all four recti muscles. The muscles themselves are not dissected to avoid further trauma.

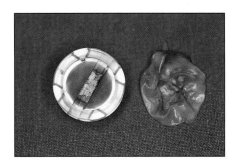

**Figure 25.10**
A Castroviejo implant removed with its fibrous capsule.

If an implant is present, this must be very carefully dissected from the surrounding tissues. A Castroviejo/Roper Hall type of implant is relatively easy to remove and yields very good results following an implant exchange as the recti are easily identified and preserved. The implant capsule should be carefully dissected from the socket (Figure 25.10). Other types of implant are not as straightforward to remove.

The appropriate size of orbital implant is determined with the use of sizing spheres. If the Tenon's fascia cannot be closed over the surface of the sizing sphere without undue tension, a smaller sphere should be substituted. The implant of appropriate size is then wrapped in the material which has been selected by the patient during the preoperative consultation, e.g. donor sclera, Vicryl mesh, autogenous fascia lata, temporalis fascia. It is then inserted into the intraconal fat space using a Carter sphere injector. The Vicryl sutures are attached to the implant as far anteriorly as possible.

A patch graft of donor sclera or autogenous fascia is then placed over the suture line to reduce any risk of implant exposure. Anterior Tenon's fascia is then closed with interrupted 7/0 Vicryl sutures, and finally the conjunctiva is closed likewise.

A sterile surgical conformer of appropriate size and shape is inserted into the conjunctival sac, ensuring that the eyelids will close passively over the conformer without creating tension on the conjunctival suture line. If there is any concern about the possibility of excessive postoperative swelling, a temporary suture tarsorrhaphy should be undertaken using a central 4/0 nylon suture passed through tarsorrhaphy tubing. A retrobulbar injection of 5 ml of 0.5% Marcain (bupivacaine) and 1:200,000 units of adrenaline is given to aid postoperative analgesia. An intravenous injection of a broad-spectrum antibiotic is given along with an anti-inflammatory agent and an opiate analgesic. Topical antibiotic ointment is instilled into the conjunctival sac and a pressure dressing and bandage are applied. These are not removed for a minimum of 5 days.

# Postoperative management

The patient is discharged on 1 week's course of systemic antibiotic, a 2-week course of a systemic anti-inflammatory agent and an analgesic. Topical antibiotics are instilled for 4 weeks after removal of the dressing 5–7 days postoperatively. The patient should not be fitted with an artificial eye until a minimum of 8 weeks have passed to allow sufficient wound healing and complete resolution of postoperative oedema. If the artificial eye is fitted too soon after surgery the risk of implant exposure is increased. In addition, the artificial eye will not fit the socket properly once complete resolution of postoperative orbital oedema has occurred.

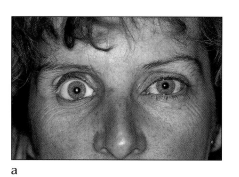

a

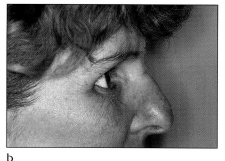

b

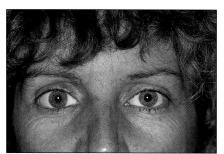

c

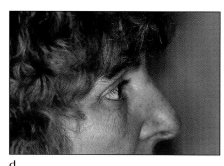

d

**Figure 25.11**
(a) A patient without an orbital implant who has a typical post-enucleation socket syndrome. (b) A lateral view of the patient reveals a typical backward tilt of the artificial eye. (c) The patient following the placement of a secondary orbital implant. (d) A lateral view of the patient demonstrates that the artificial eye lies within the correct plane.

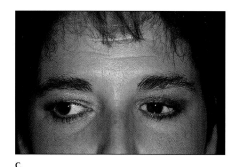

a

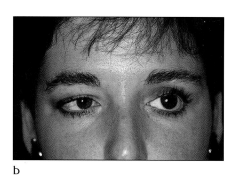

b

c

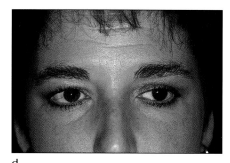

d

**Figure 25.12**
(a,b) A patient with a Castroviejo orbital implant who complained of a poor cosmesis, chronic socket pain and discharge. (c,d) The patient following removal of the Castroviejo orbital implant which was exchanged for an hydroxyapatite orbital implant. The patient is seen following placement of a motility peg 12 months following implantation.

The degree of movement of the implant may be poor initially as a consequence of neuropraxia or direct trauma to the extraocular muscles. This frequently improves over the course of the next few months.

The improvement in the features of a post-enucleation socket syndrome following placement of a secondary orbital implant is demonstrated in Figure 25.11. The improvement gained by the exchange of a Castroviejo for an hydroxyapatite orbital implant is demonstrated in Figure 25.12.

# Dermis fat graft

A 25 mm circle is outlined on the inferior quadrant of the abdomen or on the upper outer quadrant of the buttock. The circle is extended to form an ellipse to facilitate wound closure. A volume of 3 ml of 0.5% Marcain with 1:200,000 units of adrenaline is injected subconjunctivally in the socket and a further 10 ml is injected intradermally in the anterior abdominal wall at the proposed site of the graft excision to create a peau d'orange appearance.

Next, an epidermal incision is made around the circular mark and the epidermis shaved off the proposed graft using a No. 15 Bard Parker blade. An incision is made through one edge of the dermis and the dermis fat graft is removed using curved scissors. The skin is then incised along the elliptical mark and further tissue excised to create an elliptical wound. The wound is closed using interrupted subcutaneous 4/0 Vicryl sutures and interrupted 4/0 nylon sutures for the skin.

The socket is prepared and dissected as for a secondary spherical implant. The dermis fat graft is then inserted into the socket and the Vicryl sutures are attached to the anterior surface of the graft. If there is a conjunctival lining deficit, the sutures are positioned closer to the edge of the graft in order to leave a central bare area of graft exposed; this epithelializes gradually. As the sutures are tied, the fat is reduced into the intraconal fat space. The conjunctiva is sutured to the front surface of the graft with interrupted 7/0 Vicryl sutures, leaving an area of the graft bare in the presence of socket contracture. In the absence of a lining deficit, the conjunctiva is closed over the dermis fat graft.

A sterile surgical conformer of appropriate size and shape is inserted into the conjunctival sac, ensuring that the eyelids will close passively over the conformer without creating tension on the conjunctival suture line. If there is any concern about the possibility of excessive postoperative swelling, a temporary suture tarsorrhaphy should be undertaken using a central 4/0 nylon suture passed through tarsorrhaphy tubing. A retrobulbar injection of 5 ml of 0.5% Marcain and 1:200,000 units of adrenaline is given to aid postoperative analgesia. An intravenous injection of a broad-spectrum antibiotic is given along with an anti-inflammatory agent and an opiate analgesic. Topical antibiotic ointment is instilled into the conjunctival sac and a pressure dressing and bandage are applied. These are not removed for a minimum of 5 days.

# *Postoperative management*

The patient is discharged on 1 week's course of systemic antibiotic, a 2–week course of a systemic anti-inflammatory agent and an analgesic. Topical antibiotics are instilled for 4 weeks after removal of the dressing 5–7 days postoperatively. The patient should not be fitted with an artificial eye until a minimum of 8 weeks have passed to allow sufficient wound healing and complete resolution of postoperative oedema.

# Correction of a residual orbital volume deficiency

If the patient has a residual orbital volume deficiency in spite of the insertion of a secondary orbital implant of adequate size, the next option is to proceed with the placement of a subperiosteal implant. Although there are a number of implant options, such as autogenous bone (e.g. calvarial bone graft), acrylic, homologous cartilage, silicone blocks and porous polyethylene, Proplast 2 remains the author's implant of choice. This synthetic implant is porous, which allows fibrovascular ingrowth. It is malleable, and easy to shape and insert through a small incision. It is well tolerated with excellent long-term results. Medpor (porous polyethylene) is also a very suitable implant material and can be easily cut into pieces and placed as separate pieces into the subperiosteal space.

Alternative or additional options are:

- A contralateral camouflage blepharoplasty
- A dermis fat graft insertion in the upper eyelid sulcus

A contralateral blepharoplasty may be performed on the opposite upper eyelid to provide a more symmetrical appearance in a patient who has an upper lid sulcus deformity but who does not wish to undergo a subperiosteal implant procedure. The patient must appreciate the small risks involved in such surgery performed around an only eye.

A small dermis fat graft can be inserted after exposing the orbital roof via a skin crease incision. The dermis is sutured to the periosteum of the orbital roof while the fat is placed in such a position as to mimic the preaponeurotic fat. The dermis fat graft is oversized to allow for postoperative atrophy. If the graft remains oversized it can be easily debulked.

# Subperiosteal orbital implant: surgical technique

A lateral canthal incision is marked along a skin crease using gentian violet. A volume of 3 ml of 0.5% Marcain with 1:200,000 units of adrenaline is injected subcutaneously. A lateral canthal skin incision is made using a Colorado needle leaving the lateral commissure intact. The soft tissues are dissected down to the periosteum. The periosteum of the lateral orbital margin is exposed by blunt dissection with a Freer periosteal elevator and a 2–3 cm vertical incision is made with the Colorado needle. The periosteum is raised and reflected from the lateral orbital wall and from the lateral aspect of the orbital floor, taking care not to extend to the region of the infraorbital nerve. The zygomatic vessels are cauterized.

Next, the Proplast implant is shaped with a No. 15 Bard Parker blade into a smooth contour with the bulk of the implant posteriorly. It is then divided into two or three pieces which are impregnated with gentamicin 80 mg in a 50 ml syringe filled with sterile saline. A finger is placed over the tip of the syringe while the plunger is alternately depressed and withdrawn until the air has been expelled from the implant and the gentamicin solution has permeated the pores (Figure 25.13).

The pieces are then inserted into the subperiosteal space side by side and the effect on the upper lid sulcus and the conjunctival sac is observed (Figure 25.14).

It is important not to overcorrect the volume replacement. The anterior aspect of the implant should not compromise the inferior fornix and should remain posterior to the inferior orbital margin. It should not be visible or palpable. The skin wound is closed using interrupted 5/0 Vicryl sutures for the subcutaneous layer and a continuous 7/0 Vicryl for the skin. A sterile surgical conformer of appropriate size and shape is inserted into the conjunctival sac, ensuring that the eyelids will close passively over the conformer. If the patient shows significant lower eyelid laxity, the operation can be combined with a lateral tarsal strip procedure.

An intravenous injection of a broad-spectrum antibiotic is given along with an anti-inflammatory agent. A pressure dressing and bandage are applied for 3 days.

## Postoperative management

The patient is discharged on 1 week's course of systemic antibiotic, a 2-week course of a systemic anti-inflammatory agent and an analgesic. The dressing is removed 3 days postoperatively and topical antibiotic is applied to the wound for 1 week. The patient should not be fitted with an artificial eye until a minimum of 4 weeks have passed to allow sufficient wound healing and complete resolution of postoperative oedema. The improvement in the features of a severe post-enucleation socket syndrome following the use of a secondary orbital implant and a subperiosteal implant is demonstrated in Figure 25.15.

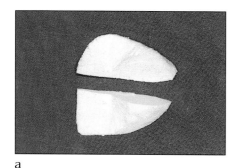
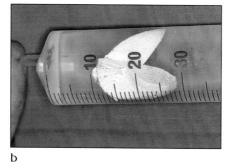
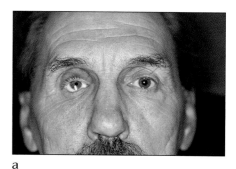

**Figure 25.13**
(a) A Proplast implant divided into two separate pieces for implantation. (b) The pieces have been inserted into a 50 ml syringe containing gentamicin.

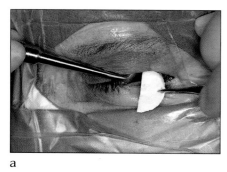
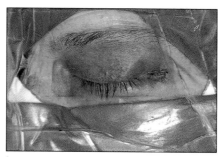
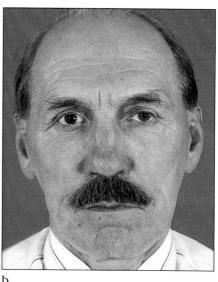

**Figure 25.14**
(a) A piece of Proplast is inserted through a small lateral canthal incision. (b) The appearance following wound closure.

**Figure 25.15**
(a) A patient with a severe post-enucleation socket syndrome. (b) The patient following placement of a secondary orbital implant and a subperiosteal orbital implant.

# Lower eyelid laxity

Lower eyelid laxity in the anophthalmic patient can be managed with a lateral tarsal strip procedure in most cases. The artificial eye should not be worn for at least 4 weeks following the surgery. If the medial canthal tendon is very lax it is preferable to place a lower eyelid fascial sling.

## *Lower lid fascia sling: surgical technique*

A lateral canthal incision is marked along a skin crease using gentian violet. A small incision is also marked over the medial canthal tendon and three 2 mm subciliary incisions marked in the lower eyelid. A volume of 3 ml of 0.5% Marcain with 1:200,000 units of adrenaline is injected subcutaneously. A lateral canthal skin incision is made using a Colorado needle. The soft tissues are dissected down to the periosteum. The periosteum of the lateral orbital margin is exposed by blunt dissection with a Freer periosteal eleva-

tor and a 2–3 cm vertical incision is made with the Colorado needle. The periosteum is raised and reflected from the anterior portion of the lateral orbital wall. A 2 mm hole is drilled through the bone at the level of the lateral canthal tendon.

A small incision is made using the Colorado needle at the medial canthus, and the medial canthal tendon is exposed. A 2 mm strip of autogenous fascia lata or temporalis fascia is threaded around the anterior limb of the medial canthal tendon close to its insertion, taking care not to damage the canaliculi (Figure 25.16).

This is threaded along the lower eyelid in front of the tarsal plate close to the eyelid margin via a series of small skin incisions using a Wright's ptosis needle. The fascia is threaded through the hole and through a hole made in the periosteum. The fascia is then tied to itself with 5/0 Ethibond sutures (Figure 25.17).

The lateral canthal wound is closed using interrupted 5/0 Vicryl sutures for the subcutaneous layer and continuous 7/0 Vicryl sutures for the skin. The other wounds are closed with interrupted 7/0 Vicryl sutures. A sterile surgical conformer of appropriate size and shape is inserted into the conjunctival sac. A compressive dressing is placed for a minimum period of 5 days. The ocular prosthesis is not replaced for at least 4 weeks.

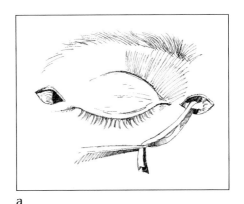

a

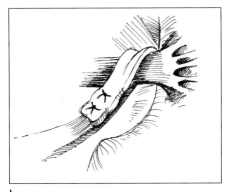

b

**Figure 25.16**
(a) The medial canthal tendon is exposed by blunt dissection and the fascia looped around it. (b) The fascia is sutured to itself below the tendon.

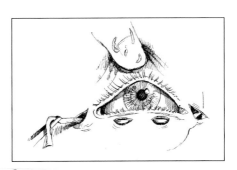

a

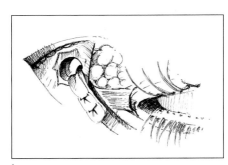

b

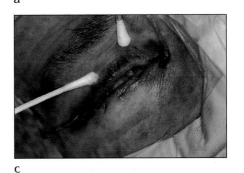

c

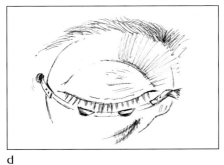

d

**Figure 25.17**
(a) The fascia is threaded along the lower eyelid via a series of small skin incisions. (b) The fascia is threaded through a small drill hole in the lateral orbital margin and tied to itself. (c) An intraoperative photograph of the fascial sling. (d) A diagram demonstrating the desired position of the sling.

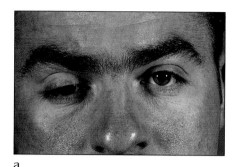
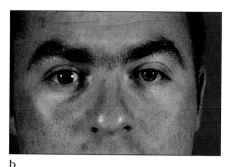
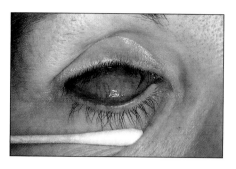

a

b

**Figure 25.18**
(a) An anophthalmic patient with a marked right ptosis. (b) The patient following a right levator aponeurosis advancement procedure.

**Figure 25.19**
Marked shallowing of the inferior fornix due to the presence of an orbital implant placed too low within the socket.

# Ptosis

The ptosis should be evaluated after the orbital volume deficit has been corrected, any lower eyelid tightening has been performed, and a new ocular prosthesis has been fitted. A temporary ptosis is common following any socket surgery and time should be allowed for spontaneous recovery. The ocularist may be able to correct small degrees of ptosis by manipulating the ocular prosthesis.

Any residual ptosis is then evaluated and managed as it would be in the presence of a normal eye (Figure 25.18).

The patient must, however, appreciate that any ptosis procedure will inevitably compromise the patient's reflex blink, necessitating the long term use of topical lubricants and the possible requirement for more frequent polishing of the artificial eye.

# Shallowing of the inferior fornix

The inferior fornix may shallow and cause instability of ocular prosthesis for three reasons:

1.  The suspensory ligament of the inferior fornix has been damaged
2.  There is contracture of the conjunctiva of the inferior fornix
3.  A socket or subperiosteal implant has been placed incorrectly or has migrated (Figure 25.19)

## *Management*

If the suspensory ligament is damaged but the conjunctival lining is normal, the inferior fornix can be reformed using fornix-deepening sutures in conjunction with a silicone explant (usually used in retinal reattachment procedures). This may be combined with a horizontal eyelid-shortening procedure. It is important to ascertain that there is sufficient conjunctival lining present by holding the eyelid forward. The fornix will automatically reform if there is no shortage of conjunctiva. If there is conjunctival contracture, a mucous membrane graft will be required. An incorrectly placed implant will usually have to be removed and repositioned.

## *Fornix-deepening sutures: surgical technique*

A volume of 3 ml of 0.5% Marcain and 1:200,000 units of adrenaline is injected subconjunctivally into the inferior fornix. A silicone retinal explant (276) is trimmed to a suitable size. A 4/0 nylon suture is passed through the explant and through the conjunctiva in the proposed position of the depth of the inferior fornix centrally. The needle should engage the periosteum of the inferior orbital margin and then exit the skin at the level of the inferior orbital margin. The second needle of the double-armed suture is then passed in the same fashion 2 mm medial or lateral to the first needle. The needles are then passed through a small piece of silicone explant and tied externally (Figure 25.20). Additional sutures are placed medial and lateral to this suture.

A surgical conformer of appropriate size and shape is placed and a compressive dressing applied for 5 days. Topical antibiotic is used for 2 weeks. The sutures and explant are removed after a period of 6 weeks. Another surgical conformer is fitted to ensure that the fornix is maintained. An artificial eye is fitted without delay.

# Management of implant complications
## *Orbital implant exposure*

The risk of exposure of an orbital implant should be minimized by:

1.  Careful patient selection
2.  Avoiding an oversized implant

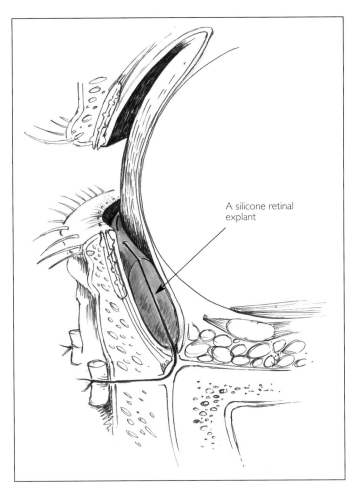

**Figure 25.20**
A silicone retinal explant is placed and sutured into the inferior fornix.

3. The use of a suitable wrapping material and a patch graft
4. Meticulous intraoperative haemostasis
5. Meticulous surgical technique
6. Strict attention to asepsis
7. The use of a compressive dressing postoperatively
8. Ensuring good quality ocular prosthetic aftercare at the appropriate time postoperatively

Implant exposure should be a rare problem. It can be classified into early and late exposure.

## Early exposure

If the orbital implant becomes exposed it is important to correct the defect as soon as possible to prevent further exposure and infection. The patient's ocular prosthesis should be removed and replaced with a surgical conformer which is vaulted anteriorly to ensure no contact with the area of exposure. A topical antibiotic/steroid is prescribed. The conjunctiva is gently undermined over the area of exposure and the edges revised with Westcott scissors. A temporalis fascial patch graft is harvested and two circular pieces are shaped. These are inserted to lie over the defect beneath the conjunctiva, one on top of the other. The conjunctival edges are then sutured to the graft with interrupted 8/0 Vicryl sutures. The conformer is replaced and a compressive dressing is left in place for 7 days. The ocular prosthesis is not replaced until the graft has epithelialized fully. Donor sclera is more convenient to use but its use is now rarely acceptable to patients.

## Late exposure

The management of late implant exposure depends on the area of exposure and the health of the adjacent conjunctiva. A relatively small area of exposure can be managed with a temporalis fascial patch graft, a small hard palate mucosal graft (Figure 25.21) or a small dermal graft. The implant surface should be burred away using a small diamond burr before placing the graft.

An alternative solution is to remove the implant and place it deeper within the socket if this was not done at the time of the initial implantation. Procedures that involve the use of local tarsoconjunctival flaps should be avoided as these can cause secondary eyelid problems or socket contracture.

If there is a large area of implant exposure with unhealthy adjacent conjunctiva or evidence of chronic infection, the implant should be removed and exchanged for a dermis fat graft.

## Implant malposition

An implant placed secondarily may become malpositioned in the socket and cause shallowing of a fornix. The ocularist may then have difficulty fitting the ocular prosthesis. A CT scan should be

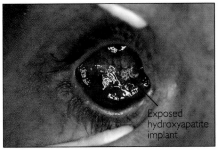

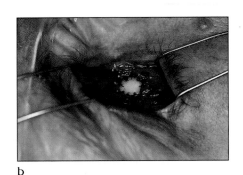

**Figure 25.21**
(a) A small area of exposure of an hydroxyapatite orbital implant. (b) The exposed area has been covered with a small hard palate mucosal graft.

a

b

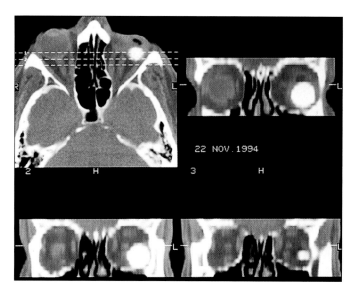
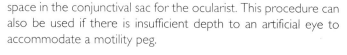

**Figure 25.22**
A CT scan demonstrating a malpositioned hydroxyapatite orbital implant.

performed to demonstrate the relationship of the implant to the extraocular muscles (Figure 25.22). The implant should then be removed and repositioned.

## Oversized orbital implant

It is not uncommon for the ocularist to find that there is an apparent overcorrection of the orbital volume deficit when he/she comes to fit the ocular prosthesis. It is wise to defer fitting of the ocular prosthesis for a few more weeks to allow further resolution of oedema. If the implant position remains too anterior leaving insufficient room for the ocular prosthesis, there are three options:

- Remove the implant and replace it with smaller implant
- Burr down the surface of the implant
- Decompress the lateral orbital wall

Of these options a lateral orbital decompression is preferred. This causes the least disruption of the socket with a faster postoperative recovery and does not risk implant exposure. The lateral orbital wall is approached as described for a subperiosteal implant procedure. A diamond burr is used to burr down the internal aspect of the lateral orbital wall, which creates more

space in the conjunctival sac for the ocularist. This procedure can also be used if there is insufficient depth to an artificial eye to accommodate a motility peg.

## Management of socket contracture

A contracted socket may be congenital or acquired. The management of congenital socket contracture is particularly difficult and is beyond the scope of this book. Acquired socket contracture may be classified as mild, moderate or severe. If possible, it is important to attempt to remedy the underlying cause before proceeding with surgical reconstruction. There are many factors that may contribute to the development of socket contracture:

1. Burns – chemical, thermal, irradiation
2. Trauma
3. Chronic infections
4. Previous socket surgery, e.g. implant extrusion
5. Socket inflammation/infection
6. Poor maintenance of the ocular prosthesis
7. Cicatrizing conjunctival disease, e.g. pemphigoid

## Mild socket contracture

A patient with a mild degree of socket contracture may have lagophthalmos with discomfort and socket discharge. The patient should be encouraged to lubricate the ocular prosthesis regularly. The ocular prosthesis should be polished every 6 months. Any associated papillary conjunctivitis should be treated with topical steroids. A mild degree of upper eyelid entropion can be managed with an anterior lamellar reposition. This procedure is discussed in Chapter 4 (Upper Eyelid Entropion). A small linear conjunctival scar can be managed with a Z-plasty.

## Moderate socket contracture

More severe degrees of socket contracture require the use of mucous membrane grafts (Figure 25.23). These are harvested from the lower lip and, if required, the upper lip. If there is

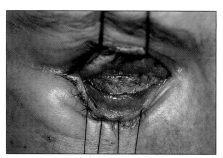
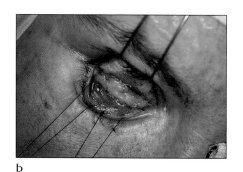

**Figure 25.23**
(a) A contracted inferior fornix has been dissected free of scar tissue and prepared for a mucous membrane graft. (b) A labial mucous membrane graft has been placed into the inferior fornix.

a                    b

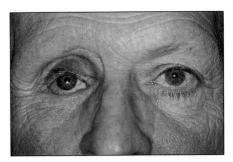

**Figure 25.24**
This patient has both socket contracture and a volume deficit. The inferior fornix has contracted, leading to a lower eyelid cicatricial entropion. This patient would be best managed with the use of a dermis fat graft.

insufficient mucous membrane available at these sites, buccal mucosa can be used, taking care not to damage the parotid duct. If a contracted socket is also volume deficient, a dermis fat graft may be placed with the dermis left exposed (Figure 25.24). This gradually becomes covered by conjunctiva, thus replacing both volume and conjunctival lining.

These patients will often have a cicatricial entropion, which may require additional eyelid surgery at the same time. If the tarsal plate in the upper eyelid has been markedly foreshortened, it may be necessary to place an auricular cartilage graft at the same time that mucous membrane grafts are placed. The upper

eyelid retractors must be recessed. In some patients the anterior lamella of the upper eyelid will be chronically foreshortened and may require a skin graft or local skin–muscle transposition flap to lengthen it.

# Fornix-deepening sutures and mucous membrane graft: surgical technique

The procedure is described for reconstruction of the inferior fornix. It can be applied equally to the superior fornix but great care must be taken not to damage the levator aponeurosis/muscle.

The procedure is performed under general anaesthesia. A throat pack is placed and the anaesthetist is asked to position the endotracheal tube to one corner of the mouth. A volume is 3–5 ml of 0.5% Marcain and 1:200,000 units of adrenaline is injected subcutaneously and subconjunctivally in the lower eyelid/fornix. A 4/0 silk traction suture is inserted through the grey line and the eyelid everted over a Desmarres retractor. A horizontal incision is made through the conjunctiva along the whole length of the lower border of the tarsus with a No. 15 blade. The inferior margin of the tarsus is freed from the lid retractors and the orbital septum, then, a template is taken of the conjunctival defect.

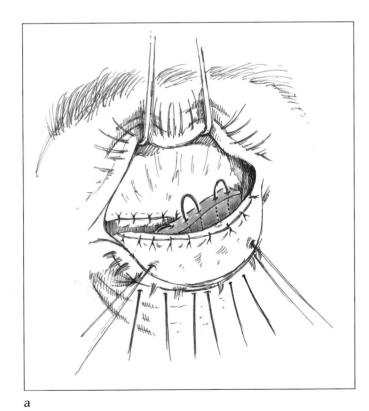

a

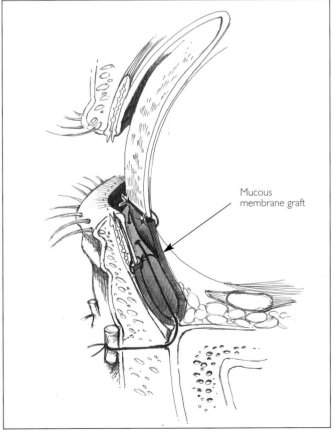

Mucous membrane graft

b

**Figure 25.25**
(a) The silicone retinal explant is placed and sutured after placement of the graft. (b) A diagrammatic view of the graft, explant and suture placement.

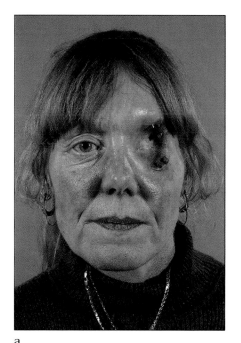 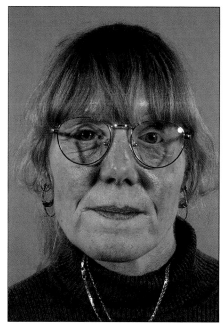

a                    b

**Figure 25.26**
(a) A patient who had severe socket contracture following subtotal exenteration and placement of osseointegrated implants. (b) The patient wearing her orbital prosthesis.

Next, the lower lip mucosa is injected with 5 ml of 0.5% Marcain and 1:200,000 units of adrenaline. Atraumatic bowel clamps are used to evert the lower lip. The template is transferred to the lower lip mucosa, avoiding the vermillion border. This is outlined with gentian violet. The graft is harvested either with a mucotome or free hand using a No. 15 Bard Parker blade and blunt-tipped Westcott scissors. The bowel clamps are removed and the graft donor site is treated with topical 1:1,000 adrenaline on a swab. The lip mucosa does not require sutures. The buccal site should be sutured with 6/0 Vicryl sutures.

The graft is shaped with Westcott scissors and sutured into place with interrupted 7/0 Vicryl sutures. A silicone explant is shaped and fornix-deepening sutures are passed (Figure 25.25). A sterile surgical conformer is placed. A compressive dressing is applied for 7 days.

## Postoperative management

The fornix-deepening sutures should not be removed for at least 6 weeks. Topical antibiotic is used for 2 weeks. The conformer must be left in place. The ocular prosthesis is fitted once the sutures and silicone explant have been removed. The patient is instructed to take a soft diet for 2 weeks. An oral antiseptic agent is prescribed for 10 days postoperatively.

## Severe socket contracture

The patient should be carefully counselled about the surgical difficulties posed by severe socket contracture. It may not be possible to achieve a result that is satisfactory for the patient. Options should be considered that take into account the patient's age, general health, occupation, social interests, procedure costs, etc. It may be more appropriate to consider the option of performing a conservative subtotal exenteration with the use of an orbital prosthesis. The patient may be a suitable candidate for osseointegrated orbital implants, which may yield a far superior cosmetic result (Figure 25.26) but at far greater financial cost.

## Further reading

1.  Ataullah S, Whitehouse RW, Stelmach M, Shah S, Leatherbarrow B. Missed orbital wall blowout fracture as a cause of post-enucleation socket syndrome. *Eye* (1999) **13**:541–4.
2.  Beaver HA, Patrinely JR, Holds JB, Soper MP. Periocular autografts in socket reconstruction. *Ophthalmology* (1996) **103**:1498–502.
3.  Smit TJ, Koornneef L, Zonneveld FW, Groet E, Otto AJ. Computed tomography in the assessment of the post enucleation socket syndrome. *Ophthalmology* (1990) **97**:1347–51.
4.  Nerad JA, Carter KD, LaVelle WE, Fyler A. Branemark PI. The osseointegration technique for the rehabilitation of the exenterated orbit. *Arch Ophthalmol* (1991) **109**:1032–8.

# 26

# The use of autogenous grafts in ophthalmic plastic surgery

## Introduction

Autogenous grafts have widespread application in ophthalmic plastic surgery. In contrast, homologous material such as donor sclera, although very convenient to use, is no longer acceptable to the vast majority of patients because of the small risk of transmissible disease. For this reason the use of homologous material should be avoided if possible. If the surgeon feels it is in the best interests of the patient to use homologous material, the risks must be explained to the patient and fully informed consent for its use obtained.

## Skin grafts

Skin grafts may be full-thickness or split-thickness grafts. A split-thickness skin graft contains only a portion of the dermis and the graft is harvested using a dermatome (Figure 26.1), the thickness of the graft being varied by adjustments made on the device. In contrast, a full-thickness skin graft is harvested free hand. Split-thickness skin grafts contract and have a poor colour match with adjacent skin. Full-thickness skin grafts are more commonly utilized in ophthalmic plastic surgery.

## *Indications*

### Full-thickness skin graft

- Repair of cicatricial ectropion
- Eyelid reconstruction
- Scar revision surgery

### Partial thickness skin graft

- Reconstruction of the exenterated socket
- Skin coverage of large facial skin defects (Figure 26.2)

## *Full-thickness skin graft*

There are a number of potential donor sites for full-thickness skin grafts:

- Upper eyelid
- Postauricular area
- Preauricular area
- Upper inner arm
- Supraclavicular fossa

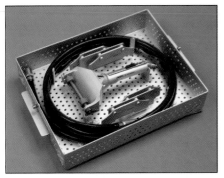

a

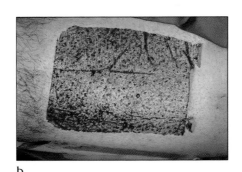

b

**Figure 26.1**
(a) A Zimmer dermatome. (b) The appearance of the donor site after removal of a split-thickness skin graft.

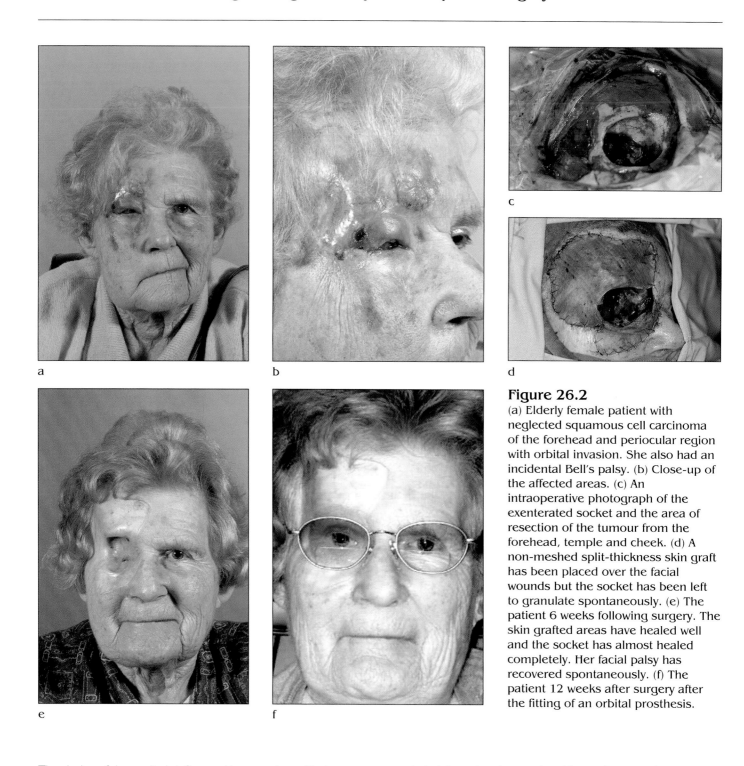

a

b

c

d

e

f

**Figure 26.2**
(a) Elderly female patient with neglected squamous cell carcinoma of the forehead and periocular region with orbital invasion. She also had an incidental Bell's palsy. (b) Close-up of the affected areas. (c) An intraoperative photograph of the exenterated socket and the area of resection of the tumour from the forehead, temple and cheek. (d) A non-meshed split-thickness skin graft has been placed over the facial wounds but the socket has been left to granulate spontaneously. (e) The patient 6 weeks following surgery. The skin grafted areas have healed well and the socket has almost healed completely. Her facial palsy has recovered spontaneously. (f) The patient 12 weeks after surgery after the fitting of an orbital prosthesis.

The choice of donor site is influenced by a number of factors, e.g. the patient's age, the size of graft required, the degree of solar damage of the skin.

The upper eyelid skin is easy to harvest, provides a good colour and texture match for eyelid defects and has no subcutaneous fat. This site does not yield much skin, however, except in older patients with dermatochalasis. Removing too much skin may cause lagophthalmos. It may also leave the patient with an asymmetrical appearance. The skin above the skin crease is removed in a similar fashion to a blepharoplasty. Alternatively, the skin may be removed temporally just beneath the eyebrow.

Postauricular skin provides a relatively good colour and texture match for eyelid and canthal defects. Its use may be precluded by solar damage in older patients or the use of a hearing aid. The skin to be removed is shared between the ear and the scalp in the mastoid area. The removal of large grafts can leave the ear closer to the skull. Preauricular skin is more accessible but may not yield sufficient skin for large defects. It is a poor site to use in patients who have very greasy skin with prominent sebaceous glands. Such skin is prone to a 'pin cushion' effect, particularly when used for medial canthal defects.

The upper inner arm affords a number of advantages. The skin is not solar damaged. It is readily accessible and can yield large grafts. The resultant scar is hidden from view. The graft can be taken and the donor site sutured by an assistant while the graft is being placed by the surgeon. The graft colour and texture match is relatively good, although it can appear very pale in patients who have a very ruddy complexion. The patient's arm is placed at 45 degrees to the body on an arm board and prepared with undiluted iodine solution.

The supraclavicular fossa is easily accessible but is rarely required. The resultant scar can be obtrusive, particularly in female patients.

## Surgical technique

Meticulous attention to detail is required in order to obtain a good result from a skin graft without complications.

1. The recipient bed must be prepared carefully and all bleeding stopped. The defect should be exaggerated in the eyelids by placing traction sutures through the grey line and placing the eyelid on traction. It must be remembered that it is frequently necessary to tighten the lower eyelid before placing a skin graft.

2. A piece of Steri-Drape is placed over the defect and outlined with a marker pen (Figure 26.3). This is cut to the exact size and shape of the defect and used as a template.
3. The template is then transferred to the donor site, where it is outlined with the marker pen (Figure 26.4a).
4. The donor site is then injected subcutaneously with 0.5% Marcain (bupivacaine) with 1:200,000 units of adrenaline.
5. The marked incision line is incised with a No. 15 scalpel blade and the graft removed using forceps and the scalpel blade (Figure 26.4b). Alternatively, Westcott scissors may be used. The defect may need to be converted to an ellipse to effect adequate closure of the wound.
6. The graft is protected in a gauze swab moistened with saline. This must be stored carefully to avoid inadvertent loss of the graft.
7. The donor site is closed with a continuous simple or blanket suture.

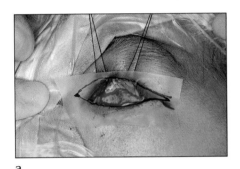

a

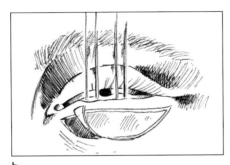

b

**Figure 26.3**
(a) A piece of Steri-drape is used to mark a template. (b) The template is cut to size and placed into the defect to ensure the fit is exact.

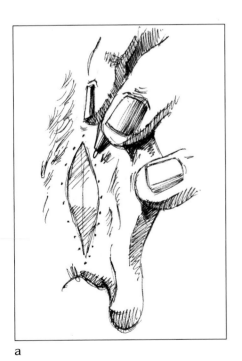

a

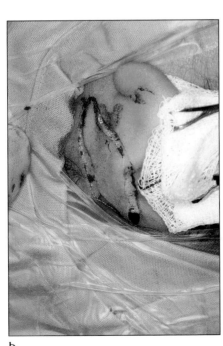

b

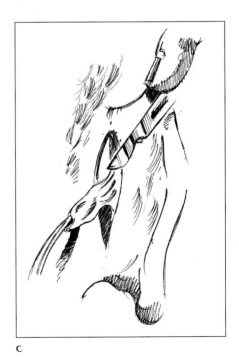

c

**Figure 26.4**
(a) The template has been placed behind the ear. The template is marked to share the skin equally between the mastoid area and the ear. (b) The ear is held forward with Babcock's clamps and an incision made with a No. 15 Bard Parker blade. (c) The skin graft is removed using a sweeping action with the blade.

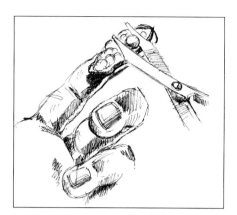

**Figure 26.5**
A skin graft being thinned.

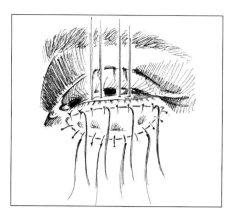

**Figure 26.6**
The skin graft is sutured to the recipient skin using 7/0 Vicryl sutures; 6/0 silk sutures are used as bolster sutures.

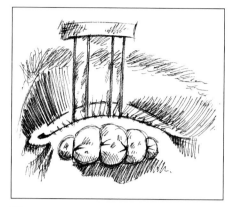

**Figure 26.7**
The 6/0 silk sutures are tied over a sponge bolster.

8. All subcutaneous tissue is completely removed with Westcott scissors while holding the graft over the index finger of the non-dominant hand (Figure 26.5). Large skin grafts are perforated with the scalpel blade.

9. The graft is then placed on the recipient bed and four interrupted 6/0 silk sutures are placed. The sutures are passed from graft to recipient skin edge. Interrupted 7/0 Vicryl sutures are placed between the silk sutures (Figure 26.6).

10. A piece of sterile sponge is then cut to the size and shape of the graft using the original template. This is covered with Vaseline gauze and placed onto the graft. The silk sutures are tied to each other over the sponge to act as a bolster (Figure 26.7). This prevents the accumulation of serous fluid or blood under the graft, which will act as a barrier to vascularization.

11. In the case of an eyelid skin graft, the grey line silk suture is left in place and used to keep the graft stretched and the globe protected. The skin of the cheek or forehead is treated with a small amount of tincture of benzoin applied with a swab to dry the skin. The silk suture is taped to the cheek in the case of an upper lid graft or to the forehead in the case of a lower lid graft using Steri-strips.

12. A pressure dressing is applied and reinforced with a head bandage. The dressings are maintained in place for 7 days. The silk sutures are then removed. The Vicryl sutures may be left in place and removed 2–3 weeks later. The sutures are removed from the donor site.

13. Aftercare of the skin graft is very important. The patient should avoid sun exposure for a period of a few weeks to minimize colour changes in the graft. Antibiotic ointment should be applied to the graft three times per day for 2 weeks and massage of the graft commenced after 2 weeks. Massage prevents contracture and thickening of the graft and should be continued for 2–3 months. Lacri-Lube (liquid paraffin) ointment is applied to the graft prior to massage.

# Split-thickness skin graft

The usual donor site for a split-thickness skin graft is the thigh.

## Surgical technique

1. The thigh is prepared with undiluted iodine solution and the area draped.

2. A light coating of glycerine is applied to the thigh for lubrication.

3. The dermatome is prepared with a blade of an appropriate size and the desired thickness of the graft set on the dermatome (usually 1/16 inch). The dermatome is checked to ensure it is working correctly.

4. The assistant places a small wooden board across the thigh in front of the dermatome in order to flatten the contour of the thigh (Figure 26.8).

5. The dermatome is applied to the thigh at a shallow angle and slowly advanced .

6. An assistant holds the skin as it emerges from the dermatome. Once the desired amount of skin has been harvested, the dermatome is stopped and the skin attachment to the thigh is cut with scissors.

7. The thigh wound is covered with a Granuflex (hydrocolloid) dressing. A piece of Gamgee and a bandage are also applied to aid haemostasis and to reduce the amount of exudate.

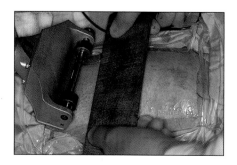

**Figure 26.8**
An assistant is flattening the skin of the thigh ahead of the dermatome.

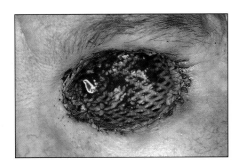

**Figure 26.9**
A meshed split-thickness skin graft placed into an exenterated socket.

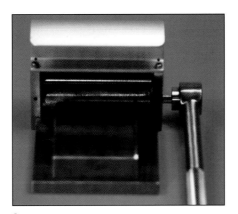

a

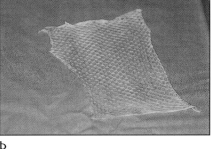

b

**Figure 26.10**
(a) A skin graft mesher. (b) A meshed split-thickness skin graft.

This dressing should be changed if any exudate leaks from it. Once the wound is dry, a non-adherent dry dressing can be used to protect the area from clothing. The area should be massaged with Vaseline.

8. The skin graft is then cut and shaped according to the defect and sutured into place as described for a full-thickness skin graft.
9. The patient requires appropriate postoperative analgesia.
10. Most split-thickness skin grafts in oculoplastic surgery are used to line an exenterated socket (Figure 26.9).
11. Such grafts are first placed in a skin graft mesher (Figure 26.10).

This effectively enlarges the graft, reducing the size of the donor site. It also ensures egress of serosanguinous fluid. The graft is inserted into the socket and the edges of the graft are sutured to the skin edges around the socket. The socket cavity is packed with Lyofoam and a compressive dressing applied, which is left undisturbed for 7 days.

Once the dressing has been removed, the socket is cleaned and Lyofoam again used if the socket is wet or if there is a fistula to a paranasal sinus. This is changed twice a week. In the absence of a sinus fistula, alginate sheet dressings can be used and changed twice a week until the socket has healed. Any adherent debris can be removed with hydrogen peroxide.

# Mucous membrane graft

A mucous membrane graft can be removed free-hand or with the aid of a mucotome. It is generally easier and safer to remove such a graft free-hand. The donor sites are the lower lip, upper lip and the buccal mucosa. The lower lip is preferred. The access is easier and no sutures are required for the wound. The buccal mucosa yields more graft material but normally has to be sutured and is not as accessible. Care must be taken to avoid the parotid duct.

## Indications

- Conjunctival replacement following an enucleation
- Fornix reconstruction

- Severe upper eyelid entropion
- Symblepharon

Any patient who is to undergo an enucleation who has conjunctival scarring from previous surgery or trauma may require a mucous membrane graft. The patient should be counselled about this possibility prior to surgery and the anaesthetist should be informed. The anaesthetist should place a throat pack after induction of anaesthesia and should place the endotracheal tube to one side of the mouth. The donor site is injected with 0.5% Marcain with 1:200,000 units of adrenaline before the patient is prepared and draped for surgery.

## *Surgical technique*

1. The recipient bed must be prepared carefully and all bleeding stopped.
2. A piece of Steri-Drape is placed over the defect and outlined with a marker pen. This is cut to the exact size and shape of the defect and used as a template.
3. Babcock's bowel clamps are placed over the edge of the lower lip, which is protected with gauze swabs moistened with saline. The vermillion border of the lip is included in the clamps, ensuring that this area cannot be included in the graft.
4. The template is then transferred to the donor site, where it is outlined with the marker pen after the mucosa has been dried.
5. The donor site is then injected with saline (Figure 26.11). This is repeated at intervals, as it aids the dissection of the graft.

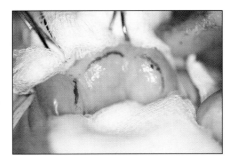

**Figure 26.11**
The lower lip has been marked and injected with saline in preparation for the removal of a mucous membrane graft.

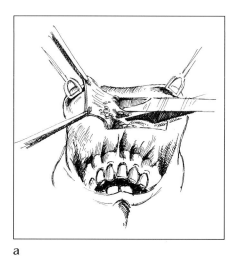

a

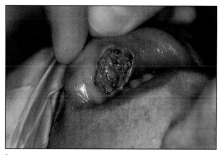

b

**Figure 26.12**
(a) The mucous membrane graft is harvested with blunt-tipped Westcott scissors. (b) The appearance of the donor site after the use of bipolar cautery to secure haemostasis.

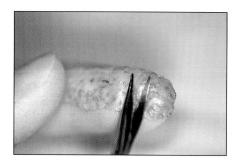

**Figure 26.13**
The graft is thinned with blunt-tipped Westcott scissors.

6. The marked incision line is gently incised with a No. 15 scalpel blade and the graft removed very carefully using blunt-tipped Westcott scissors and small-toothed forceps (Figure 26.12). The Westcott scissors should be kept just under the surface of the graft with the edge of the graft drawn horizontally to ensure that the graft is not inadvertently perforated and that the dissection is not taken too deep. Dissection in a deeper plane risks leaving areas of the lip with sensory loss. Alternatively, a mucotome may be used.

7. The graft is protected in a gauze swab moistened with saline. This must be stored carefully to avoid inadvertent loss of the graft.

8. A swab gently moistened with 1:1000 units of adrenaline is held over the donor site for 5 min and any bleeding vessels are cauterized.

9. The graft is carefully thinned with Westcott scissors while holding the graft over the index finger of the non-dominant hand (Figure 26.13).

10. The graft is then placed on the recipient bed and interrupted 7/0 Vicryl sutures are placed from the graft edge to the recipient conjunctival edge (Figure 26.14).

11. The graft must be maintained in position with the use of a symblepharon ring or a conformer of an appropriate size and shape.

The patient should be prescribed an antiseptic mouthwash for 7–10 days and should have a soft bland diet. The donor site re-epithelializes with 2–3 weeks.

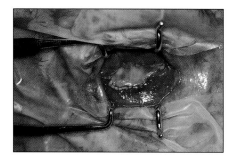

**Figure 26.14**
The mucous membrane graft has been sutured into a conjunctival defect in the socket.

# Hard palate graft

Hard palate mucosa is more rigid than lip or buccal mucosa but has a rougher surface. It does not tend to shrink more than 1–2 mm postoperatively. As a general rule it should not be used in the upper eyelid where it may abrade the cornea except in the anophthalmic patient. The anaesthetist should place a throat pack after induction of anaesthesia. The donor site is injected with 0.5% Marcain with 1:200,000 units of adrenaline before the patient is prepared and draped for surgery.

## *Indications*

- A spacer in lower lid retractor recession
- A posterior lamellar graft in lower eyelid reconstruction
- A graft in severe lower eyelid cicatricial entropion surgery
- A graft for the reconstruction of a contracted socket

## *Surgical technique*

1. A Boyles–Davis (or similar) retractor is carefully placed, ensuring that the endotracheal tube is not displaced.
2. The hard palate is dried.
3. The graft size to be harvested is measured and the margins marked on the hard palate, avoiding the gingival border, the midline and the soft palate (Figure 26.15a).
4. An incision is made with a No. 15 Bard Parker blade through the surface epithelium and into the adipose layer beneath. The periosteum should not be disturbed.
5. The graft is then removed using a No. 66 Beaver blade keeping the dissection plane within the firm adipose layer (Figure 26.15b). Westcott scissors may aid the dissection once the plane has been established with the No. 66 blade.
6. The graft is protected in a gauze swab moistened with saline. This must be stored carefully to avoid inadvertent loss of the graft.

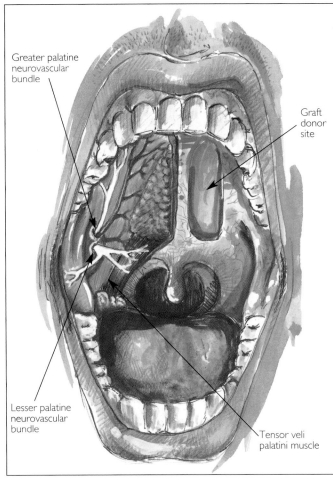

Greater palatine
neurovascular
bundle

Graft
donor
site

Lesser palatine
neurovascular
bundle

Tensor veli
palatini muscle

a

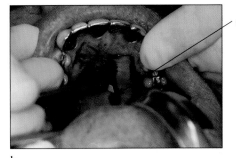

66 Beaver blade

b

**Figure 26.15**
(a) The area of the hard palate from which a graft can be
safely harvested. (b) The graft is carefully undermined with
a No. 66 Beaver blade.

7. A patty gently moistened with 1:1000 units of adrenaline is
held over the donor site for 5 min and any bleeding vessels
are cauterized.
8. Excess adipose tissue is removed with Westcott scissors
while holding the graft over the index finger of the non-
dominant hand.
9. The graft is then placed on the recipient bed and interrupted
7/0 Vicryl sutures are placed from the graft edge, to the
recipient conjunctival edge, ensuring that the sutures are
buried (Figure 26.16).

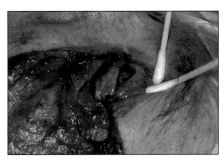

**Figure 26.16**
A hard palate graft used as a posterior lamellar
replacement in a total lower eyelid reconstruction in
conjunction with a cheek rotation flap.

The patient should be prescribed an antiseptic mouthwash for
7–10 days and should have a soft bland diet. Edentulous
patients may replace clean dentures after 2 days. This increases
patient comfort and provides a mechanical barrier for the
healing area. The donor site granulates and re-epithelializes
within 2–3 weeks.

# Upper eyelid tarsal graft

A free tarsal graft is harvested from the upper eyelid. Caution
should be exercised, however, in the use of such a graft as the
tarsus provides structural support for the upper eyelid and the
adjacent conjunctiva contains accessory lacrimal tissue. It is
important to evert the upper eyelid and to ensure that the height
of the tarsus is adequate. A minimum of 3.5 mm of tarsus from
the eyelid margin should be left undisturbed.

## Indications

- A posterior lamellar graft in eyelid reconstruction
- A graft in severe upper or lower eyelid cicatricial entropion
surgery

## Surgical technique

1. The eyelid is everted over a Desmarres retractor and 0.5%
Marcain with 1:200,000 units of adrenaline is injected
subconjunctivally at the upper border of the tarsus.
2. The tarsus is dried and a horizontal incision marked 3.5 mm
from the eyelid margin.
3. The required width of the graft is also marked on the tarsus
(Figure 26.17).
4. The tarsus is incised centrally along the horizontal mark with
a No. 15 Bard Parker blade and the remainder of the incision
is made with blunt-tipped Westcott scissors.

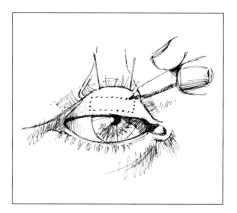

**Figure 26.17**
The upper eyelid is everted over a Desmarres retractor and the area of the tarsal graft is marked, ensuring that a minimum of 3.5 mm is left intact between the eyelid margin and the inferior incision.

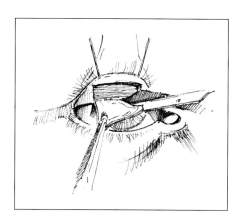

**Figure 26.18**
The tarsal graft is easily removed with blunt-tipped Westcott scissors.

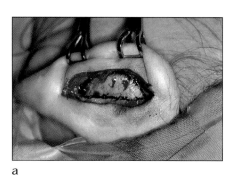

a

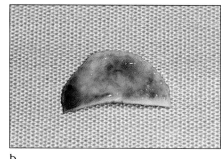

b

**Figure 26.19**
(a) The auricular cartilage has been exposed via an incision on the posterior surface of the pinna and marked out with gentian violet to the desired size and shape. (b) The appearance of the auricular cartilage graft.

**Figure 26.20**
Two dental rolls are used to compress the ear to prevent a haematoma.

5. Vertical relieving incisions are made and the tarsus dissected from the underlying orbicularis muscle with blunt-tipped Westcott scissors. The graft is then cut free and removed (Figure 26.18).
6. The donor area is left to heal spontaneously.

# Auricular cartilage graft

The auricular cartilage graft has a number of indications but its use is limited by the anatomical size and shape of an individual patient's pinna. In contrast to the hard palate graft, the auricular cartilage graft has the disadvantage of lacking a mucosal surface.

# *Indications*

- A tarsal replacement in upper eyelid reconstruction, e.g. as part of a Cutler–Beard procedure.
- A tarsal replacement in upper eyelid entropion surgery, e.g. following overly aggressive tarsal excision during a Fasanella–Servat procedure.
- A tarsal replacement in lower eyelid reconstruction.

# *Surgical technique*

1. The pinna is injected subcutaneously with 0.5% Marcain with 1:200,000 units of adrenaline both anteriorly and posteriorly.
2. Babcock's bowel clamps are placed on the edge of the pinna over a swab (Figure 26.19a).
3. A skin incision is made with a No. 15 Bard Parker blade over the posterior aspect of the pinna centrally. This is deepened to the auricular cartilage with blunt-tipped Westcott scissors.
4. The overlying tissues are dissected from the cartilage until sufficient cartilage has been exposed to enable a graft of sufficient size to be harvested.
5. Next, the graft size is marked out with a gentian violet marker (Figure 26.19a).
6. An incision is made with a No. 15 Bard Parker blade through the cartilage and the rest of the excision is completed with blunt-tipped Westcott scissors (Figure 26.19b).
7. The graft is stored carefully in a moistened swab to prevent inadvertent loss.
8. The skin incision is closed with a continuous 4/0 nylon suture.
9. Two 4/0 nylon sutures are then passed through the pinna and tied over two dental rolls covered in Vaseline gauze to prevent a haematoma (Figure 26.20). These sutures are left in place for 1 week.

10. The graft is then cleaned of any overlying soft tissue and sutured into its recipient bed with interrupted 5/0 Vicryl sutures. Any undulations in the graft can be improved by gentle partial-thickness vertical scoring of the graft with a No. 15 Bard Parker blade.

## Nasal septal cartilage graft

A nasal septal cartilage graft makes an ideal posterior lamellar replacement for lower eyelid reconstruction where the whole of the lower eyelid has been resected. It is usually used in conjunction with a Mustardé cheek rotation flap.

## *Surgical technique*

1. An injection of 0.5% Marcain with 1:200,000 units of adrenaline is given submucosally on one side of the nasal septum to aid separation of the mucosa from the perichondrium. This facilitates removal of the graft without the risk of perforation of the mucosa. Perforation should be avoided as this can lead to whistling and nasal crusting. The same solution is injected submucosally just above the base of the nasal septum on the opposite side in the region of the planned incision.
2. A nasal epistaxis tampon is placed into each nostril and moistened with 5% cocaine solution. This is removed after 5 min.
3. An incision in the naso-alar fold is made and the nostril lifted if insufficient exposure can be obtained with a nasal speculum alone.
4. An area measuring approximately 10–15 mm × 5–8 mm is outlined with a No. 15 Bard Parker blade in the mucosa. It is important to leave approximately 0.8 mm of cartilage anteriorly to avoid collapse of the nasal strut (Figure 26.21).
5. A superficial incision is made through the inferior aspect of the septum, leaving a strut measuring approximately 0.5 mm above the columella. This incision is then extended with a Freer periosteal elevator, taking care not to perforate the mucosa on the opposite side.
6. The blunt end of the Freer elevator is then slipped between the nasal septal cartilage and the overlying mucoperichondrium. The elevator is kept against the cartilage and used to sweep the mucosa away.
7. Vertical cuts are then made with straight blunt-tipped scissors and the most proximal attachment of the mucosa and cartilage is severed with a No. 66 Beaver blade.
8. The graft is stored carefully in a moistened swab.
9. Any nasal incision is sutured internally with 5/0 Vicryl and the skin closed with 6/0 nylon.
10. A fresh nasal epistaxis tampon, lightly coated with antibiotic ointment is inserted into each nostril and left overnight. It is gently soaked with saline before being gently removed. The nose is gently irrigated with a nasal douche twice a day for 1 week.

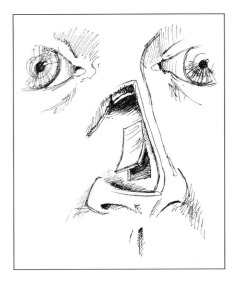

**Figure 26.21**
The area of the nasal septal cartilage from which a graft is typically harvested.

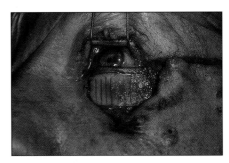

**Figure 26.22**
A nasal septal cartilage graft. A frill of mucosa has been left proud on the superior surface of the graft and the cartilage has been scored vertically with a blade.

11. The graft is very carefully prepared. The nasal cartilage is gently thinned by shaving excess cartilage away using a No. 15 Bard Parker blade. A small strip of cartilage is removed from the border, which will lie against the globe, enabling a strip of mucoperichondrium to be carried over the edge of the cartilage, thereby creating a new eyelid margin (Figure 26.22).
12. The cartilage may be gently scored vertically to enable the graft to bend towards the globe.

## Dermis fat graft

Fat can be used to replace volume and to prevent adhesions. Dermis is left attached to the fat to provide a blood supply, but postoperative fat atrophy is very variable. Hair follicles and sebaceous units which may be left within the graft usually atrophy but may be responsible for the formation of cysts and the growth of hair. The graft is usually harvested from the upper outer quadrant of the buttock but it is easier and more comfortable for adult patients for the graft to be taken from the lower abdominal wall. The graft may be completely buried but the surface is left partially exposed when it is used in a volume-deficient socket which also lacks conjunctival lining. The exposed dermis epithelializes spontaneously over a period of 3–4 weeks.

## Indications

- A primary or secondary orbital implant
- A primary or secondary orbital implant when socket lining is also required
- A replacement orbital implant in the management of an extruding orbital implant
- Prevention/management of adhesions following periorbital trauma/infection
- Camouflage of upper eyelid sulcus deformity in post-enucleation socket syndrome

## Surgical technique

1. The size of graft required is outlined on the skin with a skin marker pen (Figure 26.23). A graft to be used as an orbital implant is taken as a circular graft, whereas one to be used within the eyelid is taken as an ellipse (Figure 26.24).

2. A volume of 0.5% Marcain with 1:200,000 units of adrenaline is injected subcutaneously in the marked area.

3. Saline is injected into the epidermis under pressure using a 10 ml syringe and a fine-gauge needle to create a 'peau d'orange' appearance (Figure 26.25). This is repeated as required.

4. An incision is made through the epidermis with a No. 15 Bard Parker blade. The edge of the epidermis is grasped with toothed forceps and drawn away as the blade is used to sweep under the epidermis, separating it from the dermis (Figure 26.26a). The dermis should appear quite pale with multiple bleeding points (Figure 26.26b). No fat should be visible. The epidermis should be removed in a single sheet.

5. A small incision is made through one edge of the dermis with the blade and the rest of the incision completed with Stevens scissors (Figure 26.27a). The fat is dissected to an approximate depth of 2–3 cm and removed with the overlying dermis (Figure 26.27b) The graft is stored safely in a moistened swab.

6. The donor site is closed with subcutaneous 4/0 Vicryl sutures and interrupted 4/0 nylon sutures passed in a vertical mattress fashion for the skin closure.

7. The graft is compressed in a dry swab before it is sutured into the recipient site. In the socket the extraocular muscles are sutured to the edge of the graft and the conjunctiva

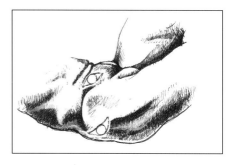

**Figure 26.23**
The typical donor sites for a dermis fat graft.

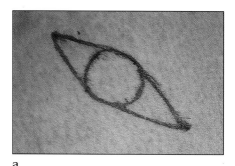

a                                          b

**Figure 26.24**
(a) The typical configuration of a dermis fat graft to be harvested from the abdominal wall. (b) The typical configuration of a dermis fat graft to be harvested from the buttock.

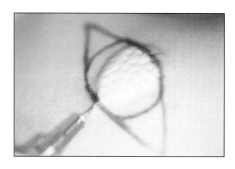

**Figure 26.25**
Saline is injected into the skin to create a 'peau d'orange' appearance.

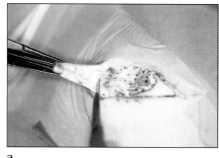

a                                          b

**Figure 26.26**
(a) The epidermis is removed with a No. 15 Bard Parker blade, with a sweeping action, the epidermis being stretched away from the blade. (b) The appearance of the dermis with the epidermis removed. There are multiple bleeding points and a white appearance to the dermis. No fat is exposed.

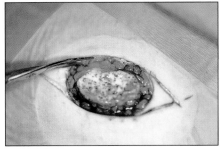

a

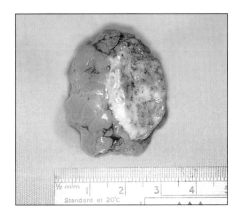

b

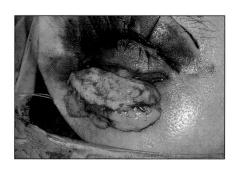

**Figure 26.27**
(a) The dermis fat graft is removed with Stevens scissors. (b) The typical appearance of a dermis fat graft to be used for an orbital implant in an anophthalmic socket reconstruction.

**Figure 26.28**
An elliptical dermis fat graft being used to prevent readhesion of the lower eyelid to the inferior orbital margin following trauma. The dermis will be inserted into the wound to lie against periosteum. The fat is positioned to lie anteriorly.

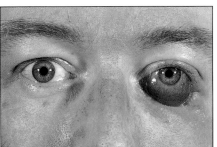

a

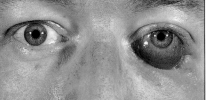

b

**Figure 26.29**
(a) A patient referred with an extruding silicone orbital floor implant, scarring and retraction of the lower eyelid into the orbit and chemosis. (b) The patient following removal of the implant, release of eyelid adhesions and placement of a dermis fat graft visible as a residual bulge in the lower eyelid.

either closed over the graft or sutured to its surface, leaving part of the dermis exposed. In the eyelid the dermis is positioned against the periosteum to which it is sutured with 5/0 Vicryl sutures. The fat is positioned to mimic the anatomical location of the preaponeurotic fat (Figures 26.28 and 26.29).

## Fascia lata graft

Fascia lata is harvested from the lateral aspect of the thigh. Its use can lead to some herniation of the vastus lateralis muscle and an obtrusive scar. It is usually harvested via an incision in the lower aspect of the thigh, although it may be removed via an incision in the superior aspect of the thigh.

## Indications

- Frontalis suspension surgery
- Lower eyelid suspension
- Patch grafting of exposed orbital implant
- Wrapping of orbital implant

## Surgical technique

1. A 4–5 cm incision is marked approximately 10 cm above the knee joint along a line drawn from the head of the fibula to the anterior superior iliac spine (Figure 26.30).
2. The area is injected subcutaneously with 0.5% Marcain with 1:200,000 units of adrenaline.
3. A skin incision is made with a No. 15 Bard Parker blade.

The anterior
superior iliac spine

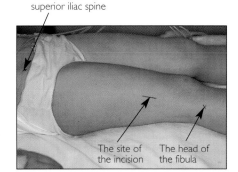

The site of    The head of
the incision    the fibula

**Figure 26.30**
The incision for the removal of fascia lata lies on a line running between the anterior superior iliac spine and the head of the fibula.

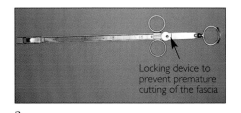
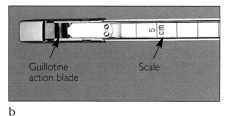
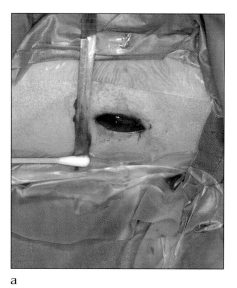

a

**Figure 26.31**
(a) Crawford fascia lata stripper. (b) Close-up of the cutting end of the stripper.

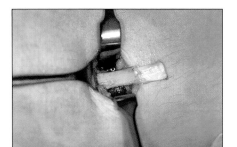
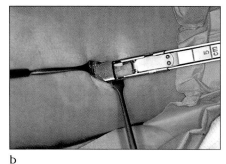
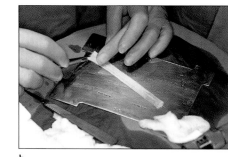

a                              b                              b

**Figure 26.32**
(a) The leading strip of fascia lata is dissected free. (b) The inferior end of the fascia lata is inserted into the stripper.

**Figure 26.33**
(a) The appearance of the fascia lata removed with the stripper. (b) The fascia is cleaned of any attached muscle and fat.

4. Blunt-tipped scissors are passed beneath the fascia and the fascia is separated from the underlying muscle.
5. The inferior aspect of the fascia is then cut and the end is introduced into a Crawford fascia lata stripper (Figures 26.31 and 26.32).
6. The stripper is passed along the line of the fascia, ensuring that the end of the stripper is passed under the horizontal investing fascia. It is imperative to ensure that the cutting mechanism is locked before the stripper is passed along the fascia.
7. Once the stripper has been passed along the fascia to the desired length, as measured on the stripper, the cutting mechanism is unlocked and activated to cut the superior aspect of the fascia.
8. The fascia and the stripper are removed and external pressure applied to the thigh (Figure 26.33).
9. The fascia is carefully stored in a moistened swab.
10. The thigh wound is closed with subcutaneous 4/0 Vicryl sutures and the skin is closed with interrupted 4/0 nylon sutures passed in a vertical mattress fashion.
11. A pressure dressing and bandage are applied.

# Temporalis fascia graft

Temporalis fascia is readily accessible and its removal leaves a scar hidden behind the hair. This site does not, however, yield the quantity of fascia which is obtainable from the thigh.

## *Indications*

- Lower eyelid suspension
- Patch grafting of exposed orbital implant
- Surface wrapping of orbital implant

## *Surgical technique*

1. The patient's hair is thoroughly cleaned over the temporal fossa with Hibiscrub (chlorhexidine) and parted with a comb posterior to the superficial temporal artery.

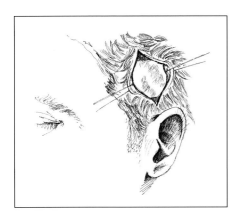

**Figure 26.34**
The placement of the incision for a temporalis fascia harvest.

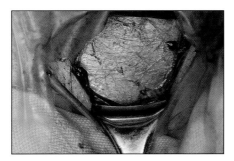

**Figure 26.35**
The appearance of deep temporal fascia.

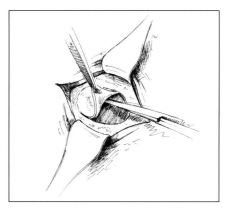

**Figure 26.36**
The fascia is removed with Stevens and Werb scissors, exposing the underlying temporalis muscle.

2.  A volume of 0.5% Marcain with 1:200,000 units of adrenaline is injected subcutaneously into the area of the proposed incision.
3.  A 3–4 cm incision is made with a No. 15 Bard Parker blade through the skin (Figure 26.34).
4.  The incision is deepened with Stevens tenotomy scissors until the glistening fibres of the deep temporal fascia are visible (Figure 26.35).
5.  The fascia is widely exposed with blunt dissection.
6.  Desmarres retractors are inserted and the wound edges moved around to expose the fascia as required.
7.  The fascia is incised with a No. 15 Bard Parker blade. The fascia is then dissected free with Stevens scissors (Figure 26.36). Werb scissors are very useful for cutting the peripheral margins of the fascia.
8.  The fascia is stored carefully in a moistened swab.
9.  The wound is closed with subcutaneous 5/0 Vicryl sutures and the skin is closed with staples. These are removed after 7 days.

# Eyelid composite graft

Approximately one-third of the upper eyelid in an older patient may be resected without altering the appearance and function of the eyelid. In patients with marked eyelid laxity an even greater proportion may be removed. The tissue can be used for the reconstruction of a contralateral upper eyelid defect which cannot be closed directly with a lateral canthotomy and cantholysis. The same technique can be used for the lower eyelid. The technique can yield very good cosmetic and functional results but the eyelashes rarely survive.

## Surgical technique

1.  The eyelids are injected with 0.5% Marcain with 1:200,000 units of adrenaline.
2.  A full-thickness wedge resection of the upper eyelid is performed (Figure 26.37). The defect is closed directly.
3.  The skin and orbicularis muscle are removed from the tarsus with Westcott scissors (Figure 26.38).
4.  The remaining tarsus with its lid margin and eyelashes are transplanted into the opposite upper eyelid defect. The tarsus is sutured edge to edge with 5/0 Vicryl sutures (Figure 26.39).
5.  The lid margin is sutured with 6/0 Vicryl sutures in a vertical mattress fashion.
6.  A local skin–muscle flap is fashioned to advance or rotate over the graft to provide a blood supply.

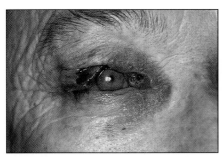

a

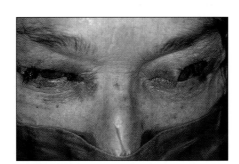

b

**Figure 26.37**
(a) A large right upper eyelid defect following a Mohs' micrographic surgery resection of a squamous cell carcinoma. (b) A wedge resection has been performed on the contralateral upper eyelid.

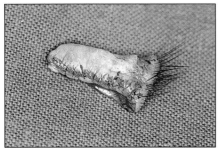

a

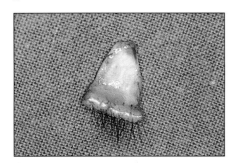

c

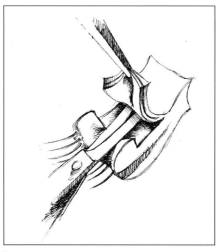

b

**Figure 26.38**
(a) The wedge resection of upper eyelid. (b) The skin and orbicularis muscle are removed. (c) The appearance of the composite graft.

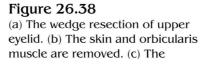

**Figure 26.39**
The eyelid composite graft sutured into place.

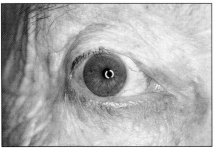

a

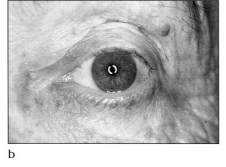

b

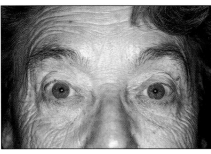

c

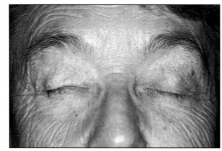

d

**Figure 26.40**
(a) Appearance of the reconstructed eyelid 5 years following surgery. The eyelashes have not survived.
(b) Appearance of the donor eyelid.
(c) The patient has a symmetrical appearance. (d) There is no lagophthalmos.

# Bone graft

With the improvement of alloplastic materials now available for the reconstruction of orbital bony defects there is rarely an indication to use bone grafts. The following sites may be used for harvesting bone:

- Cranium
- Rib
- Iliac crest

The outer table of the skull yields bone that does not tend to show much resorption. It has the disadvantage, however, of being rigid and brittle. It is very difficult to contour when used for orbital wall defects. It can be stacked piecemeal for simple orbital volume augmentation. The bone can be split from the outer table of the skull in the parietal area using a burr and a curved osteotome. Alternatively, the inner table can be split from a full-thickness piece of calvarium, e.g. following a frontal craniotomy, and used to reconstruct the orbital roof following its removal to gain access to the orbital apex.

Rib grafts can be split, curved and contoured but show more resorption. The potential donor site morbidity must be considered.

The iliac crest can yield relatively large quantities of corticocancellous bone. The bone does not contour well, however, and also may show resorption. The patient may experience considerable postoperative pain at the donor site.

# Further reading

1. Bartley GB, Kay PP. Posterior lamellar eyelid reconstruction with a hard palate mucosal graft. *Am J Ophthalmol* (1989) **107**:609–12.

2. Hawes MJ. Free autogenous grafts in eyelid tarsoconjunctival reconstruction. *Ophthalmic Surg* 1897;**18**:37–41.

3. Leone CR, Jr. Nasal septal cartilage for eyelid reconstruction. *Ophthalmic Surg* (1973) **4**:68–71.

4. Levin PS, Stewart WB, Toth BA. The technique of cranial bone grafts in the correction of posttraumatic orbital deformities. *Ophthal Plast Reconstr Surg* (1987) **3**:77–82.

5. Lisman RD, Smith BC. Dermis-fat grafting. In: Smith BC, ed., *Ophthalmic plastic and reconstructive surgery*. St. Louis: CV Mosby Co, 1987, pp. 1308–20.

6. Putterman AM. Viable composite grafting in eyelid reconstruction: a new method of upper and lower eyelid reconstruction. *Am J Ophthalmol* (1978) **85**:237–41.

# Index